Pediatric Interventional Radiology

Michael Temple • Francis E. Marshalleck
Editors

Pediatric Interventional Radiology

Handbook of Vascular and Non-Vascular Interventions

Springer

Editors
Michael Temple
Hospital for Sick Children
University of Toronto
Toronto, ON, Canada

Francis E. Marshalleck
Riley Hospital for Children-Indiana
University Health
Indianapolis, IN, USA

ISBN 978-1-4419-5855-6 ISBN 978-1-4419-5856-3 (eBook)
DOI 10.1007/978-1-4419-5856-3
Springer New York Heidelberg Dordrecht London

Library of Congress Control Number: 2014934667

Printed on acid-free paper

Springer is part of Springer Science+Business Media (www.springer.com)

Foreword

Following Seldinger's approach to intravascular catheterization for first diagnostic angiography and then for catheter-based interventions, it was realized that this technique could provide access for catheter placement in other anatomical spaces besides blood vessels.

From this adult world, it was appreciated by the early pioneers in the yet-to-be recognized speciality of pediatric interventional radiology that, with modification, these procedures could be adapted to children.

The early days before ultrasound, which were later followed by computed tomography and magnetic resonance imaging, saw the development of pediatric angiography for diagnosis. It was recognized that, as in the adult practice, therapeutic catheter techniques could be adopted for children leading to seminal procedures including bronchial artery therapy for massive and otherwise fatal hemoptysis from cystic fibrosis.

Drainage and biopsy techniques developed alongside the evolution of diagnostic and catheter-based therapies in children.

Whereas procedures of angioplasty, thermal ablation, and laser therapy were adopted from the adult IR world, the new speciality of vascular anomaly diagnosis and therapy is primarily pediatric, so much so that a pediatric interventionalist with special expertise may be the lead physician in a vascular anomalies speciality group and moreover be using therapies which do not require image guidance.

A reputation for excellence in pediatric interventional radiology particularly with vascular anomalies and other specialized therapies will attract patients beyond the normal referral areas.

As this book emphasizes, pediatric interventional radiology is very much a consultation service involved in clinical care with early morning rounds with a team including residents and nurse practitioners working long hours into the evening providing a care that is either unique to the speciality or can compete very favorably with surgical specialities in terms of economy, service, and outcomes.

With a changing health care system, pediatric interventional radiology services provide safe, prompt service by dedicated, trained practitioners. They will continue to expand and evolve with the adaptation of new techniques and technologies.

Pediatric interventional radiology makes a difference.

Los Angeles, California, USA — Philip Stanley

Preface

About 25 years ago, a few pioneering radiologists began performing "special procedures" in pediatric patients. Since that time, the practice of pediatric interventional radiology (PIR) has come a long way. It has spread throughout children's hospitals around the world; dedicated fellowship programs have been developed; the number of pediatric interventional radiologists continues to grow, and the Society for Pediatric Interventional Radiology was recently created. During that time, the number and types of PIR procedures have continued to expand and evolve.

With the ongoing evolution of our specialty in mind, we welcome you to *Pediatric Interventional Radiology*: *Vascular and Non-Vascular Interventions*. To our knowledge, this is the first textbook solely dedicated to the array of interventional procedures performed in infants and children.

Our aim in creating this book was to provide concise, easy-to-read descriptions regarding the performance and periprocedural care relating to a wide array of interventional radiology procedures in infants and children.

This book is targeted at anyone who performs or wishes to obtain further knowledge on minimally invasive, image-guided procedures in infants and children. We envision that the book will be used as an educational resource for residents, fellows, adult interventionalists, and diagnostic radiologists. The book and its summary tables were created to as a reference source for both pediatric and adult interventionalists.

Book Organization

The introductory section of the book highlights the unique elements of clinical pediatric practice that are necessary to provide safe patient care. The remainder of the book covers major vascular and non vascular PIR procedures. The organization will be procedure specific with secondary area classification. Pediatric neurointerventional procedures are not included in this book.

Chapter Organization

In general, procedural chapters start with an overview of the procedure followed by chapters that highlight information important to specific indications. For example, the arteriography section begins with an overview of basic angiographic techniques and equipment. Subsequent chapters discuss renal, pulmonary, bronchial, and GI angiography.

Procedural chapters are organized using a standardized format to provide easy access to information. Chapters are organized to describe the following:

- Background information
- Indications/contraindications
- Equipment
  - Recommendations are provided for varying patient sizes when possible or applicable
- Pre-procedure work up
- Procedure technique
- Post procedure monitoring
- Follow-up

Within each chapter, images, illustrations, and tables provide quick access to information. Each chapter ends with a point form chapter summarization containing essential information in one easy-to-access location.

Toronto, ON, Canada — Michael Temple
Indianapolis, IN, USA — Francis E. Marshalleck

Contents

Contributors

Joao Amaral, M.D. Department of Medical Imaging, University of Toronto, Toronto, ON, Canada

Department of Diagnostic Imaging-Image Guided Therapy Centre, The Hospital for Sick Children, Toronto, ON, Canada

R. Torrance Andrews Swedish Medical Center and University of Washington, Seattle, WA, USA

Kevin M. Baskin, M.D. Advanced Interventional Institute, Pittsburgh, PA, USA

Leonardo R. Brandão, M.D., M.Sc. Division of Hematology/Oncology, The Hospital for Sick Children, Toronto, ON, Canada

Anne Marie Cahill, M.B., B.Ch., B.A.O. Department of Radiology, Children's Hospital of Philadelphia, Philadelphia, PA, USA

Bairbre Connolly, M.B., F.R.C.P.(C). Image Guided Therapy, Diagnostic Imaging, The Hospital for Sick Children, University of Toronto, Toronto, ON, Canada

James S. Donaldson Department of Medical Imaging, Ann & Robert H. Lurie Childrens Hospital of Chicago, Feinberg School of Medicine at Northwestern University, Chicago, IL, USA

Josée Dubois, M.D., F.R.C.P.(C)., M.Sc. Department of Medical Imaging, Sainte-Justine Mother and Child University Hospital Center, Montreal, QC, Canada

Laurent Garel, M.D. Department of Medical Imaging, Sainte-Justine Mother and Child University Hospital Center, Montreal, QC, Canada

Paul Haste, B.S., M.D. Department of Radiology, Indiana University School of Medicine, Indianapolis, IN, USA

Fredric A. Hoffer, M.D., F.A.A.P., F.S.I.R. Department of Radiology, University of Washington, Seattle, WA, USA

Mark J. Hogan, M.D. Department of Radiology, Nationwide Children's Hospital, The Ohio State University, Columbus, OH, USA

Philip John, M.B.Ch.B., D.C.H., F.R.C.R., F.R.C.P.C. Department of Diagnostic Imaging, The Hospital for Sick Children, Toronto, ON, Canada

Ganesh Krishnamurthy, M.D., D.N.B. The Children's Hospital of Philadelphia, Philadelphia, PA, USA

Kamlesh Kukreja, M.D. Department of Radiology, Cincinnati Children's Hospital Medical Center, Cincinnati, OH, USA

Krijn P. van Lienden, M.D., Ph.D. Department of Radiology, Emma Children's Hospital, Academic Medical Center Amsterdam, Amsterdam, The Netherlands

Francis E. Marshalleck, M.D. Interventional Radiology, Indiana University School of Medicine, Riley Hospital for Children, Indianapolis, IN, USA

Keira P. Mason, M.D. Department of Anesthesia, Children's Hospital Boston, Harvard Medical Center, Boston, MA, USA

Frank P. Morello, M.D. Department of Radiology, University Medical Center, University of Arizona College of Medicine, Tucson, AZ, USA

Dimitri A. Parra, M.D. Department of Medical Imaging, Image Guided Therapy, The Hospital for Sick Children, University of Toronto, Toronto, ON, Canada

John M. Racadio, M.D. Department of Radiology, Cincinnati Children's Hospital and Medical Center, Cincinnati, OH, USA

David Rea, M.D., M.Ch., M.R.S.C.I., F.F.R.R.C.S.I. Department of Radiology, Our Lady's Children Hospital, Dublin, Ireland

Rick R. van Rijn, M.D., Ph.D. Department of Radiology, Emma Children's Hospital, Academic Medical Center Amsterdam, Amsterdam, The Netherlands

William E. Shiels, D.O. Department of Radiology, Nationwide Children's Hospital, The Ohio State University College of Medicine, Columbus, OH, USA

Manrita Sidhu, M.D., F.S.I.R. Seattle Radiologists and Children's Hospital, University of Washington, Seattle, WA, USA

Michael Temple, M.D., F.R.C.P.(C). Hospital for Sick Children, University of Toronto, Toronto, ON, Canada

Sandeep S. Vaidya, M.D. Department of Radiology, Vascular and Interventional Radiology, Seattle Children's Hospital and the University of Washington, Seattle, WA, USA

Nghia-Jack Vo, M.D. Department of Radiology, Pediatric Imaging and Interventional Radiology, Children's Hospital of Wisconsin, Medical College of Wisconsin, Milwaukee, WI, USA

Section I

Patient Care

1 Overview of Pediatric Interventional Radiology: Clinical Care

Bairbre Connolly, R. Torrance Andrews, and Manrita Sidhu

Introduction

Interventional radiology techniques are increasingly being applied to children as pediatric interventional radiology (IR) services are being developed and expanded in institutions worldwide. The practice of interventional radiology (IR) within a pediatric setting shares many similarities to that in an adult practice but has some specific or unique differences [1–4]. This chapter outlines many practical considerations involved in a pediatric PIR service: the interventional suite itself, the delivery of a pediatric service and program, and the operation of a pediatric PIR clinic. The next chapter will outline various clinical aspects of care during the pre-, intra-, and post-procedure phases. Inevitably there will be some overlap between these chapters, but intentionally these will be kept to a minimum. Procedure-specific aspects of care will be addressed in each individual chapter. The examples included throughout both chapters are drawn from the authors' experience to highlight those points of difference from an adult practice and to provide examples of both common pediatric situations and uniquely pediatric clinical scenarios.

B. Connolly, M.B., F.R.C.P.(C). (✉)
Image Guided Therapy, Diagnostic Imaging, The Hospital for Sick Children, University of Toronto, 555 University Avenue, Toronto, ON, Canada M5G 1X8
e-mail: bairbre.connolly@sickkids.ca

R.T. Andrews
Swedish Medical Center and University of Washington, 747 Broadway, Seattle, WA 98122, USA
e-mail: tandrews@searad.com

M. Sidhu, M.D., F.S.I.R.
Seattle Radiologists and Children's Hospital, University of Washington, 1229 Madison Street, Suite 900, Seattle, WA 98104, USA
e-mail: msidhu@searad.com

Evolution of Pediatric IR

From the outset, interventional radiology procedures have been performed in children, even during the early years of the field of IR. For instance, the first published paper on percutaneous nephrostomy included a case report of three patients, two of whom were children [5]. Just as the field of "adult" IR developed within diagnostic radiology departments, there was a parallel evolution within several pediatric radiology departments. Pioneering pediatric radiologists sought creative minimally invasive ways to resolve urgent clinical problems, leading to early PIR procedures [6, 7]. While many PIR procedures and devices are adapted from existing "adult" techniques, pediatric interventionalists are continually modifying them to suit the needs of children. In addition, many pediatric diseases and pathologies are distinctly different from those seen in adults, so for certain pediatric clinical situations, there is no suitable adult equivalent. The development of uniquely pediatric solutions or modifications has therefore been driven by clinical need (e.g., percutaneous cecostomy for children with spina bifida and fecal incontinence) [8, 9].

M. Temple and F.E. Marshalleck (eds.), *Pediatric Interventional Radiology: Handbook of Vascular and Non-Vascular Interventions*, DOI 10.1007/978-1-4419-5856-3_1,

Originally practiced in only a handful of centers worldwide, pediatric PIR has steadily grown and is now widely—though not yet universally—available. While it is clearly a subspecialty of both pediatric diagnostic radiology and adult IR, pediatric IR is being increasingly recognized as a unique subspecialty with its own distinct opportunities and challenges. In 2007, the maturing field of PIR reached another formal milestone with the development of a new society, the Society of Pediatric Interventional Radiology (SPIR) [10].

As with any new business line (e.g., adult IR, "general" IR, or PIR), the building of a pediatric IR service requires dedicated equipment, personnel, space, resources, and a commitment on the part of the institution [2, 11, 12]. Without such resources, growth and development is extremely slow if not impossible. In addition to these physical components necessary for success, a pediatric PIR program must also assume a large element of clinical care into its practice in order to flourish and a willingness on the part of the interventionalist to be a clinician as outlined by Dotter in 1968. It is no longer adequate for an IR program—adult or pediatric—to limit itself to providing the technical aspects of care by performing its procedures in isolation [13]. Rather, there is an appropriate expectation that interventional radiologists, like other treating physicians, provide a clinical service beyond the procedural period itself. This represents a shift in focus and a new emphasis for IR practices over the last several decades, which is necessary for several reasons outlined below.

It is not medically acceptable to perform a requested procedure without ensuring that it is indicated, appropriate, and technically feasible and that its risks and benefits have been fully considered and explained to the patient. Although a referring provider may understand much of what is involved in an IR procedure, it is the IR physician who can best evaluate its applicability to a specific patient. He or she is also best qualified to evaluate the results of a procedure and to recognize the early signs of an unexpected outcome. In addition to improving the safety of procedural care, establishing IR as a consultative service rather than a technical one improves the overall medical experience for patients and their families. Better medical care is provided through longitudinal continuity of contact with the team before and after the procedure. Therefore, when assessing the requirements of a pediatric PIR service, one must include the clinical care component as a vital requirement and integral part of the program. A modern pediatric PIR service extends well beyond the procedure room to include ward rounds and an IR clinic. As a PIR service further develops into a more complete program, it includes other aspects of care such as audit, morbidity and mortality reviews, quality improvement programs, fellowship training, and education [14].

There is no one "right way" to create a pediatric PIR program. Each program will have a different style or character and will evolve to suit the environment and individual needs of the hospital and patient population it serves. Once established the pediatric interventional program must adapt and embrace change, so as to continue to survive and grow. Given the wide variety of local needs, regulations, referral patterns, and specialty services, there will necessarily be some diversity in application of the basic requirements, although the fundamental needs and structure of a clinical service do not vary. By learning from the successes of different approaches adopted, one can apply those successful features of other programs—adult or pediatric—that have applicability or are suitable to one's own environment.

Requirements for a Pediatric IR Service

Although many successful IR programs evolved from humble beginnings—using portable C-arms in operating room space, diagnostic fluoroscopy suites, or shared resources with cardiology and being staffed by physicians who worked primarily as diagnostic imagers or adult interventionalists—it is inappropriate in the modern era to contemplate starting a pediatric PIR program without dedicated resources. At a minimum, these include:

(a) IR suite – suitable procedure room(s)
(b) Equipment—appropriate imaging and procedural

(c) Personnel—physician, team, and support personnel
(d) IR clinic and longitudinal clinical care
(e) Building and growing an IR service—commitment from all stakeholders

At the other end of the spectrum, many already established IR programs are evolving with the creation of hybrid suites for combined procedures with other disciplines, e.g., surgery, cardiology, etc.

IR Suites

Room Features

The IR room(s) may be located within the diagnostic imaging department or the operating room or may be freestanding units in a separate space, depending on local factors such as available space and historic and political factors. Pediatric IR suites should be large enough to accommodate patient populations of all types, from the patient in the neonatal intensive care unit (NICU) in an incubator to the adult-sized teen in a large bed. In addition to fixed equipment (the angiographic unit, anesthesia logans, and machines), the rooms must also hold mobile equipment such as an ultrasound unit and accommodate any additional pieces of equipment that may be brought by other teams who may perform concurrent procedures in the IR suite (e.g., an endoscopy tower for combined biliary or urological interventions). Around all the fixed and mobile equipment, the IR rooms must have sufficient space for safe access to the patient by the IR team, anesthesiology, and visiting teams, which may be present. The rooms should have restricted or limited access to public traffic. Ideally, they should also meet the standards for strictly sterile procedures (e.g., for port insertions), including being compliant with the required number of air changes per hour (ACH) for operating room standards (e.g., ACH of 15/h). Of course, they must be lead lined to meet the radiation safety standards, dictated by the equipment housed in the room.

Equipment

Imaging Equipment

Ultrasound (US) plays a more significant role in pediatric PIR than it does in adult PIR. Given their lack of abdominal fat and smaller size, the neonate and child are ideally suited to the use of US for image guidance. US guidance is therefore used in many pediatric procedures, which in adults would be performed using CT guidance. Advantages of ultrasound include its inherent lack of ionizing radiation, its ability to provide real-time guidance (which increases speed), an enhanced visualization of vascular structures, and increased versatility. Therefore, the ultrasound machine itself is a major piece of equipment for pediatric PIR.

The US scanner used for pediatric PIR procedures should be a high-end machine with color Doppler capability and a wide variety of probes suitable for procedures on children of all sizes and ages (500 g neonate to >100 kg teenager). The US must be capable of providing adequate visualization of a wide range of structures, from the very superficial <1 mm vein being targeted for PICC placement in a baby to the small nodule deep in the liver of a large teenager being targeted for biopsy. It is therefore necessary that there be a wide range of probes available. Some of the most frequently used probes include:

(a) 15 MHz small "hockey stick"-type probe (e.g., for vascular access, joint and tendon injections)
(b) 8 MHz vector probe (e.g., for intercostal access/mediastinal approaches/pleural drainage, infant nephrostomy, liver and renal biopsies) [15]
(c) 5–7 Mhz curved probe (e.g., large patient organ biopsies, deep pelvic drainage)
(d) Endocavitary probe (e.g., transrectal) with a guide (e.g., for pelvic abscess drainage)
(e) 10–12 MHz linear probe (e.g., for neonatal percutaneous cholecystography, superficial pulmonary lung nodule localization and biopsy) [16, 17]

Newer equipment with sophisticated software that smoothes the ultrasound image for diagnostic purposes can, ironically, have a negative impact upon the visualization of needles used for intervention. The preset imaging parameters may therefore need to be adjusted to improve needle resolution for IR work. The capability of angled or steered beams with some of the newer technologies has the potential to overcome some of this limitation. Many US probes have attachable needle guides, the use of which can make a procedure faster and more accurate with less need for needle repositioning compared with freehand technique, depending on user experience and preference.

Many pediatric PIR services perform procedures at the bedside in the NICU or the pediatric intensive care unit (PICU). A portable US machine is invaluable for these procedures. Image quality is still of primary concern, but with improving resolution among the newer generation of small portable and even laptop-based machines, some of these devices are now adequate for the simpler type of bedside procedures. Having such a machine available (in addition to a dedicated unit in the IR suite) increases flexibility and efficiency in the IR schedule, as it can be taken to the floor without interfering with ongoing cases in the suite [18].

Endovascular ultrasound (IVUS) is a newer modality that has many potential applications for vascular diagnosis and intervention. It is a helpful adjunct in certain situations. Having such a machine available in the IR suite is ideal, but not an absolute necessity at this point in time [19, 20].

The X-ray equipment built into a pediatric IR suite should be chosen with pediatrics and radiation protection in mind (see Chap. 2). The imaging chain should be capable of low-dose fluoroscopy (e.g., 1, 3, 7 pulses/s and greater), last image hold, and electronic zoom. Many new units are capable of capturing fluoroscopy loops, which provide adequate resolution for the purpose of documentation in some situations (e.g., venous stenosis or collaterals during placement of a venous access device) but with significant radiation reduction as compared to traditional digital image acquisition. High-quality digital subtraction angiography (DSA) is necessary for evaluating large and small vessel diseases in children. Biplane imaging is very important in pediatric IR. In addition to its classic role in adults for neuroangiography and cardiac interventions, biplane is useful in a wide range of other pediatric procedures because the simultaneous acquisition of images in two planes reduces injected contrast volume and improves safety of accessing small organs (such as the stomach for G tube placement, infant kidneys for nephrostomy placement, or infant thecal sac for lumbar puncture).

The functionality and dose reduction features of X-ray equipment continue to evolve. Rotational angiography, virtual CT, and remote guides have become standard on new angiographic machines. The traditional image intensifier has been replaced with digital flat panel technology with associated benefits of dose reduction for children. However, it is important that the actual presets, parameters, and outputs of the equipment as suggested by the manufacturer are assessed and measured to ensure that the settings are optimized and tailored for children to achieve maximum dose savings with adequate image resolution [21]. Pediatric-specific protocols need to be developed for each institution. Easily accessible information is available for pediatric dose reduction in PIR, CT, and fluoroscopy at the Image Gently website, including the Step Lightly section (www.imagegently.org) [22].

Non-imaging Equipment

Each room should have adequate ambient lighting and more focused, directional task lighting at the procedure table for catheter and wire manipulation, suturing, and other technical aspects of work undertaken during a wide variety of procedures (e.g., subcuticular suturing for port insertion, mixing sclerosants or embolic agents, examining adequacy of a biopsy specimen). Each room should be equipped to provide general anesthesia to children of all ages. This includes having piped gases and suction, as well as physiological monitoring (ECG, O_2 saturation, capnography, and invasive venous or arterial pressures). An assorted range of BP cuffs appropriate for all ages is necessary for noninvasive blood pressure measuring in neonates, infants, children, and teenagers.

These physiological parameters need to be displayed in real time and visible by the operator, the anesthesia/sedation team, and others who may be involved in monitoring the patient. Ideally, the data would also be displayed on slave monitors in the control room to permit the team to step away during DSA acquisitions.

Temperature control is a very important topic in children, as their ability to control their own temperature is limited. Infants and young children can rapidly lose body heat and become profoundly hypothermic, which negatively impacts their ability to withstand stress and infection [18, 23, 24]. The temperature of most imaging rooms is designed to suit high-energy electronic equipment and the leaded, gowned operator and is thus lower than would be appropriate for pediatric applications. Temperature-preserving equipment is therefore vitally important. Devices include simple warm blankets, cloth head covers or bonnets, plastic covers for the intubated child, warm air blowers (e.g., Bair Hugger, Augustine Medical Inc., MN, USA), warm air mattresses, and chemical blankets for the very low birth weight <1.5 Kg [24]. Monitoring of the child's peripheral and/or core temperature should routinely be done for any child <1 year and for older children undergoing a procedure of any significant length. This can be done using the temperature probe on the anesthetic equipment for those under general anesthesia but must also be available independently for children having procedures under IR-administered sedation.

The room should be equipped with a variety of lead screens, above table for the head and neck region of the operators during hand injections, and lead screen skirts to protect the legs of those around the table. It is no longer adequate to have a table skirt just at the side of the table. Ideally leg protection for personnel at the top of the table is important, i.e., for the nurse or anesthesiologist who may be holding a child and for the operator standing at the head of the table, as more procedures are performed from a jugular approach. Transparent mobile lead screens are important for the anesthesiologist and other team members who may be required to stay in the room during imaging runs. A supply of personal protective devices should be available for the IR team and visitors to the suite, e.g., lead glasses (prescription, nonprescription, over personal glasses), lead gloves, and a variety of sizes of lead aprons with thyroid shields.

A fully equipped pediatric crash cart should be available nearby. It must contain a range of sizes and appropriate selection of oral airways, endotracheal tubes, masks for bag-mask ventilation, as well as resuscitation drugs with weight-based dose calculation tables. A defibrillator with both pediatric- and adult-sized paddles should also be available.

In addition to the above requirements, which are universal, there is an ever-increasing array of additional equipment that may be desirable. The specific needs of a facility will depend upon the types of cases being performed there. For example:

- Electrocautery equipment and required grounding pads are frequently part of the armamentarium of an IR suite that performs port insertions, other procedures that require a wide incision, or combined procedures with a surgical team.
- Image-guided percutaneous radiofrequency alblation (RFA) is the treatment of choice for osteoid osteomas; those facilities that perform this procedure or that use RFA to treat other tumors and lesions in other organs will require RF generators, probes, and grounding pads [25].
- Thrombolysis and thrombectomy are increasingly being used in the treatment of pediatric patients with arterial or venous occlusions. Mechanical thrombectomy procedures require dedicated catheters, pumps, and other devices [26].
- Interstitial or endovascular laser technology is finding a role in the management of vascular malformations, with a concomitant need for laser generators, optical fibers, and glasses and related protective gear [27]. Local regulations and requirements vary but the use of a laser will require compliance with all the training and safety requirements and usually the presence of a laser safety officer during the procedure.
- A variety of other devices, e.g., electric or battery-operated orthopedic drills, and a host

of other tools can be "owned" entirely by the IR suite or can be shared with other services [28]. However, in-servicing and training in the use of all auxiliary devices is necessary for the entire team, as there is potential for adverse events with any of them.

Finally, given the acuity of cases that frequently present to an IR lab, having in-room point-of-care testing capability for critical laboratory variables is highly desirable. Many test units are handheld devices that can provide a variety of results based on a tiny amount of blood (e.g., iStat, Abbott Laboratories, Abbott, IL). Different cartridges are available that will test for hemoglobin, electrolytes, glucose, blood gases, etc. These devices require regular supervision and calibration by the hospital laboratory. IR suites, which perform a significant number of cases with anticoagulation, may own or have access to an ACT machine to measure the patient's anticoagulation status.

Personnel

Personnel of the Pediatric IR Team

Making the commitment to provide IR services requires that the institution provide appropriate infrastructure and resources. A critical and difficult aspect of this obligation is recruiting and retaining the personnel who run the program. Since, as already described, IR has evolved into a broad clinical service, its staffing needs have expanded from the core team of nurse, technologist, and interventionalist to include midlevel practitioners, hospitalists, Child Life specialists, pediatric vascular access specialists, sedation specialists, administrative personnel, etc. [2, 3, 29].

The core team that actually performs IR procedures includes nurses, medical radiology technologists, interventional radiologists, and, in the pediatric environment, anesthesiologists. At some institutions, nurses and technologists rotate through IR from other modalities, thus providing a broad pool of individuals with various specialized expertise in other imaging modalities (e.g., CT). Other institutions utilize a team of nurses and technologists who are specifically assigned to IR. The latter fosters a cohesive team spirit and enhances the expertise and comfort level with procedures and devices that are unique to IR. There is no single credentialing process for nurses and technologists who wish to become members of the pediatric PIR team. Most come with related prior experience, and they train on the job to acquire the unique set of skills needed. Ideally a nursing background might include experience in a high-acuity area, such as NICU or PICU, or emergency department (ER) nursing.

Like their nurse and technology colleagues, the physicians who enter the field of pediatric interventional radiology do so without a single specific credentialing pathway. Some do fellowships in diagnostic pediatric radiology, others in adult interventional radiology, and many have done both [30]. This varied training is often reflected in their subsequent practices, which may include both diagnostic and interventional radiology or a combination of adult and pediatric IR. These mixed interests and skill sets are actually quite beneficial during the building phase of a pediatric PIR program, when the case volume may initially be too low to support a dedicated pediatric interventionalist. Conversely, having some degree of cross coverage by primarily diagnostic pediatric radiologists or by adult IRs is very helpful in sharing otherwise onerous call coverage and has the added benefit of providing additional expertise and skills which might be difficult for a solo pediatric interventionalist to achieve in an isolated practice [30].

It is clearly understood that children undergoing painful or unfamiliar procedures may be frightened and unable to cooperate fully. Therefore, providing conscious sedation, such as in a child undergoing PICC placement, or, more often, deep sedation or general anesthesia is an indispensable component of a pediatric IR practice. The specific process for delivery of sedation will vary by institution, with some using nurse-administered sedation under IR supervision, others using OR-based anesthesiologists, and still others using ICU, ER, or roving sedation teams [30, 31]. Irrespective of the approach used, it is imperative that those administering sedation have the knowledge, skill, and judgment to do so safely and that they be capable of managing the pediatric patient who experiences respiratory compromise or other complications of sedation. Usually this requires PALS certification. The topic of sedation is dealt with in detail in another chapter (Chap. 3).

Other important team members are the Child Life specialists who provide unique service to the pediatric patient during procedures using a variety of distraction techniques [32]. They provide the child with coping mechanisms that empower them and maximize their ability to cooperate, thereby reducing the need for sedation. These individuals can make the difference between success and failure during an interventional procedure. Furthermore, by improving the quality of a patient's experience during a given procedure, the participation of a Child Life specialist can significantly reduce the fears of children who must undergo subsequent repeat procedures.

The longitudinal clinical work required outside the IR suite may be performed primarily by a member of the core IR team (interventionalist, IR fellow, or IR nurse) or by an additional IR staff person such as nurse practitioner. Having an individual dedicated to clinical management allows that effort to occur in parallel with the procedural work, thereby reducing disruptions to the daily schedule. In many cases, the salary of this person can be paid through the billable work that he or she provides. Patients who are admitted to the hospital for observation or recovery after a procedure are, in many institutions, managed by the IR service alone, while in others they are admitted to a hospitalist service with the IR team following. Each facility needs to arrive at a system that best suits its patient population and procedure mix. Irrespective of the approach adopted, the inclusion of adequate staff, time, and resources to provide longitudinal clinical participation and ward rounds into the IR practice is now a standard of care requirement [2, 3].

Other important but commonly overlooked members of the IR team are the staff who schedule cases and those who maintain and turn over the procedure rooms. The daily schedule in an IR suite is usually a fluid one, with frequent adjustments being necessary to accommodate urgent procedures. In most active centers, such "add-on" cases constitute more than half of a day's workload. It is imperative that the individuals who manage this schedule have a good understanding of the procedures being requested and maintain close communication with the operating team. Similarly, those who turn over a room between procedures—quickly cleaning and restocking it—are integral to the overall efficiency of the practice. The competency and skill level of these team members are crucial to the efficiency of the IR service. As respected and integral members of the team, these individuals have a role that can be rewarding and fulfilling, with opportunities to interact with patients and their families.

Despite all the different roles described above, it is critical for patient safety and quality of care that the successful IR team function as a unit [33]. Different tasks are suited to different unique professional roles, but the highest quality care can only be achieved through mutual respect and a shared ownership of the overall effort by all team members.

Pediatric IR Clinic and Longitudinal Care

Members of the IR team are the group of healthcare professionals most knowledgeable about the risks and complications of their procedures. The IR team therefore must play a pivotal role in the periprocedural care of its patients. It is the IR service that should determine and organize the necessary preprocedure investigations tailored to the planned IR procedure (e.g., blood work, imaging, anesthesia consults, etc.). Similarly, it is the IR team which should directly manage or, at the very least, actively follow its patients post procedure to ensure that complications are recognized and appropriately addressed. This activity does not have to be done in isolation, but may be done in conjunction with a hospitalist or specialty services as needed [1, 33]. Although initially daunting for many interventional radiologists, assuming this broad clinical role can be assimilated gradually, over time becoming the routine way of practice. Just as embracing the philosophy of ward rounds pre and post procedure was a change for many proceduralists, so too the development of a clinic-based practice, providing longitudinal and excellent patient care, is a natural evolution. The development of a pediatric PIR clinic is a natural outgrowth of this endeavor [34–36].

While a few simple image-guided procedures can be scheduled and performed without consultation by the IR service (e.g., cecostomy (C), gastrostomy (G), gastrojejunostomy (GJ) tube checks and changes), most require some level of IR evaluation prior to treatment. At one end of this consultation continuum is brief assessment by the extended IR team if available, such as a member of a vascular access service prior to venous access device placement or removal, or by an enterostomy team or IR nurse for G tube assessment. More complex patients may require physician consultation with the referring requesting service and include a ward visit or a mapping ultrasound pre procedure, prior to booking (e.g., fluoroscopy and ultrasound mapping to assess technical feasibility of a G tube placement in an infant with complex abdominal anatomy). Still more complex patients—especially outpatients —require a full and detailed IR evaluation. Procedures carrying material risk, those in which the IR procedure is the major therapy responsible for an admission, high-risk procedures, and low-risk procedures on high-risk patients should be preceded by a visit to the IR clinic.

During the IR clinic visit, the interventionalist obtains a detailed history and physical assessment, discusses with the family the alternatives for treatment, explains the intended procedure, creates a management plan, organizes further consultations or preprocedure investigations that may be required, and obtains informed consent. If appropriate, the interventionalist might also use the clinic visit to perform some of his/her own imaging to assist in planning. For instance, if the planned procedure is an ultrasound-guided biopsy, he or she may use office-based ultrasound to assess the acoustic window, judge the safety of access (presence of overlying vessels and adjacent critical structures), and determine the ease or difficulty of the intended procedure [3].

The IR clinic visit also provides an opportunity to ensure that all procedures planned under the same general anesthetic/sedation episode are coordinated. This "one-stop shopping" concept is very important in pediatrics, where numerous unrelated procedures may be planned for the same anesthetic event in an effort to reduce the total number of such events. Although this can be logistically challenging for the various services that may be involved, parents and children appreciate the efforts of health-care professionals to coordinate all of the involved teams and their necessary equipment. Timing of the separate procedures during a "one-stop shopping" visit, or sequencing of events in a combined procedure, must be thought through to ensure one procedure does not negatively impact the ability to perform another. IR can lead this initiative and invite the other specialties to perform their procedure in their IR suites. IR can advocate for the patient and be a catalyst for change in the delivery of pediatric care. In addition to the safety aspect of minimizing the episodes of anesthesia for a child, this can also minimize parent or guardian time lost from work and patient time lost from school. One factor that impacts the success of pediatric medical care is the impact on and support for the family. For this reason, consideration of family issues, as in the philosophy of "family-centered care," is very important as it has been shown to improve clinical success of pediatric interventions as well as family and staff satisfaction [37].

In addition to facilitating the coordination of clinical issues, a preprocedure clinic visit has other benefits. It offers the patient and family a valuable opportunity to meet members of the team, thereby creating a physician–patient relationship without the stress that exists on the day of a procedure, and allows time for the family to assimilate all the information provided. Furthermore, the clinic setting conforms to the expectation that patients have of meeting their physicians in an office setting. This is how they interact with other clinical specialties, and it should also be the norm for IR. Thus, as the pediatric IR clinic becomes established in a program, it becomes the gateway for most patients into the IR system [2].

The IR clinic also plays a valuable long-term role as the setting for follow-up after procedures (e.g., RFA of osteoid osteomas). During these visits, the IR team is able to assess for complications or problems (e.g., reassessment of a pseudoaneurysm post thrombin injection) and to discuss and arrange subsequent procedures that might be required (e.g., further interventions for a vascular malformation). Follow-up clinic visits also provide a forum for further education and may thereby prevent future problems (e.g., management of a new C tube so as to prevent tube, site, or bowel problems). Often they can be linked to imaging studies to assess the status of a device (e.g., biliary or ureteric drains, follow-up and evaluation of an abscess with a persistent fistula), thereby keeping the number of repeat hospital visits minimum. This provides assurance for families that they are not abandoned by the system but have ongoing resources available to them.

The specific needs of each IR clinic will vary with the volume of the IR practice, the nature and type of its cases, and the clinical setting of the institution. However, for a pediatric PIR clinic, sufficient space must be available to accommodate the family (usually at least the patient and two parents), a child's stroller or wheelchair, and the toys and distraction tools necessary to occupy a child. Some advocate that IR clinics should be physically located with other outpatient clinics, sharing common space with other specialties. The advantage of such a configuration is that IR is then viewed by peers and patients' families as a full clinical service on par with other specialties. A very different option is to create clinic space within or adjacent to the IR suite itself. This proximity allows clinic visits to be integrated with the IR procedure schedule and seamlessly provide any imaging that may be required. Yet another arrangement is to establish multidisciplinary clinics targeting specific pathologies (e.g., combined IR–plastic surgery clinic for vascular malformations). Such clinics facilitate complex treatment planning and reduce the time burden on patients and families. Ultimately, the physical arrangement chosen is of less importance than is creation of the IR clinic itself, no matter how simple or humble its beginnings.

The time allocated to IR clinic activities will depend on the nature of the practice and the availability of physician extenders. Clinic activities need to be incorporated into the physician schedule to ensure there is sufficient time for both new patient consults and return visits. Published figures from adult IR and general pediatric clinics suggest time allocations of 60 and 15–30 min, respectively, for these appointments [2, 38].

Documenting the clinic visit is of critical importance. It creates a record of the IR team's assessment of the clinical situation, outlines the rationale for a treatment plan, and may be indispensible in communicating that information to other providers and to the patient's insurance company. Radiologists are accustomed to dictating radiology reports and to the use of radiology information systems and PACS, but they are not generally familiar with direct medical correspondence. Yet while detailed radiology reports are invaluable in documenting a procedure and may reveal some clinical involvement, a personal letter written to a referring physician, outlining the patient's IR clinic visit and the resulting management plan, is an extremely powerful tool [2, 3]. A letter is recommended over a radiology report for clarity and quality of care and for marketing and communication with other medical colleagues and referring physicians.

IR Clinic Coordinator

While the final decision-maker in treatment planning for patients in the IR clinic may be a physician, the person responsible for day-to-day operation of the clinic and the main point of contact for patients and their families is more likely to be a nurse or midlevel provider. The role of a pediatric PIR clinic coordinator is a valuable and rewarding one and can be tailored to the specific IR clinic population. The IR clinic coordinator is involved at all stages of interaction with the patient, pre, peri, and post procedure. He/she plays an important role in taking the history, performing the physical assessment, and organizing any relevant investigations prior to the procedure. During a visit, it is often the coordinator who explains any planned procedure, in terms the child can understand, and allays as much anxiety as possible. He or she can give a virtual tour of the procedure suite through pictures or computer images, so the child understands what to expect.

The coordinator/nurse can discuss coping strategies and pain medications beforehand (e.g., Child Life, distraction techniques using videos, music, ipod, etc.). He/she also is an important contact for the patient after discharge should any need arise. Many clinics use these individuals to make post-procedure phone calls to enquire about patient progress following invasive procedures. In this way, any unexpected issues can be identified early and triaged for referral to the interventionalist as needed.

As the IR clinic evolves, the IR clinic coordinator has the opportunity to be involved with creating information pamphlets for patients and their families. Through firsthand experience, the coordinator knows the common concerns, the frequently asked questions, and the common pieces of advice that are required. Some may find it fulfilling and rewarding to create paper pamphlets or electronic web-based information tools for procedural information, preparation, consent, and informed discharge. Such patient guides provide the families with take-home documentation and ensures consistency of message between different practitioners.

Building and Growing an IR Service

Interventional radiology is unique as a medical specialty in that much of its contribution to an institution, through the minimally invasive approaches it employs, is in costs saved rather than charges generated. Reduced morbidity, shortened hospital stays, and decreased use of higher-cost procedures done in an operating room (OR), impact strongly on a balance sheet, but their specific dollar value is not readily quantified. Nor can one put an exact price upon the enhanced prestige that accrues to an institution when it offers truly comprehensive pediatric care and the greater willingness of outside referrers to send patients to such an institution. To be sure, elective outpatient procedures done by a pediatric PIR service can and do produce high-dollar billing opportunities that might not otherwise exist, but to focus solely upon those opportunities is to vastly undervalue the whole of the pediatric PIR service.

Considering these points, and also bearing in mind the relatively high capital costs of equipping a pediatric IR service, it is evident that having the support of administration is of vital importance. Building a good business case is essential, but beyond that the approach required to leverage support from administrative leaders will depend upon the individual institution and the health-care system of the country in question. While some administrators will recognize the larger picture that includes revenues generated and costs saved, others will not see beyond the business case, billing, and expected profit. Both groups may be concerned about the issue of turf conflicts with other specialties (e.g., vascular surgery), with other disciplines, and even with the IRs' own diagnostic colleagues. For those reasons, a newly proposed IR service is far more likely to meet with administrative approval if it targets a need unmet by existing competitors than if it seeks to share an existing patient population. It may be necessary to begin with a smaller and narrower focus than one hopes to achieve in the longer term. Are patients going to the OR for open biopsies? If so, propose a CT- or ultrasound-guided biopsy alternative. Are they being sent to another facility for embolization of vascular malformations or for RFA of liver masses? If so, start there. Even the most limited patient group can, over time, form a strong foundation from which the value of the service becomes evident and the case for expansion can be made.

When starting a service or during times of growth, it also behooves the interventionalist(s) to have input from, and the support of, other members of the team, especially anesthesiology, nursing, and technology. These people should be actively involved in planning, design, choice of equipment, construction, and finally equipment installation. The planners should cultivate a good working relationship with medical engineering and plant and environmental services during any construction or renovation project. Time must be made in the day to attend frequent planning meetings. The representatives of the team must actively participate at the planning meetings to ensure their influence is felt. Infection control needs to be consulted for advice at various steps along the way. Physical space for the suite should be fought for, and given the large numbers of health-care workers and sometimes different teams involved in combined procedures, as much space as possible should be acquired for the IR room(s).

Even if the physical space has already been allocated, developing an IR service requires hard work in a multipronged approach, at various levels. It requires active liaison with referring teams; willingness to assume the clinical roles and responsibilities, by paying due diligence for patient care pre, peri, and post procedure; collaborating with surgical and medical colleagues on difficult cases; attending radiology–clinical rounds; and an openness to considering new strategies for treatments. It also involves advocating for IR at hospital committee and administrative levels whenever the opportunity arises, as well as creating the opportunities for such interactions. All these measures assist in the move towards creating an effective service and, eventually, a fully operational clinical IR program.

A more developed pediatric PIR program likely will include various supportive networks or systems, which provide the infrastructure to run the program efficiently. These might include such things as a vascular access service (for triaging and troubleshooting vascular access issues), an enterostomy service (for triaging and troubleshooting G and gastrojejunostomy issues), a vascular malformation service (combined expertise with plastic surgery, dermatology, IR), a sedation service, dedicated IR morbidity and mortality reviews, IR educational/lecture series, IR fellowships, a quality improvement program or QI rounds including radiation protection, and research and development, to mention just a few [14, 39]. All these aspects will draw from different areas within the hospital and from different disciplines (e.g., dietitians, quality and risk, medical physics, etc.). In this way resources are shared and a growing IR service does not need to "reinvent the wheel" at every step. Growth and development can be achieved by continually striving for excellence in clinical care and new or better ways to do things.

Challenges

The challenges faced by IR will vary from center to center. Some of these are specific to an institution or region, but many are shared common issues. Examples include workforce shortages and the recruitment and retention of staff. A workforce survey of PIR published in 2007 demonstrated a high level of reported burnout due to call frequency, lack of department and institutional support, and severe difficulty in finding and recruiting qualified PIRs [30]. Others struggle with an institutional commitment that may vary from day to day, with change in leadership, budget constraints, and competing draws on resources. For others, it is the problem of finding the funding for optimum equipment, establishing admitting privileges, addressing turf issues, and sharing procedural space with other services that do similar procedures (e.g., general surgical service). Pediatric interventionalists face additional challenges that are unique to pediatrics, such as having reliable access to ancillary services, e.g., Child Life services and anesthesiology. Those who work in pediatric hospitals must also identify adult practitioners who are willing and able to take over the management of chronic patients (e.g., children with epidermolysis bullosa, C tubes, and vascular anomalies) once they have "graduated" or passed the upper age limit for the institution. Avoiding burnout is a common challenge as one struggles with any of these issues. Having a determined, respectful, consistent approach to these issues, with a clear business case delivered to the correct people at the relevant level, is critical for success.

Summary

Creation, development, or expansion of a pediatric IR service is a multifaceted challenge. The main driver or goal is the provision of high-quality patient care. This can evolve from simple beginnings and grow with time and considerable effort into a major program. Attention to equipment, space, and personnel is key. Creation of a committed and competent team is vital.

Acknowledgment of the clinical role in terms of preprocedure assessment and post-procedure follow-up is important. Support of the administration is crucial to ongoing growth and development. Willingness to adapt to change and embrace new challenges and opportunities is necessary for survival and to avoid stagnation.

References

1. Lord D. The practice of pediatric interventional radiology. Tech Vasc Interv Radiol. 2011;14(1):2–7.
2. Collaborative statement from the American College of Radiology, the American Society of Interventional and Therapeutic Neuroradiology, and the Society of Interventional Radiology. Practice guideline for interventional clinical practice. J Vasc Interv Radiol. 2005; 16:149–55.
3. Baskin K, Hogan M, Sidhu M, et al. Developing a clinical pediatric interventional practice: a joint clinical practice guideline from the Society of Interventional Radiology and the Society for Pediatric Radiology. J Vasc Interv Radiol. 2011;22(12):1647–55.
4. Tsapaki V, Ahmed NA, AlSuwaidi JS, et al. Radiation exposure to patients during interventional procedures in 20 countries: initial IAEA project results. Am J Roentgenol. 2009;193(2):559–69.
5. Babcock Jr JR, Shkolnik A, Cook WA. Ultrasound-guided percutaneous nephrostomy in the pediatric patient. Urology. 1979;121(3):327–9.
6. Towbin RB. Removal of foreign bodies from the upper gastrointestinal tract of children. Curr Opin Radiol. 1990;2(6):904–8.
7. Towbin R. Interventional procedures in pediatrics. Semin Pediatr Surg. 1992;1(4):296–307.
8. Chait PG, Shandling B, Richards HM, Connolly BL. Fecal incontinence in children: treatment with percutaneous cecostomy tube placement—a prospective study. Radiology. 1997;203(3):621–4.
9. Shandling B, Chait PG, Richards HF. Percutaneous cecostomy: a new technique in the management of fecal incontinence. J Pediatr Surg. 1996;31(4):534–7.
10. www.spirweb.org
11. Baerlocher MO, Asch MR. The future interventional radiologist: clinician or hired gun? J Vasc Interv Radiol. 2004;15(12):1385–90.
12. American College of Radiology White Paper. Clinical practice of interventional radiology and neurointerventional radiology (White Paper). 2003. http://www.acr.org/dyna/?doc=departments/stand_accred/standards/ir_white_paper.html
13. Murphy TP. Introduction to clinical interventional radiology. Semin Intervent Radiol. 2005;22(1):3–5.
14. Tuong B, Shnitzer Z, Pehora C, Choi P, Levine M, Krishnamurthy G, Chait P, et al. The experience of conducting mortality and morbidity reviews in a pediatric interventional radiology service: a retrospective study. J Vasc Interv Radiol. 2009;20(1): 77–86.
15. McCrone L, Alexander S, Karsli C, et al. Ultrasound guided percutaneous needle biopsy of anterior mediastinal masses in children. Pediatr Radiol. 2012; 42(1):40–9.
16. Fontalvo LF, Amaral JG, Temple M, Chait PG, John P, Krishnamuthy G, Smith C, Connolly B. Percutaneous US-guided biopsies of peripheral pulmonary lesions in children. Pediatr Radiol. 2006; 36(6):491–7.
17. Nwomeh BC, Caniano DA, Hogan M. Definitive exclusion of biliary atresia in infants with cholestatic jaundice: the role of percutaneous cholecysto-cholangiography. Pediatr Surg Int. 2007;23(9):845–9.
18. Coley BD, Hogan MJ. Image-guided interventions in neonates. Eur J Radiol. 2006;60(2):208–20. Epub 2006 Sep 8.
19. Roebuck D, et al. ESPR proceedings. Pediatr Radiol. 2007;37 Suppl 1:46–70.
20. Roebuck D, et al. ESPR proceedings. Pediatr Radiol. 2009;39 Suppl 3:496–507.
21. Strauss KJ. Interventional suite and equipment management: cradle to grave. Pediatr Radiol. 2006;36 Suppl 2:221–36.
22. www.imagegently.org
23. Knobel R, Holditch-Davis D. Thermoregulation and heat loss prevention after birth and during neonatal intensive-care unit stabilization of extremely low-birth weight infants. J Obstet Gynecol Neonatal Nurs. 2007;36(3):280–7.
24. Laffan EE, McNamara PJ, Amaral J, Whyte H, L'Herault J, Temple M, John P, Connolly BL. Review of interventional procedures in the very low birth-weight infant (<1.5 kg): complications, lessons learned and current practice. Pediatr Radiol. 2009; 39(8):781–90.
25. Donkol RH, Al-Nammi A, Moghazi K. Efficacy of percutaneous radiofrequency ablation of osteoid osteoma in children. Pediatr Radiol. 2008;38(2):180–5.
26. Kukreja K, Vaidya S. Venous interventions in children. Tech Vasc Interv Radiol. 2011;14(1):16–21.
27. Sidhu MK, Perkins JA, Shaw DW, Bittles MA, Andrews RT. Ultrasound-guided endovenous diode laser in the treatment of congenital venous malformations: preliminary experience. J Vasc Interv Radiol. 2005;16(6):879–84.
28. Johnson ND, Racadio JM. IR challenges in the MSK system. Pediatr Radiol. 2010;40(4):474–7.
29. Rosenberg SM, Rosenthal DA, Rajan DK, Millward SF, Baum RA, Silberzweig JE, Tuite CM, Cardella JF, American Academy of Physician Assistants. Position statement: the role of physician assistants in interventional radiology. J Vasc Interv Radiol. 2009;20(7 Suppl): S337–41.
30. Sidhu MK, James CA, Harned II RK, Connolly BL, Dubois J, Morello FP, Kaye R, Siddiqui NJ, Roberson PK, Seidel KD. Pediatric interventional radiology workforce survey summary. Pediatr Radiol. 2007; 37(1):113–5.

31. Mason KP. The pediatric sedation service: who is appropriate to sedate, which medications should I use, who should prescribe the drugs, how do I bill? Pediatr Radiol. 2008;38 Suppl 2:S218–24.
32. Bandstra NF, Skinner L, Leblanc C, Chambers CT, Hollon EC, Brennan D, Beaver C. The role of child life in pediatric pain management: a survey of child life specialists. J Pain. 2008;9(4):320–9. Epub 2008 Jan 16.
33. Agency for Healthcare Research and Quality (AHRQ). Medical teamwork and patient safety: the evidence based relation. (www.ahrq.gov/qual/medteam/medteamref.htm)
34. Connolly B, Mahant S. The pediatric hospitalist and interventional radiologist: a model for clinical care in pediatric interventional radiology. J Vasc Interv Radiol. 2006;17(11 Pt 1):1733–8.
35. Cardella JF, et al. Society of Interventional Radiology clinical practice guidelines. J Vasc Interv Radiol. 2009;20 Suppl 7:189–91.
36. Siskin GP, Bagla S, Sansivero GE, Mitchell NL. The interventional radiology clinic: key ingredients for success. J Vasc Interv Radiol. 2004;15(7):681–8.
37. American Academy of Pediatrics. Policy statement: family centered care and the pediatricians role. Pediatrics. 2003;112(3):691–6.
38. ACR–SIR–SNIS. Practice guidelines for interventional clinical practice. 2009; (Res 24*):1–9.
39. Steele JR, Wallace MJ, Hovsepian DM, James BC, Kundu S, Miller DL, Rose SC, Sacks D, Shah SS, Cardella JF. Guidelines for establishing a quality improvement program in interventional radiology. J Vasc Interv Radiol. 2010;21:617–25.

Periprocedural Care in Pediatric Interventional Radiology

2

Bairbre Connolly, R. Torrance Andrews, and Manrita Sidhu

Introduction

This chapter will focus on the clinical aspects of delivery of patient care, from periprocedural assessment to discharge. Practices will vary from institution to institution so several different approaches and options are presented in this chapter. Many examples from pediatric interventional radiology (PIR), drawn from the authors' experience, are interspersed throughout the text to explain a point or to highlight differences between pediatrics and adult practices. Several tables are included, intended to be useful for quick reference, such as definitions of relevant clinical terms for PIR (Tables 2.1, 2.2, 2.3, 2.4, 2.5, 2.6, 2.7, 2.8, 2.9, and 2.10).

As outlined in Chap. 1, it is no longer standard of care for interventional radiology (IR) physicians to perform procedures and leave the entire care of the patient to their referring team [1–4]. Increasingly IRs are actively involved in the continuum of patient care, following their patients pre- and post-procedure, either in the capacity of a consulting service or assuming full responsibility with admitting privileges. Many IRs without admitting privileges are actively seeking to obtain such privileges.

Details of specific procedures are dealt with in individual chapters. This chapter will address the following general aspects of periprocedural care:

(a) Pre-procedure clinical care
(b) Clinical care during the procedure
(c) Post-procedure care

Pre-procedure Clinical Care

Patient Assessment

The requirement for pre-procedure assessment depends on the nature of the procedure to be undertaken and ranges from minimal (such as for a gastrostomy tube check) to full IR pre-procedure evaluation, as in a patient with complex vascular malformation seen in a multidisciplinary clinic (see Chap. 1). Much of the IR workload can be considered "service work," in which case IR provides a valuable supportive service for a large number of patients referred from a variety of specialties, for example, when providing central venous access for surgical and oncologic patients. In other instances, IR provides the definitive therapeutic

B. Connolly, M.B., F.R.C.P.(C). (✉)
Image Guided Therapy, Diagnostic Imaging, The Hospital for Sick Children, University of Toronto, 555 University Avenue, Toronto, ON, Canada M5G 1X8
e-mail: bairbre.connolly@sickkids.ca

R.T. Andrews
Swedish Medical Center and University of Washington, 747 Broadway, Seattle, WA 98122, USA
e-mail: tandrews@searad.com

M. Sidhu, M.D., F.S.I.R.
Seattle Radiologists and Children's Hospital, University of Washington, 1229 Madison Street, Suite 900, Seattle, WA 98104, USA
e-mail: msidhu@searad.com

M. Temple and F.E. Marshalleck (eds.), *Pediatric Interventional Radiology: Handbook of Vascular and Non-Vascular Interventions*, DOI 10.1007/978-1-4419-5856-3_2,

Table 2.1 Common terms, definitions, and calculations used in a pediatric practice

Term	Term	37 completed weeks to 41 weeks and 6 days
Premature	Preterm	<37 weeks
Low birth weight	LBW	<2,500 g
Very low birth weight	VLBW	<1,500 g
Extreme low birth weight	ELBW	<1,000 g
Small for gestational age	SGA	BW <10th percentile for GA
Large for gestational age	LGA	BW >90th percentile for GA
Absolute neutrophil count	ANC	White cell count *x*% that are neutrophils
Severe neutropenia		ANC $<0.5 \times 10^9$/L
Normal urine output		Infants and young children: 1.5–2 mL/kg/h
		Older children and adolescents: 1 mL/kg/h
Estimated body weight (in kg) based on child's age		Children 1–9 years: (age in years × 2) + 8
		Children >10 years: age in years × 3.3
Endotracheal tube size (internal diameter in mm)		Infants <1 year: 3.5 mm (uncuffed)
		Children 1–2 years: 4 mm (uncuffed)
		Children 2–10 years: 4 + (age/4) (uncuffed)
		Children 2–10: 3.5 + (age/4) (cuffed)
Hypothermia		Core temperature <35 °C

Table 2.2 American Society of Anesthesia—a physical status classification system [6]

ASA 1	Normal healthy patient
ASA 2	A patient with mild systemic disease
ASA 3	A patient with severe systemic disease
ASA 4	A patient with severe systemic disease that is a constant threat to life
ASA 5	A moribund patient who is not expected to survive without the operation
ASA 6	A declared brain-dead patient whose organs are being removed for donor purposes
Prefix "e"	Emergency

Table 2.3 Variations in laboratory values with maturity and age [8]

Test name	Age	Reference values
Activated partial thromboplastin time (APTT)	<3 month	25–35 s
	>3 month	23–35 s
INR	<3 month	0.9–1.6
	>3 month	0.9–1.1
Hemoglobin	<30 days	140–200 g/L
	1 month	115–180 g/L
	2 months	90–135 g/L
	3–11 months	100–140 g/L
	1–4 years	110–140 g/L
	5–13 years	120–160 g/L
	≥14 years female	120–153 g/L
	≥14 years male	140–175 g/L
Creatinine	≤6 days	19–90 µmol/L
	7–60 days	10–56 µmol/L
	2 months–5 years	<36 µmol/L
	6–9 years	<53 µmol/L
	10–13 years	<79 µmol/L
	≥14 years	<98 µmol/L
Glucose *	<1 year	2.5–5.5 mmol/L
	1–2 years	2.5–5.0 mmol/L
	3–11 years	2.8–6.1 mmol/L
	≥12 years	3.3–6.1 mmol/L

* 1 mmol/L = 18 mg/dL

procedure for a variety of conditions, such as embolization of an arteriovenous malformation. Irrespective of the type of procedure considered, clearly it is important to ensure that the IR procedure requested is indicated and appropriate for that individual patient and to weigh the risk factors or contraindications prior to undertaking the procedure. Making this assessment may necessitate an IR clinic or multidisciplinary clinic visit. At such a visit, a clinical history is taken, physical examination is performed, necessary imaging is reviewed, and any required specialty consultation, imaging, or blood work is organized.

Evaluation of Imaging

Careful evaluation of available imaging is important in order to confirm that the procedure, for example, a biopsy or abscess drainage, is technically possible and clinically appropriate. If there is any uncertainty about access, choice of modal-

Table 2.4 Fasting guidelines for GA or sedation (may vary slightly from institution to institution) [8]

Clear fluids	2 h
Breast milk	4 h
Infant formula/cow's milk	6 h
Solids	8 h

Table 2.5 Example "time-out" checklist

All team members to stop what they are doing and take part in time-out
• Staff present
– Operator(s)
– Anesthesiologist
– Nurse
– Technologist
• Patient name
• Patient identification
• Patient diagnosis/history
• Procedure to be performed
• Procedures by other services to be performed
• Written consent
• Correct site and correct side marked (on patient)
• Patient allergies
• Blood work reviewed
• Last menstrual period/pregnancy test results
• Prophylactic antibiotics
• Correct name on imaging equipment
• Correct orientation on equipment
• Correct side markers in place on equipment
• Radiation protection equipment in place
• Grid in/out
• Any potential adverse events expected
• Equipment for adverse events inside/outside of room
– Crash cart
– Blood warmer
– Blood products
– Warming lights/blankets for neonates
• Equipment for procedure in room
• Any other concerns or comments from any team member in room?

ity to be used, or suitability for the planned procedure, this can be resolved by pre-procedure "mapping" imaging, ideally performed by an interventionalist, with the very specific and focused questions below in mind (different than those asked in a standard diagnostic imaging exam):

(a) Is the lesion well visualized with this imaging modality, or is another modality required?
(b) Can the lesion be safely accessed percutaneously, avoiding interposed vessels and other relevant structures, such as bowel or pleura?
(c) What are the risks and benefits of different trajectories or angles?
(d) What level of sedation/anesthesia is required for this patient for this procedure?

Mapping imaging may involve ultrasound, fluoroscopy, CT, or a combination of imaging modalities (e.g., combination of US and fluoroscopy mapping to assess the feasibility of placing a gastrostomy tube in an infant with distorted abdominal anatomy post diaphragmatic hernia repair). Mapping will determine the imaging required (e.g., should US or CT be used to access a small peripheral pulmonary nodule for biopsy) [5]. Time taken for pre-procedural mapping is time well spent, as it improves the accuracy of procedure planning, decreases the need for last-minute changes to the plan, enables the case to be scheduled with the most suitable equipment (e.g., CT scanner if needed), and avoids the situation where the patient must be moved during a case or, even, the procedure canceled. In addition, an appointment for mapping gives the parents and child an opportunity to visit the IR department and meet members of the team. The results of the mapping imaging are shared with the referring physician and the family, and a plan to proceed (or not proceed) is reached. This visit also provides an opportunity to obtain informed consent well in advance of the procedure, which is preferable to obtaining written consent immediately prior to the procedure, as the more relaxed setting allows a more adequate consent process for the family.

Consultations

Specialty consultation may need to be arranged prior to a procedure. Most commonly this involves an anesthesia consultation, usually indicated in children with known airway difficulties, complex cardiopulmonary problems, or American Society of Anesthesiology (ASA) Class 4 or 5 (Table 2.2) [6]. Additional investigations if required by the anesthesiologist are arranged in advance of the

Table 2.6 Age-appropriate normal estimates of weight, endotracheal tube size, and vital signs [8, 24]

Age	Weight (kg) (approx)	HR awake	HR sleeping	RR	BP	ETT size
Birth	3.5	85–205	80–160	30–60	65/40	3.0–3.5
6 months	7.5	110–160	80–160	24–38	85/50	3.5–4.0
1 year	10	90–150	75–160	22–30	90/55	4.0
3 years	14	80–125	60–90	22–30	92/55	4.5
5 years	18	70–115	60–90	20–24	95/58	5.0–5.5
10 years	30–32	60–100	50–90	16–22	100/62	6.0–6.5
12 years	40	60–100	50–90	16–22	106/62	6.5
14 years	45	60–100	50–90	14–20	110/66	6.5–7.0

Table 2.7 Abnormal vital signs in infants and children [8, 24]

Age	Pulse rate/min	Blood pressure (systolic)	Respiratory rate/min
≤3 months	<80 or >200	<60 mmHg	<30 or >60
3–12 months	<80 or >180	<65 mmHg	<24 or >50
1–10 years	<60 or >150	<70 + (2 × age in years)	<22 or >40
• 10 years	<60 or >120	<90 mmHg	<12 or >30

procedure (e.g., in an acute setting, an ECG, cardiology consultation, and echocardiography in a patient with a large anterior mediastinal mass pre-biopsy to evaluate pulmonary artery and venous flows, vascular compression, as well as the cardiac ejection fraction) [7]. Other examples include an ophthalmology consultation to evaluate eyes/vision prior to management of a periorbital vascular malformation or a cardiology consult in a child with cardiac symptoms or signs.

Blood Analyses

Blood work is frequently requested as part of the pre-procedure workup, individualized to the patient and procedure risk factors. Common examples pertinent to a pediatric practice are included, and the normal, abnormal and variations of values with age are shown in Table 2.3 [8].

Hematology

- Complete blood count (hemoglobin, platelet, neutrophil counts): Normal ranges of hemoglobin vary with patient age and gestation, as well as with local laboratory ranges (sample values Table 2.3). Severe neutropenia (absolute neutrophil count $<0.5 \times 10^9$/L) in an immunosuppressed child may represent a relative contraindication for certain procedures, e.g., gastrostomy tube insertion.
- Coagulation screen (PTT, INR): Coagulation parameters vary with patient age and gestation (Table 2.3). Guidelines for acceptable values have been drafted for IR procedures in adults [9].
- Sickle cell testing for sickle cell disease: May be required to plan for pre-procedure hydration, oxygenation +/– transfusion [10].
- Blood products: Consider type and screen if bleeding is a recognized complication (e.g., liver or kidney biopsy), or cross-match for units of packed red blood cells if greater risk of significant bleeding (e.g., angioplasty). Repeat type and screen is necessary after 3 days, or if blood products have been given in the interim. Blood products (e.g., FFP, platelets, cryoprecipitate) must be organized to be available if needed, and ideally only used if necessary, to avoid the potential for adverse reactions and disease transmission to the patient [11].

Biochemistry

- Electrolytes: In certain patients, assessment of the patient's electrolyte levels is indicated. For example, abnormal serum K^+, Ca^{2+}, and Mag^+ levels may need to be corrected to reduce the risk of wire-induced cardiac arrhythmia.

Table 2.8 Commonly used drugs (in alphabetical order)

Name	Dose
Acetaminophen	15 mg/kg PO
Adenosine	0.1 mg/kg/dose IV rapidly
Cefazolin	30 mg/kg/dose IV
Cefoxitin	30 mg/kg/dose IV
Diphenhydramine	1–2 mg/kg/dose IV (anaphylaxis)
Fentanyl	1 μg/kg/dose IV
Flumazenil	10 μg/kg IV over 15 s. Wait 1–3 min. Repeat up to four times
Glucagon	0.02–0.03 mg/kg/dose. Max dose 0.5 mg <20 kg; 1 mg>20 kg
Heparin	50–100 units/kg to max 5,000 units loading dose
Ketamine	0.25 mg/kg/dose IV
Midazolam	0.05 mg/kg/dose IV; 0.5 mg/kg/dose PO <20 kg; 0.3 mg/kg/dose >20 kg
Morphine	0.05 mg/kg IV dose
Naloxone	0.001–0.01 mg/kg/dose for narcotic reversal in sedated patients
Sucrose	23–32 weeks: up to 0.5 mL PO 2 min prior to procedure
	32–37 weeks: up to 1 mL PO 2 min prior to procedure
	>37 weeks: up to 2 mL PO 2 min prior to procedure
	All infants who are NPO: up to 0.5 mL PO 2 min prior to procedure. Dose may be administered in increments of 2-min intervals for prolonged procedures; divided or repeated to the maximum daily dose. Maximum daily dose: four times in 24 h
Topical anesthetic	Lidocaine (Maxilene) topical anesthetic cream: 2 %—thin layer to skin
	Tetracaine (Ametop) 4 % cream/patch—thin layer to skin

- Creatinine: The creatinine level is important prior to the use of large volumes of iodinated contrast (Table 2.3).

Other

For invasive procedures in patients with complex conditions (e.g., hemophilia or diabetes mellitus), blood work is usually managed in cooperation with the referring teams to determine adequate coagulation factor levels, serum glucose, fibrinogen, etc.

Table 2.9 IV Fluid maintenance and bolus guidelines

Maintenance		
Weight	Daily volume	Hourly volume
1–10 kg	100 mL/kg/day	4 mL/kg/h
11–20 kg	50 mL/kg/day	2 mL/kg/h
>20 kg	20 mL/kg/day	1 mL/kg/h
Bolus		
Hypovolemic shock	20 mL/kg bolus, repeat prn	Give rapidly over 5–10 min
Cardiogenic shock	5–10 mL/kg bolus, repeat prn	Give slowly over 10–20 min

Examples:
Maintenance 23 kg child daily: 1000 mL+500 mL+60 mL = 1560 mL/day (~65 mL/h)
Maintenance 23 kg child hourly: 40 mL+20 mL+3 mL=63 mL/h (~1512 mL/day)

Medications

Review of the patient's medications is important to ensure that specific medications are discontinued (e.g., antiplatelet agents for 5 days prior to the procedure, anticoagulants for required time interval, etc.) [9]. Parents will need advice regarding continuation of vital oral medications to be taken the morning of the procedure with the minimal amount of water possible (e.g., antiseizure medications). Preparatory medications must be planned, e.g., bowel-cleansing agents (Pico-Salax, Ferring Inc., North York, Ontario, Canada) and clear fluid diet for 48 h pre-cecostomy tube insertion, steroid premedication for radiographic contrast allergy, and timing of tetracycline pre-bone biopsy for bone histomorphometry in osteoporosis [12–14].

"One-Stop Shopping"

In the pediatric population, it is worthwhile from the perspectives of resource utilization and patient safety and convenience to plan for several procedures under one sedation. This needs to be addressed during the work-up period and takes foresight and effort to coordinate. It is important to ensure that all the planned procedures are compatible together and that the order of procedures is optimal, i.e., that the performance of one does not prevent or interfere with the next procedure (e.g., a US-guided abdominal procedure should precede introduction of intraperitoneal gas during a laparoscopic procedure).

Table 2.10 Sodium recommended in routine post-procedure fluids

Fluid	Na^+ mmol/L	K^+ mmol/L	Dextrose g/100 mL	Tonicity
D5W (dextrose 5 % in water)	0	0	5	Hypotonic
D10W (dextrose 10 % in water)	0	0	10	Hypotonic
NS (normal saline, 0.9 % NaCl)	154	0	0	Isotonic
½ NS (half normal saline, 0.45 % NaCl)	77	0	0	Half-isotonic
$\frac{2}{3}:\frac{1}{3}\left(\frac{2}{3}\text{ dextrose and }\frac{1}{3}\text{ saline}\right)$	45	0	3.33	Hypotonic
Ringers lactate	130	4	0	Isotonic

Informed Consent

Informed consent before an interventional case is a significant part of any IR practice, but especially so in pediatrics. The consent process may take longer and be significantly more detailed than adults. It is usually obtained from a substitute decision maker (SDM) such as a parent or guardian. Obtaining adequate and appropriate consent is truly a process rather than a single event or a form-filling exercise [15, 16]. Adequate time spent on the consent process, in addition to being an ethical imperative, is invaluable in increasing compliance with the preparation, procedure, and follow-up, in patient and family satisfaction, and in establishing rapport prior to the case in the event of complication. Sometimes the parents need to meet on more than one occasion, in order to fully accept their child's condition and understand treatment options. They should meet a member of the team in the IR clinic or during an assessment on the ward, and have the opportunity to ask their relevant questions and consider all the options, before signing consent. Parents are frequently too stressed immediately before a procedure to comprehend a detailed explanation of a procedure and its risks. Ideally therefore, when time permits, informed consent should be obtained in advance of the procedure in a separate encounter with the parents, even if separated by a few hours or the day before, rather than immediately prior to the patient entering the IR suite. Sitting with them, explaining in understandable terms, and providing diagrams and written material in advance of the procedure time are all strategies to ensure a SDM has the best opportunity to absorb the content fully which in turn supports informed decision making [17–19]. At the time of the procedure, they may wish to revisit some issues previously discussed, to refresh or clarify their understanding.

The responsibility of the interventionalist is to outline material risk [15]: those risks that are common but may be minor (e.g., site problems with a gastrostomy tube), those that are rare but severe (e.g., death), as well as the recognized risks in the range between that the average person would wish to know (e.g., central venous catheter-related thrombosis, infection). It is also important when possible to involve the pediatric patient in the discussion to the extent that is appropriate for their age, obtain a verbal assent, and address the child's worries or concerns [20]. It is necessary to document the risks that were discussed. A signed written consent must be obtained from the SDM and placed in the medical record.

Atypical Situations for Consent

In difficult clinical/psychosocial situations, where it is not clear what the proper or advisable course of action is, it may be helpful to contact the Bioethics Department or even the Risk Management Department for advice:

Age. In some jurisdictions there is no lower limit of age for consent, and the concept of maturity has replaced chronological age [15]. In these jurisdictions, as long as the patient has an understanding of the procedure, its implications, and the alternatives, they may sign. Some older teenagers prefer to sign their own consent, which is legally valid in some jurisdictions. In other jurisdictions, the patient must be over 18 years to sign. In common practice, however, most parents or guardians provide written consent, even for teenage patients [20–22].

Legal status. In pediatrics, obtaining consent through SDM (parents and guardians) may pose specific additional ethical/legal difficulties. It is important to clarify that the person giving consent is in fact the legal guardian (e.g., in blended families, grandparents with signing authority). Procedures planned for children who are in the care of child protection services require that the consent is obtained through their case worker. Informing and involving the biological parent is, however, usually appropriate, even if they do not actually sign the consent.

Cultures. In certain families, the parent may dictate that the child is not informed or given minimal information about the procedure. This may prove stressful for the physician obtaining the consent. A balance needs to be achieved between the child's right to know and the parent's opinions.

Religious. Religious beliefs may influence consent, especially with respect to giving of blood products or DNR status. In most institutions, legally approved consent forms are available that have been approved by representatives or religious elders of the group, such as Jehovah's Witness.

Telephone. Consent may have to be obtained over the telephone if person-to-person consent is not possible. This is not uncommon in the case of a newborn where the mother is at an obstetric facility or parents are at home looking after siblings. Distance adds an emotional strain for the parents when giving consent. It is good practice, and in many facilities required, that a witness (another health-care professional such as a nurse or IR team member) cosign the consent form with the interventionalist, attesting that the person has understood what has been explained and that they give approval to proceed.

Emergency. In cases of emergency without parents present, the referring physician or two physicians in some jurisdictions may give consent. He or she must document and sign to that effect in the medical records [22].

Off-label. Parents must be informed of any use of devices or drugs that are not approved, special access, or "off label," e.g., intrasalivary injections of Botox for drooling in children with cerebral palsy [23].

Alterations. Some parents may wish to change part of the institution's consent form, e.g., dictate that no fellow be involved in the procedure. In academic institutions, this can be challenging. It is usually not advisable that the form be altered and it is prudent to seek advice from the Risk Management Team or the hospital's lawyers in such situations.

Information Pamphlets

Information pamphlets, which provide parents with simple, direct, clear facts either in paper or online format, are valuable resources in terms of increasing access to information and providing consistent information. Parents usually welcome as much information as possible and appreciate the ability to review it at their own pace. Diagrams and sketches are helpful to explain many concepts or procedures.

Fasting Status

The guidelines for fasting vary slightly from institution to institution and it is important to operate within them. In general, the guidelines for sedation are similar to those for general anesthetic. Although fasting from midnight may be suitable for adults undergoing an anesthetic, this is inappropriately long for most young children. Prolonged fasting for solids or liquids may result in dehydration and/or hypoglycemia. A commonly used and simple to remember recommendation is the "2, 4, 6, 8 rule" (Table 2.4). Vital medications (e.g., antiseizure) may be given with a small amount of water.

Clinical Care During Procedure

Sedation and anesthesia are dealt with in Chap. 3. Specific aspects of clinical care pertinent to each different procedure type are also addressed in detail in individual chapters. This section deals with the more general principles/aspects of clinical care during a procedure.

Even for the most minor of cases (e.g., gastrostomy tube change), it is imperative that the room is equipped with suction, oxygen, and masks for bag-mask ventilation and that these are checked, available, and functioning at the start of each day. Consideration should be given as to whether the parent will be in the room, distraction techniques (DVDs, etc.), and the need for a Child Life worker to be with the child. In the event of an adverse outcome during a procedure, there is increasing evidence to support that the parent or family member stay during the resuscitation [24]. It is often helpful for the family to be present. Parents of chronically ill children are usually comfortable with medical equipment and emergency procedures. It has generally been found not to be disruptive or stressful for the staff [24]. In the event of such an occurrence, there needs to be a person assigned to be with the parent, to explain, comfort, and support the family—and should the need arise to respectfully ask the family to leave if their presence is considered detrimental to the resuscitation.

Checklists and Time-Out

In recent years the use of safety measures including pre-procedure "huddles," checklists, time-outs, and others has become the norm prior to an invasive procedure [25–27]. The "huddle" is valuable prior to bringing a patient into the suite, to discuss patient-specific issues, review the plan for the procedure(s), ensure that all necessary equipment is available, including blood if necessary. It is also important to share with the team pre-procedure information such as the side of the table one plans to work at as it may influence room set up (e.g., a left-sided empyema for pleural drainage), the need for bladder catheterization, or the need for an NG tube.

At the time-out, personnel in the room ensure that all necessary aspects of the case/concerns are known, the correct patient is present, the correct procedure is going to be done, the correct site has been identified and marked, informed consent for all procedure(s) has been obtained, allergies are noted, need for pre-procedure prophylactic antibiotics is determined (noting that to be effective, prophylactic antibiotics must be given within 1 h of "knife/needle-to-skin"), pregnancy status determined (date of last menstrual period, pregnancy test result), the correct name is on the imaging monitors, radiation protection equipment is in place (e.g., table skirt), grid is in or out, and orientation of imaging is correct (e.g., when performing CT fluoroscopy, correct patient orientation is selected, prone or supine, head or feet first, and the working side of the table). All members of the team in the room should stop momentarily to listen and participate in the time-out. Any anticipated adverse events should be raised (e.g., known airway compromise, expected blood loss, possible bradycardia/asystole during mechanical thrombectomy) and the presence of the necessary equipment in the room is ensured (e.g., flexible bronchoscope, blood products, correct French size, and length of double J stent). Some centers insist on a team introduction during the time-out (see Table 2.5) [25].

Organs with laterality (e.g., kidney) or those with multiple options (e.g., joints in hands or feet) should be marked pre-procedure [27]. It is imperative to mark the correct sites before the child is sedated, with involvement and agreement of the parents. The marking should be with a safe skin marker and using the operators' initials rather than an "X" or "*."

At the end of the procedure, another "time-out" ensures that the correct specimens have been labeled and sent to the laboratory as required, allergic dressings are avoided, and all the requested procedures have been done before the child is awakened [25]. This is especially relevant in the "one-stop shopping model," to ensure that all the teams have attended. The team(s) must discuss post-procedure orders to ensure that there is no conflict between orders from different teams.

Monitoring

The level of monitoring during a case depends not just on the level of sedation or anesthesia but also on the invasiveness of the procedure. For example, a liver biopsy under local anesthetic, even without sedation, still carries the risk of significant bleeding and therefore monitoring and documentation of blood pressure and pulse is important during the procedure; drainage of a large volume of ascites requires monitoring of pulse, blood pressure, and respirations because of fluid shifts. Usually the minimum requirement is electronic heart tracing, continuous oxygen saturation measurements, pulse rate, and intermittent blood pressure records. These values must be interpreted within the norms for the child's age (6, 7) and within the trend for the individual patient. Temperature monitoring is especially important in the younger child, who can rapidly lose body heat. Hypothermia is defined as a core temperature <35 °C, and temperatures <36 °C should be avoided especially in the neonate [28]. Equipment requirements for such monitoring are discussed in Chap. 1. Documentation of monitoring during the procedure is imperative, in the form of an anesthetic record, sedation record, or another monitoring record for cases done under local anesthetic, such as PICC insertion or paracentesis. The record provides a pattern or trend of the child's vital signs for comparison in the recovery phase (Table 2.6).

Medications/Fluid Management Pre-, Per-, and Post-procedure

As pediatric patients come in all sizes and weights, medication dosages must be calculated according to patient weight. Some drugs frequently used in PIR are shown in Table 2.8. With respect to intravenous fluids, consideration must be given to fluid regimens (Tables 2.9 and 2.10). There are standard maintenance fluid regimens calculated according to patients' weights (Table 2.9). These are suitable for the majority of children. However, in specific groups of children, these may be harmful, in volume and/or constituents. Some of these clinical situations will be beyond the expertise of many pediatric interventionalists; it is incumbent on the IR team to seek advice from those most expert in that specific fluid management. Examples of such circumstances are shown:

- Renal impairment—fluid restriction, impaired potassium, and sodium balance: the advised fluid management should be discussed with the referring or attending nephrologists.
- Cardiac disease—unable to tolerate routine fluid maintenance volumes without causing cardiac decompensation: fluids should be given cautiously and ideally with advice from cardiologists.
- Metabolic disorders—unique needs for chemical composition and volume requirements pre- and post-procedure, e.g., avoidance of hypoglycemia in glycogen storage disorder type 1. These become especially challenging if fasting is expected to extend post-procedure, e.g., post-gastrostomy tube insertion.
- Diabetes mellitus—usually successfully managed by the consulting endocrinology service who manages their insulin and IV fluids.
- Diabetes insipidus—has large fluid and sodium requirements, should be the first case of the day, should have their urine output monitored during the procedure (if necessary via bladder catheter), and should have care taken to avoid hypovolemia and serious sodium shifts.
- Ketogenic diet for intractable seizures—is maintained within a tight range of ketosis and requires avoidance of sugar in most situations.
- Hemoglobinuria—double fluid maintenance is usually required.

In addition to general considerations of fluid volumes, there is concern with respect to the amount of sodium recommended in routine post-procedure fluids. Traditionally a glucose-containing solution with little salt (hypotonic) was employed in the past, e.g., Dextrose 5 % and 2/3:1/3—hypotonic fluids (see Table 2.10) [29]. However, cases of severe iatrogenic hyponatremia with resulting morbidity and mortality have been reported in hospitalized children, especially in the post-procedure period [30]. With recognition of the adverse effects of hyponatremia in children, a salt-containing isotonic solution during the periprocedural period is now recommended in pediatrics to avoid the effects of low sodium [31]. Use of glucagon during IR procedures can lead to transient rise in blood sugar followed by a rebound hypoglycemia. Therefore, IV fluid maintenance with a glucose-containing solution is important and checking serum glucose may be necessary post-glucagon [32].

Volume of iodinated contrast given is important especially in the young child. Although 3 mL/kg. is considered the conservative limit in diagnostic imaging procedures, this can be exceeded to approximately 6 mL/kg. when spread over the period of time during an IR procedure, e.g., angiography [33]. Careful recording of the volume of contrast administered throughout the entire procedure is necessary, both in terms of hand and pump injections. Use of dilute contrast (50:50) will frequently be adequate for visualization and results in less contrast load. The recorder, either the nurse or the technologist in the room, should alert the operator intermittently to the total contrast volume used. Use of small volume syringes (e.g., 3 cm^3) to draw up the contrast helps avoid inadvertent administration of excessive amounts in small children and minimizes wastage.

Radiation Protection

The topic of radiation protection can be approached from a departmental perspective of optimum equipment, applications, and safety devices (Chap. 1), as well as from an individual patient/procedure perspective, including patient and occupational dose [34, 35]. The responsibility for radiation protection at the individual level is a shared one resting to a major degree with the interventional radiologist and the technologist. Radiation awareness is the most important first step—awareness about dose for the patient and scatter radiation for the whole team. Whenever possible, imaging modalities that do not involve radiation should be employed, but when X-ray imaging is required, there is a responsibility to use all available radiation protection options and strategies especially in pediatric patients and personal protective devices for the team (Table 2.11). The following are some of the steps the individual provider should consider during a procedure [36].

Fluoroscopy

Keeping the "beam on time" to a minimum is the operator's most effective method to reduce patient dose—stepping as infrequently and briefly as possible on the fluoroscopy pedal, as the Image Gentle "Step Lightly" Initiative advocates [37]. Choosing the lowest pulse rate available which enables the procedure to be completed

Table 2.11 Abbreviated and modified from the Image Gently "Step Lightly" checklist*

	Patient protection	Personnel protection
General	Awareness of patient radiation history	Vigilant about personal fitted lead aprons, thyroid, glasses
US vs. X-ray	Use ultrasound, if possible	
DSA	Plan each run carefully	Use pump injection > hand injection if possible
	Avoid improper runs	Maximize distance from primary beam
	Min # frames/s	Use table skirt and hanging shields
	Short a run as possible	
	Minimize overlapping fields	
Fluoroscopy	Set pulse rate as low as possible	Use table skirt and hanging shields
	Minimize time with foot on pedal	Keep hands out of primary beam
	Review and use image saves	when using X-ray (fluoroscopy)
	Keep magnification to a minimum	Angle away from hands
	Use post-processing zoom	Heed alerts re-fluoroscopy time
	Collimate, without fluoroscopy if possible, excluding radiosensitive organs	

Occupational dose is related to patient dose. Steps to reduce patient dose also reduce occupational dose
* *Source*: www.imagegently.org
With permission: The Alliance for Radiation Safety in Pediatric Imaging

(e.g., 3 pulses/s) should be used. Optimum imaging is not always required for many procedures (e.g., gastrostomy tube change), where the "good enough" concept is more applicable. Smoothing of the image on current generation equipment enables a very low pulse rate to be used without a visible staccato effect. In equipment that has a removable grid, it is important to remove or insert the grid as one switches from a small to a large child. Use of collimation limits exposure to organs outside of the region of interest and can dramatically reduce the patient's effective dose. Newer equipment allows positioning without fluoroscopy and collimating on a last image hold—both excellent ways to reduce patient dose. Even without state-of-the-art equipment, careful manual positioning, avoidance of panning in search of the correct area, and collimation that is continuously adjusted as the procedure progresses, all assist in keeping patient dose to as low as reasonably achievable, ALARA [34–37]. Judicious use of magnification when needed, remembering to switch back down in magnification when not necessary, and +/– use of post-processing zoom are important factors in minimizing dose. The technologists play a major role in promoting dose reduction by taking the necessary steps to protect the patient and the team, alerting the operator who is otherwise absorbed and focused on the procedure about magnification and fluoroscopy time [34, 36]. A useful checklist is available on the Image Gently—Step Lightly web site for use (see Table 2.10) [37–39]. Ultimately, reducing radiation dose comes down to careful practice habits.

Exposures

Single spot exposures or angiographic runs are used if detailed image acquisition is required. Careful planning before a run is imperative to ensure that the position is correct, collimation is appropriately tight, magnification is as low as needed, frame rate is suitably adjusted to the rate of flow (venous or arterial), and contrast volume and pump settings are chosen properly. These will avoid aborted runs or the need to repeat a run [33, 36]. Newer equipment permits archiving of fluoroscopy runs, which may be of adequate quality to avoid the need for DSA in some circumstances. There is evidence that, for complex lesions, the use of rotational angiography results in dose savings, compared with repeated imaging in different projections [40, 41]. An additional clinical advantage of biplane imaging or rotational angiography in the pediatric setting is the need for less contrast. If and when CT is required, use of low-dose protocols is imperative, with significant gains possible by the adjustment of parameters including mA, KVp, number slices, and area covered [42, 43].

Occupational Dose

As occupational dose is largely influenced by the scatter dose from the patient, practices aimed at reducing patient dose also reduces scatter radiation to the team [36, 44]. Availability and use of personal protective devices is obligatory (see Chap. 1). In addition to the use of protective devices, careful personal practices and behaviors influence occupational dose for the individual and the whole team. Use of the inverse square law for distance from the source is a powerful tool to reduce dose to personnel. Approximation of the image intensifier or flat plate detector to the patient is another example of a technique to reduce occupational dose.

Supplies

For certain conditions, the creation of specific supply "kits" can be a very practical and helpful aid in the clinical management of the patient. Although there is a trend toward creating completely latex-free environments in pediatric facilities, it is helpful to have a "latex-free box" which can be brought in for a patient who is latex allergic; all contents are latex-free, so there is no doubt as to the whether certain dressings or devices contain latex or not [45]. In another example, children with epidermolysis bullosa are now living longer and therefore increasingly being referred for IR-type procedures (e.g., esophageal dilatation, gastrostomy placement, and venous access devices). The creation of an "epidermolysis bullosa box" contains all the appropriate types of dressings that are suitable for their skin [46].

Communication and Hand-Off

At the end of the procedure, a note must be written in the chart and an appropriate IR team member speaks to the parents. Necessary precautions for post-procedure recovery are reviewed with the recovery team and floor nursing staff (e.g., patient positioning, serum glucose level checks, etc.). Post-procedure orders are written to communicate issues of monitoring, fluid intake (oral or IV), antibiotics, time for discharge, etc. A phone call to the referring physician is clinically worthwhile and promotes good clinical relations. A radiology report is dictated as soon as possible.

Post-procedure Care

During the immediate post-procedure phase, nursing care involves patient monitoring during recovery from the effects of sedation, anesthesia, and the procedure, as requested in the post-procedure orders—vital signs (pulse, blood pressure, respiratory rate, temperature, pain score) and urine output (see Tables 2.1, 2.6, and 2.7). Later a member of the IR team should review the patient for his/her general well-being. In addition the procedural site is examined and signs of procedure-specific complications should be sought (e.g., swelling/bleeding at port insertion site; pallor, coolness, presence of pedal pulses post-angiography; macroscopic hematuria post-renal biopsy; hemoglobinuria post-thrombectomy). A written note of the visit should be made in the chart, dated, timed, and signed. If the patient is well, the IR team may sign off or choose to follow with subsequent visits. If the patient is due to go home, discharge information for the family is required (see below).

In the event of a complication or concern, the IR team takes the appropriate measures, relevant orders are placed, and the patient remains on the list for further follow-up. The IR team may need to consult other specialties to assist in the management of a complication (e.g., general surgery in case of a bowel perforation, plastic surgery in the event of skin ischemia/ulceration). The IR team should assume this responsibility and directly liaise with the other specialists as needed.

Follow-Up

The state-of-the-art interventionalist is a clinician who follows his or her patients outside of the IR suite. Either the interventionalist or an appropriate member of the IR team (e.g., physician extender) should review the patient post-procedure [2, 47, 48]. Whether this is driven by desire to practice good medicine, institutional expectations, demands of clinical colleagues, billing, or local regulatory requirements, this development is a positive one. At minimum an inpatient should be seen on the ward later in the day of the procedure, and an outpatient should be seen before discharge. Further follow-up is necessary for some of the IR procedures (e.g., radiofrequency ablation of osteoid osteoma) as outlined in Chap. 1. The benefits of follow-up—including timely recognition of complications and appropriate longitudinal care—are also discussed in Chap. 1.

Early Follow-Up: Inpatient

In addition to the immediate ward visit following the procedure, subsequent single or ongoing daily post-procedure ward visits are indicated for certain groups of patients. They may include those with a possibility of a late/delayed complication (e.g., high-risk transjugular liver biopsy, peritonitis post-gastrostomy tube insertion, fluctuating hypertension post-renal angioplasty), as well as those who have a catheter or drain in situ following their IR procedure (e.g., post-empyema drainage). The latter patients should be followed until resolution of the problem (e.g., gastrostomy achieving full feeds) or removal of a device (e.g., chest drain removal post-empyema). The IR team should advise and plan for any subsequent measures required, such as the timing and type of repeat imaging, the use of tissue plasminogen activator (tPA), and the decision when to remove the drain. The IR team should remove the drain (e.g., transrectal drain on resolution of pelvic collection). Subsequent follow-up depends on the nature of the procedure. Service-type procedures such as image-guided percutaneous biopsies and placement of vascular access devices do not usually require further visits beyond the immediate post-procedure time. Some exceptions may apply, e.g., repeat packing of a wound following a port removal for purulent port pocket infection. Other cases require longer-term follow-up in an outpatient setting, to ensure they are not lost to follow-up (see below).

Informed Discharge

Informing patients and families about what to expect post-procedure, what signs and symptoms to look out for as indicators of a complication, and instructions regarding bathing, activity, and dressings can be done verbally but more appropriately should be with written discharge instructions, or information pamphlets, including names and telephone numbers of whom to contact in the event of a problem. The provision of informed discharge should be documented in the medical records. Some centers prefer to use an informed discharge form, which the parents sign, a copy of which is then placed in the medical record, to document that the parent/guardian has received the necessary instructions. The printed discharge information is also useful for any subsequent visits to the Emergency Department, as it documents the procedure and device (e.g., post-intrasalivary Botox injections for drooling; intramuscular Botox for spasticity; size and type of vascular access device) [49, 50].

Early Follow-Up: Outpatient

Many IR procedures are performed in the outpatient setting, which is efficient in terms of health-care resources and is emotionally and psychologically better for many children. Along with an outpatient IR service, or early discharge of inpatients, comes a responsibility to address aftercare and follow-up. Informed discharge is discussed above. For the outpatient, a follow-up phone call by a member of the IR team (e.g., clinic nurse) is one way to provide continuity of clinical care. It provides support for families and a means to answer their questions (e.g., management of PleurX catheters in malignant effusions). It also provides reassurance for the IR team regarding the procedure and the patient's well-being. For those procedures in which IR is providing a major component of treatment (e.g., radiofrequency ablation of a lesion), a return visit to the IR clinic ensures the patient is not lost to follow-up [2–4]. It provides the opportunity for assessment of treatment efficacy, any unexpected developments (e.g., purulent discharge/infection at site), and ongoing education (e.g., irrigation and bowel management post-cecostomy tube insertion). Some groups of procedures may be followed in a multidisciplinary clinic organized with another specialty (e.g., with plastic surgery for vascular anomalies, with urology for angiomyolipoma post-embolization) (see Chap. 1).

Late Follow-Up

For those in whom the IR treatment is the definitive therapy (e.g., varicocele embolization), arrangement for late follow-up is necessary. Depending on the procedure, this will vary both in timing (e.g., a few weeks following ablation of an osteoid osteoma, 3–6 months post-varicocele embolization) and in location (e.g., in the IR clinic or in a multidisciplinary clinic). The IR team is responsible to plan for and schedule follow-up procedures required for their devices (e.g., exchange of a long-term biliary or ureteric stent, removal of a transgastric pancreatic pseudocyst drain, and follow-up of a fistula). This is especially true for those devices that are only internal, with no external reminder for the patient or the physician that there is a device that warrants attention (e.g., IVC filter). The IR team is the health-care team most knowledgeable about the subsequent management required and has a responsibility to ensure the patient is not lost to follow-up.

Rather than considering the clinical roles outlined above as daunting for the interventional team, it can be embraced and incorporated into daily practice, as it is a significant step forward in providing excellent patient care.

References

1. American College of Radiology, The American Society of Interventional and Therapeutic Neuroradiology, The Society of Interventional Radiology. Practice guideline for interventional clinical practice. J Vasc Interv Radiol. 2005;16:149–55.
2. Baskin K, Hogan M, Sidhu M, et al. Developing a clinical pediatric interventional practice: a joint clinical practice guideline from the society if interventional radiology and the society for pediatric radiology. J Vasc Interv Radiol. 2011;22:1647–55.
3. American College of Radiology White Paper: Clinical Practice of Interventional Radiology and Neurointerventional Radiology White Paper. 2003. http// www.acr.org/dyna/?doc=departments/stand_accred/standards/ir_white_paper
4. Siskin GP, Bagla S, Sansivero GE, Mitchell NL. The interventional radiology clinic: key ingredients for success. J Vasc Interv Radiol. 2004;15(7):681–8.
5. Fontalvo LF, Amaral JG, Temple M, Chait PG, John P, Krishnamuthy G, Smith C, Connolly B. Percutaneous US-guided biopsies of peripheral pulmonary lesions in children. Pediatr Radiol. 2006; 36(6):491–7.
6. Daabiss M. American Society of Anaesthesiologists physical status classification. Indian J Anaesth. 2011; 55:111–5.
7. McCrone L, Alexander S, Karsli C, Taylor G, Amaral JG, Parra D, et al. US-guided percutaneous needle biopsy of anterior mediastinal masses in children. Pediatr Radiol. 2012;42(1):40–9. doi:10.1007/s00247-011-2204-2. Epub 2011 Aug 24.
8. Dipchand A, Jeremy Friedman J, editors. The Hospital for Sick Children. Handbook of pediatrics. 11th ed. Ed: Section III Laboratory References Values by Alabdulrazzaq, Adeli and Lau. W B Saunders Co Canada Ltd, Toronto. 1997;810–82.
9. Malloy PC, Grassi CJ, Kundu S, Gervais DA, Miller DL, Osnis RB, Postoak DW, Rajan DK, Sacks D, Schwartzberg MS, Zuckerman DA, Cardella JF, for the Standards of Practice Committee with Cardiovascular and Interventional Radiological Society of Europe (CIRSE) Endorsement. Consensus guidelines for periprocedural management of coagulation status and hemostasis risk in percutaneous image-guided interventions. J Vasc Interv Radiol. 2009;20:S240–9.
10. Firth PG, McMillan KN, Haberkern CM, Yaster M, Bender MA, Goodwin SR. A survey of perioperative management of sickle cell disease in North America. Paediatr Anaesth. 2011;21(1):43–9. doi:10.1111/j.1460-9592.2010.03415.x. Epub 2010 Sep 29.
11. Lavoie J. Blood transfusion risks and alternative strategies in pediatric patients. Paediatr Anaesth. 2011; 21(1):14–24.
12. Chait PG, Shlomovitz E, Connolly BL, Temple MJ, Restrepo R, Amaral JG, Muraca S, Richards HF, Ein SH. Percutaneous cecostomy: updates in technique and patient care. Radiology. 2003;227(1):246–50. Epub 2003 Feb 11.
13. Rauch F. Bone biopsy: indications and methods. Endocr Dev. 2009;16:49–57. Epub 2009 Jun 3.
14. Thomsen HS. European Society of Urogenital Radiology (ESUR) guidelines on the safe use of iodinated contrast media. Eur J Radiol. 2006;60(3): 307–13. Epub 2006 Sep 11.
15. Evans KG. Consent: a guide for Canadian physicians. 4th ed. Ottawa: The Canadian Medical Protective Association; 2006.
16. Temple-Doig L, Gordon M, Buckenham T, Roake J, Lewis D. Informed consent for vascular intervention. N Z Med J. 2005;118(1221):U1630.
17. Davies L. The consent process in interventional radiology: the role of specialist nurses. Clin Radiol. 2004;59:246–52.
18. Foglia MB. A quality improvement approach to improving informed consent practices in pediatric research. J Clin Ethics. 2009;20(4):343–52.
19. Braddock C. "Surgery is certainly one good option": quality and time-efficiency of informed decision-making in surgery. J Bone Joint Surg. 2008; 90:1830–8.
20. Canadian Paediatric Society. Treatment decisions regarding infants, children, and adolescents. http://www.cps.ca/english/statements/B/b04-01.htm
21. Bello BA. Dignity and informed consent in the treatment of mature minors. J Int Bioethique. 2010; 21(4):103–22, 164–5.
22. Committee on Pediatric Emergency Medicine and Committee on Bioethics. Policy statement—consent for emergency medical services for children and adolescents. Pediatrics 2011;128:427–33.
23. SIR Policy on Off-Label Use. http://www.sirweb.org/clinical/policy.shtml
24. Kleinman ME, Schexnayder SM, Samson RA, et al. Pediatric advanced life support: 2010 American heart association guidelines for cardiopulmonary resuscitation and emergency cardiovascular care. Circulation. 2010;122:S876–908.
25. Gawande A. The checklist manifesto: how to get things right. New York: Metropolitan Books; 2009.
26. Norton EK, Rangel SJ. Implementing a pediatric surgical safety checklist in the OR and beyond. AORN J. 2010;92(1):61–71.
27. Angle JF, Nemcek AA Jr, Cohen AM, et al, for the SIR Standards Division. Quality improvement guidelines for preventing wrong site, wrong procedure, and wrong person errors: application of the Joint Commission "Universal Protocol for Preventing

Wrong Site, Wrong Procedure, Wrong Person Surgery" to the practice of interventional radiology. J Vasc Interv Radiol. 2008;19:1145–51.
28. Laffan EE, McNamara PJ, Amaral J, Whyte H, L'Herault J, Temple M, John P, Connolly BL. Pediatr Radiol. 2009;39(8):781–90.
29. Moritz ML, Ayus JC. Review of interventional procedures in the very low birth-weight infant (<1.5 kg): complications, lessons learned and current practice. Prevention of hospital-acquired hyponatremia: a case for using isotonic saline. Pediatrics. 2003;111(2): 227–30.
30. Eulmesekian PG, Pérez A, Minces PG, Bohn D. Hospital-acquired hyponatremia in postoperative pediatric patients: prospective observational study. Pediatr Crit Care Med. 2010;11(4):479–83.
31. Moritz ML, Ayus JC. Intravenous fluid management for the acutely ill child. Curr Opin Pediatr. 2011; 23(2):186–93.
32. Bernhard N1, McAlpine K, Moineddin R, Connolly BL.Variations in blood glucose levels following gastrostomy tube insertion in a paediatric population. Pediatr Radiol. 2014 Feb 18. [Epub ahead of print].
33. Heran MK, Marshalleck F, Temple M, Grassi CJ, Connolly B, Towbin RB, Baskin KM, Dubois J, Hogan MJ, Kundu S, Miller DL, Roebuck DJ, Rose SC, Sacks D, Sidhu M, Wallace MJ, Zuckerman DA, Cardella JF, Society of Interventional Radiology Standards of Practice Committee, Society of Pediatric Radiology Interventional Radiology Committee. Joint quality improvement guidelines for pediatric arterial access and arteriography: from the societies of interventional radiology and pediatric radiology. Pediatr Radiol. 2010;40(2):237–50.
34. Strauss KJ, Kaste SC. The ALARA (as low as reasonably achievable) concept in pediatric interventional and fluoroscopic imaging: striving to keep radiation doses as low as possible during fluoroscopy of pediatric patients—a white paper executive summary. Pediatr Radiol. 2006;36 Suppl 2:110–2.
35. Strauss KJ. Interventional suite and equipment management: cradle to grave. Pediatr Radiol. 2006;36 Suppl 2:221–36.
36. Connolly B, Racadio J, Towbin R. Practice of ALARA in the pediatric interventional suite. Pediatr Radiol. 2006;36 Suppl 2:163–7.
37. www.imagegently.org
38. Sidhu M, Strauss K, Connolly B, et al. Radiation safety in pediatric interventional radiology. Tech Vasc Interv Radiol. 2010;13(4):205.
39. Sidhu M, Coley B, Goske M, et al. Image gently, *step lightly*: increasing radiation dose awareness in pediatric interventional radiology. Pediatr Radiol. 2009; 39(10):1135–8.
40. Wielands JY, et al. Effective dose analysis of three dimensional rotational angiography during catheter ablation procedures. Phys Med Biol. 2010;55(3): 563–79.
41. Bridcut RR, Murphy E, Workman A, Flynn P, Winder RJ. Patient dose from 3D rotational neurovascular studies. Br J Radiol. 2007;80(953):362–6.
42. Parra DA, Chan M, Krishnamurthy G, Spiegel L, Amaral JG, Temple MJ, John PR, Connolly BL. Use and accuracy of US guidance for image-guided injections of the temporomandibular joints in children with arthritis. Pediatr Radiol. 2010;40(9):1498–504.
43. Zhu X, Felice M, Johnson L, Sarmiento M, Cahill AM. Developing low-dose C-arm CT imaging for temporomandibular joint (TMJ) disorder in interventional radiology. Pediatr Radiol. 2011;41(4):476–82.
44. Dauer LT, Thornton RH, Solomon SB, St GJ. Unprotected operator eye lens doses in oncologic interventional radiology are clinically significant: estimation from patient kerma-area-product data. J Vasc Interv Radiol. 2010;21(12):1859–61.
45. Taylor JS, Erkek E. Latex allergy: diagnosis and management. Dermatol Ther. 2004;17(4):289–301.
46. Mavili E, Amaral J, Healey A, Karsli C, Pope E, Connolly B. Percutaneous interventional radiology procedures in patients with epidermolysis bullosa: modifications and challenges. AJR Am J Roentgenol. 2010;195(2):468–75.
47. Connolly B, Mahant S. The pediatric hospitalist and interventional radiologist: a model for clinical care in pediatric interventional radiology. J Vasc Interv Radiol. 2006;17(11 Pt 1):1733–8.
48. Rosenberg SM, Rosenthal DA, Rajan DK, Millward SF, Baum RA, Silberzweig JE, Tuite CM, Cardella JF. Position statement: the role of physician assistants in interventional radiology. American Academy of Physician Assistants. J Vasc Interv Radiol. 2009; 20(7 Suppl):S337–41.
49. Khan WU, Campisi P, Nadarajah S, Shakur YA, Khan N, Semenuk D, McCann C, Roske L, McConney-Ellis S, Joseph M, Parra D, Amaral J, John P, Temple M, Connolly B. Botulinum toxin A for treatment of sialorrhea in children: an effective, minimally invasive approach. Arch Otolaryngol Head Neck Surg. 2011; 137(4):339–44. Epub 2011 Jan 17.
50. Ellies M, Rohrbach-Volland S, Arglebe C, Wilken B, Laskawi R, Hanefeld F. Successful management of drooling with botulinum toxin A in neurologically disabled children. Neuropediatrics. 2002;33(6): 327–30.

Pediatric Anesthesia and Sedation for Interventional Radiology

3

Keira P. Mason

Introduction

As interventional radiology evolves, the emerging technological advances and increased complexity of procedures challenge the anesthetic technique. In infants and children, even the simplest procedures may require a general anesthetic to provide safe and motionless conditions. Indications for general anesthesia or sedation, aside from the inability to remain motionless on one's own, include the need for intermittent breath holding during image acquisition. Further indications for an endotracheal intubation may include those situations in which there is a risk of vasospasm (cerebral angiography and embolization). In these circumstances, controlled ventilation with purposeful hypercarbia can promote vasodilatation.

Interventional techniques include nonvascular and vascular intervention [1]. Biopsies, insertion and/or repositioning of drainage catheters, and insertion of catheters for central intravenous access often represent the majority of procedures and may be managed with a straightforward anesthetic or sedation. In some circumstances, regional anesthesia may provide a viable alternative. Intercostal nerve blocks may be very useful for lung or rib biopsies, chest tubes, biliary or subphrenic drainage procedures, and insertion of biliary stents.

The vascular interventions can range from straightforward angiography to complex procedures. Embolization and sclerotherapy for vascular malformations and anomalies tend to represent the more complex interventional vascular procedures. Percutaneous transluminal angioplasty and fibrinolytic therapy have been shown to benefit from procedural sedation or anesthesia [2]. The basic indications for embolization are occlusion of vascular malformations, management of uncontrollable hemorrhage, medical renal ablation, and presurgical embolization of hypervascular masses.

Sedation Strategies for Radiological Imaging Studies

Interventional radiological procedures for pediatric patients frequently require either general anesthesia or deep sedation for successful completion. Procedures that in adults would normally be performed with minimal sedation or local anesthesia often demand deep sedation or anesthesia in children.

K.P. Mason, M.D. (✉)
Department of Anesthesia, Children's Hospital Boston, Harvard Medical Center,
300 Longwood Avenue, Boston, MA 02115, USA
e-mail: keira.mason@childrens.harvard.edu

M. Temple and F.E. Marshalleck (eds.), *Pediatric Interventional Radiology: Handbook of Vascular and Non-Vascular Interventions*, DOI 10.1007/978-1-4419-5856-3_3,

Patient Selection

A thorough medical history and review of systems should be completed and documented prior to scheduling a patient, in addition to relevant clinical consults and laboratory studies. A list of medical conditions that would immediately contraindicate non-anesthesiologist-delivered sedation can help guide this triage process as well as ensure consistency of decision-making (Table 3.1). Prior to the scheduled study, all families should receive a prescreen telephone call to confirm if there have been recent changes in medical history along with the nil per os (NPO) instructions. In most circumstances, families are instructed to administer the child's routine morning medications with a sip of clear fluid.

The patients scheduled for non-anesthesiologist-delivered sedation are typically American Society of Anesthesiologists level 1 or level 2 but rarely level 3 (Table 3.2).

Table 3.1 Red flags for sedation

1. Apnea
2. Full-term infant less than 1 month of age (unless an inpatient admitted to the hospital)
3. Respiratory compromised patients
4. Uncontrolled/unpredictable gastroesophageal reflux or vomiting that poses an aspiration risk
5. Craniofacial abnormality that may make it difficult to establish effective mask airway
6. Cyanotic cardiac disease or unstable cardiac status
7. Painful procedure that may be challenging to provide adequate analgesia without a general anesthetic
8. High-risk procedure that may require presence of an anesthesiologist for resuscitation
9. Procedure that requires absolute immobility only achievable with a general anesthetic
10. Procedure being performed in remote location that is so removed that immediate emergency backup assistance would be virtually impossible
11. Inadequate qualified personnel available to provide safe procedural sedation

With permission from Mason KP. Pediatric Sedation for Radiological Imaging Studies. In: Ray CE, ed. Pain Management in Interventional Radiology. New York, NY: Cambridge University Press; 2008:270

In the United States, the delivery of deep sedation by non-anesthesiologists should be administered according to the American Society of Anesthesiologists Guidelines [3]. Under these guidelines, registered nurses are no longer qualified to administer deep sedation. The sedation provider must be a physician, nurse anesthetist, or anesthesia assistant. Specifically, the sedation care provider is expected to be experienced in the delivery of positive pressure ventilation via a facemask, endotracheal intubation, and insertion of laryngeal mask airways along with placement of nasal and oropharyngeal airways. A minimum of 35 patients or simulated cases must be performed in order to demonstrate competence. Recently, the Center for Medicaid and Medicare Services published their guidelines which are consistent with the American Society of Anesthesiologist's qualification requirements for sedation providers [4].

In the event that there are questions regarding the medical status or appropriateness of a child for sedation, a liaison from the Department of Anesthesia can facilitate the evaluation process by reviewing the history and, if appropriate, requesting consultations with appropriate specialty services (cardiac anesthesia, otolaryngology, surgery, nephrology, cardiology, or endocrinology). If the patient is deemed appropriate to receive sedation, then personal discussion between the consulting physician and sedation care provider is helpful to maximize safe care.

Table 3.2 ASA physical status classification

1. A normal healthy patient
2. A patient with mild systemic disease
3. A patient with severe systemic disease
4. A patient with severe systemic disease that is a constant threat to life
5. A moribund patient who is not expected to survive without the operation
6. A declared brain-dead patient whose organs are being removed for donor purposes

With permission from Mason KP. Pediatric Sedation for Radiological Imaging Studies. In: Ray CE, ed. Pain Management in Interventional Radiology. New York, NY: Cambridge University Press; 2008:270

It is important for the practitioner responsible for sedation to have a thorough understanding of the procedure requested. For example, the same patient may be medically appropriate to undergo sedation for an MRI scan but may be an inappropriate sedation candidate for a nephrostomy tube, placed with the patient prone in interventional radiology. Although a patient may meet the medical criteria for sedation, a collaborative discussion between the practitioners responsible for the sedation and the radiologist will ensure that the procedure and patient lend itself to sedation. In the event that the procedure is deemed high risk (e.g., cerebral embolization), associated with significant pain (e.g., sclerotherapy with doxycycline), or long in duration, the patient is usually best referred to general anesthesia for management. Additional, important, considerations should be the physical layout of the procedure room and its geographical proximity to the operating rooms. In the event of an emergency and the need for a "code team," the physical layout is important. If the radiological suites are physically isolated and distant from backup assistance, the more conservative approach will be to request anesthesia services prior to the initiation of a high-risk procedure.

Patient Sedation Guidelines

To minimize the chance of drug delivery error or miscalculation, it is helpful to have preprinted order sheets that should be approved by the Hospital Sedation Committee as recommended by JCAHO. The practice standards adopted by the American Society of Anesthesiologists in 1986 for basic intraoperative monitoring apply as well to extramural locations. Practice standards and guidelines promulgated by the American Academy of Pediatrics [5] are exceeded by established practice standards in anesthesiology [6]. Significant variances may exist when non-anesthesiologists sedate [7]. Practice Standards for Nonanesthetizing Locations were adopted by the American Society of Anesthesiologists in 1994 [8]. Recent practice standards by the American Society of Anesthesiologists for deep sedation by non-anesthesiologists stipulate monitoring which includes electrocardiogram, pulse oximetry, capnography, and noninvasive blood pressure monitoring [3].

A director of anesthesia services for a busy extramural radiology site will facilitate the delivery and coordination of anesthesia and sedation services. By being available to answer questions, do on-site consults, examine patients, and provide backup support or emergency airway expertise, the anesthesiologist is critical to the viability of a non-anesthesiologist-delivered sedation program. In addition to the American Society of Anesthesiologist, the Joint Commission on Accreditation of Healthcare Organizations (JCAHO) Anesthesia and Sedation Manual has set guidelines for credentialing of all personnel who administer sedation [3, 9].

Medications

The selection of a sedation agent depends on the patient's underlying medical condition, age, drug tolerance, and anticipated procedure. Each medication has its own property which can include a hypnotic, anxiolytic, and/or analgesic. In order to appropriately make a sedation plan for each procedure, it is important to understand the properties of each medication and its potential synergistic actions with adjuvant medication. The more common sedatives administered for light, moderate, and deep sedation will be reviewed below.

Ketoralac

Ketoroloac (Toradol; Abbott labs, N. Chicago, IL) is an analgesic. It does not have sedative, hypnotic, or amnestic properties. Ketorolac tromethamine can be administered intravenously every 6 h with a maximum of 72 h of administration. It is useful for onetime administration to provide analgesia for short procedures such as biopsies. As a nonsteroidal anti-inflammatory agent, ketorolac may inhibit platelet aggregation and prolong bleeding time, which may be an undesirable effect for some interventional procedures. Agreement to administer a nonsteroidal should be obtained from the interventional radiologist prior to administration. Alternative analgesics could include narcotics or ketamine.

Narcotics

The choice of narcotic should depend on the duration of the procedure and the extent of analgesia required. Morphine (Baxter Healthcare Corp, Deerfield, IL) and fentanyl (Baxter) are the more popular narcotics. Morphine requires approximately 10 min for effect and can provide analgesia for up to 2 h. Fentanyl works within minutes and has 100 times the potency of morphine. It generally needs to be redosed every 30–60 min, depending on the procedure. Narcotics work best when administered prior to (in anticipation of) the painful stimulus so that adequate analgesia is present at the time of the stimulus.

Ketamine

Ketamine, 2-(o-chlorophenyl)-2-(methylamino) cyclohexane, a phencyclidine and cyclohexamine derivative, was developed and introduced into clinical anesthesia practice in the 1960s. It may be administered via intravenous, intramuscular, oral, rectal, nasal, epidural, or intrathecal routes. The use of ketamine for pediatric sedation and analgesia has been described in various non-operating room settings that include emergency departments [10], gastroenterology [11], oncology [12], dental [13], and radiology suites [14, 15]. Ketamine produces rapid onset of deep sedation and analgesia with minimal respiratory depression and cardiovascular side effects [16–21]. A review of the literature reveals that despite the widespread use of ketamine by non-anesthesiologists, there is no consistent protocol for ketamine administration. Mason et al. describe the intravenous or intramuscular administration of ketamine, up to 2 mg/kg, for interventional radiological procedures. The intravenous dosage is followed by a continuous infusion of up to 125 μg/kg/h ketamine until the procedure is completed [17, 18]. When given in small bolus doses, it provides analgesia for an average of 30 min. As an infusion, ketamine can produce a continuous state of analgesia that may be titrated up and down in response to (or in anticipation of) the painful stimulus. It is especially useful for patients who are going to undergo an exceptionally painful procedure (doxycycline sclerotherapy, chest tube), are on chronic opioids, or have a high tolerance to opiates. The coadministration of ketamine with an anticholinergic is no longer recommended [19]. Ketamine provides an effective alternative to narcotics in some patients.

Hallucinations, delusions, nightmares, and emergence delirium are phenomenon most commonly described as a potential side effect of ketamine; these are more commonly noted in adults [22, 23]. The presence of these adverse events in the pediatric population is controversial [13, 24]. In adults, the concomitant administration of benzodiazepines (midazolam or diazepam) with ketamine has been shown to decrease the incidence of these events. Again, the utility of benzodiazepines in reducing these events in children is controversial [25–27]. Some reports indicate that the addition of benzodiazepines leads to an increased incidence of oxygen desaturation events [28]. Under age five, there is no definitive evidence that benzodiazepine administration will reduce the hallucinations, delusions, and excitatory behavior that can occur with ketamine. Children over age five may in fact benefit from concomitant benzodiazepine administration. Although ketamine administration and supervision by interventional radiologists is not a widely recognized technique, it offers an alternative agent for children who require profound analgesia albeit the risk of dissociative side effects.

Collaboration between the Departments of Anesthesiology and Radiology can provide for the radiologist-supervised administration of ketamine by nurses for interventional procedures, liver and renal biopsies included, in pediatric patients who might otherwise have required a general anesthetic. With sufficient triage and careful review of the medical history as well as relative and absolute contraindications to ketamine administration, radiologists can safely incorporate ketamine into their sedation armamentarium (Tables 3.3 and 3.4). Patients and parents are often relieved and grateful to avoid general anesthesia.

Table 3.3 Exclusion criteria for ketamine induced sedation

1. Active pulmonary infection or disease
2. Known or potential (i.e., risk of) airway compromise
3. Pulmonary hypertension
4. Age of 3 months or younger
5. History of apnea or obstructive sleep apnea
6. Craniofacial defect that would make mask ventilation difficult
7. Complex cardiac disease
8. Acute globe injury
9. Prior adverse reaction to ketamine
10. History of bipolar disease or schizophrenia
11. Head injury associated with loss of consciousness, altered mental status, or emesis
12. Intracranial hypertension (i.e., CNS mass lesions, hydrocephalus, head injuries associated with increased intracranial pressure): if there is any doubt, please have radiologist consult ordering physician to determine whether there is increased intracranial pressure risk
13. Any child in whom there is a question of increased intracranial pressure
14. Child with potential ventriculoperitoneal shunt malfunction
15. Increased intraocular pressure
16. Patient or parent refusal

With permission from Mason KP, Padua H, Fontaine P, Zurakowski D. Radiologist Supervised Ketamine Sedation for Solid Organ Biopsies in Children and Adolescents. AJR Am J Roentgenol 2009;192(5):1265 (requested permission from American Roentgen Ray Society)

Table 3.4 Adverse events and parent and patient satisfaction

Variable	Total cohort ($n=65$)	Liver biopsy ($n=35$)	Renal biopsy ($n=30$)
Adverse events (no. of patients)			
During sedation	2[a]	0	2
During recovery	8[b]	6	2
24 h after procedure	4[c]	2	2
7 day after procedure	0	0	0
Sedation failure (no.)	0	0	0
Satisfaction (%)[d]			
Dissatisfied	0	0	0
Neutral	8	6	10
Satisfied	58	60	57
Very satisfied	34	34	33

[a] Renal biopsy: range ($n=1$), marked hypertension ($n=1$)
[b] Liver biopsy, need for supplemental oxygen ($n=1$), need for inhalers ($n=1$), vomiting or nausea (or both) ($n=4$); renal biopsy, agitation ($n=1$), vomiting and nausea ($n=1$)
[c] Liver biopsy, rash ($n=1$), vomiting ($n=1$); renal biopsy, irritability ($n=1$), drowsiness ($n=1$)
[d] Parent- and patient-based assessment

With permission from Mason KP, Padua H, Fontaine P, Zurakowski D. Radiologist Supervised Ketamine Sedation for Solid Organ Biopsies in Children and Adolescents. Am J Roentgenol 2009;192(5):1263 (requested permission from American Roentgen Ray Society)

Preparing for Emergencies in Areas Distant to the Operating Room

There are three particularly challenging scenarios that may occur in nonoperating room (off-site) locations: (1) the child with a known difficult airway, (2) the child with an unrecognized difficult airway, and (3) cardiovascular arrest. Each challenging situation will be addressed in order and in detail below. Most interventional radiology suites are remote to the operating room, to skilled and knowledgeable airway (otolaryngology, anesthesia, and surgery) assistance, and to backup airway support (bronchoscopes and alternative airway devices). Fiber-optic equipment and procedures are not routine in outfield areas and thus, when anticipated, should be reserved for the operating room environment. It is suggested that the "potential difficult airway" be managed first in the operating room and, after the airway is secured, the patient can then be transported to the radiological suites.

In the operating room, there are appropriate backup support and supplies if needed. Remember that each extramural anesthetizing location is unique with regard to conducting resuscitation. Redundancy of monitoring devices and equipment is important; one should not be limited to a single item that could malfunction at the time of resuscitation. The physicians, nurses, anesthesiologists, technologists, and support personnel must know the location of emergency equipment. In addition, a hard board to be placed under the patient during resuscitation should be readily available. Mock codes and simulation of emergencies should be performed regularly to ensure adequate flow, teamwork, and delineation of responsibilities.

The administration of iodine-containing contrast for interventional procedures necessitates a complete knowledge of risk factors for anaphylaxis and appropriate prophylaxis and intervention (Table 3.5). Patients with multiple allergies, shellfish allergies, or atopic disease are at increased risk of exhibiting anaphylaxis to iodine-containing contrast. These patients may benefit from pretreatment with steroids and antihistamines.

The unrecognized and unanticipated difficult airway should be a scenario for which alternate airway devices, such as laryngeal mask airways and even tracheostomy sets, are routinely available and stocked in off-site locations. In the event that the child cannot be ventilated nor intubated, the laryngeal mask airway may be life saving [29, 30]. Transfusion requirements are rare in extramural locations, yet preprocedural anemia, accidental perforation of vascular structures, or medical transfusion requirements, such as sickle cell disease or prematurity, may require transfusion therapy. Equipment consistent with that available in the operating room must be available in these off-site locations.

Table 3.5 Management of acute reactions in children

Urticaria • No treatment needed in most cases • Give H_1-receptor blocker: diphenhydramine PO, IM, or IV 1–2 mg/kg, up to 50 mg • If severe or widely disseminated, give α-agonist, epinephrine SC (1:1,000) 0.01 mL/kg
Facial edema • Give O_2 6–10 L/min (via mask, face tent, or blow-by stream) administered at 2 times the maintenance rate in order to monitor electrocardiogram, O_2 saturation (pulse oximeter), and blood pressure • Give α-agonist: epinephrine SC or IM (1:1,000) 0.01 mL/kg/, up to 0.3 mL/dose. Repeat in 15–30 min as needed • Give H_1-receptor blocker: diphenhydramine IM or IV 1–2 mg/kg, up to 50 mg • If no response to therapy, seek appropriate assistance (e.g., cardiopulmonary arrest response team)
Laryngeal edema or bronchospasm • Give O_2 6–10 L/min (via mask, face tent, or blow-by stream). Monitor electrocardiogram, O_2 saturation (pulse oximeter), and blood pressure • Give β-agonist inhalers: bronchodilators, such as metaproterenol, terbutaline, or albuterol 2–3 puffs. Repeat as necessary • Give epinephrine SC or IM (1:1,000) 0.1 mL/kg, maximum 3 mL/dose. Repeat in 3–5 min as needed • Call for assistance (e.g., cardiopulmonary arrest response team) for severe bronchospasm or if O_2 saturation <88 % persists
Pulmonary edema • Give O_2 6–10 L/min (via mask, face tent, or blow-by stream). Monitor electrocardiogram, O_2 saturation (pulse oximeter), and blood pressure • Give diuretic: furosemide IV 1–2 mg/kg • Call for assistance (e.g., cardiopulmonary arrest response team)
Hypotension with tachycardia • Give O_2 6–10 L/min (via mask, face tent, or blow-by stream). Monitor electrocardiogram, O_2 saturation (pulse oximeter), and blood pressure • Legs elevated 60° or more (preferred) or Trendelenburg position • Keep patient warm • Give IV or IO normal saline or lactated Ringer's solution 20 mL/kg over 5–10 min. Bolus infusion over 10–20 min in patients with myocardial dysfunction • Seek appropriate assistance (e.g., cardiopulmonary arrest response team)
Hypotension with bradycardia (vagal reaction) • Give O_2 6–10 L/min (via mask). Monitor electrocardiogram, O_2 saturation (pulse oximeter), and blood pressure • Legs elevated 60° or more (preferred) or Trendelenburg position • Keep patient warm • Give IV or IO normal saline or lactated Ringer's solution 20 mL/kg over 5–10 min. Give infusion over 10–20 min in patients with myocardial dysfunction • Give atropine IV 0.02 mg/kg if patient does not respond quickly to steps 2, 3, and 4. Minimum initial dose of 0.1 mg. Maximum initial dose of 0.5 mg (infant/child), 1 mg (adolescent). Atropine dose may be doubled for second administration • Seek appropriate assistance (e.g., cardiopulmonary arrest response team)

IM intramuscular, *IO* intraosseous, *IV* intravenous, *SC* subcutaneous, *PO* per os (orally)

With permission from Mason KP, Holzman RS. Anesthesia and Sedation for Pediatric Procedures Outside the Operating Room. In: Davis PJ, Caldis FP, Motoyama EK eds. Smith's Anesthesia for Infants and Children. 8th ed. Philadelphia, PA: Mosby, Elsevier Science; 2011. Box 33-2. © Elsevier 2011

Summary

The demand for anesthesia and sedation services in sites distant to the operating room can be challenging and with extra risk. Although the incidence of adverse outcomes for anesthesia and sedation in these radiological areas has not been reported, reports from office-based and ambulatory surgery centers have extrapolated risks. In Florida, the incidence of adverse events is higher in office-based versus outpatient surgical centers [31]. Although these outcomes cannot be directly compared with off-site anesthetizing locations, it prompts the consideration of the level of added risk in the off-site location. Sedation, monitored anesthesia care, and general anesthesia are all choices that carry risks. Historically, an avoidance of a general anesthesia has been thought to minimize the risk of adverse outcome. Closed-claims analysis demonstrates that monitored anesthesia care poses an equal risk to general anesthesia with respect to severity of injury, death, and permanent brain damage. Twenty-four percentage of all monitored anesthesia care claims involve oversedation and respiratory depression [32]. Anesthesia and sedation providers must recognize that a careful risk analysis is critical when selecting patients and formulating a plan of care.

This chapter has reviewed some general issues and some specific and challenging situations that anesthesiologists and radiologists must be prepared for in the interventional radiology suite. These guidelines will be best tailored to the unique setup, support, and equipment available at each facility. As the American Society of Anesthesiologists and Center for Medicaid and Medicare Services continue to present guidelines for deep sedation, it is likely that the involvement of anesthesiologists in caring for children outside of the operating room will burgeon.

Special Topics: Anesthesia for Vascular Anomalies

The anesthetic management of patients with vascular malformations can be challenging. Vascular malformations are congenital aberrant connections between vessels, which may be comprised of lymphatics, arteries, capillaries, and veins. These lesions, although present at birth, may not become clinically apparent until the child grows. A rapid proliferative phase may occur in response to hormonal changes (pregnancy and puberty), trauma, or other stimuli [33]. Vascular malformations may present high-flow or low-flow lesions. High-flow lesions include arteriovenous fistulas, some large hemangiomas, and arteriovenous malformations. Extensive lesions with an arterial component may create a high-output cardiac failure with resultant congestive heart failure and the potential for pulmonary edema. Low-flow lesions, those with venous, intramuscular venous, and lymphatic malformations, do not present such a risk. Surgical resection of symptomatic vascular malformations presents risks of significant intraoperative bleeding and coagulopathy, in addition to surgical and anesthetic risk. For this reason, invasive angiography and embolization have become popular alternatives to surgical resection when possible.

Because vascular malformations tend to grow, even those lesions that are asymptomatic may someday require intervention. Accompanying clinical conditions can include pain, tissue ulceration, disfigurement, multiorgan compromise, impairment of limb function, coagulopathy, claudication, hemorrhage, and progressive nerve degeneration or palsy.

A dedicated anesthesia team committed to interventional radiology has an advantage: in addition to gaining a familiarity with the procedures and the radiologists, nurses, and technologists, the patients and parents often return for multiple procedures and are comforted by seeing familiar anesthesiologists. Especially with these complicated patients, familiarity with the patient, their vascular lesion, the procedures involved, and the interventional radiologist all benefit from a core group of anesthesiologists. Vascular embolization may be used as a bridge to surgical resection and may decrease the risk of intraoperative bleeding.

When embolizing vascular malformations, radiologists may use various techniques and agents: ethanol, stainless steel coils, antibiotics, absorbable gelatin pledgets and powder, polyvinyl alcohol foam, glues, thread, and ethanol. The choice of agent depends on the clinical situation and the size of the blood vessel. When permanent occlusion is the goal, polyvinyl alcohol foam and ethanol are often employed as they both occlude at the level of the arterioles and capillaries. Medium- to small-sized arteries may be occluded with coils, which are the surgical equivalent of ligation. In trauma situations, when only temporary (days) occlusion is the goal, absorbable gelatin pledgets or powder is employed [34]. Absolute ethanol (99.9 % alcohol) is a powerful sclerosing agent, which has particular implications for the anesthesiologist and perioperative care provider.

Ethanol can cause thrombosis of the vascular endothelium, which can extend to the capillary bed. A powerful sclerosant, it is particularly useful in the embolization of symptomatic vascular malformations. For that reason, using selective catheterization and direct percutaneous puncture, normal blood vessels are avoided. Ethanol causes denaturation of blood proteins and may produce a coagulum of blood with endothelial necrosis [35]. Sclerotherapy or embolization with absolute (99.9 %) ethanol may elicit a post-procedure coagulopathy [36] marked by positive d-dimers, elevated prothrombin time, and decreased platelets. Extensive ethanol injections (usually considered to be >0.5 mL/kg) can cause hematuria and should require the placement of a Foley catheter during the procedure for careful monitoring of urine output throughout and in recovery. On average, it has been our practice to administer between 50 and 100 mL/kg intravenous fluids over the course of the procedure. When hemoglobinuria is noted during the procedure, the anesthesiologist should notify the radiologist so that the need for continued injections of ethanol is reevaluated. Aggressive and immediate treatment of hematuria is essential as soon as it is recognized to minimize the risk of renal damage. Inadequate hydration with subsequent hemolysis has resulted in renal failure with subsequent hemodialysis (personal correspondence). Hemoglobinuria may not occur until the end of the procedure, particularly when a large volume of ethanol is injected towards the end of the procedure or with procedures that involve the injection of lower extremity lesions below a tourniquet. With tourniquets, hemoglobinuria should be expected within 10 min of deflation. In anticipation of hematuria following tourniquet deflation, generous fluid replacement should be initiated prior to deflation and continued thereafter in order to mitigate hematuria. Furosemide intravenous (0.5–1.0 mg/kg) promotes diuresis and a faster resolution of gross hematuria (personal experience). It is important to recognize that the appearance of hemoglobinuria may be delayed and can present up to 1–2 h after completion of the procedure. It is suggested that following large injections of ethanol, patients be observed for a minimum of 2 h for hematuria in recovery prior to discharge to the floor. Fluid administration should be balanced with urine output. At our institution, persistent hemoglobinuria is treated with sodium bicarbonate (75 mEq/L in 5 % dextrose and water), which is administered at a rate of 2 times the maintenance in order to alkalinize the urine and minimize the risk of hemoglobin precipitating in the renal tubules [37]. All hematurias should be resolved prior to discharge from post-anesthesia recovery room.

Administration of ethanol has the potential for severe complications. Albeit infrequent, there is a risk of cardiovascular collapse, which is generally preceded by hypoxemia and bradycardia. Most reported cases of cardiovascular collapse involved lower extremity malformations [38]. The etiology of the cardiovascular collapse associated with ethanol is unclear, although its occurrence has been reported coincident with the injection of ethanol into the systemic veins or after the release of lower extremity tourniquets after ethanol injection. It is critical that the radiologist communicate with the anesthesiologist whenever ethanol is being injected and before the deflation of the tourniquet. In our practice, sudden desaturation without arrhythmia or hypotension has occurred with ethanol administration, without cardiovascular sequela. Alternatively, pulmonary embolism from thrombus dislodgement at the site of the vascular malformation has occurred with mild (mid 80 % to low 90 %) oxygen desaturation and prolonged (24–48 h) hypoxemia, presumably from micro-thromboembolism.

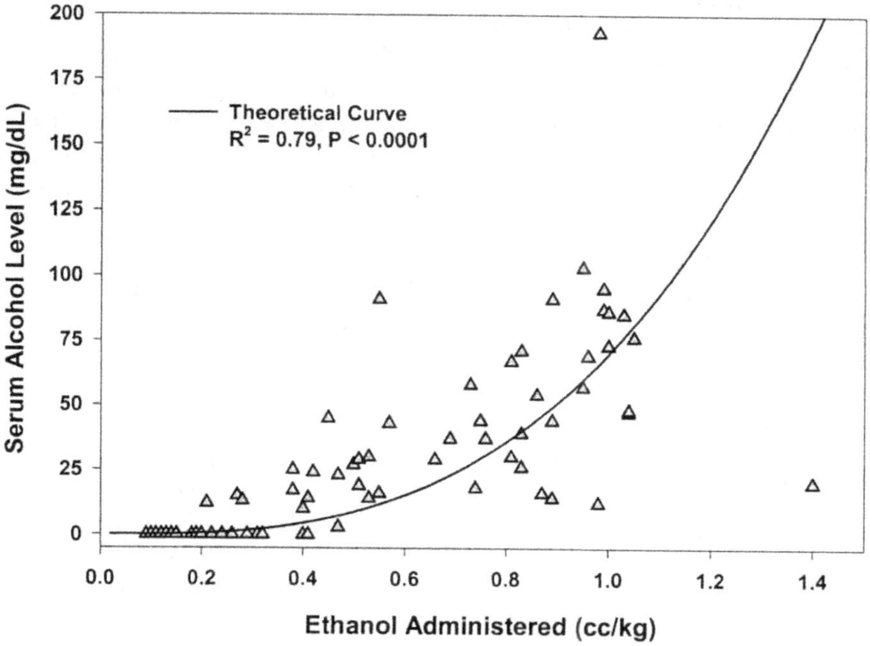

Fig. 3.1 Graph shows the positive relationship between serum ethanol level and amount of ethanol administered in all 71 patients. *Solid line* indicates the theoretic curve based on the nonlinear exponential power model *y* 5 70*x*3, where *x* is the amount of ethanol administered and *y* is the predicted serum ethanol level. *Triangles* represent empirical values. Theoretic curve demonstrates the most accurate fit compared with all other linear and nonlinear models tested. *Reprinted with permission from Mason KP, Michna E, Zurakowski D,* et al. *Serum Ethanol levels in children and adults after ethanol embolization or sclerotherapy for vascular anomalies. Radiology 2000;217:127-132 © Radiological Society of North America*

These patients benefit from systemic anticoagulation without long-term sequelae.

In addition to neuropathy and tissue necrosis, if not injected selectively, ethanol can produce a state of intoxication. The ethanol used for embolization and sclerotherapy is concentrated to 95–98 %. Patients who receive >0.75 mL/kg can be clinically intoxicated. Blood levels correlate with the volume of ethanol administered, regardless of the location or type of vascular malformation (Fig. 3.1).

On extubation, particularly following large injections of ethanol, patients can display extremes of behavior ranging from significant agitation to extreme somnolence. In both situations, narcotics, if needed, should be administered with caution, as these patients tend to be slow to emerge from anesthesia (some even have strong odor of alcohol on their breath). High serum levels of ethanol provide analgesia. Narcotics may produce a synergistic effect with the potential for respiratory depression. Until the extent of pain is assessed, narcotics should be titrated in small, conservative doses. Ketorolac can provide analgesia in those who are not at risk of developing a coagulopathy or a post-procedure bleed.

Large hemangiomas may be associated with a coagulopathic condition called Kasabach–Merritt syndrome. In this condition, the hemangioma traps and destroys platelets and clotting factors, resulting in thrombocytopenia and an increased risk of hemorrhage. As the hemangioma involutes, the coagulation status tends to improve [39]. A condition described as systemic intravascular coagulation can occur after the embolization of extensive vascular malformations. Systemic intravascular coagulation is a condition similar to disseminated intravascular coagulation (DIC) but specific for the coagulopathy, which results from embolizations: an elevated prothrombin time with a decrease in coagulation factors and platelets. Other patients with vascular malformations, particularly venous malformations, can have preexisting coagulation disturbances that resemble DIC [40–44]. A hematology consult should be obtained for those patients with laboratory values consistent with a consumptive coagulopathy. They may be initiated on heparin for 2 weeks before the procedure in order to replenish their fibrinogen levels. During extensive embolizations, cryoprecipitate or platelets may be administered to promote clotting and successful sclerosis. The use of ethanol for sclerosis or embolization can elicit a coagulation disturbance that resembles DIC. There is a statistical relationship between the amount (mL/kg) of ethanol administered and the degree of coagulation disturbance elicited [36]. The coagulopathy is generally not symptomatic, resolves in about 5 days, and does not require additional cryoprecipitate or fresh frozen plasma transfusions. Major surgery is usually deferred until the coagulation parameters have normalized.

There are a number of concerns and perioperative issues. Following extensive embolization procedures, these patients frequently experience pain from the tissue necrosis and swelling. A variety of analgesic techniques should be considered. Steroids, although they do not have analgesic properties, may reduce edema and postembolic neuritis with resultant analgesia. Postembolic swelling will impact the perioperative airway management following procedures in the head and neck. Pediatric patients in particular may need to remain intubated after such procedures, particularly when edema in the floor of the mouth, tongue, hypopharynx or oropharynx, or anterior neck could compromise a patent airway. An additional post-procedure concern is that vomiting may, because of the Valsalva maneuver, increase venous blood pressure and aggravate bleeding and swelling at puncture sites or cause swelling and airway obstruction following the head and neck procedures. Hypothermia is a risk in interventional radiology, particularly with long procedures. Heating lamps and body surface warming devices may be used when safe and appropriate. Finally, with the use of iodine-containing radiocontrast media, sclerosing, and embolizing agents, consideration must be given to adequate volume resuscitation, the risk of a contrast reaction, and bladder catheterization for detection of oliguria, polyuria, or hematuria.

Special Topics: Anesthesia and Angiography

Cerebral angiography typically requires endotracheal intubation. Hypercarbia to end tidal CO_2 >50 mmHg will promote vasodilation to allow better access and visualization of cerebral vasculature (Fig. 3.1). Orogastric, nasogastric tubes, esophageal stethoscopes, and esophageal temperature probes should be avoided during cerebral angiography as they can create artifacts on the angiographic images. Cerebral studies may be indicated in the work-up or postoperative follow-up of vascular malformation or tumor resections, stroke, hemorrhagic events, vascular disease, and unexplained mental status changes. It is important to know the indications for the cerebral angiography, as these indications may guide the perioperative management. For example, any child requiring a study for the potential or confirmed diagnosis of moyamoya should be treated with utmost precaution, with anesthetic techniques that minimize the risk of transient ischemic attacks and stroke during the procedure [45]. The recommended anesthetic technique is to hydrate with 10 mL/kg intravenous fluid prior to anesthetic induction to reduce the risk of hypotension (and potential cerebral ischemia) with induction. Inhalational inductions are generally discouraged in favor of a well-controlled intravenous induction with concomitant hemodynamic stability. Hypocarbia should be avoided to minimize risk of cerebral vasoconstriction and normocarbia is generally the goal throughout. In the event of vasospasm or difficult access of small, torturous vessels, the interventional radiologist can administer (through the intravascular catheter) nitroglycerin in small doses (25–50 μg) to promote vasodilation and improve visualization and access. Small doses of nitroglycerin are generally successful in vasodilating specific discrete and local areas and do not have a clinically relevant effect on systemic blood pressure.

Angiographic imaging of the abdomen or pelvis may be enhanced through the use of glucagon, administered in divided doses of 0.25 mg to a maximum of 1.0 mg intravenously. Glucagon is efficacious for digital subtraction angiography, visceral angiography, and selective arterial injection in the viscera. Risks with glucagon include hyperglycemia, vomiting (particularly when given rapidly), gastric hypotonia with post-procedure vomiting, anaphylaxis with rapid administration, and physiologic signs (tachycardia and hypertension) that mimic pheochromocytoma [46–48]. Antiemetics may be considered prophylactically or as a treatment in the recovery room.

Imaging of the lower extremities and pelvis may involve the added challenge of positioning the patient in reverse position on the fluoroscopy table, the addition of extra long ventilator tubing, and the added awareness that the patient's airway is distant to the anesthesia machine and anesthesiologist. Particularly in these circumstances, the anesthesiologist should determine a plan of action in the event of an airway emergency. Unless the patient can be repositioned quickly with the head at the head of the bed adjacent to the anesthesiologist, emergency anesthesia assistance should be heralded immediately and the ancillary medical staff (nurses and radiologists) should be trained to assist as help is summoned.

References

1. Towbin RB, Ball Jr WS. Pediatric interventional radiology. Radiol Clin North Am. 1988;26(2):419–40.
2. Diament MJ, Boechat MI, Kangarloo H. Interventional radiology in infants and children: clinical and technical aspects. Radiology. 1985;154(2):359–61.
3. Yakes WF et al. Ethanol embolization of arteriovenous fistulas: a primary mode of therapy. J Vasc Interv Radiol. 1990;1(1):89–96.
4. Bin Abdul Rahman S et al. East Asia Review, 1973. 5. Malaysia. Stud Fam Plann. 1974;5(5):158–9.
5. American Academy of Pediatrics Committee on Drugs. Guidelines for monitoring and management of pediatric patients during and after sedation for diagnostic and therapeutic procedures. Pediatrics. 1992;89(6 Pt 1):1110–5.
6. Hackel A et al. Guidelines for the pediatric perioperative anesthesia environment. American Academy of Pediatrics. Section on Anesthesiology. Pediatrics. 1999;103(2):512–5.
7. Keeter S et al. Sedation in pediatric CT: national survey of current practice. Radiology. 1990;175(3):745–52.
8. Boll DT, Merkle EM, Lewin JS. MR-guided percutaneous sclerotherapy of low-flow vascular malformations in the head and neck. Magn Reson Imaging Clin N Am. 2005;13(3):595–600.
9. Tyagi I, Syal R, Goyal A. Management of low-flow vascular malformations of upper aero digestive system-role of N-butyl cyanoacrylate in peroperative devascularization. J Oral Maxillofac Surg. 2006;44(2):152–6.
10. Dachs RJ, Innes GM. Intravenous ketamine sedation of pediatric patients in the emergency department. Ann Emerg Med. 1997;29(1):146–50.
11. Kirberg A et al. Ketamine for pediatric endoscopic procedures and as a sedation complement for adult patients. Gastrointest Endosc. 2005;61(3):501–2.
12. Marx CM et al. Ketamine-midazolam versus meperidine-midazolam for painful procedures in pediatric oncology patients. J Clin Oncol. 1997;15(1):94–102.
13. Roelofse JA, Joubert JJ, Roelofse PG. A double-blind randomized comparison of midazolam alone and midazolam combined with ketamine for sedation of pediatric dental patients. J Oral Maxillofac Surg. 1996;54(7):838–44; discussion 845-6.
14. Bennett JA, Bullimore JA. The use of ketamine hydrochloride anaesthesia for radiotherapy in young children. Br J Anaesth. 1973;45(2):197–201.
15. Cotsen MR et al. Efficacy of ketamine hydrochloride sedation in children for interventional radiologic procedures. AJR Am J Roentgenol. 1997;169(4):1019–22.
16. Huang YL et al. Rescue of cardiopulmonary collapse in anterior mediastinal tumor: case presentation and review of literature. Pediatr Emerg Care. 2010;26(4):296–8.
17. Mason KP et al. Radiologist-supervised ketamine sedation for solid organ biopsies in children and adolescents. AJR Am J Roentgenol. 2009;192(5):1261–5.
18. Mason KP et al. Evolution of a protocol for ketamine-induced sedation as an alternative to general anesthesia for interventional radiologic procedures in pediatric patients. Radiology. 2002;225(2):457–65.
19. Green SM, Roback MG, Krauss B. Anticholinergics and ketamine sedation in children: a secondary analysis of atropine versus glycopyrrolate. Acad Emerg Med. 2010;17(2):157–62.
20. Green SM et al. Predictors of airway and respiratory adverse events with ketamine sedation in the emergency department: an individual-patient data

meta-analysis of 8,282 children. Ann Emerg Med. 2009;54(2):158–68; e1-4.
21. Green SM, Cote CJ. Ketamine and neurotoxicity: clinical perspectives and implications for emergency medicine. Ann Emerg Med. 2009;54(2):181–90.
22. Fine J, Finestone SC. Sensory disturbances following ketamine anesthesia: recurrent hallucinations. Anesth Analg. 1973;52(3):428–30.
23. Meyers EF, Charles P. Prolonged adverse reactions to ketamine in children. Anesthesiology. 1978;49(1): 39–40.
24. Sherwin TS et al. Does adjunctive midazolam reduce recovery agitation after ketamine sedation for pediatric procedures? A randomized, double-blind, placebo-controlled trial. Ann Emerg Med. 2000;35(3):229–38.
25. Green SM, Johnson NE. Ketamine sedation for pediatric procedures: part 2, review and implications. Ann Emerg Med. 1990;19(9):1033–46.
26. Hollister GR, Burn JM. Side effects of ketamine in pediatric anesthesia. Anesth Analg. 1974;53(2):264–7.
27. Wathen JE et al. Does midazolam alter the clinical effects of intravenous ketamine sedation in children? A double-blind, randomized, controlled, emergency department trial. Ann Emerg Med. 2000;36(6):579–88.
28. Sussman DR. A comparative evaluation of ketamine anesthesia in children and adults. Anesthesiology. 1974;40(5):459–64.
29. Hansen TG et al. Laryngeal mask airway guided tracheal intubation in a neonate with the Pierre Robin syndrome. Acta Anaesthesiol Scand. 1995;39(1):129–31.
30. Haxby EJ, Liban JB. Fibreoptic intubation via a laryngeal mask in an infant with Goldenhar syndrome. Anaesth Intensive Care. 1995;23(6):753.
31. Vila Jr H et al. Comparative outcomes analysis of procedures performed in physician offices and ambulatory surgery centers. Arch Surg. 2003;138(9):991–5.
32. Bhananker SM et al. Injury and liability associated with monitored anesthesia care: a closed claims analysis. Anesthesiology. 2006;104(2):228–34.
33. Jackson IT et al. Hemangiomas, vascular malformations, and lymphovenous malformations: classification and methods of treatment. Plast Reconstr Surg. 1993;91(7):1216–30.
34. Coldwell DM, Stokes KR, Yakes WF. Embolotherapy: agents, clinical applications, and techniques. Radiographics. 1994;14(3):623–43; quiz 645-6.
35. Mason KP et al. Serum ethanol levels in children and adults after ethanol embolization or sclerotherapy for vascular anomalies. Radiology. 2000;217(1):127–32.
36. Mason KP et al. Coagulation abnormalities in pediatric and adult patients after sclerotherapy or embolization of vascular anomalies. AJR Am J Roentgenol. 2001;177(6):1359–63.
37. Burrows PE, Mason KP. Percutaneous treatment of low flow vascular malformations. J Vasc Interv Radiol. 2004;15(5):431–45.
38. Yakes WF, Baker R. Cardiopulmonary collapse: sequelae of ethanol embolotherapy. Radiology. 1993;189:145–7.
39. Mulliken J, Anthony Y. Vascular birthmarks, hemangiomas, and malformations. Philadelphia: Saunders; 1988.
40. Aronoff DM, Roshon M. Severe hemorrhage complicating the Klippel-Trenaunay-Weber syndrome. South Med J. 1998;91(11):1073–5.
41. D'Amico JA, Hoffman GC, Dyment PG. Klippel-Trenaunay syndrome associated with chronic disseminated intravascular coagulation and massive osteolysis. Cleve Clin Q. 1977;44(4):181–8.
42. Dube B et al. Blood coagulation studies in children with surface hemangiomas. Int Surg. 1975;60(10): 524–5.
43. Neubert AG, Golden MA, Rose NC. Kasabach-Merritt coagulopathy complicating Klippel-Trenaunay-Weber syndrome in pregnancy. Obstet Gynecol. 1995;85(5 Pt 2):831–3.
44. Yamamoto H et al. Lower leg fracture with Parkes-Weber syndrome complicated by disseminated intravascular coagulation. J Orthop Trauma. 1995; 9(5):449–52.
45. Soriano SG, Sethna NF, Scott RM. Anesthetic management of children with moyamoya syndrome. Anesth Analg. 1993;77(5):1066–70.
46. Chernish SM, Maglinte DD. Glucagon: common untoward reactions–review and recommendations. Radiology. 1990;177(1):145–6.
47. Jehenson PM. Reducing doses of glucagon used in radiologic examinations. Radiology. 1991;179(1): 286–7.
48. McLoughlin MJ, Langer B, Wilson DR. Life-threatening reaction to glucagon in a patient with pheochromocytoma. Radiology. 1981;140(3):841–5.

Section II

Vascular Interventions: Arterial

Pediatric Angiography

4

Francis E. Marshalleck

Background/Indications

Current techniques in magnetic resonance (MR) angiography, computed tomographic (CT) angiography, and Doppler ultrasound have made it possible to diagnose a plethora of vascular diseases in the child precluding the use of catheter-directed angiography in most cases. Catheter-directed angiography may be required in the diagnosis of intracerebral vascular diseases, renovascular hypertension, gastrointestinal vascular pathology, and in the setting of trauma [1–3]. In the majority of instances, the diagnosis is known and angiography is done at the time of intervention. Importantly, the development of new devices has now made it possible for arterial interventions such as angioplasty, peripheral embolization, and endoneurovascular procedures to be performed in children [4, 5].

Contraindications

If the desired information can be obtained using noninvasive imaging, then catheter-directed angiography is contraindicated. Most contraindications are relative and include conditions such as severe contrast allergy, severe hypertension, coagulopathy, renal insufficiency, significant volume restrictions or metabolic disease, skin infection at the intended access site, and sepsis. A patient with active vasculitis or collagen vascular disease would be prone to vessel injury and would therefore need to be on treatment and in remission prior to angiography. A hypertensive crisis can be precipitated in patients with a known pheochromocytoma.

Preprocedure Evaluation

As with any procedure the indications must be valid. Specific allergies, abnormal renal function, or laboratory parameters need to be treated or corrected as in the adult population. Laboratory values vary within the pediatric population. Neonates (age <28 days), usually hypercoagulable, can have prolonged values. It is generally accepted that angiography can be performed safely with a platelet count of greater than 50,000/μL, prothrombin time of less than 18 s, partial thromboplastin time of less than 32 s, and an International Normalized Ratio (INR) of less than 1.2 (elective cases) or 1.5 (urgent cases). Coagulopathies may need to be corrected with fresh frozen plasma, vitamin K, or platelet transfusion [1]. A full physical examination of the patient is warranted along with evaluation of extremity pulses. In the majority of cases, angiography will be performed with the use of general anesthesia with conscious sedation being

F.E. Marshalleck, M.D. (✉)
Interventional Radiology, Indiana University School of Medicine, Riley Hospital for Children, 705 Riley Hospital Drive, Room 1053, Indianapolis, IN 46202, USA
e-mail: frmarsha@iupui.edu

M. Temple and F.E. Marshalleck (eds.), *Pediatric Interventional Radiology: Handbook of Vascular and Non-Vascular Interventions*, DOI 10.1007/978-1-4419-5856-3_4,

used for older patients. Chapters 2 and 3 of this handbook discuss radiation safety and pediatric sedation, respectively. In addition, Chap. 3 includes a description of special anesthesia considerations for angiography.

Technique

Depending on the size of the patient, obtaining arterial access may prove to be a challenge. Vessels are more superficial especially in neonates and infants and are more prone to vasospasm, thrombosis, and occlusion. This is seen especially in children weighing less than 15 kg [1, 6, 7].

The standard approach in obtaining arterial access is with palpation. This can become challenging in a neonate, young infant, or very obese child. As a result, using ultrasound guidance to obtain access should be considered to allow access to be quick and limited to a single-needle puncture. Ultrasound guidance would also be useful in the pediatric patient with a history of multiple prior angiograms where peripheral pulses may be more difficult to palpate. As in the adult population, access is obtained below the inguinal ligament with the common femoral artery being the standard access site. Ultrasound allows the interventionalist to determine the site of bifurcation of the femoral artery to allow for appropriate puncture above the bifurcation. Other sites can be chosen for access. These include axillary, brachial, and umbilical access [2, 6–9]. The umbilical artery can be used for up to 5 days after birth and represents an excellent alternate to femoral puncture to avoid potential access site complications [2, 9]. Axillary access is indicated in patients with occluded femoral arteries.

Double- or single-wall access can be done safely. Starting with a smaller gauge needle and floppy wire combination, e.g., 21-Ga/0.018-in. guidewire is advantageous primarily in smaller patients. Conversion to a 0.035-in. system is then performed with a 4- or 5-Fr micropuncture sheath depending on patient size. The routine use of a vascular sheath is operator dependent; however, it is recommended that a vascular sheath be used if there will be multiple catheter exchanges or manipulations [1]. Vascular sheaths and angiographic catheters are available as small as 3-Fr in size. In patients weighing greater than 10 kg, 4-Fr angiographic catheters can be used for diagnostic angiography with 3-Fr catheters used in patients under 10 kg in weight [7]. If a microcatheter is going to be used, it can be placed directly through an indwelling 3- or 4-Fr vascular sheath. In fact, if the intent is to perform an embolization procedure, 4-Fr 0.038-in. inner diameter catheters are widely available to accommodate a coaxially placed microcatheter thereby limiting the size of the vascular sheath to 4-Fr.

Table 4.1 Pediatric dosing of medications used during angiography

Nitroglycerin	1–3 μg/kg intra-arterial in 1 μg/kg aliquots
Heparin	75–100 IU/kg intravenous
Protamine	10 mg intravenous per 1,000-IU heparin
Glucagon	20–300 (max 200 in neonates) μg/kg IV/IA max 1 mg
Papaverine	1 mg/kg intra-arterial

It is generally recommended for patients weighing less than 15 kg; intraprocedural systemic heparin should be administered to prevent access site thrombosis. A dose of 75–100 IU/kg is typically used. In prolonged cases, activated clotting time can be useful to determine the appropriate level of anticoagulation [1]. The common medications that can be administered during angiography are listed in Table 4.1.

As opposed to the adult population, vessels within the pediatric population are not tortuous making catheter selection and advancement easier. Since pediatric vessels are prone to vasospasm, leading with a wire is suggested. Also, careful attention to the volume of flushes and contrast administered is important to avoid volume overload. It is recommended that the volume of contrast used in neonates should be less than 5 mL/kg and 6–8 mL/kg in patients outside the neonatal age group [1, 2]. These limits can be exceeded depending on the necessity of intervention, complexity of the procedure, and the overall procedure time. Contrast injection rates vary depending upon the weight of the patient as seen

Table 4.2 Contrast injection rates and volumes in pediatric angiography

	Patient weight (kg)			
Artery	<10	10–20	20–50	>50
Aorta	[b]	5–10 for 8–15	10–20 for 20–40	20–25 for 25–50
Celiac	[b]	2–3 for 10–20	3–5 for 15–30	5–8 for 30–60
Splenic	[b]	2–3 for 20–15	3–5 for 15–20	5–8 for 20–50
Hepatic	[b]	2–3 for 5–10	3–5 for 10–15	5–8 for 15–25
SMA	[b]	2–3 for 10–15	3–5 for 15–30	5–8 for 30–50
IMA	[b]	[b]	1–3 for 6–9	2–3 for 10–15
Renal	[b]	2–4 for 3–5	3–5 for 6–9	5–8 for 10–15
Adrenal	[b]	[b]	[b]	[b]
Subclavian	[b]	2–3 for 4–6	3–4 for 6–15	5–8 for 15–25
Common carotid	[b]	2–3 for 3–5	4–6 for 5–10	6–8 for 10–15
Internal carotid	[b]	1–2 for 3–5	2–4 for 5–8	4–5 for 6–10
External carotid	[b]	[b]	[b]	2–3 for 6–9
Vertebral	[b]	[b]	2–5 for 4–6	4–7 for 6–9

Note: values presented as rates in mL/s for total volumes in mL. No consensus is available on injection rates or volumes, and these figures serve as suggested reference ranges only. Improvements in imaging, contrast agents, and injector pumps, as well as use of medications (e.g., bowel paralytic agents or vasodilators), may result in significant variability from institution to institution. Pump injections are often required for arteriography performed in regions requiring high flow rates (e.g., aorta); however, many pediatric angiographers prefer hand injections for selective arteriography, or in arteriography in neonates and small infants, to maximize control of arterial bed opacification and minimize contrast agent reflux or excessive injection rates

IMA inferior mesenteric artery, *SMA* superior mesenteric artery

[a]Low rates and volumes recommended in each weight category for those toward the lower limit of the range, whereas higher rates and volumes are recommended for those toward the upper limit of each weight category. Arterial phase imaging of 3–4 frames per second is suggested, whereas injection imaging into venous phase (e.g., splenoportography) will likely require greater contrast medium volumes and slower imaging (i.e., down to 1 frame per second)

[b]Hand injection recommended

With permission from Heran MK, Marshalleck FE, Temple M et al. *Joint quality improvement guidelines for pediatric arterial access and arteriography: from the Societies of Interventional Radiology and Pediatric Radiology. Pediatr Radiol (2010)40:238-250* [1]

in Table 4.2 [1, 6, 10, 11]. In smaller patients, most selected vessels are interrogated with hand injection of contrast especially in patients weighing less than 15 kg. Closure devices are not recommended in the pediatric population due to the smaller size of vessels that are already prone to spasm and injury. Hemostasis patches have been shown to be useful in reducing post-angiography hematoma formation and compression times in children undergoing cardiac catheterization [12].

Complications

Although low, the rate of complications increases in patients with less than 15 kg in weight. The development of smaller profile devices has helped to further decrease the complication rate. In adults, the overall complication rate of angiography is less than 1 % and can be as high as 10 % within the pediatric age group especially in children less than 1 year of age [13, 14]. Puncture site complications can be as high as 25 % in patients less than 15 kg when arterial interventions are performed. These include hematoma, dissection, thrombosis, occlusion, pseudoaneurysm, and arteriovenous fistula formation. The major of access site complications are self-limiting and require no further intervention. The number of examinations, larger sheath size, and alternative access sites such as the axillary or brachial artery can lead to increased risk. US guidance will limit access to a single puncture resulting in a decreased complication rate.

As in the adult population, nitroglycerin at a dose of 1–3 μg/kg can be administered intra-arterially in 1 μg/kg aliquots to treat or prevent vasospasm. Concomitant administration of systemic heparin at a dose of 75–100 μg/kg will prevent thrombosis primarily in patients under 15 kg in weight. Treatment of arterial thrombosis includes keeping the extremity warm with blankets and heparin infusion to keep PTT twice normal [1]. Importantly, because children will develop good collaterals, it is uncommon for claudication or leg length discrepancy to develop in the future [15]. Thrombolysis and thrombectomy of arterial thrombosis are described in Chap. 15.

Hypoglycemia and hypothermia are more prevalent in the neonate age group primarily within premature patients. Prevention of hypothermia is discussed in Chap. 2 of this handbook. Hypoglycemia can be treated with boluses of 5–10 % glucose peripheral with higher dose used centrally [1].

The risk of contrast nephropathy in adults varies from 7 to 25 % depending on preexisting risk factors such as renal insufficiency, diabetes, vascular disease, and nephrotoxic medications. The risk can be decreased, as in adult population, with the use of low osmolar or diluted contrast medium, preprocedure hydration, and with the use of alternative contrast agents such as carbon dioxide [16].

Postprocedure Care

Immediately after the examination, the peripheral pulses are felt and the groin reexamined in the recovery room for any evidence of hematoma. Inpatients are reevaluated the next day on the ward. Outpatients will be contacted with a follow-up phone call within 24 h.

Chapter Summary

Indications

- Diagnostic indications now uncommon
  - Intracerebral vascular disease
  - Renovascular hypertension
  - Gastrointestinal bleeding
  - Trauma
- Therapeutic
  - Embolization
  - Angioplasty

Contraindications

- Noninvasive method of diagnosis
- Contrast allergy
- Severe hypertension
- Coagulopathy
- Renal insufficiency
- Volume restrictions
- Skin infection
- Active vasculitis or collagen vascular disease
- Pheochromocytoma

Preprocedure workup

- Bloodwork
  - CBC, PTT, INR
  - BUN, creatinine

Equipment

- Access
  - Micropuncture set (especially for smaller infants)
  - 19-G single-wall puncture needle for larger infants
- 3–7-Fr vascular sheath, long or short
- Angiographic catheters: 3–7-Fr microcatheters
- Drugs: see Table 4.1, page X

Technique

- US for access
- Consider heparin for <15 kg
- Considerations
  - Maximum contrast dose: <5 mL/kg in neonates, 6–8 mL/kg in others
  - Avoid volume overload
  - Appropriate warming techniques
- Closure devices NOT recommended

Complications

- Higher in smaller patients
- Puncture site complications
  - Hematoma
  - Dissection
  - Thrombosis
  - Pseudoaneurysm
  - Arteriovenous fistula
- Hypothermia
- Hypoglycemia
- Contrast nephropathy

Postprocedure care

- Monitor peripheral pulses
- Follow-up phone call within 24 h

References

1. Heran MK, Marshalleck FE, Temple M, et al. Joint quality improvement guidelines for pediatric arterial access and arteriography: from the Societies of Interventional Radiology and Pediatric Radiology. Pediatr Radiol. 2010;40:238–50.
2. Borrows PF, Robertson RL, Barnes PD. Angiography and the evaluation of cerebrovascular disease in

childhood. Neuroimaging Clin N Am. 1996;6: 561–88.
3. Christensen R. Invasive radiology for pediatric trauma. Semin Pediatr Surg. 2001;10:7–11.
4. Sadd DF, Gow KW, Redd D, et al. Renal artery pseudoaneurysm secondary to blunt trauma treated with microcoil embolization. J Pediatr Surg. 2005;40:e65–7.
5. McLaren CA, Roebuck DJ. Interventional radiology for renovascular hypertension in children. Tech Vasc Interv Radiol. 2003;6:150–7.
6. Stanley P. Pediatric angiography. Baltimore: Williams & Wilkins; 1982.
7. Chait P. Future directions in interventional pediatric radiology. Pediatr Clin North Am. 1997;44:763–82.
8. Gauderer MW. Vascular access techniques and devices in the pediatric patient. Surg Clin North Am. 1992;72:1267–84.
9. Weber HS. Transumbilical artery interventions in the neonate. J Invasive Cardiol. 2001;12:39–43.
10. Kirks DR, Fitz CR, Harwood-Nash DC, et al. Pediatric abdominal angiography: practical guide to catheter selection, flow rates and contrast dosage. Pediatr Radiol. 1976;5:19–23.
11. Kandarpa K, Aruny JE. Handbook of interventional radiologic procedures. 3rd ed. Philadelphia: Lippincott Williams & Williams; 2010.
12. Nader RG, Garcia JC, Drashal K, Pesek T. Clinical evaluation of the Syvek Patch in consecutive patients undergoing interventional EPS and diagnostic cardiac catheterization procedure. J Invasive Cardiol. 2002; 14:305–7.
13. Hessel SJ, Adams DF, Abrams HL. Complications of angiography. Radiology. 1981;138:273–81.
14. Vitiello R, McCrindle BW, Nykanen D, et al. Complications associated with pediatric cardiac catheterization. J Am Coll Cardiol. 1998;32:1433–40.
15. Nehler MR, Taylor Jr LM, Porter JM. Iatrogenic vascular trauma. Semin Vasc Surg. 1998;11: 283–93.
16. Kriss VM, Cottrill CM, Gurley JC. Carbon dioxide (CO_2) angiography in children. Pediatr Radiol. 1997; 27:807–10.

5 Renal Arteriography and Interventions

James S. Donaldson

Indications for Renal Arteriography

Includes evaluation for:
Vascular cause of hypertension
Cause of hematuria
Vasculitis
Bleeding in setting of trauma
Bleeding following renal biopsy

Hypertension Evaluation

One to five percent of children are hypertensive and, of those, it is not well known how many will have an arterial cause but this number ranges from 5 to 25 %. It is beyond the scope of this chapter to assess the complex issue of children with hypertension and how the different modalities (US, Doppler, CTA, MRA) should be used in the workup. The renal arteriogram remains the gold standard in identifying or excluding an arterial abnormality as the cause of hypertension.

J.S. Donaldson (✉)
Department of Medical Imaging, Ann & Robert H. Lurie Childrens Hospital of Chicago, Feinberg School of Medicine at Northwestern University, Chicago, IL, USA
e-mail: JDonaldson@luriechildrens.org

Indications for Arteriography

Hypertension >99th percentile for age and requiring more than two drugs for control. Shahdadpuri reported that angiograms were positive 43 % of the time in patients who met these criteria.

Special Considerations

In very small infants (under 18 month of age), the ability to treat a lesion with angioplasty or embolization even if identified is small. It is preferred not to do an arteriogram under this age if the hypertension can be managed medically. Our recommendation is to wait until the child is at least 2 or 3 years of age before doing an arteriogram.

Etiology

Etiology can include any of the following long lists of disorders:

Fibromuscular dysplasia (approximately 60–80 % of all causes) (Figs. 5.1 and 5.2)
Neurofibromatosis I (Figs. 5.3–5.5)
Midaortic syndrome (Fig. 5.6)
William's syndrome
Takayasu's arteritis (Fig. 5.7)
Polyarteritis nodosa
Radiation therapy
Trauma (Fig. 5.8)

M. Temple and F.E. Marshalleck (eds.), *Pediatric Interventional Radiology: Handbook of Vascular and Non-Vascular Interventions*, DOI 10.1007/978-1-4419-5856-3_5,

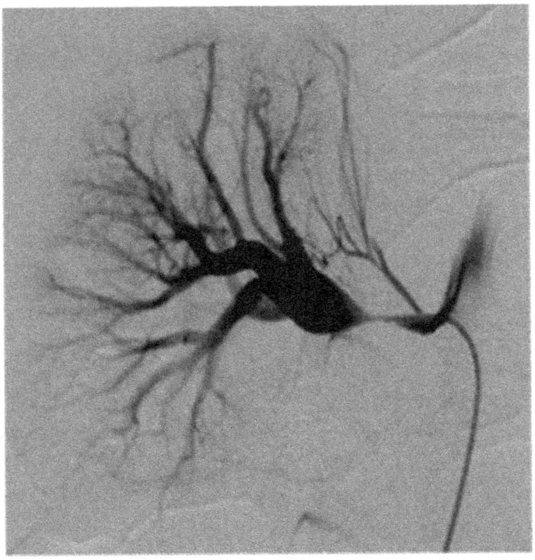

Fig. 5.1 FMD in a 12-year-old with hypertension. Angiographic findings typical for the intimal fibroplasia type of FMD

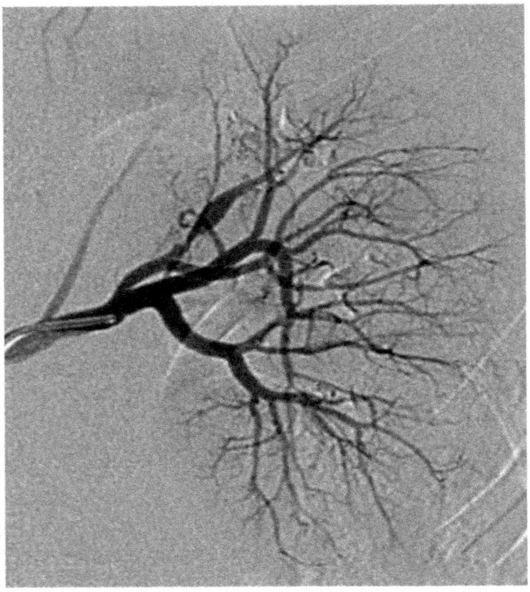

Fig. 5.2 FMD in a 4-year-old with hypertension. Angiographic findings reveal long-segment smooth stenosis with post-stenotic dilation of an intrarenal segmental artery

Congenital rubella syndrome
Tuberous sclerosis
Marfan's syndrome
Klippel-Trenaunay-Weber
Epidermal nevus syndrome
Tumor encasement (neuroblastoma)

Technique

Preprocedure

Hypertensive medications are generally not withheld even if treatment is to be undertaken. Renal function should be known with BUN and creatinine levels checked within last 30 days.

Anesthesia

General anesthesia is recommended for all diagnostic and interventional procedures. General anesthesia can provide apnea eliminating respiratory motion and also provides for longer procedures.

Access

The femoral artery is most often used for access and is always using ultrasound guidance with a 4.5 Fr vascular sheath inserted. We have on occasion used brachial artery or even carotid artery access (with assistance of cardiovascular surgery) for patients in whom unfavorable renal artery or aorta anatomy makes cephalad access preferable.

Anticoagulation

Heparin, 50–100 units/kg, is given after insertion of the vascular sheath.

Aortogram

Aortogram is almost always performed first. This provides an assessment of the main renal arteries prior to any guidewire or catheter instrumentation of the renal artery that may produce spasm and mimic a stenosis (Fig. 5.9). A 4 Fr pigtail catheter is preferred and positioned below the superior mesenteric artery to avoid reflux into overlying arteries. Renal arteries usually arise at the level of L1–L2.

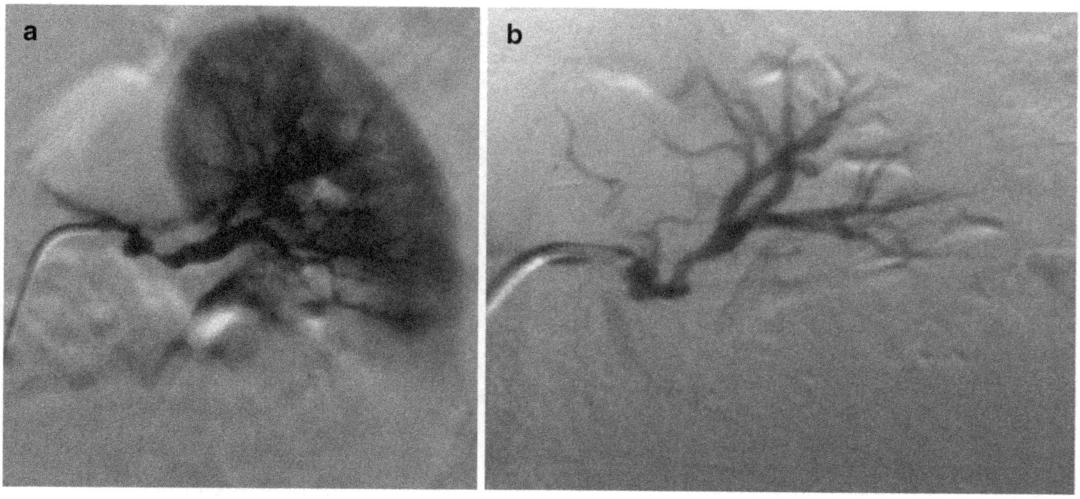

Fig. 5.3 NF1 and severe renal artery stenosis. (**a**) Angiogram of left kidney reveals irregular main renal artery with stenosis. (**b**) Post angioplasty reveals slight improvement but considerable narrowing and irregularity persists. Patient had some improvement but developed restenosis 2 years later requiring repeat angioplasty

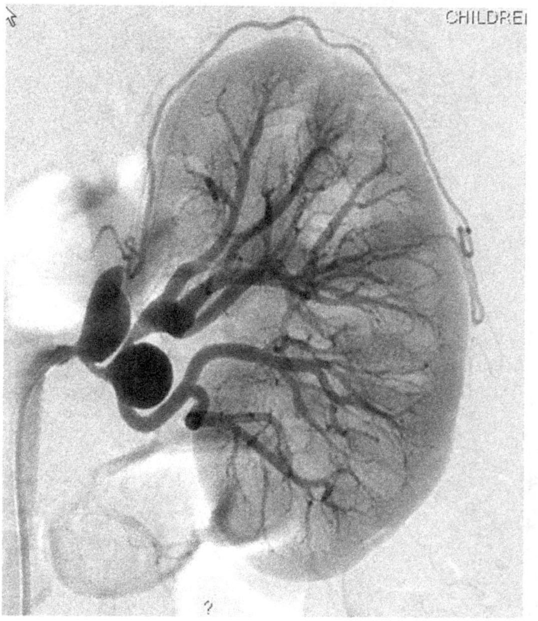

Fig. 5.4 NF1 and hypertension. Angiogram of the left kidney reveals multiple aneurysms in the renal hilum. No endovascular options were considered in this patient

Contrast volume: As a general rule, the volume necessary for an upper abdominal aortogram is 1 cm^3/kg. Below the celiac artery and SMA, 0.8 cm^3/kg up to an adult volume of 25 cm^3 should be adequate.

Flow rate should be such that entire volume is injected over 1–1.5 s. Most 4 Fr pigtail catheters have a limit of 17 cm^3/s maximum rate at 1,200 psi.

Selective Arteriography

Every renal arteriogram should have selective catheterizations to evaluate for small lesions that may be missed on the aortogram (Fig. 5.10). A 4 Fr reverse curve (Sos 1 or 2) catheter is preferred to catheterize each renal artery. Cobra-shaped catheters will often recoil out of the renal artery; thus, the reverse curve shapes are preferred. Thirty to forty percentage of patients will have multiple renal arteries and each should be selectively catheterized.

Hand injections are often performed in small children with volumes of 3–5 cm^3. Large adolescent children will require adult rates of 6–8 cm^3/s and volumes of 10–15 cm^3.

DSA imaging is required with apnea. Rapid sequences of 4 frames/s for the aortogram are desired. Three frames/s during the selective angiograms are used. Two oblique views are obtained with approximately 5 and 25° of angulation toward the ipsilateral side.

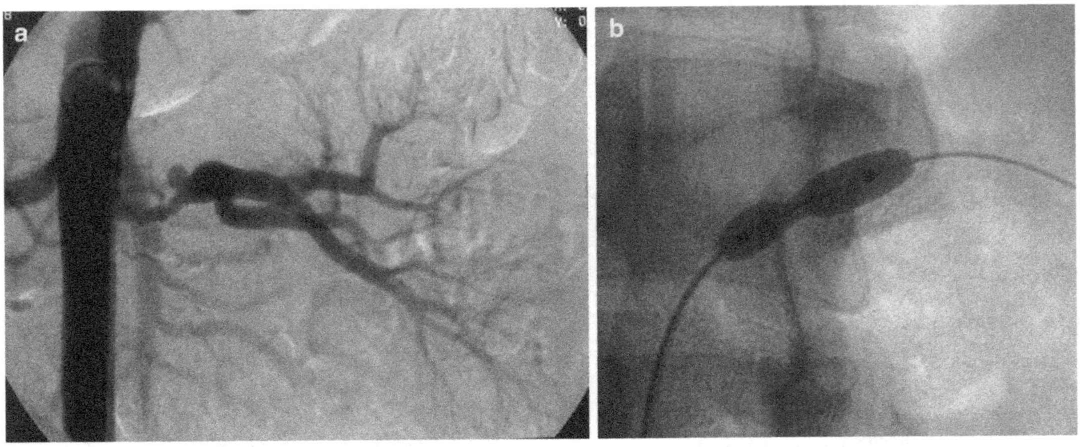

Fig. 5.5 NF1 with difficult balloon dilation. Angiogram reveals irregularity and narrowing of the main renal artery. Balloon waist persists during dilation

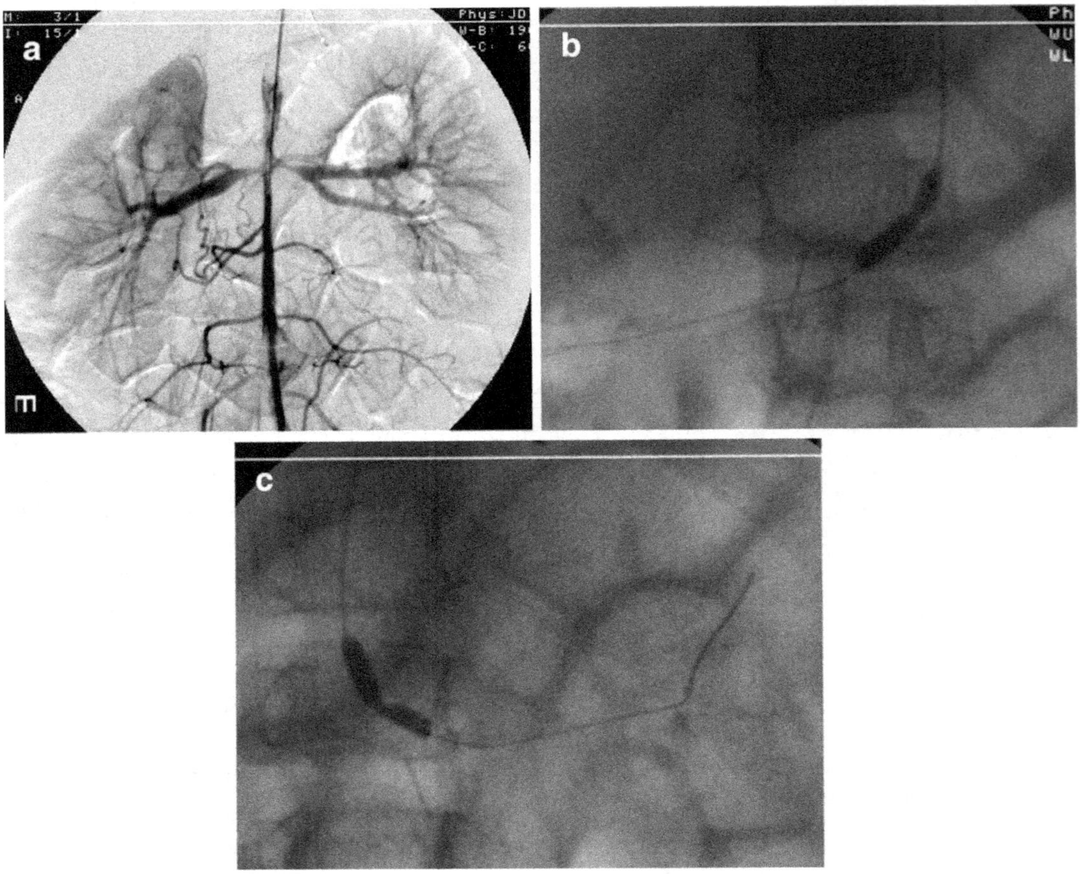

Fig. 5.6 Midaortic syndrome with bilateral renal artery stenosis. (**a**) Angiogram reveals narrowing of the aorta and proximal renal arteries. (**b**, **c**) Brachial access used for bilateral angioplasties

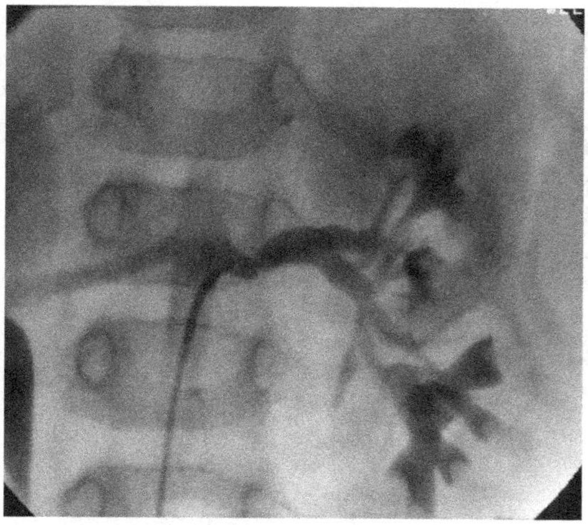

Fig. 5.7 Takayasu's arteritis. Focal narrowing and ectasia of the main and segmental renal arteries are seen in this patient found to have large vessel abnormalities throughout the upper extremities and thoracic vessels as well

The diagnostic arteriogram should be undertaken with the most careful technique so that isolated small intrarenal lesions are not overlooked.

Angiographic Findings

There can be a number of direct and indirect findings indicating the presence of a significant vascular lesion:

Stenosis

Stenosis may be seen secondary to a number of causes listed above. The most common etiology is fibromuscular disease (FMD) which is an idiopathic angiopathy characterized by noninflammatory fibrodysplastic narrowing of medium-size arteries. FMD has been classified into intimal, medial, and perimedial subtypes. Lesions with intimal fibroplasia generally demonstrate highly stenotic localized lesions often with post-stenotic dilation. Perimedial fibroplasia is characterized by severe focal stenoses and mild beading. Medial fibroplasia is characterized by more typical beaded appearance. Approximately 50 % of children with renal artery stenosis will have main renal artery disease, and the other half may have isolated intrarenal stenoses. This underscores the need for careful evaluation of the selective renal artery injections (Fig. 5.11).

Post-stenotic Dilation

Post-stenotic dilation may be the only abnormality seen and should prompt additional views be obtained to try and identify a subtle stenosis or web (Figs. 5.12 and 5.13).

Intrarenal Collateral Vessels

Intrarenal collateral vessels are seen in approximately 50 % of patients with stenotic lesions. Identification of collaterals should lead to thorough assessment of entire arterial anatomy as the stenoses may be subtle and readily seen. Careful angiography with additional oblique projections or rotational angiography may be necessary to identify subtle stenoses (Figs. 5.14 and 5.15).

Aneurysms

Aneurysms can be seen in 28 % of patients with FMD and NF1 patients (Fig. 5.4).

Delayed Contrast Perfusion

Delayed contrast perfusion of renal parenchyma may be seen as result of a large stenosis.

Distribution of Renal Artery Stenosis Lesions

The stenoses encountered in the renal vasculature can be seen from the ostium of the main renal artery to the parenchyma. In a series by Srinivasan of 43 patients with renal artery stenosis, ostial stenoses were present 33 % of the time. Bilateral disease was seen in 30 % of patients.

An important distribution of renal lesions noted in two separate studies by Deal and Vo is that in

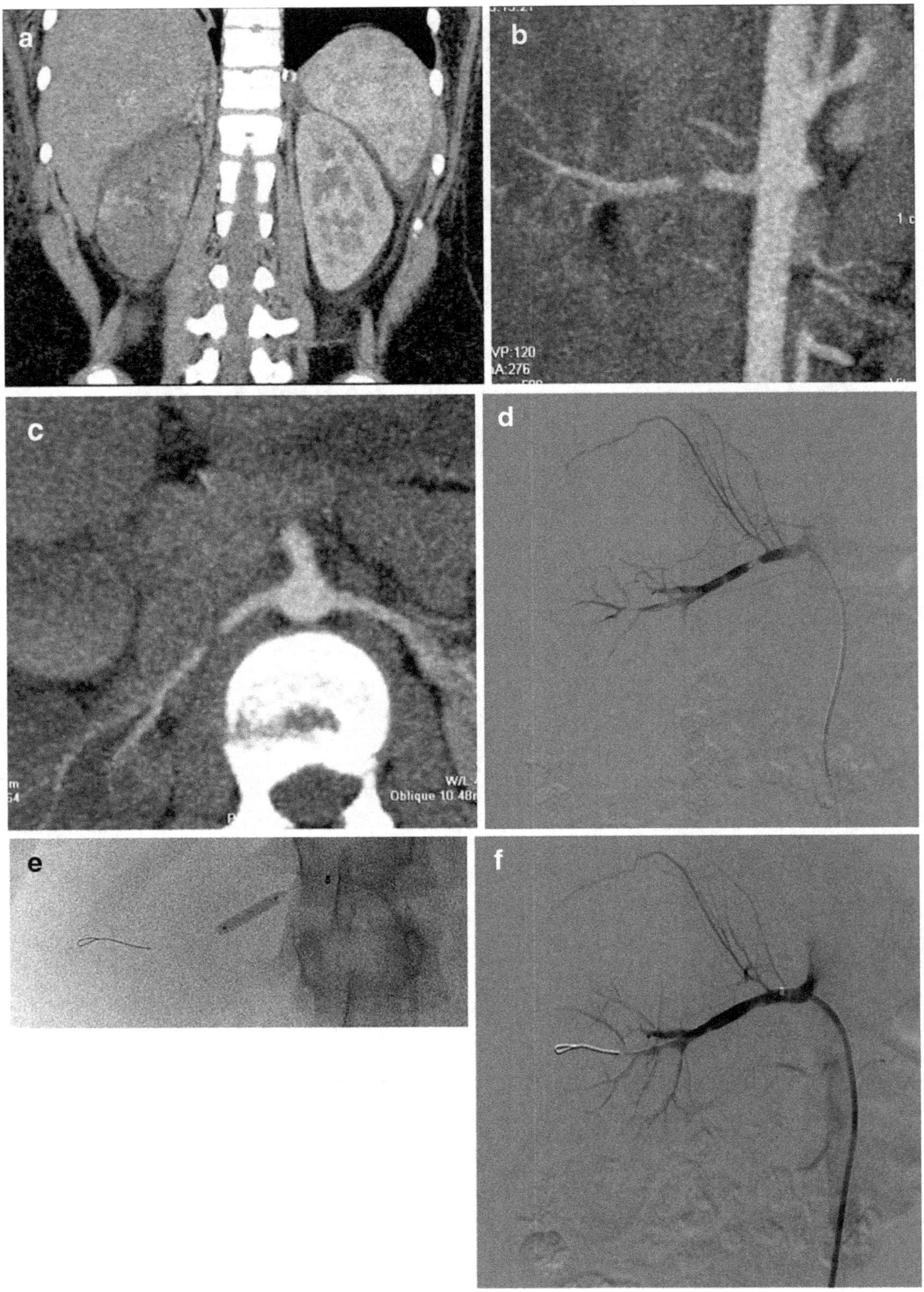

Fig. 5.8 Traumatic injury of the renal artery from motor vehicle accident. (**a**, **b**, **c**) CTA reveals poor perfusion of the right kidney, and reconstructions show a mid-renal artery lesion. (**d**) Selective angiography shows an intimal dissection of the mid-renal artery. (**e**) Angioplasty was successful in revascularizing the kidney

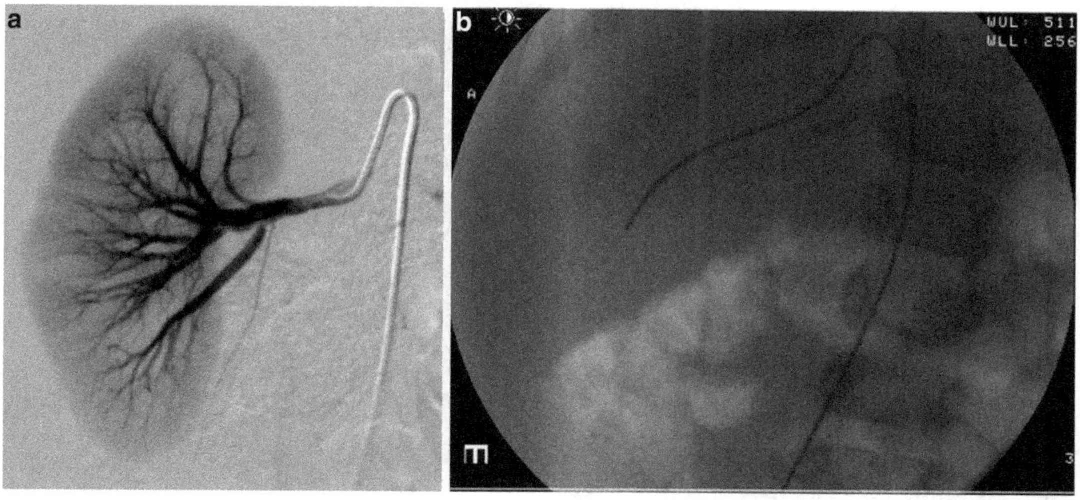

Fig. 5.9 Selective arteriogram of right kidney reveals an area of spasm in the lower pole branch not present on the aortogram. (**b**) During selective catheterization the guide wire advanced into the lower pole artery causing spasm

approximately 50 % of patients the stenoses were found exclusively in second order and smaller renal arteries and did not involve the main renal artery (Fig. 5.16). This underscores the need for careful selective arteriography to look for such lesions. It is also important to keep this in mind when judging the validity or sensitivity of noninvasive imaging modalities (Doppler, CTA, MRA, captopril renography) to detect such lesions.

Vasculitis

Inflammation of vessels can affect all vessels of the body including the kidney. Diagnosis usually requires a biopsy and only rarely requires angiography. Intrarenal aneurysms and irregularity of small vessels is seen with polyarteritis nodosa (Fig. 5.17). Takayasu's arteritis, uncommonly seen in first and second decades of life, involves large vessels but can involve renal arteries in 25–40 % of patients.

Trauma

Pseudoaneurysms, arteriovenous shunting, arterial occlusion, and communication with the collecting system may all be seen following trauma including following biopsies. Angiography is indicated if therapeutic intervention is considered.

Interventions

Hypertension

Revascularization of the compromised renal vasculature can be curative and allay serious sequelae of hypertension such as nephrosclerosis and cerebrovascular, cardiac, or retinal injury. If not curative, revascularization can reduce the polypharmacy requirements in a significant number of patients. When a stenotic lesion is identified, there are a number of questions that need to be addressed:

1. Is the lesion significant and does it need to be treated? Based on the improved clinical results following angioplasty and embolization of the very smallest of lesions, it appears that any stenosis in the setting of hypertension deserves an attempt at correction.
2. What is the best method: open surgery or via endovascular techniques? Surgery has for years been successful at autotransplantion of kidneys for main renal artery lesions. "Bench" surgery has also been shown to be effective at partial nephrectomy sparing normal renal parenchyma. However, improved materials have made endovascular techniques highly successful and in most centers would be considered the preferred primary approach.
3. When should the lesion be corrected? If a small child's hypertension is well controlled

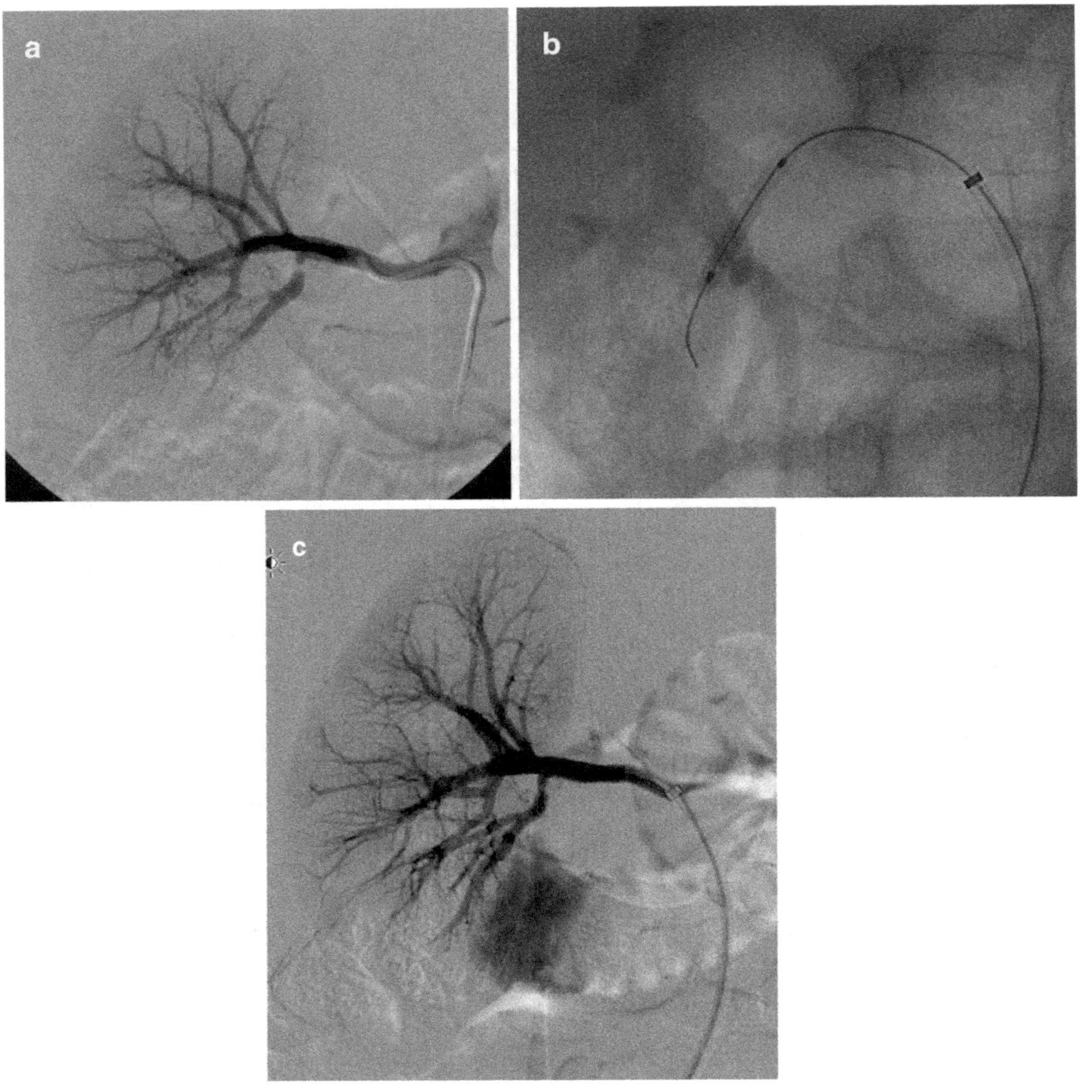

Fig. 5.10 Segmental stenosis of right lower pole branch seen on selective angiogram. This lesion was not apparent on the aortogram performed with a flush catheter from the abdominal aorta. (**a**) lower pole stenosis demonstrated. (**b**) Following angioplasty. (**c**) improved lower pole blood flow was seen

medically, it is preferred to defer attempts to correct a lesion until the child is 3–4 years old. This will make any procedure technically easier, likely more successful, and probably safer.

4. Should bilateral lesions be treated at the same setting? Doing procedures on both kidneys raises the risk, but if the first procedure has gone smoothly and the desired result has been achieved, I would recommend proceeding with the contralateral side.

Percutaneous Transluminal Angioplasty

Percutaneous transluminal angioplasty (PTA) has gained acceptance as first-line treatment in adults with RAS and is should be considered first-line treatment for children as well. Stents, readily used in adults, should be avoided in children except as a last resort to salvage a kidney.

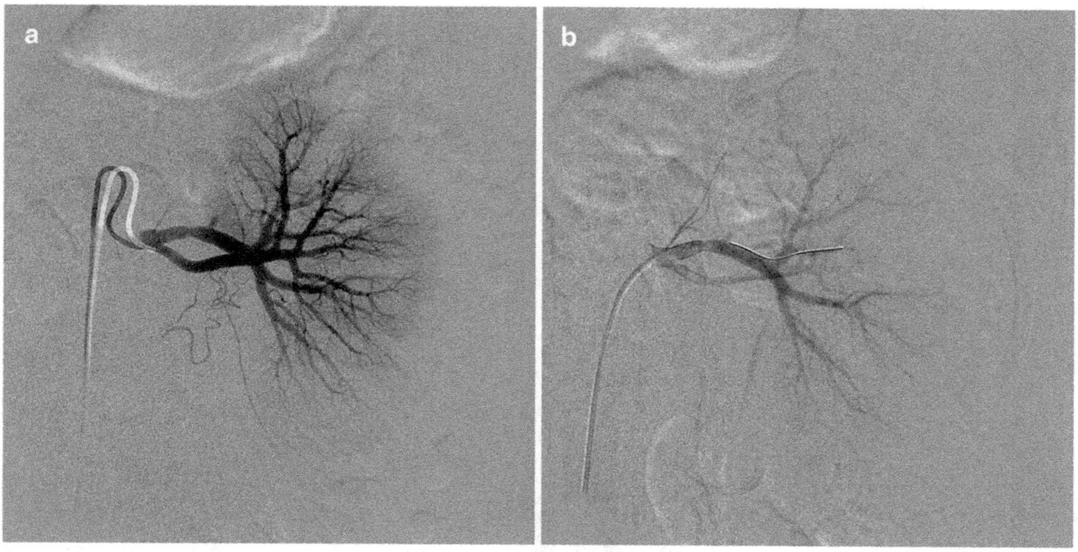

Fig. 5.11 FMD in a 5-year-old patient with hypertension. (**a**) Selective angiography reveals a relatively focal narrowing of the upper pole main renal artery. (**b**) Post angioplasty (4-mm balloon) with guidewire still across the area of dilation, an angiogram reveals the improved angiographic results

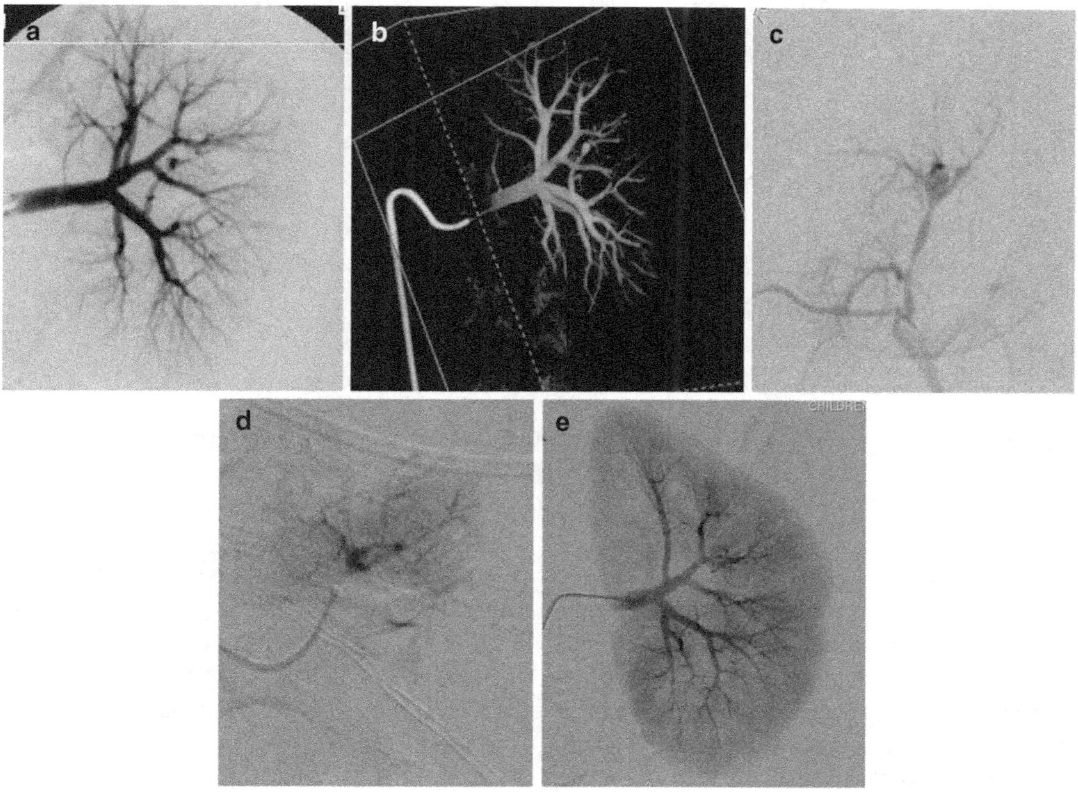

Fig. 5.12 A 6-year-old with hypertension. (**a**) Selective angiogram reveals a suspicious "dilated" vessel in the mid-polar region of the left kidney. (**b**) Following additional oblique projection angiograms, a rotational angiogram with 3D reformations was performed confirming a stenosis with post-stenotic dilation of a small lower pole interlobular artery. (**c**) Selective catheterization of this vessel was performed with microcatheter and the segmental artery embolized with ethanol (4 mL). Post-embolization angiogram reveals occlusion of the artery. The patient's hypertension resolved

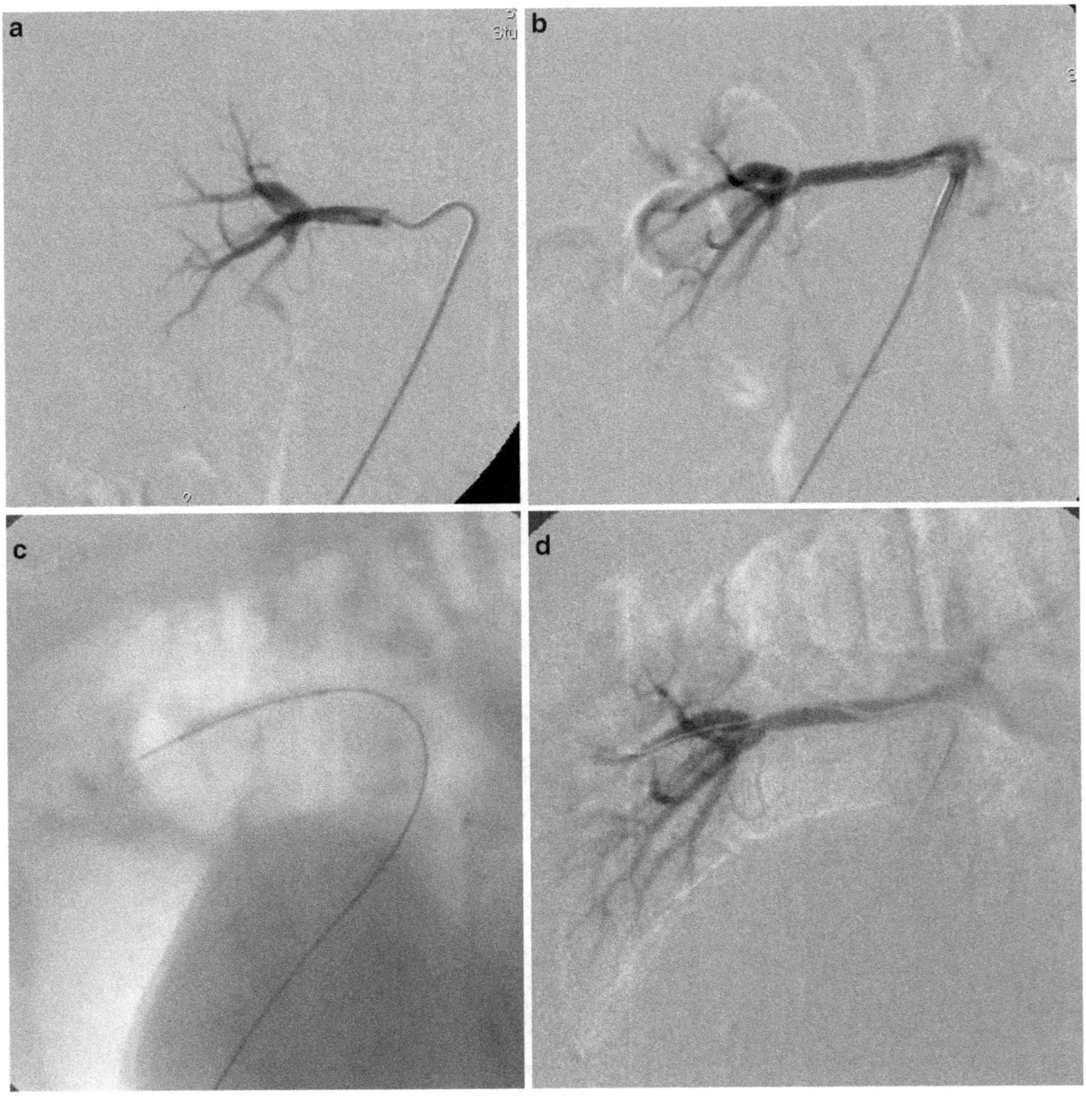

Fig. 5.13 Upper pole stenosis with post-stenotic dilation. The initial finding was the mildly ectatic (post-stenotic dilation) upper pole vessel. A web stenosis was only seen after several oblique projections were done

PTA Technique

Heparin 100 units/kg is administered. Nitroglycerin 1–2 μg/kg is administered directly into the renal artery. After selecting the renal artery with an appropriate guidewire, a guiding sheath (5–6 Fr) is advanced to the ostium. Use of a guiding sheath may not be possible in small children or infants. The stenosis can be crossed with either a 0.035″ wire or a microwire 0.018″ or smaller. Coronary balloons (2–6 mm) used with microwires are suited to treat lesions in small children. Cutting balloons have been used in resistant stenoses with success. Follow-up angiograms are performed following balloon dilation through the guide sheath while leaving the guidewire across the stenosis.

Use of two simultaneous wires may be desired for treatment of multiple intrarenal lesions.

Postprocedure Care

After angioplasty, patients are admitted for careful monitoring of blood pressure. This may be best done in an ICU setting particularly if a cutting balloon was used or if a dissection was noted during the angioplasty. Heparin is continued over-

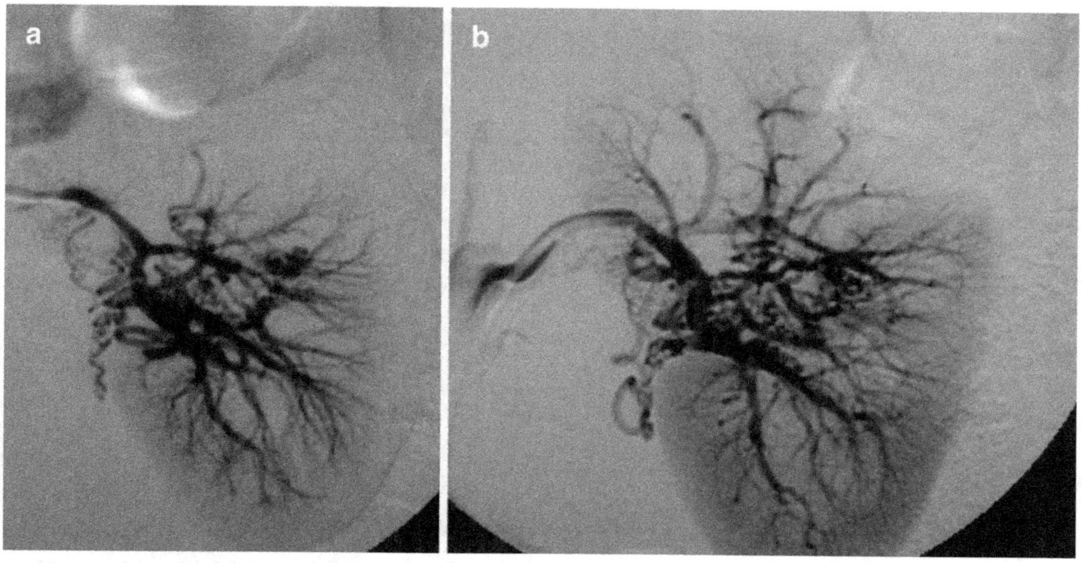

Fig. 5.14 Intrarenal segmental arterial occlusion with collaterals and delayed upper pole artery filling. (**a**) An early arterial phase angiogram reveals extensive collateral vessels in the mid-portion of the kidney and nonvisualization of normal upper pole arteries. (**b**) A delayed image reveals the upper pole artery filling solely through the intrarenal collaterals. Angioplasty and embolization options were unsuccessful in this patient

night at 20 units/kg/h. An ultrasound examination with Doppler is performed the following morning. Clopidogrel bisulfate (75-mg loading dose and a half tablet of 37.5 mg daily) or aspirin (81 mg daily) should be administered for 6 weeks.

Results

Technical results following angioplasty range from 85 to 95 %. Cure of hypertension can be expected in 40 % of patients. Overall clinical improvement is seen from 50 to 80 % of patients. Restenosis can be expected in 25 % of patients.

Embolization

Embolization of Intrarenal Stenoses

Renal-sparing angioplasty should always be the desired approach. If angioplasty is not technically feasible because of occlusion of an intrarenal artery, unfavorable anatomy or a very tiny vessel embolization of a segment of renal parenchyma may cause infarction of the renin-producing tissue and improve the hypertension. Liquid agents (ethanol) are preferred over coils or particles because of the possibility of collaterals forming around the more central occlusion. Liquid agents ideally will perfuse and cause tissue destruction of the parenchyma thus precluding the formation of collaterals. Since embolization of small intrarenal vessels cannot be done with a protective balloon, the infusion of alcohol must be done slowly to avoid reflux unless the catheter is occlusive and a more forceful injection is thought to be safe. A theoretical limitation of this technique is that alcohol may occlude a feeding vessel quickly and not perfuse the parenchymal tissue adequately to avoid watershed zones of ischemia around the targeted tissue.

If the vessel feeding the ischemic parenchyma is completely occluded, microcatheterization of a collateral vessel may allow embolization of the target parenchyma through the collateral.

Postprocedure Care

Following embolization, hospitalization for blood pressure monitoring is necessary, but heparin and antiplatelet agents are not.

Results

There are a number of case reports and small series of children with successful segmental

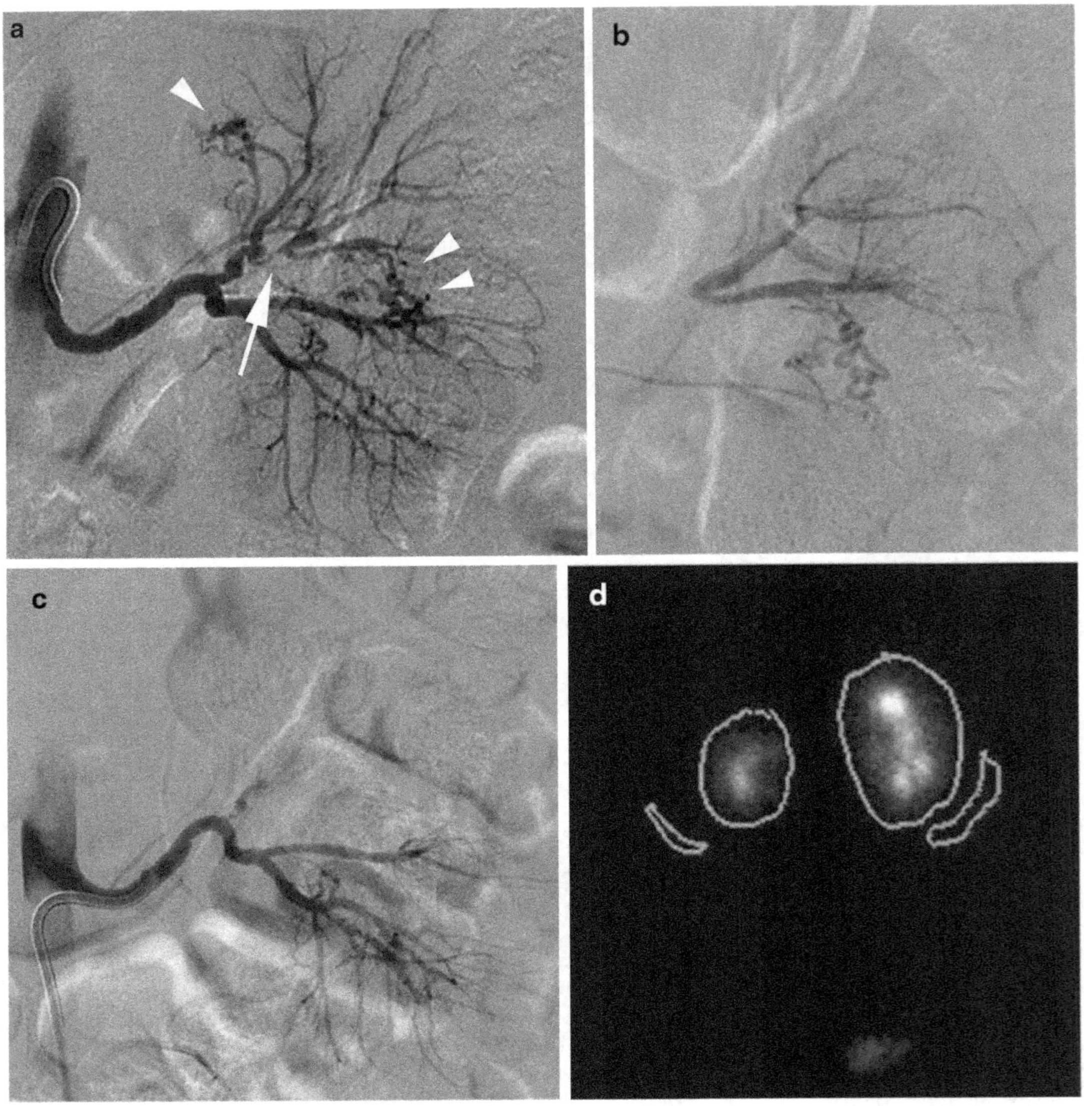

Fig. 5.15 An 18-month-old with hypertension. (**a**) Selective angiogram reveals an intra-renal stenosis (*arrow*) and several tortuous collateral vessels (*arrowheads*). Initial attempts to cross the tight stenosis failed. (**b**) The patient returned a year later and the stenosis could still not be crossed. A collateral vessel was engaged with a microcatheter (*arrow*) and the sequestered segment embolized with ethanol. (**c**) Post-embolization angiogram reveals embolization of the upper pole of the kidney. (**d**) A renogram performed several months later (posterior image) reveals only 25 % residual function of the left kidney. Hypertension, however, was significantly improved

artery embolization for hypertension. No large pediatric series have been published.

Stents

The use of stents is generally discouraged in children because of the long life expectancy and expected growth of the renal arteries (Fig. 5.18). Stents have been used when angioplasty has failed and there is no reasonable alternative kidney sparing treatment. Shroff reported a series of 33 patients with renal artery stenosis in whom 10, with poor angioplasty results, had stents placed. They report 37 % stenosis rate after stent deployment.

Embolization for Post-biopsy Hemorrhage

Significant hemorrhage following renal biopsy occurs from 1.5 to 3 % of the time (Fig. 5.19). If hematuria persists, embolization may be indicated. Selective catheterization with microcatheters and

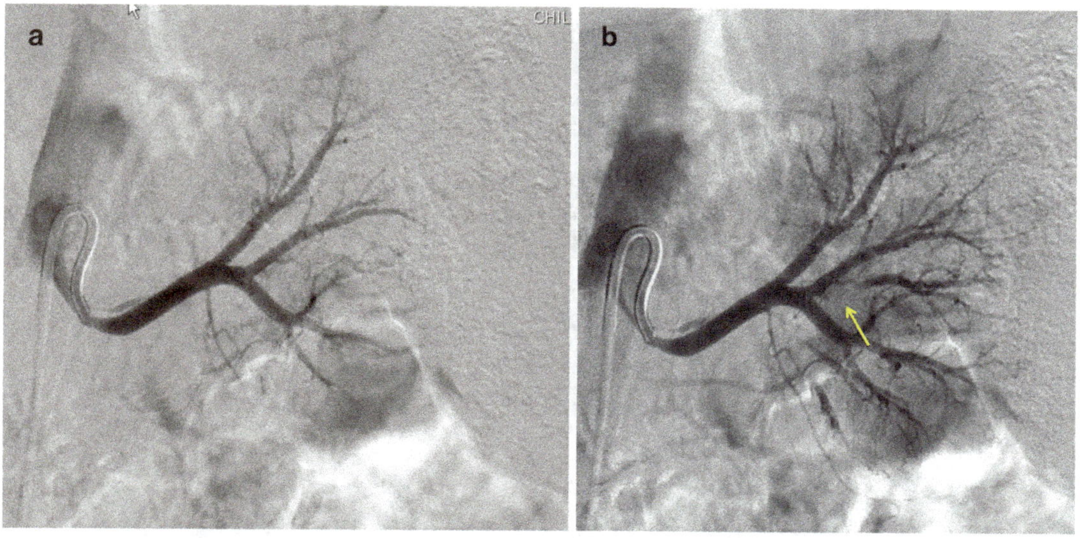

Fig. 5.16 A 5-month-old with hypertension. (**a**) Early angiogram reveals no obvious arterial stenoses. (**b**) Late arterial phase reveals a mid-polar artery (*arrow*) filling via collateral vessels. The artery was completely occluded and attempts to revascularize the artery were unsuccessful. Embolization via collaterals has not been attempted

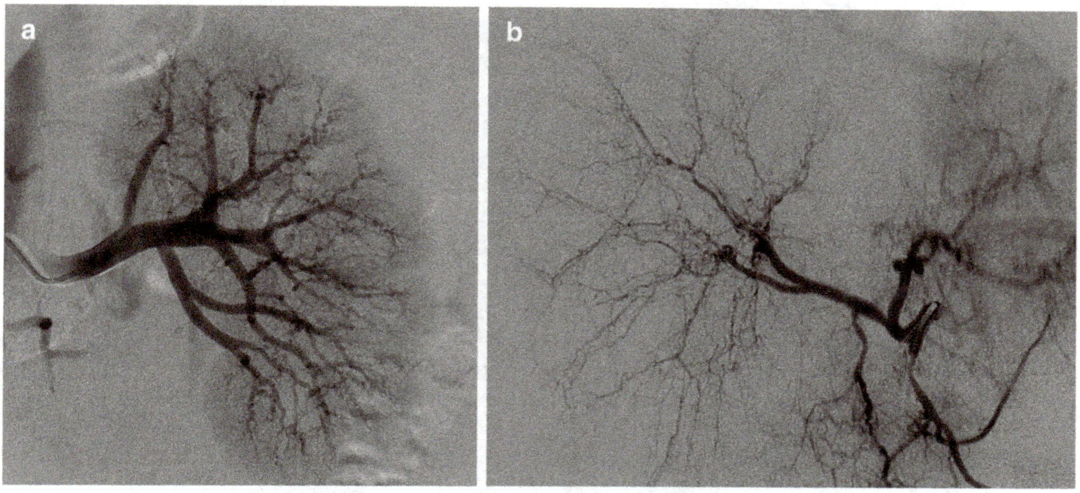

Fig. 5.17 A 7-year-old with hypertension. (**a**) Angiogram reveals marked small vessel intrarenal artery irregularity with small aneurysms throughout the both kidneys. (**b**) Hepatic artery angiogram reveals vessel irregularity with aneurysms in the liver typical of polyarteritis nodosa

embolization with microcoils are preferred in order to minimize the amount of normal renal parenchyma that is embolized in the process of occluding the site of bleeding.

Embolization of Arteriovenous Fistulas

Embolization of arteriovenous fistulas occurs up to 9 % of the time following biopsies of both native and transplant kidneys. Fistulae may be clinically silent and be detected on routine renal imaging or may compromise renal function by stealing blood flow from the rest of the kidney (Fig. 5.20). Coils are the preferred embolic materials.

Embolization of Angiomyolipoma

Angiomyolipomata are found in patients with tuberous sclerosis generally after the first

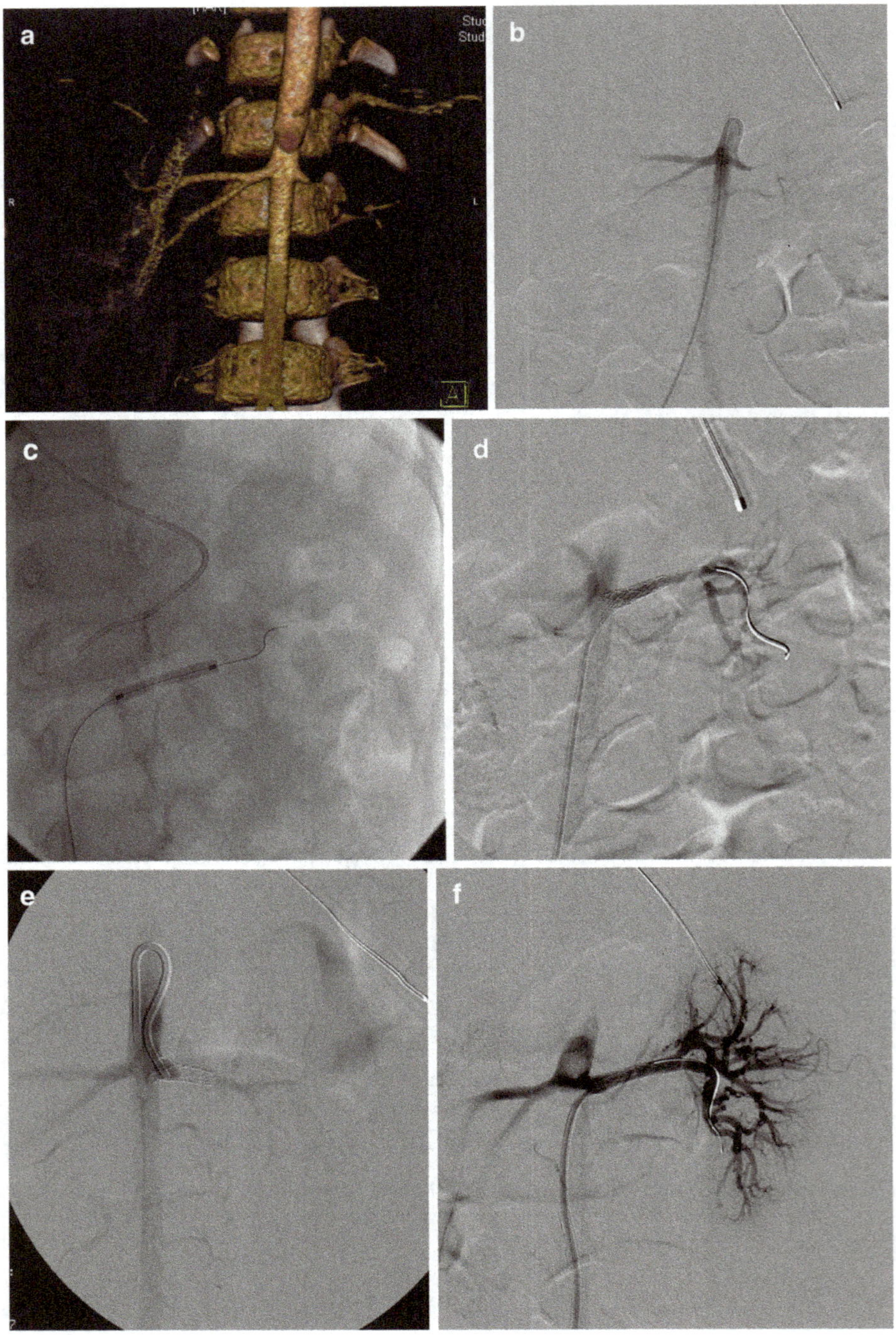

Fig. 5.18 A 2-month-old with seizures and severe hypertension. (**a**) CTA reformatted image reveals occlusion of the left renal artery. (**b**) Angiogram confirms occlusion of the artery. (**c**) Successful recanalization of the artery was performed with angioplasty but recurrent occlusion occurred. (**d**) As there was no surgical option feasible, decision was made to place a stent. (**e**) Several months later, the stent was shown to be occluded, and a second stent was deployed inside and slightly distal to the first stent. (**f**) Angiogram following the second stent insertion shows revascularization of the kidney. Stent placement is considered a procedure of last resort

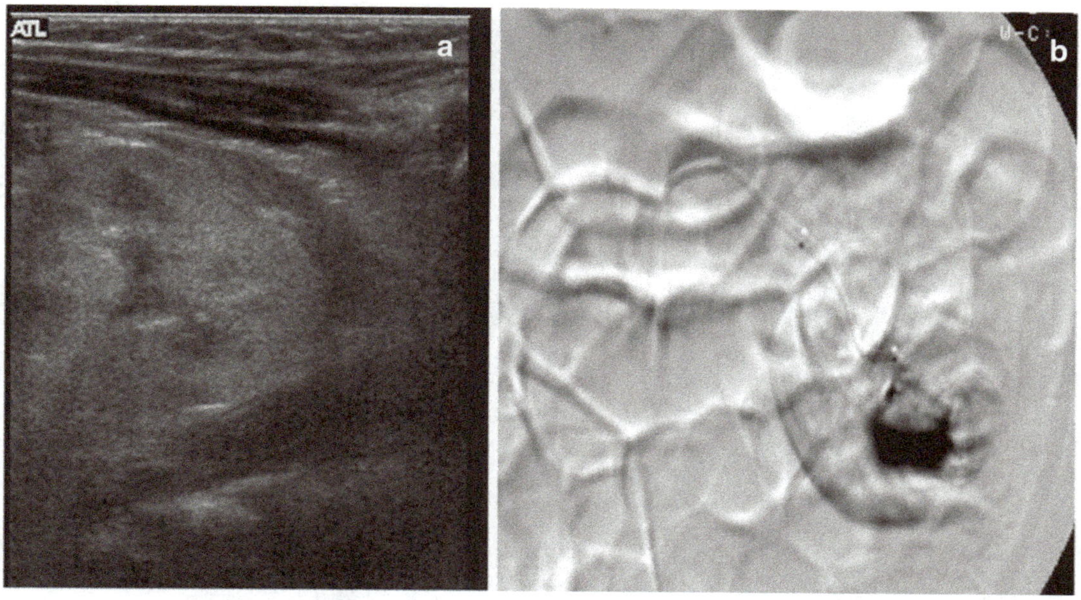

Fig. 5.19 A 3-month-old with gross hematuria s/p needle biopsy several hours earlier. (**a**) US reveals clot formation in the bladder. (**b**) Selective angiogram with microcatheter reveals contrast opacification of the collecting system. Microcoils were successful embolizing the bleeder

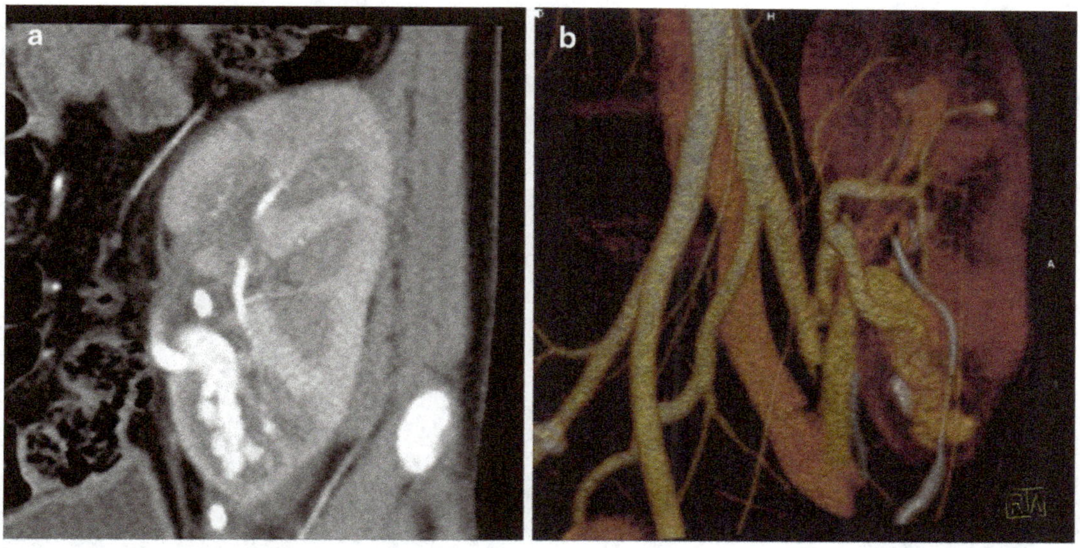

Fig. 5.20 A 15-year-old with decreasing renal function 1 year post renal transplant. (**a**, **b**) CTA with 3D reconstructions reveals an arteriovenous fistula in the lower pole of the transplant kidney. (**c**) Angiogram confirms the AV fistula. (**d**) Post-coil embolization angiogram reveals successful occlusion of the fistula

decade of life. Angiomyolipomata can reduce renal reserve and lead to insufficiency and failure. As the lesions enlarge, they may bleed and require emergent embolization. They may also be embolized preemptively to avoid acute bleeding episode (Fig. 5.21). Embolizing lesions larger than 4 cm the risk of hemorrhage is reduced. Selective embolization preserves renal parenchyma in these patients at risk for further renal events.

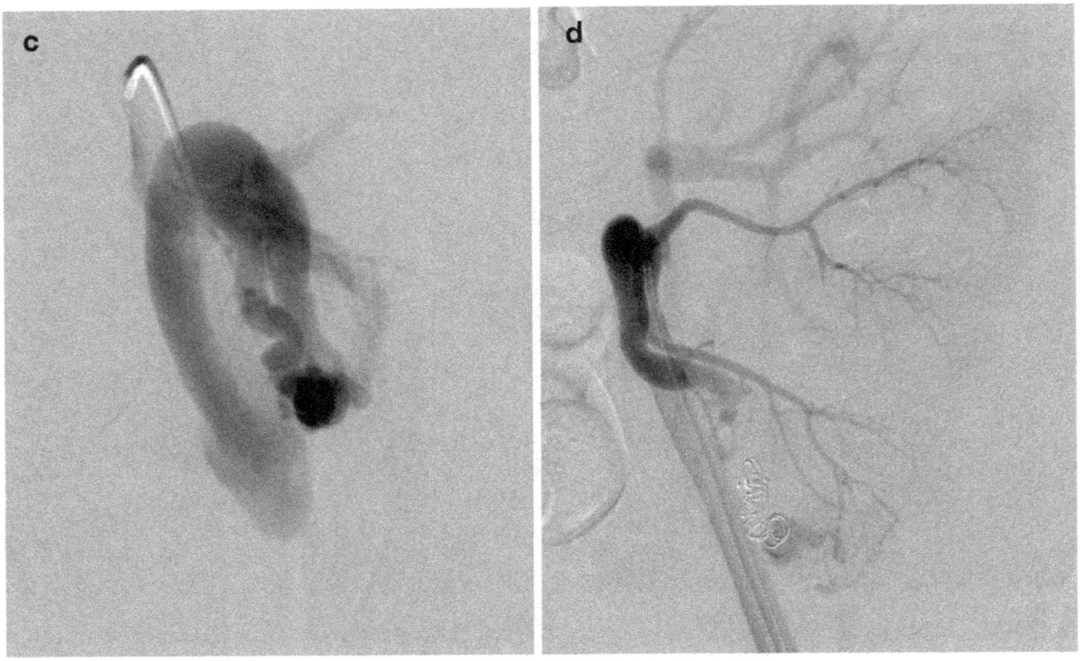

Fig. 5.20 (continued)

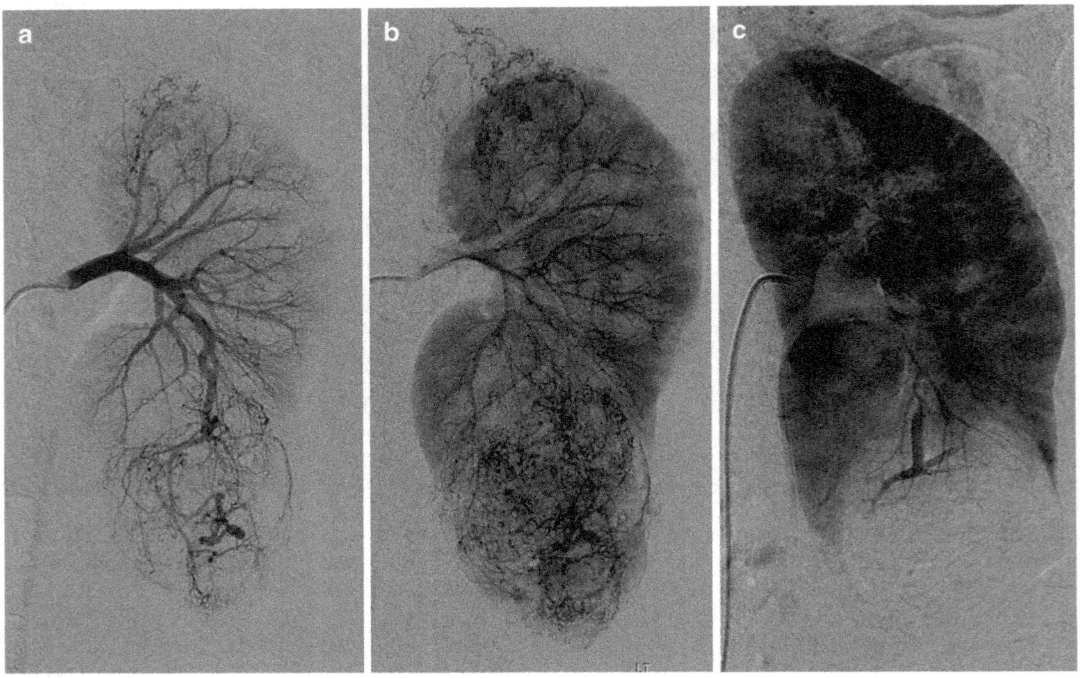

Fig. 5.21 Teenager with tuberous sclerosis and hematuria. (**a**, **b**) Early and late angiograms reveal a hypervascular angiomyolipoma in the lower pole of the kidney. (**c**) Post-selective embolization of the lower pole of the kidney reveals devascularization of the neoplasm. Case courtesy of John Racadio, MD

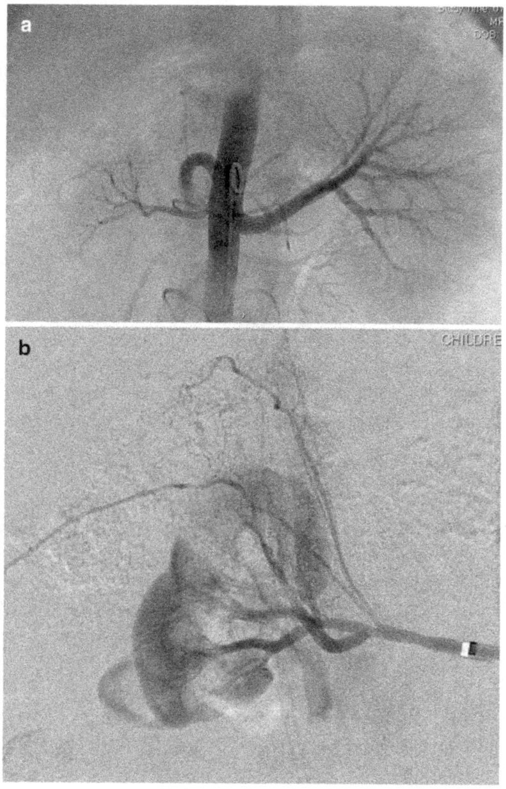

Fig. 5.22 A 17-year-old football player with hypertension that developed after fractured kidney the prior year. (**a**) Angiogram reveals a small right kidney consistent with Page kidney. (**b**) Ethanol ablation was performed and hypertension resolved

Renal Ablation with Ethanol

Select cases are reported in the literature where complete renal ablation can be performed with ethanol. Hidaka reported renal ablation of benign renal conditions using ethanol intra-arterially and sclerotherapy of the collecting system via percutaneous nephrostomy. Laparoscopic techniques have significantly reduced the morbidity of a nephrectomy procedure probably reducing the advantage for endovascular techniques. Nevertheless, ablating the kidneys with ethanol should still be considered an option in children needing nephrectomy to control hypertension. A small kidney, such as a Page kidney, can be easily treated with ethanol ablation with little post-embolization morbidity (Fig. 5.22).

Chapter Summary

Indications

- Hypertension
  - Hypertension >99th percentile; requiring more than two drugs
- Hematuria
- Vasculitis
  - Usually biopsy proven, angiography rarely required
- Trauma
- Post biopsy

Equipment

- 4 Fr vascular sheath
- Catheters
  - Pigtail
  - Sos
  - Cobra

Preprocedure Workup

- Continue medications
- BUN, creatinine

Technique

- GA
- Heparin: 50–100 units/kg
- Aortogram
- Selective catheterization
  - Multiple renal arteries in 30–40 %
- DSA with apnea, AP and 5- and 25° ipsilateral oblique angulation
- Findings
  - Stenosis
  - Post-stenotic dilation
  - Intrarenal collaterals
  - Aneurysm
  - Delayed opacification
- PTA
  - Heparin ± nitroglycerin
  - 5–6 Fr long guiding sheath
  - 0.014–0.035″ wire
  - Balloons
    - Rapid exchange or over the wire.
    - Cutting balloons have been used.
  - Repeat angiogram with wire in place
- Embolization
  - Renal ablation: focal or diffuse

- Ethanol preferred
- Slow injection to avoid reflux
- Consider embolization of collateral
- Post-biopsy hemorrhage
  - Microcoils as peripheral as possible
- Arteriovenous fistulae
  - Coils preferred when treatment necessary
- Angiomyolipoma
  - Lesions larger than 4 cm (artery >3 mm) prone to bleeding
- Stents
  - Avoid in children whenever possible.

Postprocedure Care

- PTA
  - Hospital admission for BP monitoring
    - Consider ICU especially if complicated
  - Heparin: 20 units/kg/h
  - Ultrasound following day
  - Antiplatelet agent
- Embolization/ablation
  - Hospital admission for BP monitoring

Suggested Reading

1. Corbetta JP, Durán V, Burek C, Weller S, Sager C, Dingevan R, Lopez JC. Renal autotransplantation for the treatment of renovascular hypertension in the pediatric population. J Pediatr Urol. 2011;7(3):378–82; Epub 2011 Apr 27.
2. Kimura H, Sato O, Deguchi JO, Miyata T. Surgical treatment and long-term outcome of renovascular hypertension in children and adolescents. Eur J Vasc Endovasc Surg. 2010;39(6):731–7; Epub 2010 Apr 28.
3. Lindblad B. Renovascular hypertension in children: time to further centralise handling? Eur J Vasc Endovasc Surg. 2011;41(6):778–9; Epub 2011 Mar 24.
4. Marshalleck F. Pediatric arterial interventions. Tech Vasc Interv Radiol. 2010;13(4):238–43.
5. Shroff R, Roebuck DJ, Gordon I, Davies R, Stephens S, Marks S, Chan M, Barkovics M, McLaren CA, Shah V, Dillon MJ, Tullus K. Angioplasty for renovascular hypertension in children: 20-year experience. Pediatrics. 2006;118(1):268–75.
6. Srinivasan A, Krishnamurthy G, Fontalvo-Herazo L, Nijs E, Keller MS, Meyers K, Kaplan B, Cahill AM. Angioplasty for renal artery stenosis in pediatric patients: an 11-year retrospective experience. J Vasc Interv Radiol. 2010;21(11):1672–80; Epub 2010 Sep 29.
7. Srinivasan A, Krishnamurthy G, Fontalvo-Herazo L, Nijs E, Meyers K, Kaplan B, Cahill AM. Spectrum of renal findings in pediatric fibromuscular dysplasia and neurofibromatosis type 1. Pediatr Radiol. 2011;41(3):308–16; Epub 2010 Oct 16.
8. Tullus K. Renal artery stenosis: is angiography still the gold standard in 2011? Pediatr Nephrol. 2011;26(6):833–7; Epub 2011 Jan 30.
9. Vo NJ, Hammelman BD, Racadio JM, Strife CF, Johnson ND, Racadio JM. Anatomic distribution of renal artery stenosis in children: implications for imaging. Pediatr Radiol. 2006;36(10):1032–6; Epub 2006 Jul 4.
10. Williams JM, Racadio JM, Johnson ND, Donnelly LF, Bissler JJ. Embolization of renal angiomyolipomata in patients with tuberous sclerosis complex. Am J Kidney Dis. 2006;47(1):95–102.
11. Shahdadpuri J, Frank R, Gauthier BG, Siegel DN, Trachtman H. Yield of renal arteriography in the evaluation of pediatric hypertension. Pediatr Nephrol. 2000;14(8–9):816–9.
12. Hidaka T, Daiyukai General Hospital, et al. Renal ablation by transcatheter renal arterial embolization in the treatment of benign renal disease. Nippo Igaku Hoshasen Gakkai Zasshi. 1994;54(12):1107–15.

Bronchial Artery Interventions in Children

6

Mark J. Hogan

General/Background Information

Hemoptysis, defined as the expectoration of blood or bloody sputum, is rare in children. It must be differentiated from mimics such as gastrointestinal bleeding and nosebleeds [1]. While there are many etiologies for pulmonary hemorrhage (Table 6.5), cystic fibrosis (CF) is the most common cause of severe hemoptysis in the western hemisphere and developed countries [1–6].

The pathophysiology of pulmonary hemorrhage in CF patients is chronic inflammation leading to blood vessel hypertrophy, increased pulmonary artery pressure, arteriovenous fistulas, and angiogenesis [4, 7, 8]. These tortuous, thin-walled arteries supply bronchopulmonary anastomoses in peribronchial granulation tissue and are easily injured during coughing and active inflammation [6, 9]. The inciting causes are hypoxic vasoconstriction, intravascular thrombosis, and vasculitis at the pulmonary arteriole level [2, 5]. In addition, these patients are often coagulopathic with a relative vitamin K deficiency due to poor intestinal absorption, liver disease, and the use of penicillins [1, 4, 8].

Hemoptysis occurs in 5–61 % of adults with CF but is less common in children with an incidence of approximately 1 % [4, 8]. Hemoptysis is mild and self-limited. Massive hemoptysis occurs in 5–7 % of patients, increases in incidence over time (only 8 % of these are less than 10 years old), [10] and has a yearly incidence of 1 % in the CF population with a median age of onset in the third decade [1, 4, 7, 9, 11–14]. 75 % of patients with massive hemoptysis have mild to moderate lung disease as defined by their forced expiratory volume at 1 s (FEV1) being at 50–75 % of expected [14]. This can cause death in up to 75 % of patients, usually as a result of asphyxiation [7, 9, 13, 15]. The mortality rate with surgical treatment is 35 % [2, 13]. The presence of hemoptysis is a poor prognostic factor and is associated with a lower quality of life [1, 12]. Vidal et al. reported on CF patients with hemoptysis requiring treatment with embolization and compared them to matched controls who did not have hemoptysis [12]. The embolization group had greater decrease in pulmonary function, a greater incidence of transplantation, and lower survival showing the detrimental effect on prognosis in patients with hemoptysis despite treatment.

The classification of the severity of hemoptysis varies by authors. One classification scheme divides hemoptysis into massive, moderate, and mild (Table 6.1) [1, 5, 6, 8, 11]. Another classification

M.J. Hogan, M.D. (✉)
Department of Radiology, Nationwide Children's Hospital, The Ohio State University, 700 Children's Drive, Columbus, OH 45205, USA
e-mail: mark.hogan@nationwidechildrens.org

M. Temple and F.E. Marshalleck (eds.), *Pediatric Interventional Radiology: Handbook of Vascular and Non-Vascular Interventions*, DOI 10.1007/978-1-4419-5856-3_6,

Table 6.1 One classification scheme divides hemoptysis into massive, moderate, and mild

1. Massive	> 300 mL/24 h
2. Moderate	> 3 episodes of > 100 mL/day in one week
3. Mild	< 100 mL/day × 3 per week

Table 6.2 Another classification uses the terms "major or significant" and mild

1. Major or significant	>240 mL/24 h >100 mL/day, recurrent <100 mL/day, but chronic or recurrent + Interferes with lifestyle Prevents effective physiotherapy Prevents home management
2. Mild	Does not fit above criteria

Table 6.3 A postmortem study showed 80 % of cases arise from the aorta at the 6th–7th thoracic vertebral level and had the following distribution [19]

41 %	One right	Two left
21 %	One common	
21 %	Two right	Two left
10 %	One right	One left

Table 6.4 An angiographic study by Uflacker showed the following distribution [20]

31 %	One right intercostal bronchial trunk (RICBT)	One left
25 %	One RICBT	One common trunk
13 %	One RICBT	Two left
11 %	One RICBT	One right, one left

uses the terms "major or significant" and mild (Table 6.2) [2, 4, 13]. A weight-based definition uses hemorrhage of >8 mL/kg in 24 h [1].

Most authors agree that massive hemoptysis requires intervention due to the risk of death. However, consensus is not present on the treatment of chronic or recurrent hemoptysis. Chronic or recurrent hemoptysis is debilitating, interferes with chest physiotherapy and aerosol treatment, and is related to an increased number of exacerbations and lung destruction. Chronic recurrent bleeding is more common in patients with severe lung disease (FEV1<50 %) [14, 15].

Initial therapy in patients with hemoptysis is medical. CF patients are typically admitted, chest physiotherapy is discontinued along with penicillins and nonsteroidal anti-inflammatory drugs, and patients receive vitamin K and antibiotics [1, 4, 8, 9]. Blood transfusions may be given if indicated. Holsclaw et al. described 19 patients with massive hemoptysis that received medical management [16]. There was 32 % mortality, and 50 % of the survivors had repetitive hemoptysis with total mortality over 6 months of 68.4 %. A somewhat later study by Stern showed 100 % survival with medical management in the setting of massive hemoptysis, with a 45 % rebleed rate [17]. Tranexamic acid is a fibrinolysis inhibitor that has been used for medical management [1, 4, 18]. The typical dose for massive hemoptysis is 15–25 mg/kg IV every 6 h for four doses. For less severe hemoptysis, it can be given orally at a dose of 1 g three times a day for 5–6 days [1, 8]. Vasopressin and octreotide (a selective bronchial artery vasoconstrictor) have also been tried in the past [1, 8]. A recent report described the use of factor VII in treating refractory hemoptysis [13].

Endoscopic treatments include cautery or laser, balloon occlusion of the bronchus, topical drugs such as epinephrine, and selective intubation [1, 3, 6]. Surgical options include lobectomy and extrapleural bronchial artery ligation [1, 3, 11]. However, angiography and embolization have mostly replaced these options as a first-line treatment of hemoptysis [2, 3, 11, 13].

Arterial supply to the lung is primarily from the pulmonary arteries (99 %) with the bronchial arteries supplying the remainder of the flow (1 %) predominately to the mediastinum, airways, lymph nodes, and visceral pleura [5]. While the pulmonary arteries have a lower pressure, bronchial arteries have systemic blood pressure. These bronchial arteries are the cause of hemoptysis in 90 % of patients with CF and are the most common source of hemoptysis in patients with other inflammatory conditions and tumors due to their hypertrophy and angiogenesis [2, 5].

Bronchial artery anatomy is variable, but knowledge of these arteries and their possible communications is critical in treating patients with hemoptysis [1, 3]. A postmortem study showed 80 % of bronchial arteries arise from the

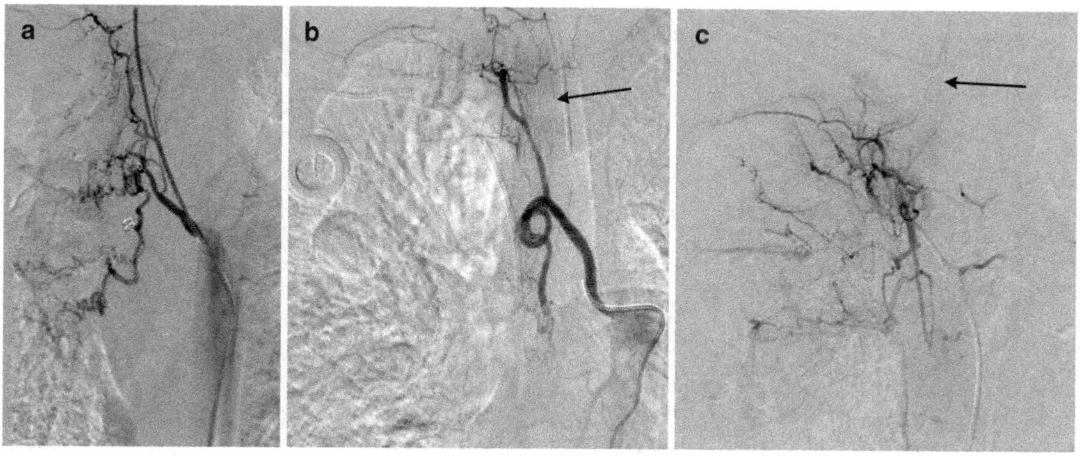

Fig. 6.1 These are three examples of the right intercostal bronchial trunk. In the last two images, anterior medullary radicular arteries are identified feeding spinal artery branches (*arrows*)

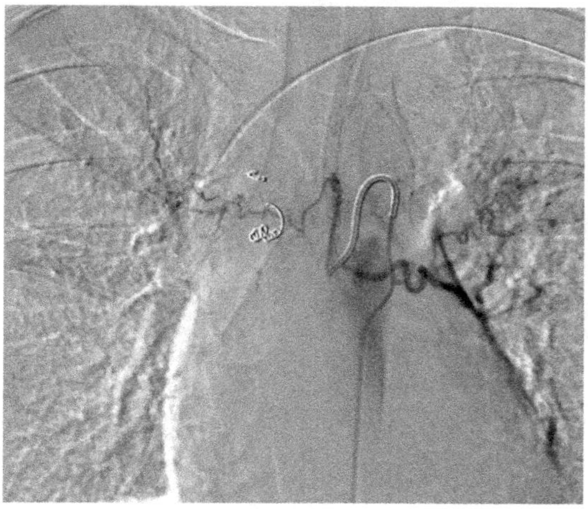

Fig. 6.2 Common bronchial artery trunk

aorta at the 6th–7th thoracic vertebral level (see Table 6.3 for distribution) [19]. Table 6.4 shows the distribution from an angiographic study by Uflacker et al. [20] (Fig. 6.2).

The origin of the RICBT is typically posterolateral, the right bronchial artery is lateral to anterior, the common trunk arises anteriorly, and the left bronchial artery may be anterior, anterolateral, or from the aortic arch. The RICBT supplies the right lung in 80 % of patients. It occasionally supplies the left lung and the superior intercostal artery and provides supply to the spinal artery in 5 % of patients (Fig. 6.1a–c) [5]. In addition, the RICBT may have collaterals to the subclavian artery, the mid-esophagus, the pericardium, and the coronary arteries [20].

In addition to these variations, there are aberrant origins of the bronchial arteries including the subclavian arteries and their branches (internal mammary artery (IMA), thyrocervical artery, costocervical artery, lateral thoracic artery), the superior intercostal artery, the inferior phrenic artery, the left gastric artery, and esophageal artery branches (Figs. 6.3a–e) [5, 20]. There are often recruited transpleural collaterals from the subclavian artery and its branches as well that can be identified by their supply to the pleura and subsequent filling of intrapulmonary branches (Fig. 6.4) [1, 2, 5].

As stated above, the RICBT may provide supply to the anterior spinal artery, and other branches may supply the anterior spinal artery as well via anterior segmental medullary arteries. These are identified by a classic hairpin turn and the largest of these is named the artery of Adamkiewicz which usually originates at the T9–12 level [1, 5, 6]. Identification of these arteries is crucial during the embolization procedure, as inadvertent embolization can cause spinal cord ischemia [6, 11].

There are many connections between the bronchial arteries, aberrant bronchial arteries,

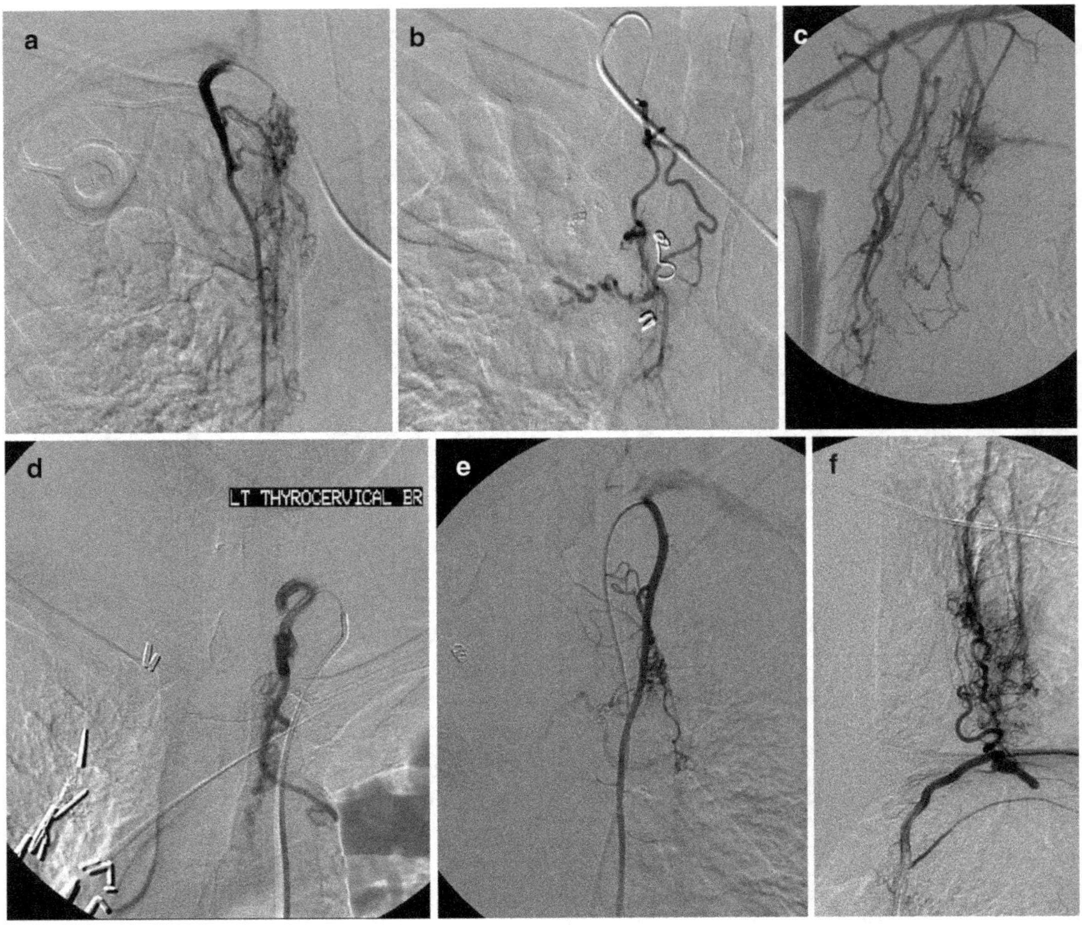

Fig. 6.3 Multiple aberrant origins of the bronchial arteries including the right internal mammary artery (**a**), right thyrocervical artery (**b**), right lateral thoracic artery (**c**), left thyrocervical artery (**d**), left internal mammary artery (**e**), and left phrenic artery (**f**)

and the transpleural collaterals; therefore, any artery may potentially supply the spinal artery or connect with the subclavian artery and its branches (Fig. 6.5) [21]. One third of arteries responsible for hemoptysis are non-bronchial systemic collaterals [3, 7, 11].

Bronchial artery embolization was first described by Remy in 1974 [22]. The use of this technique for treating hemoptysis has been described in many studies [1–8, 11, 12, 17, 23–26]. The goal of the procedure is to reduce the pressure to the site of hemorrhage allowing the artery to heal while avoiding tissue destruction [1]. A key goal is to allow a pathway for retreatment if necessary as these patients typically have an ongoing disease process, and recurrent hemoptysis is common.

While there have been no controlled studies comparing embolic agents, reported materials include gelatin sponge, polyvinyl alcohol (PVA) particles, spherical embolics, coils, and *n*-butyl cyanoacrylate (n-BCNA) [1–5, 7, 9, 11, 12, 23, 27]. Gelatin sponge can be quite effective but is a temporary agent [1, 9]. PVA is a permanent agent, although the occlusion is not permanent [1, 2]. The size of the embolic material is more uniform than with gelatin sponge. Shunts to the pulmonary circulation as large as 325 μm have been described, and therefore, the particles used are usually greater than 350 μm in size [5, 27]. Spherical agents have been used, but they need to be sized larger than PVA as they compress and can more easily pass through shunts to the pulmonary veins or arteries [1, 12]. N-BCNA has been described in

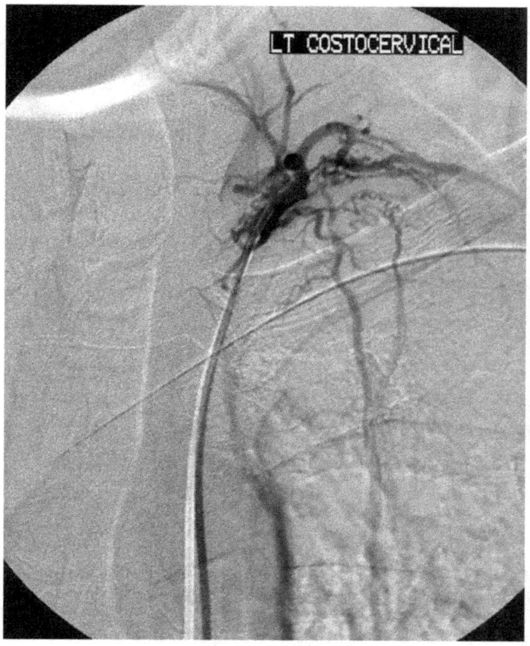

Fig. 6.4 This is a transpleural collateral from the left subclavian artery. Noted is filling of the pulmonary veins

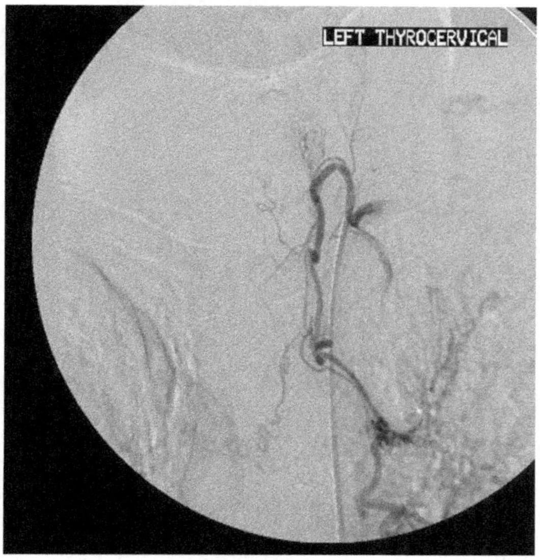

Fig. 6.5 Injection of the left thyrocervical artery demonstrates collateralization with right and left bronchial arteries and multiple mediastinal branches

some studies and is permanent, but the delivery may be more difficult [1]. It may have a lower rate of rebleeding. Coils are contraindicated for proximal occlusion but may be useful for distal arteries in a patient with recurrent hemoptysis or in excluding a nontarget artery [1, 6, 7]. Prior reports using gelatin sponge powder and ethanol have had unacceptable incidences of bronchial necrosis and other complications [1, 6, 8].

Indications/Contraindications

Indications for treatment include those patients with massive or moderate hemoptysis when medical management has failed. Embolization of chronic and recurrent hemoptysis may be indicated when [7]:

1. They have had mild hemoptysis leading to massive hemoptysis before.
2. They have hemoptysis within 2 weeks after completing recent optimal medical management.
3. Hemoptysis continues despite a trial of optimal medical management.
4. Embolization is performed to stop hemoptysis as a bridge to transplantation.

As described above, there are multiple other causes of hemoptysis in addition to CF (Figs. 6.6 and 6.7).

Consultation with the patient, family, and referring physicians is imperative including potential risks such as hemorrhage, anaphylaxis, vascular injury, stroke, and spinal cord injury, and possible alternative therapies should be discussed. Standard contraindications to angiography are valid in this setting [28].

Pre-procedural Evaluation

Prior to performing bronchial arteriography for potential embolization, attempts to localize the site of bleeding have been performed. The patient may indicate where they feel a "gurgling" or other sensation. Plain radiographs may show new areas of airspace disease representing hemorrhage (useful in 17–80 % of patients), and a CT scan may be more sensitive and can identify the bronchial arteries [1, 5, 6, 29, 30]. Bronchoscopy may identify the site or side of bleeding in 10–91 % of patients; however, it may fail as blood may be present throughout the bronchi due to coughing [5]. The site cannot be identified in 20–30 % of patients [2].

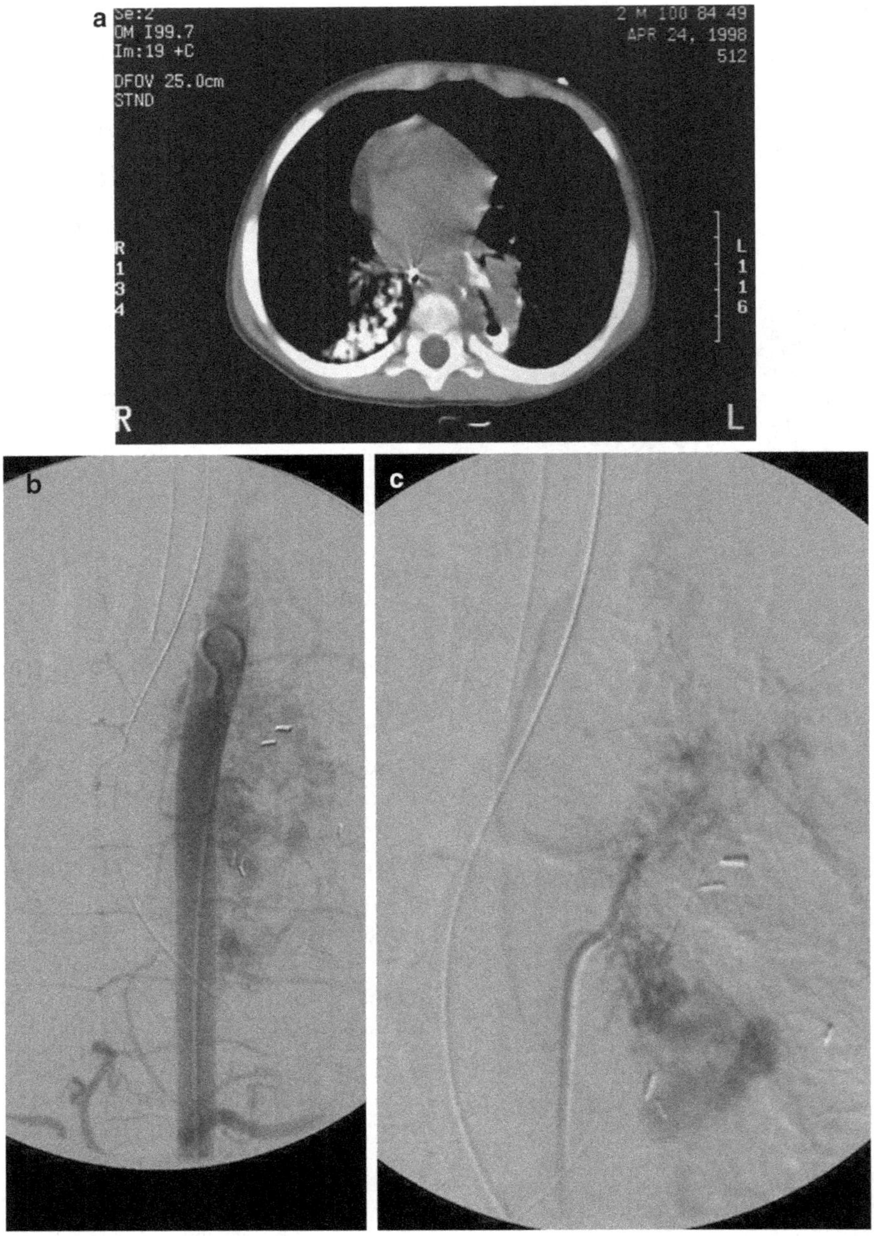

Fig. 6.6 This patient had hemoptysis after resection of the superior segment of the left lower lobe. A CT scan shows stump dehiscence with a contained leak (**a**). Subsequent aortogram (**b**) shows an extensive vascular blush in the left paraspinal region with resolution after embolization (**c**)

Routine hematology and coagulation tests should be performed, and the patient's medical treatment should be optimized including the cessation of penicillins or NSAIDs. Vitamin K should be administered [1, 2]. Where available, tranexamic acid may be given.

Procedure Technique

Sedation or anesthesia is paramount as these procedures may be lengthy [9]. General anesthesia with intubation allows for apnea during

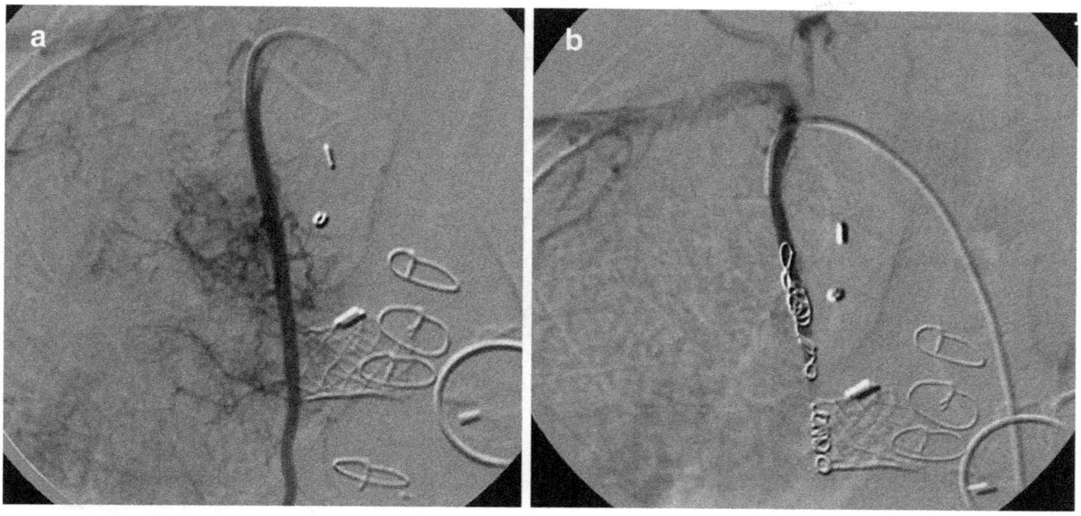

Fig. 6.7 Three-year-old patient with recurrent hemoptysis after surgery for congenital heart disease. In (**a**), an injection of the right internal mammary artery shows innumerable collaterals to the lungs. PVA and coil embolization excluded this artery (**b**), and with the embolization of multiple other pulmonary artery collaterals, the hemoptysis ceased

imaging and better images; however, there have been reports of death during induction of anesthesia for CF patients with hemoptysis [1, 10, 14, 31]. Sedation can be used for cooperative patients [32]. It is generally well tolerated, and the patient can be instructed when to breath-hold. However, intermittent coughing can be a problem that may occasionally lead to catheter dislodgement and poor images. In younger children, anesthesia is mandatory as they do not have the capacity to cooperate. We routinely use anesthesia for any patient less than 16 years old for this procedure and consider it for the older patients.

A 4 or 5 Fr femoral sheath is placed with the initial puncture under ultrasound guidance. We typically use 4 Fr sheaths in patients less than 10 years old as flush catheters of this size are sufficient for aortography, while a 5 Fr flush catheter may be better for larger patients.

Some authors prefer to perform an aortogram as the initial study [1]. The argument for this approach is that the bronchial arteries may be identified at the outset and therefore easier to access. However, this uses a large amount of contrast at the beginning of the study, and contrast limits (up to 5–7 mL/kg) may be reached prior to completion of the procedure [28]. In addition, the initial aortogram may not show collaterals which may be more apparent after embolization of the main bronchial arteries (Fig. 6.8). In our practice, we perform aortography at the end of the procedure if there is enough contrast available in order to identify any previously missed bronchial arteries or collaterals.

Abnormalities predisposing to hemorrhage are described as bronchial artery size >1.5–2.5 mm in diameter, the presence of shunts to the pulmonary vein or artery (usually 0.5–1 mm in size), aneurysms, tortuosity, and extravasation (rare) [1–3, 5, 6].

In our approach, we target the subclavian artery branches initially. The rationale behind this technique is to occlude any potential pathways that might lead to inadvertent embolization to the vertebral or carotid arteries via collaterals from the subclavian distribution. If the main bronchial arteries are treated initially, there may be reversal of flow toward the subclavian distribution via these collaterals after the distal parenchymal bronchial arteries are occluded. Angled catheters such as a vertebral catheter are typically

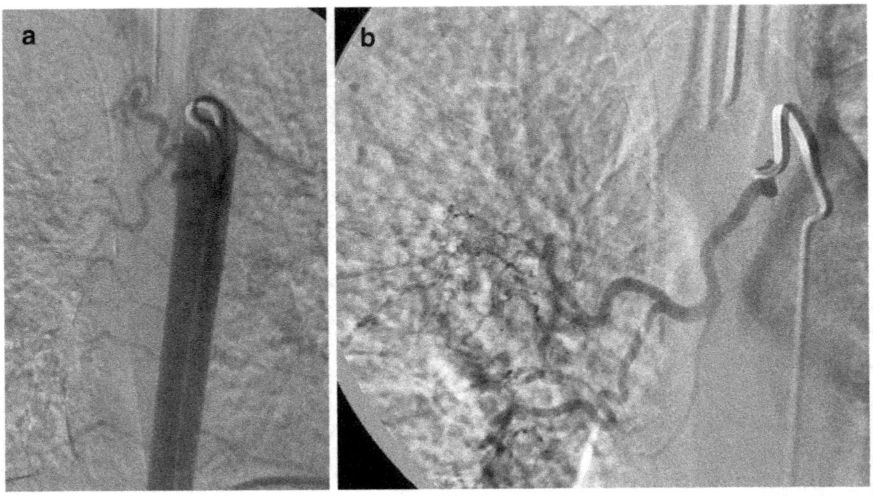

Fig. 6.8 Massive hemoptysis in a CF patient. After performing embolization of all previously identified bronchial arteries and collaterals, a follow-up aortogram demonstrated an untreated bronchial artery (**a**). This was successfully cannulated and embolized (**b**)

used. Arteriography is performed in the main subclavian artery and then in any and all branches that appear to provide flow to the bronchial arteries. If significant flow is present to the lungs (subjective), and the artery can be safely accessed, a microcatheter is advanced to provide greater control and delivery of the embolic agents [2, 3, 5, 6]. Extreme care is taken to evaluate for spinal artery collaterals and nontarget vessels. If present, this is not necessarily a contraindication to embolization. If the microcatheter can be advanced past the origin of the spinal or nontarget artery, embolization can be safely performed if done with great care [3].

Embolization is then performed with PVA particles, typically 300–500 μm in size mixed with a 50:50 contrast/saline solution. If sizable shunts to the pulmonary veins are seen, larger particles may be used up to 1,000 μm (Fig. 6.9). Embolization is performed under a negative "roadmap" technique to better visualize the flow, particularly any flow toward a spinal artery or a

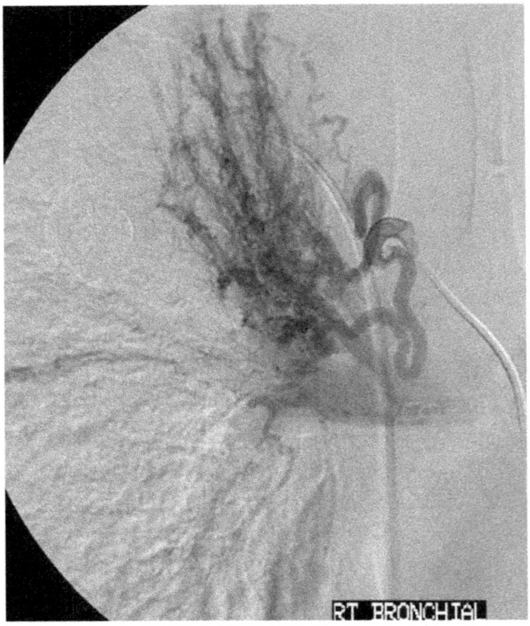

Fig. 6.9 Extensive shunting into the pulmonary vein is identified during injection of the right bronchial artery necessitating a change to larger PVA particles, 500 μm and greater in size

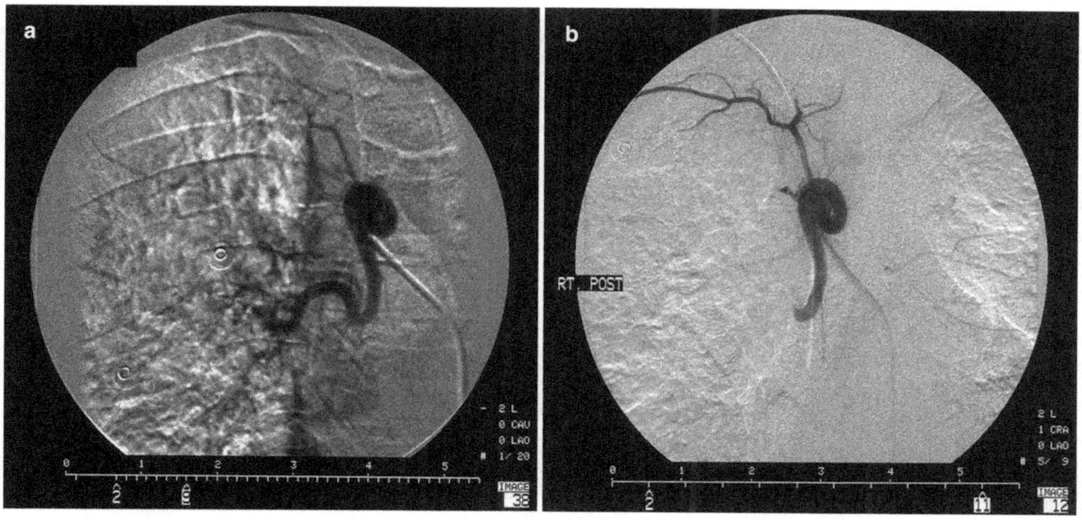

Fig. 6.10 Patient with CF and hemoptysis. The right bronchial artery is enlarged and tortuous (**a**). Note the misregistration artifact as the patient holds his breath. There is cessation of flow after PVA embolization (**b**)

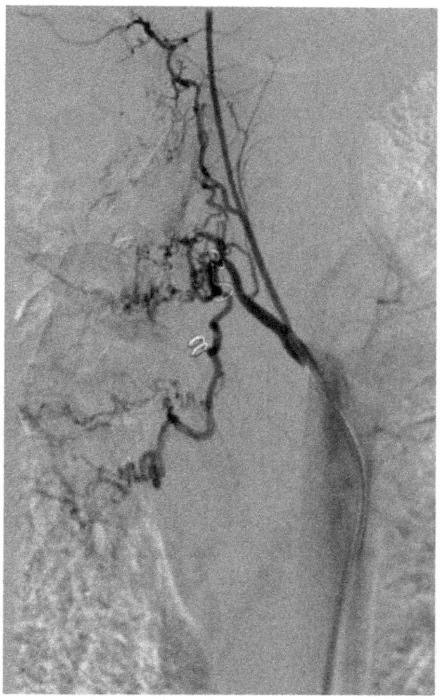

Fig. 6.11 This CF patient had frequent recurrent hemoptysis. Coil embolization has been performed distally. The bronchial artery origin remains patent and accessible should further treatment be indicated

nontarget vessel [1]. Embolization is performed to the point of flow cessation and when the intraparenchymal branches no longer opacify (Fig. 6.10a, b). In our practice, all arteries that can be safely treated are embolized. Coils are seldom indicated; however, they can be used to occlude and protect nontarget arteries. Coils are occasionally placed if the microcatheter is quite distal and the patient is having frequent (every 6 month) recurrent hemoptysis in an attempt to better control these episodes (Fig. 6.11). Coils are never placed if they preclude reaccessing the supplying artery.

Once the subclavian collaterals and aberrant bronchial arteries are treated, the catheter is placed into the thoracic aorta at a level just below the carina, and the RICBT is accessed. This may require the use of a different angled or even a reverse curve catheter. Once accessed, careful arteriography is performed. Again, any spinal branches or nontarget arteries are evaluated. If safe, arteriography and embolization can then be performed through a microcatheter with the same technique as described above.

Additional bronchial arteries are sought and treated as above when safe. We attempt to treat all possible bronchial arteries and collaterals as it cannot be reliably ascertained where the hemorrhage originated or where the patient may hemorrhage from next.

At the completion of the study, an aortogram is performed to identify any significant arteries not found during the study. If present, they are accessed and embolized as above.

Table 6.5 Causes of hemoptysis—"Battlecamp"

B	Bronchitis, bronchiectasis
A	Aspergillosis, alveolar hemorrhage
T	Tumor, trauma
T	Tuberculosis
L	Lung abscess
E	Emboli
C	Coagulopathy
A	Autoimmune, AVM
M	Mitral stenosis
P	Pneumonia
Others	Tracheostomy related, foreign bodies, aortopulmonary collaterals

Postprocedure Care

After the procedure, hemoptysis usually tapers during the next 1–2 days, as the patient coughs up the residual blood. Narcotics may be needed due to the chest pain that may accompany the procedure [2, 5, 9, 12]. Chest physiotherapy can recommence in 2 days, with the patient usually being discharged 2 days after the procedure.

Expected Outcomes and Complications

As described previously, embolization is successful in controlling hemoptysis in greater than 90 % of cases regardless of etiology [1–5, 7, 8, 11–14]. Recurrences are common and can be due to initial incomplete embolization, recanalization of the supplying arteries, disease progression, or development of new collaterals [2–5, 7, 11–13, 33]. Up to 75 % of recurrent bleeding is from collaterals [5, 7]. In the CF population, the overall incidence of recurrence is up to 60 % until resolution occurs secondary to transplantation or death [2–4, 7, 11, 12, 33]. Repeat angiography and embolization can be performed [2].

In a study by Antonelli et al., patients with non-massive hemoptysis were either treated with embolization or with conservative medical therapy [4]. The patients having embolization had significantly fewer recurrent bleeds, had less of a decline in functional status, and reported a higher quality of life. Pulmonary function deterioration was not significantly changed nor was the frequency of pulmonary exacerbations.

Complications can occur in 10–40 % of patients [1–5, 7, 8, 11, 12]. The most worrisome is death. However, this is quite rare and usually reported to be a complication of intubation and positive pressure ventilation [10, 14, 31]. Spinal cord ischemia occurs in less than 1 % of patients, presents as a transverse myelitis, and is usually self-limited [3, 5, 11]. Experimental studies have shown that this is unlikely when using particles 100 μm or larger in size, as animals below this size had paralysis, but only weakness when using larger particles [34]. Most cases of postprocedural transverse myelitis were reported with the use of ionic contrast which may have been the critical factor [6, 27].

Other reported complications include chest pain (up to 40 % of cases), dysphagia, broncho-esophageal fistula, pulmonary or bronchial infarction (with ethanol or gelatin sponge powder), stroke and cortical blindness, phrenic nerve palsy, myocardial infarction (presumably due to coronary artery collaterals), ischemic colitis, arterial dissection (up to 6.3 % of cases), and peripheral ischemia [1–8, 11, 12, 22].

Chapter Summary

Background

- CF most common cause of hemoptysis (see Table 6.5)
- Medical therapy often successful:
  - Stop chest physiotherapy and penicillin
  - Vitamin K, tranexamic acid
  - Vasopressin, octreotide
  - Antibiotics
- Endoscopic and surgical treatment possible
- Embolization—first-line treatment
- Systemic supply usually:
  - Bronchial—variable anatomy
  - Collaterals:
    - Subclavian branches
    - Intercostal
    - Phrenic
    - Left gastric
    - Esophageal
- Shunts possible:
  - Spinal cord, carotid/vertebral circulation
  - Up to 325 μm in size

Indications

- Medical management failed
- Massive/moderate hemoptysis
- Consider in chronic/recurrent when:
  - Previous massive hemoptysis
  - Recurrent hemoptysis <2 weeks post-treatment
  - Not responding to treatment
  - Bridge to transplantation

Preprocedure Evaluation

- Hematology and coagulation profile
- Attempt to identify site:
  - Clinical history
  - Imaging—CXR, CT
  - Bronchoscopy

Equipment

- Catheters, 4–5 Fr:
  - Reverse curve (Sos, Simmons, etc.)
  - Angled (vertebral)
  - Microcatheters
  - Pigtail
- Embolic agent:
  - PVA, gelatin sponge, spherical, glue
  - Coils not recommended unless very distal
- 4–5 Fr vascular sheath

Technique

- Usually GA (especially younger patients)
- Femoral access
- Author's suggested order of investigation:
  - Bilateral subclavian arteries and branches (if indicated)
  - Right intercostal bronchial trunk (switch to reverse curve catheter if necessary)
  - Other bronchial arteries
  - Aortogram
- PVA common embolic material:
  - 300–500 μm size
  - Up to 1,000 μm used when large shunts seen
- Monitor for collaterals to spine and cerebral circulation (consider higher fluoroscopy rate during embolization)

Postprocedure Care

- Supportive care
- Post-embolization syndrome can occur
- D/C home average 2 days post

Outcomes/Complications

- >90 % successful
- Recurrent hemoptysis common
- Death—10–40 %
  - Often complication of anesthesia:
    - Consider potential for extracorporeal membrane oxygenation if high risk
- Nontarget embolization:
  - Spinal ischemia:
    - Can be self-limited
    - Avoid small particles!
  - Myocardial infarction
  - Stroke, cortical blindness
  - Phrenic nerve palsy
  - Ischemic colitis
  - Peripheral ischemia
- Pain
- Dysphagia
- Esophageal fistula
- Pulmonary/bronchial infarction
- Arterial dissection

References

1. Roebuck DJ, Barnacle AM. Haemoptysis and bronchial artery embolization in children. Paediatr Respir Rev. 2008;9(2):95–104.
2. Serasli E, Kalpakidis V, Iatrou K, Tsara V, Siopi D, Christaki P. Percutaneous bronchial artery embolization in the management of massive hemoptysis in chronic lung diseases. Immediate and long-term outcomes. Int Angiol. 2008;27(4):319–28.
3. Andersen PE. Imaging and interventional radiological treatment of hemoptysis. Acta Radiol. 2006;47(8):780–92.
4. Antonelli M, Midulla F, Tancredi G, Salvatori FM, Bonci E, Cimino G, Flaishman I. Bronchial artery embolization for the management of nonmassive hemoptysis in cystic fibrosis. Chest. 2002;121(3):796–801.
5. Yoon W, Kim JK, Kim YH, Chung TW, Kang HK. Bronchial and nonbronchial systemic artery embolization for life-threatening hemoptysis: a comprehensive review. Radiographics. 2002;22(6):1395–409.
6. Kalva SP. Bronchial artery embolization. Tech Vasc Interv Radiol. 2009;12(2):130–8.
7. Brinson GM, Noone PG, Mauro MA, Knowles MR, Yankaskas JR, Sandhu JS, Jaques PF. Bronchial artery embolization for the treatment of hemoptysis in patients with cystic fibrosis. Am J Respir Crit Care Med. 1998;157(6 Pt 1):1951–8.
8. Ashleigh RJ, Webb AK. Radiological intervention for haemoptysis in cystic fibrosis. J R Soc Med. 2007;100 Suppl 47:38–45.
9. Fairfax AJ, Ball J, Batten JC, Heard BE. A pathological study following bronchial artery embolization for haemoptysis in cystic fibrosis. Br J Dis Chest. 1980;74(4):345–52.
10. Barben J, Robertson D, Olinsky A, Ditchfield M. Bronchial artery embolization for hemoptysis in young patients with cystic fibrosis. Radiology. 2002;224(1):124–30.
11. Cipolli M, Perini S, Valletta EA, Mastella G. Bronchial artery embolization in the management of hemoptysis in cystic fibrosis. Pediatr Pulmonol. 1995;19(6):344–7.
12. Vidal V, Therasse E, Berthiaume Y, Bommart S, Giroux MF, Oliva VL, Abrahamowicz M, du Berger R, Jeanneret A, Soulez G. Bronchial artery embolization in adults with cystic fibrosis: impact on the clinical course and survival. J Vasc Interv Radiol. 2006;17(6):953–8.
13. Lau EM, Yozghatlian V, Kosky C, Moriarty C, Dentice R, Waugh R, Torzillo PJ, Bye PT. Recombinant activated factor VII for massive hemoptysis in patients with cystic fibrosis. Chest. 2009;136(1):277–81.
14. Barben JU, Ditchfield M, Carlin JB, Robertson CF, Robinson PJ, Olinsky A. Major haemoptysis in children with cystic fibrosis: a 20-year retrospective study. J Cyst Fibros. 2003;2(3):105–11.
15. Chun JY, Morgan R, Belli AM. Radiological management of hemoptysis: a comprehensive review of diagnostic imaging and bronchial arterial embolization. Cardiovasc Intervent Radiol. 2010;33(2):240–50.
16. Holsclaw DS, Grand RJ, Schwachman H. Massive hemoptysis in cystic fibrosis. J Pediatr. 1970;76:838.
17. Stern RC, Wood RE, Boat TF, Matthews LW, Tucker AS, Doershuk C. Treatment and prognosis of massive hemoptysis in cystic fibrosis. Am Rev Respir Dis. 1978;117:825–8.
18. Graff GR. Treatment of recurrent severe hemoptysis in cystic fibrosis with tranexamic acid. Respiration. 2001;68(1):91–4.
19. Cauldwell EW, Siekert RG, et al. The bronchial arteries: an anatomic study of 150 human cadavers. Surg Gynecol Obstet. 1948;86(4):395–412.
20. Uflacker R, Kaemmerer A, Picon PD, Rizzon CF, Neves CM, Oliveira ES, Oliveira ME, Azevedo SN, Ossanai R. Bronchial artery embolization in the management of hemoptysis: technical aspects and long-term results. Radiology. 1985;157(3):637–44.
21. Furnari ML, Salerno S, Rabiolo A, Caravello V, Pardo F. Bronchial to subclavian shunt in a CF patient. A potential pitfall for embolization. J Cyst Fibros. 2003;2(4):217–9.
22. Rémy J, Voisin C, Dupuis C, Beguery P, Tonnel AB, Denies JL, Douay B. Treatment of hemoptysis by embolization of the systemic circulation. Ann Radiol. 1974;17(1):5–16.
23. Barben J, Robertson D, Olinsky A, Ditchfield M. Bronchial artery embolization for hemoptysis in young patients with cystic fibrosis. Radiology. 2002;224(1):124–30.
24. Uflacker R, Kaemmerer A, Neves C, Picon PD. Management of massive hemoptysis by bronchial artery embolization. Radiology. 1983;146:627–34.
25. Fellows KE, Khaw KT, Schuster S, Schwachman H. Bronchial artery embolization in cystic fibrosis: technique and long-term results. J Pediatr. 1979;95:959–63.
26. Tonkin IL, Hanissian AF, Boulden TF, Baum SL, Bavant RE, Gold RE, George P, Green WJ. Bronchial arteriography and embolotherapy for hemoptysis in patients with cystic fibrosis. Cardiovasc Intervent Radiol. 1991;14:241–6.
27. Fraser KL, Grosman H, Hyland RH, Tullis DE. Transverse myelitis: a reversible complication of bronchial artery embolisation in cystic fibrosis. Thorax. 1997;52(1):99–101.
28. Heran MK, Marshalleck F, Temple M, Grassi CJ, Connolly B, Towbin RB, Baskin KM, Dubois J, Hogan MJ, Kundu S, Miller DL, Roebuck DJ, Rose SC, Sacks D, Sidhu M, Wallace MJ, Zuckerman DA, Cardella JF, Society of Interventional Radiology Standards of Practice Committee and Society of Pediatric Radiology Interventional Radiology Committee. Joint quality improvement guidelines for pediatric arterial access and arteriography: from the Societies of Interventional Radiology and Pediatric Radiology. J Vasc Interv Radiol. 2010;21(1):32–43.

29. Bruzzi JF, Rémy-Jardin M, Delhaye D, Teisseire A, Khalil C, Rémy J. Multi-detector row CT of hemoptysis. Radiographics. 2006;26(1):3–22.
30. Remy-Jardin M, Bouaziz N, Dumont P, Brillet PY, Bruzzi J, Remy J. Bronchial and nonbronchial systemic arteries at multi-detector row CT angiography: comparison with conventional angiography. Radiology. 2004;233(3):741–9.
31. McDougall RJ, Sherrington CA. Fatal pulmonary haemorrhage during anaesthesia for bronchial artery embolization in cystic fibrosis. Paediatr Anaesth. 1999;9(4):345–8.
32. Yovichevich S. Commentary on bronchial artery embolization for hemoptysis in young patients with cystic fibrosis. Radiology. 2003;228(3):903–4.
33. Bookstein JJ, Moser KM, Kalafer ME, et al. The role of bronchial arteriography and therapeutic embolization in haemoptysis. Chest. 1977;72:658.
34. Boushy SE, Helgason AH, North LB. Occlusion of the bronchial arteries by glass microspheres. Am Rev Respir Dis. 1971;103:249–63.

7 Pulmonary Artery Interventions in Children

Mark J. Hogan

General/Background Information

Pulmonary angiography is an uncommon procedure in children. While there are no controlled studies in children comparing the efficacy of pulmonary angiography versus CT angiography (CTA), data from the adult literature has been extrapolated and CTA has essentially replaced catheter arteriography for diagnosing pulmonary embolism (PE) [1, 2]. Most pulmonary angiography at this time is performed for a planned intervention, particularly in the setting of an embolized foreign body (usually a catheter fragment), for attempted thrombolysis of a pulmonary embolism, or for the treatment of pulmonary arteriovenous malformations (PAVMs).

Catheter breakage with resultant embolization of a fragment into the pulmonary arteries is uncommon but can occur in up to 4.1 % of children with central lines [3, 4]. This can occur due to catheter pinch-off from a catheter placed from any approach, catheter damage by chemotherapy drugs, separation between the catheter and the port chamber, or breakage during attempted removal [3–8]. The catheter fragment can predispose the patient to thrombosis or, if a portion remains in the right heart, can lead to an arrhythmia.

Coils, inferior vena cava (IVC) filters (or fragments from them), and other endovascular devices can also migrate into the pulmonary circulation [9]. Ventriculoperitoneal shunts and penetrating projectiles are rare causes of lung embolization [10, 11]. Angiographic techniques can be employed to remove these foreign bodies using snare devices (Fig. 7.1a, b) [9, 12, 13].

Pulmonary embolism (PE) is less common in children than adults with a reported incidence of 0.14/100,000 children (probably an underestimation) as compared to the incidence in adults of 117/100,000 in whom the mortality is approximately 10 % [14–17]. Although 84 % of children with PE are symptomatic with shortness of breath or chest pain, only 15–17 % of children with a CTA for suspected PE have confirmation of that diagnosis [1, 2, 16]. Most children have an underlying risk factor such as immobility, a central venous catheter, recent surgery, trauma, congenital heart disease, underlying coagulopathy, malignancy, obesity, or oral contraceptive use (Fig. 7.2a–d) [16].

Massive PE is defined by the presence of shock with systolic systemic blood pressure less than or equal to 90 mmHg or a drop in systemic blood pressure of >40 mmHg, which occurs in 4.2 % of all adults with PE, and these patients have an increased mortality which may be over 50 % [17–21]. Sub-massive PE is diagnosed in normotensive patients with right ventricular dysfunction and has a mortality of approximately 8 % [18, 21, 22]. No similar data are available for children.

M.J. Hogan, M.D. (✉)
Department of Radiology, Nationwide Children's Hospital, The Ohio State University, 700 Children's Drive, Columbus, OH 45205, USA
e-mail: mark.hogan@nationwidechildrens.org

M. Temple and F.E. Marshalleck (eds.), *Pediatric Interventional Radiology: Handbook of Vascular and Non-Vascular Interventions*, DOI 10.1007/978-1-4419-5856-3_7,

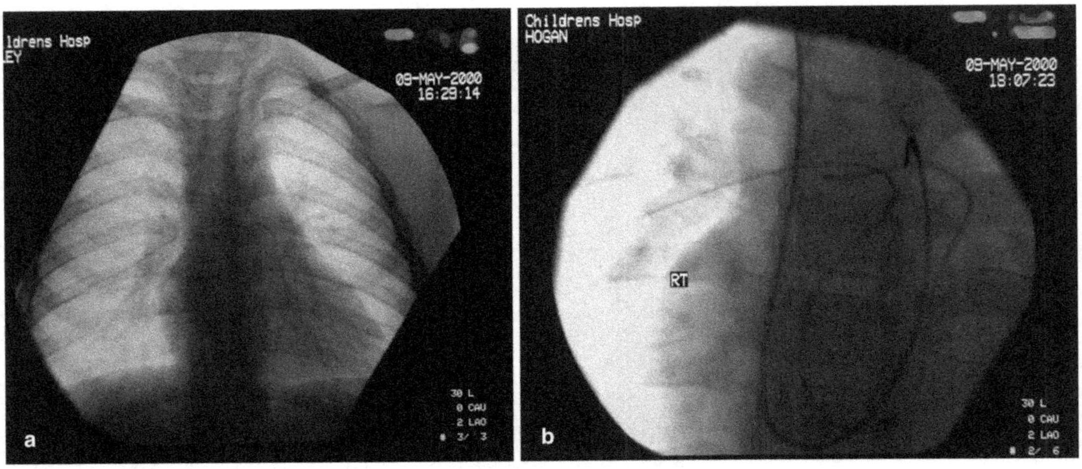

Fig. 7.1 (**a**) PICC line fragment has embolized to the pulmonary artery. Subsequently from a right brachial vein approach, a snare is advanced and used to grasp the catheter fragment for removal (**b**)

Multiple different treatment techniques have been used including systemic thrombolysis, catheter-directed thrombolysis, and the use of mechanical devices such as a rotating pigtail catheter, aspiration thrombectomy, thrombus maceration, rheolytic thrombectomy, and stent placement (Fig. 7.3a, b) [17, 21, 23–26]. There is no single accepted best treatment [21]. Systemic thrombolysis has a clinical success rate of 77 %; however, hemorrhage as a major complication is reported to occur in 20 % of patients [21]. The distal pulmonary bed has twice the volume of the proximal pulmonary arteries [27]. Therefore, theoretically, mechanical breakage of the clot will allow for a greater pulmonary bed to continue air exchange and provide a greater contact area available for pharmacological thrombolysis [21, 24].

PAVMs are abnormal fistulous connections between the pulmonary arteries and veins [22, 27–32]. Potential symptoms include hypoxia due to the right to left shunt, neurological symptoms and other ischemic events from paradoxical embolization, and hemoptysis [22, 27, 29, 30]. Hemoptysis can occur in 10–14 % of cases, and rupture is more common in pregnancy [33]. They are most commonly found in a patient with hereditary hemorrhagic telangiectasia (HHT), with 70–95 % of PAVMs occurring in this population. PAVMs occur in 25–30 % of patients with HHT [33]. The remaining 10 % are acquired lesions from systemic diseases such as hepatopulmonary syndrome [22, 29, 31]. Most do not become symptomatic until adulthood, although 4.5 % of cases will present in a child [29]. Hypoxia occurs in >70 % and paradoxical embolization in >50 % of untreated patients [29, 31]. Hypoxia is usually fairly well tolerated [29, 31]. Transthoracic echocardiography with agitated saline can be used as a screening tool to evaluate for a right to left shunt [34].

Embolization has been performed using coils (standard and detachable), detachable balloons, and the Amplatzer Vascular Plug [22, 29–32]. PAVMs are categorized as simple, complex, or diffuse depending on the distribution of feeding arteries [30, 31]. Simple lesions (85 %) have all feeding arteries arising from a single pulmonary segment, while complex lesions (5–10 %) arise from more than one segment [31]. Diffuse lesions (5 %) involve multiple segment or lobes with numerous lesions [31] (Fig. 7.4a–c).

Indications/Contraindications

Standard contraindications for angiography include contrast allergies, renal insufficiency, and coagulopathies [35]. For pulmonary angiography, left heart block is a contraindication. Complete heart block can occur if an arrhythmia is induced during right heart catheterization.

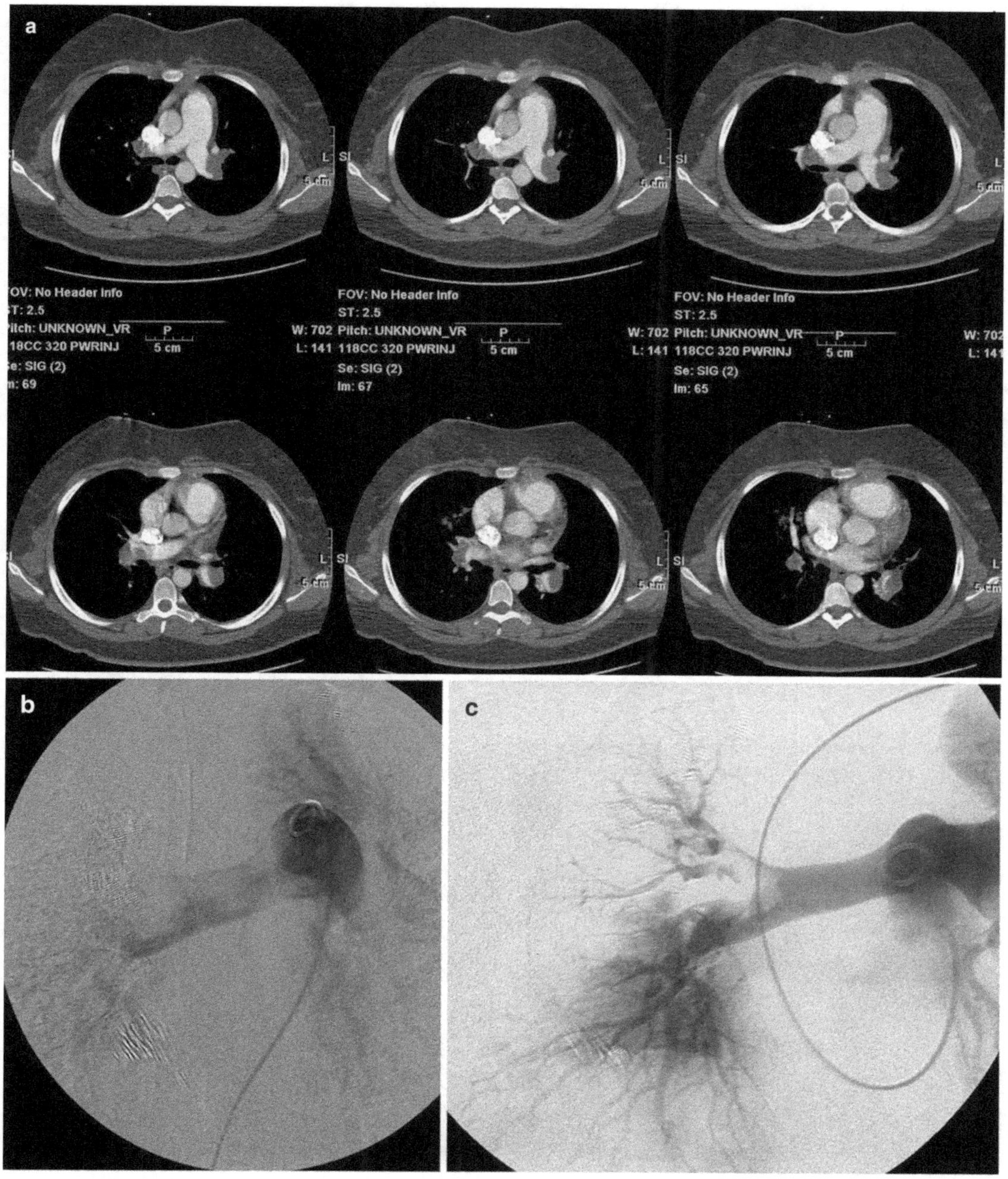

Fig. 7.2 This teenager had sudden onset of chest pain. A CT scan (**a**) shows multiple pulmonary emboli throughout the pulmonary arteries. Due to the patient being in shock, catheter-directed thrombolysis was performed. (**b**) Demonstrates a near complete occlusive thrombus in the right pulmonary artery. (**c**) The interval result after mechanical fragmentation of the thrombus shows improved flow to the right lung. Intra-arterial rt-PA was continued for 12 h. The patient improved and follow-up CT shows resolution of the pulmonary embolus (**d**)

Any foreign body in the pulmonary arteries should be removed if possible due to the risk of thrombosis and/or arrhythmia.

In adults, thrombolytic therapy is indicated in patients with massive PE due to the associated high mortality [17–21, 26]. Even though the incidence of death from PE is very low in children, recommendations for treatment are extrapolated from the experience in adults [15, 20]. The role in patients with only right ventricular dysfunction

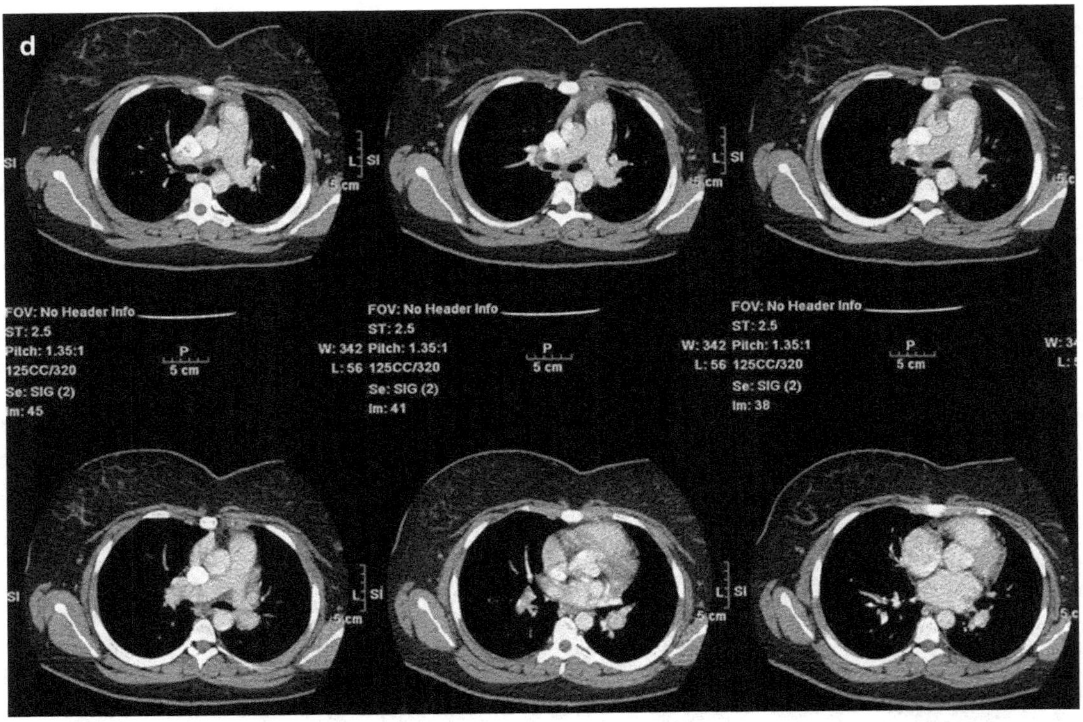

Fig. 7.2 (continued)

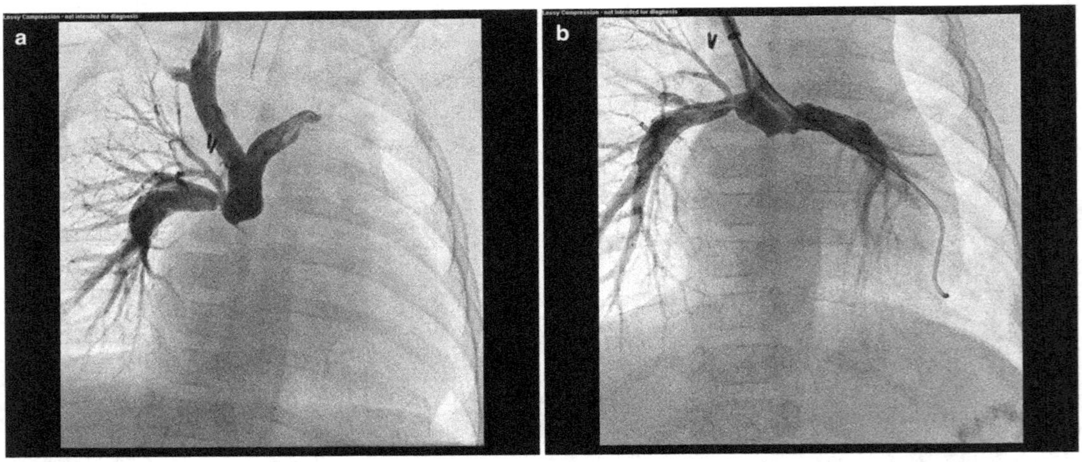

Fig. 7.3 This infant had left pulmonary thrombosis after a Glenn procedure for congenital heart disease. The clot persisted despite several days of rt-PA (**a**). Ultimately, a stent was placed across the area of thrombus restoring flow to the pulmonary artery (**b**) (Courtesy Ralf Holzer, MD)

is less clear [18, 22]. There are no studies proving the efficacy of systemic versus directed thrombolysis; however, the complications from systemic thrombolysis include a 20 % risk of major hemorrhage and a 3–5 % risk of stroke [14, 19, 21, 24, 26, 36]. Systemic pharmacological thrombolytics are a relative contraindication in patients with recent surgery, brain tumors, or stroke. However, the benefits and risks need to be assessed, and lower-dose catheter-directed pharmacological or mechanical thrombolysis may be a better option.

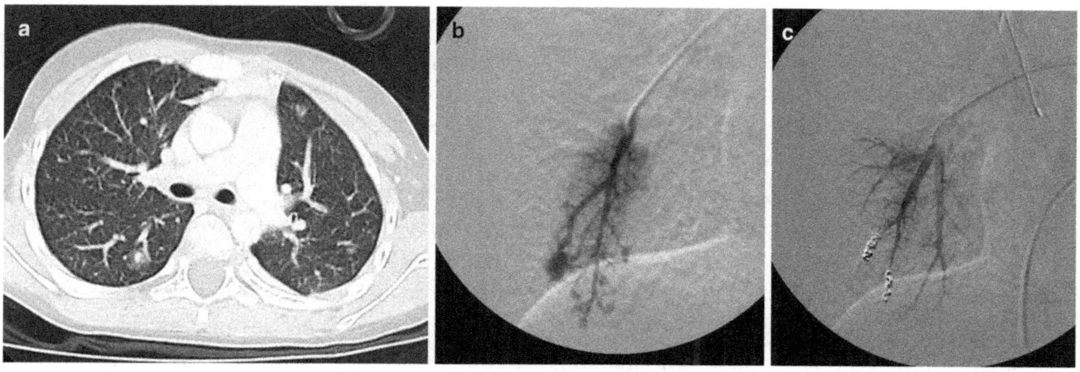

Fig. 7.4 This 6-year-old female had fatigue, exercise intolerance, and oxygen saturations in the 70 %'s. A CT (**a**) shows multiple ill-defined nodules in both lungs. The patient had a positive agitated saline echocardiogram confirming a right to left shunt. Arteriography (**b**) shows a diffuse type of pulmonary AVM. Several of the PAVMs were embolized with coils (**c**)

In adults, the use of systemic tissue plasminogen activator (rt-PA) (100 mg over 2 h) has shown to reduce pulmonary artery resistance and pressure, with improvement in mortality [14, 24]. Other protocols have given 50 mg over 2 h and then 40 mg over 4 h, or 100 mg over 7 h [24]. In children, a mean dose of 0.1–0.5 mg/kg/h of rt-PA has been used, although significant bleeding can occur in 50 % of patients [16, 37, 38].

No definite benefits have been shown using catheter-directed thrombolysis versus systemic therapy [14, 24]. Mechanical thrombolysis/thrombectomy has also been reported [14, 22, 24]. They are typically used in conjunction with fibrinolytics; however, they can be used alone if the patient has a known contraindication to pharmacological thrombolytics. These devices may provide a more rapid restoration of pulmonary flow as the clot is broken up and a greater surface area is available for contact with the fibrinolytic. Multiple devices have been described for this indication [22].

In a case study in a child, the patient had bilateral PE. The patient received a bolus of 0.05 mg/kg followed by an infusion of 0.05 mg/kg/h of rt-PA. The bolus and infusion were split into the right and left pulmonary arteries with good reperfusion of the lungs [37]. Benefits of catheter-based thrombolysis include lower dose and delivery directly into the clot [37].

For PAVMs, it is recommended that shunts that are greater than 3 mm in size be prophylactically embolized due to the risk of paradoxical embolization [22, 29, 31]. This can be determined by CTA. An additional indication for treatment is hemorrhage.

Pre-procedural Evaluation

Before performing right heart and subsequent pulmonary artery catheterization, an EKG should be performed to evaluate for arrhythmias. If the patient has a left heart block, catheter-induced right heart block may convert the patient's rhythm into complete heart block. In the presence of left heart block, cardiology should be consulted.

Retained foreign bodies in the pulmonary circulation are usually identified on plain radiographs. A CT scan may help confirm the diagnosis and localize the foreign body but is not usually indicated.

For suspected PE, CTA is now the test of choice in children, although the ventilation-perfusion nuclear medicine study is still utilized by some [1, 2, 39, 40].

If the patient is determined to have PE and be in shock (massive PE), thrombolysis is indicated. Proper patient care and monitoring are the first step, with the ICU the most appropriate place for the patient. Coagulation lab results should be obtained, and heparin should be started intravenously. The decision must then be made to perform systemic or catheter-directed thrombolysis, as they have their own benefits and risks.

In patients with suspected PAVM, workup consists of CTA [22]. This can confirm the diagnosis of a PAVM and can potentially identify the feeding arteries requiring treatment [22, 27, 41]. The patient and family should also have referral to an HHT center for further workup of that disease.

Equipment

An angiographic C-arm capable of imaging at 5 frames/s or more is recommended as is digital subtraction. Appropriate monitoring, sedation, and anesthesia equipment are mandatory [35]. Ultrasound is recommended for vascular access [35].

In children, placement of a sheath is recommended [35]. The size of the sheath is determined by the intended procedure. Diagnostic studies can be performed through a 4 Fr sheath and catheter, while larger sheaths and catheters will be required to place embolics or for thrombolysis.

Catheter, wire, and other device choices are dependent on the indications, planned procedure, and the interventionist. Pulmonary artery access can be performed via a variety of pigtail (angled or non-angled), directional, or flush catheters. There are multiple available snares for foreign body removal. They include simple loop snares and more complex and larger snares. Snare sizes range from 1 cm or less up to 3.5 cm. For mechanical thrombolysis of pulmonary emboli, the most commonly used catheter is a pigtail catheter. Additional catheters include rotating pigtail catheters and a variety of mechanical thrombectomy devices [14, 22, 24]. Appropriate sheaths, catheters, and embolic agents need to be available for treatment of PAVMs. A large sheath (8 Fr) may be required for placement of appropriate mechanical occluding devices [42].

Procedure Technique

Sedation or anesthesia is important for safety and procedural success in pediatric patients [43]. Sedation can be used for cooperative patients and is generally well tolerated, and the patient can be instructed when to breath-hold [44]. In younger children, anesthesia is mandatory as they do not have the capacity to cooperate [35].

Access can be accomplished via the femoral, jugular, or brachial veins. Ultrasound facilitates the needle puncture and can evaluate for an underlying clot. A grossly swollen leg should be avoided due to the risk of an underlying thrombosis. Once access is obtained, contrast is injected and venogram performed to exclude downstream thrombus. A wire can then be advanced and a sheath placed. The catheter is advanced over a wire into the right atrium and subsequently manipulated through the tricuspid valve, the right ventricle, and into the pulmonary artery. An assistant needs to monitor the EKG for arrhythmias during right heart catheterization. Injection rates range from approximately 5 mL/s for a 10 kg child to 20 mL/s for a teenager of adult size. Injection is over 1.5–2 s and filming should be at 5 frames/s or faster [35].

For foreign body removal, the introducer sheath must be larger than the foreign body. For a catheter fragment, the sheath needs to be at least 2 Fr sizes larger than the fragment. A selective catheter is placed into the pulmonary artery and oriented towards the foreign body. Alternatively, a long sheath or guiding catheter can be advanced over the wire into the pulmonary artery and a selective catheter introduced through this guide. A snare is then advanced through the selective catheter and a free edge of the foreign body is grasped. If this proves difficult, a pigtail catheter may be reformed around the fragment to manipulate it into another position, potentially freeing up one of the fragment ends for snare removal. The foreign body is then removed with fluoroscopic guidance to ensure that the entire fragment is removed. For larger devices, a surgical cutdown may be necessary to remove the foreign body from the circulation.

In the setting of PE, usual techniques are used to access the pulmonary artery. After measuring pulmonary pressures, if local thrombolytic therapy is indicated, the catheter and sheath of the appropriate size is advanced into the pulmonary artery. Thrombolysis can be accomplished through pharmacological means, mechanical

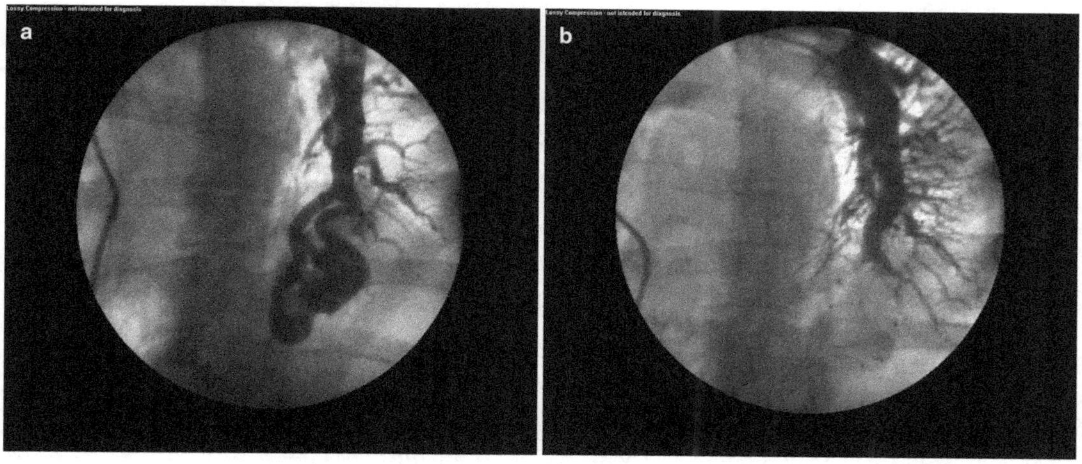

Fig. 7.5 A child with a large simple type PAVM. Arteriography demonstrates the angioarchitecture (**a**). After the placement of several Amplatzer devices, the PAVM is excluded (**b**) (Courtesy John Cheatham, MD)

devices, or a combination of these methods [22]. When using mechanical thrombolysis, anesthesia should be warned of the possibility of arrhythmias including asystole. For pharmacological fibrinolysis, the catheter needs to be in the clot itself, as a vortex in the pulmonary artery directs the fibrinolytic away from the clot if infusion is not intra-thrombus [14, 21, 24].

In adults, a described catheter-directed dose of rt-PA is a 10 mg bolus followed by 20 mg/h over 2 h, attempted clot maceration, and then another 80 mg over 2 h [24]. In children, described catheter-directed doses are 0.03–0.06 mg/kg/h [38].

Repeat angiography should be performed often to assess the degree of thrombolysis. If all of these techniques fail, placement of a stent may recanalize the occluded artery [14, 24].

For a PAVM, a pulmonary angiogram is performed to delineate the architecture of the AVM and identify the feeding artery or arteries [42]. The goal is to occlude the feeding arteries as close to the aneurysm sac as possible, sparing normal lung. The guiding sheath gives a stable platform to deploy the embolic material. The coils, balloons, or Amplatzer can then be deployed using the sheath for control angiography during the procedure (Fig. 7.4a–c). When using coils, the first portion can be deployed in a normal nearby branch to act as an anchor and secure placement (Fig. 7.5a, b) [42].

Postprocedure Care

Standard post-angiographic care should be followed including keeping the patient supine for 4–6 h after the procedure [35]. The patient should be transferred to the appropriate setting. For a foreign body removal, the patient is usually discharged that day. Patients with PE need to remain in the ICU until they are medically well enough to be sent to the general pediatric unit.

Patients with PAVM will need follow-up care and repeat imaging to exclude fistula growth or reperfusion. CTA is recommended at 6 and 12 months with thin sections no larger than 5 mm [31].

Expected Outcomes and Complications

Pulmonary angiography is well tolerated in adults with a minor complication rate of 4.8 % and major complications occurring in 0.9 % of cases [45]. Contrast nephropathy was the primary complication. Major complications were associated with pulmonary hypertension.

A meta-analysis of multiple catheter-directed studies for adult PE showed a clinical success rate of 86.5 % [21]. Potential complications of PE interventions include hemorrhage, arrhythmia, hemoglobinuria, renal insufficiency, hemoptysis, and death with an overall incidence of 7.9 % for minor and 2.4 % for major complications [21, 25]. Another study demonstrated no major hemorrhagic complications, but minor bleeds *occurred* in 25–37 % of cases [37]. Rheolytic catheters seemed to have the highest complication rate [21]. One study in children showed that 5/8 patients had some improvement in the PE with systemic thrombolysis; however, 50 % had a major hemorrhage [16].

Technical success rate with embolization of PAVMs is 88–98 % [22, 29–34]. Reperfusion of PAVMs after treatment can occur in as many as 10 % of cases [22, 31]. Failures or recurrences are thought to be due to recanalization, angiogenesis, and growth of small prior feeding arteries or recruitment of new arteries (which may be from systemic arteries) or collaterals [22, 31]. Follow-up is typically with CT, and success is identified by involution of the aneurysm sac [31]. Complications are rare at 2 % of cases and include angina and transient ischemic attacks [22, 29–34]. Chest pain can occur in up to 12 % of cases [31].

Chapter Summary

Background

- Pulmonary angiography
  - Diagnostic (but CTA often first line for diagnosis)
  - Foreign body retrieval
  - PE treatment
  - PAVM treatment

Indications

(a) Massive PE treatment (in adults)

- TPA options
  - Adults
    100 mg/2 h OR
    50 mg/2 h then 40 mg/4 h OR
    100 mg/7 h
  - Children
    0.1–0.5 mg/kg/h (significant bleeding in 50 %)

(b) PAVM >3 mm in size

Contraindications

- Contrast allergy
- Renal insufficiency
- Coagulopathy
- Left heart block

Preprocedure Evaluation

- EKG (r/o arrhythmia)
- CXR (foreign bodies)
- CT/CTA (PE, PAVM)
- Coagulation, hematology bloodwork
- Heparin (especially PE)

Equipment

- Vascular sheath
  - 4–9 Fr (depending on need)
  - Short or long
- Catheters
  - Pigtail (angled, non-angled)
  - Directional
- Snares
  - Loop, gooseneck, complex shaped
  - 5 mm to 3.5 cm
- Specialized devices
  - Thrombectomy device, infusion catheter
  - Occlusion devices—coils, balloons, vascular occlusion plug

Technique

- Sedation or GA
  - Breath holds required
- Access—femoral, jugular, brachial
  - Venogram immediately after access if thrombosis present to r/o unexpected extension
  - Sheath/catheters choice based on indication
  - Close monitoring of EKG when in heart
- DSA
  - 5 mL/s 10 kg child; 20 mL/s adult
  - 5+ frames/s
- Use “underwater technique” for PAVM work

Postprocedure Care

- Supine × 4–6 h
- Appropriate monitoring—ICU versus ward
- CTA at 6 and 12 months for PAVM patients

Outcomes/Complications

- Information limited in children
- Pulmonary angiography (adults)
  - Minor complications—4.8 %
  - Major complications—0.9 %; associated with pulmonary hypertension
- PE treatment
  - Hemorrhage, arrhythmia, hemoglobinuria, renal insufficiency, hemoptysis, death (adults)
  - Rheolytic catheters; high complication rates
  - 50 % major hemorrhage reported in children [16]
- PAVM treatment
  - 88–98 % successful
  - Recanalization, angiogenesis, and arterial growth/recruitment can cause recurrence
  - Angina, transient ischemic attacks/stroke, and chest pain reported

References

1. Kritsaneepaiboon S, Lee EY, Zurakowski D, Strauss KJ, Boiselle PM. MDCT pulmonary angiography evaluation of pulmonary embolism in children. AJR Am J Roentgenol. 2009;192(5):1246–52.
2. Lee EY, Kritsaneepaiboon S, Zurakowski D, Arellano CM, Strauss KJ, Boiselle PM. Beyond the pulmonary arteries: alternative diagnoses in children with MDCT pulmonary angiography negative for pulmonary embolism. AJR Am J Roentgenol. 2009;193(3): 888–94.
3. Ho CL, Chou CM, Chang TK, Jan SL, Lin MC, Fu YC. Dislodgment of port-a-cath catheters in children. Pediatr Neonatol. 2008;49(5):179–82.
4. Babu R, Spicer RD. Implanted vascular access devices (ports) in children: complications and their prevention. Pediatr Surg Int. 2002;18:50–3.
5. Hinke DH, Zandt-Stastny DA, Goodman LR, Quebbeman EJ, Krzywda EA, Andris DA. Pinch-off syndrome: a complication of implantable subclavian venous access devices. Radiology. 1990;177(2): 353–6.
6. Biffi R, Orsi F, Grasso F, De Braud F, Cenciarelli S, Andreoni B. Catheter rupture and distal embolisation: a rare complication of central venous ports. J Vasc Access. 2000;1(1):19–22.
7. Caruselli M, Zannini R, Giretti R, Piattellini G, Bechi P, Ventrella F, Pallotto R, Pizzi S, Pagni R. The pinch-off syndrome in a pediatric patient. Paediatr Anaesth. 2009;19(2):179–81.
8. Dinkel HP, Muhm M, Exadaktylos AK, Hoppe H, Triller J. Emergency percutaneous retrieval of a silicone port catheter fragment in pinch-off syndrome by means of an Amplatz gooseneck snare. Emerg Radiol. 2002;9(3):165–8.
9. Levi DS, Moore JW. Embolization and retrieval of the Amplatzer septal occluder. Catheter Cardiovasc Interv. 2004;61(4):543–7.
10. Keele KL, Gilbert PM, Aquisto TM, Lichtenberg R, Field TC, Lee BK. Bullet embolus to the thoracic aorta with successful endovascular snare retrieval. J Vasc Interv Radiol. 2010;21(1):157–8.
11. Morell RC, Bell WO, Hertz GE, et al. Migration of a ventriculoperitoneal shunt into the pulmonary artery. J Neurosurg Anesthesiol. 1994;6(2):132–4.
12. Hwang B, Hsieng JH, Lee BC, Lu JH, Soong WJ, Chen SJ, Meng CC. Percutaneous removal of a non-opaque silastic catheter from the pulmonary artery in two premature infants. Cardiovasc Intervent Radiol. 1997;20(4):319–21.
13. O'Neill G, Joseph SP. Pervenous retrieval of embolized catheters from the right heart and pulmonary arteries. Am Heart J. 1979;98(3):287–93.
14. Uflacker R. Interventional therapy for pulmonary embolism. J Vasc Interv Radiol. 2001;12:147–64.
15. Van Ommen CH, Peters M. Acute pulmonary embolism in childhood. Thromb Res. 2006;118:13–25.
16. Biss TT, Brandão LR, Kahr WH, Chan AK, Williams S. Clinical features and outcome of pulmonary embolism in children. Br J Haematol. 2008;142(5): 808–18.
17. Liu S, Shi HB, Gu JP, Yang ZQ, Chen L, Lou WS, He X, Zhou WZ, Zhou CG, Zhao LB, Xia JG, Li LS. Massive pulmonary embolism: treatment with the rotarex thrombectomy system. Cardiovasc Intervent Radiol. 2011;34(1):106–13.
18. Kucher N, Goldhaber SZ. Management of massive pulmonary embolism. Circulation. 2005;112:e28–32.
19. Goldhaber SZ, Visani L, De Rosa M. Acute pulmonary embolism: clinical outcomes in the International Cooperative Pulmonary Embolism Registry (ICOPER). Lancet. 1999;353:1386–9.
20. Baird JS, Killinger JS, Kalkbrenner KJ, Bye MR, Schleien CL. Massive pulmonary embolism in children. J Pediatr. 2010;156(1):148–51.
21. Kuo WT, Gould MK, Louie JD, et al. Catheter-directed therapy for the treatment of massive pulmonary embolism: systematic review and meta-analysis of modern techniques. J Vasc Interv Radiol. 2009; 20:1431–40.
22. Lee EW, Grant JD, Loh CT, et al. Bronchial and pulmonary arterial and venous interventions. Semin Respir Crit Care Med. 2008;29:395–404.
23. Nakazawa K, Tajima H, Murata S, Kumita SI, Yamamoto T, Tanaka K. Catheter fragmentation of acute massive pulmonary thromboembolism: distal embolisation and pulmonary arterial pressure elevation. Br J Radiol. 2008;81(971):848–54.
24. Uflacker R, Schönholz C. Percutaneous interventions for pulmonary embolism. J Cardiovasc Surg (Torino). 2008;49(1):3–18.
25. Krichavsky MZ, Rybicki FJ, Resnic FS. Catheter directed lysis and thrombectomy of submassive pulmonary embolism. Catheter Cardiovasc Interv. 2011; 77(1):144–7.

26. Zhou W, Shi H, Yang Z, et al. Value of percutaneous catheter fragmentation in the management of massive pulmonary embolism. Chin Med J. 2009;122: 1723–7.
27. Singhal S, Henderson R, Horsfield K, et al. Morphometry of the human pulmonary arterial tree. Circ Res. 1973;33:190–7.
28. Gossage JR, Kanj G. Pulmonary arteriovenous malformations: state of the art review. Am J Respir Crit Care Med. 1998;158:643–61.
29. White Jr RI, Pollak JS, Wirth JA. Pulmonary arteriovenous malformations: diagnosis and transcatheter embolotherapy. J Vasc Interv Radiol. 1996;7(6): 787–804.
30. Farra H, Balzer DT. Transcatheter occlusion of a large pulmonary arteriovenous malformation using the Amplatzer vascular plug. Pediatr Cardiol. 2005;26(5): 683–5.
31. Pollak JS, Saluja S, Thabet A, Henderson KJ, Denbow N, White RI Jr. Clinical and anatomic outcomes after embolotherapy of pulmonary arteriovenous malformations. J Vasc Interv Radiol. 2006;17(1):35–44; quiz 45.
32. Cil B, Canyigil M, Ozkan OS, et al. Bilateral multiple pulmonary arteriovenous malformations: endovascular treatment with the Amplatzer vascular plug. J Vasc Interv Radiol. 2006;17:141–5.
33. Andersen PE. Imaging and interventional radiological treatment of hemoptysis. Acta Radiol. 2006;47(8): 780–92.
34. Faughnan ME, Palda VA, Garcia-Tsao G, et al. International guidelines for the diagnosis and management of hereditary hemorrhagic telangiectasia. J Med Genet. 2011;48(2):73–87.
35. Heran MK, Marshalleck F, Temple M, Grassi CJ, Connolly B, Towbin RB, Baskin KM, Dubois J, Hogan MJ, Kundu S, Miller DL, Roebuck DJ, Rose SC, Sacks D, Sidhu M, Wallace MJ, Zuckerman DA, Cardella JF; Society of Interventional Radiology Standards of Practice Committee; Society of Pediatric Radiology Interventional Radiology Committee. Joint quality improvement guidelines for pediatric arterial access and arteriography: from the Societies of Interventional Radiology and Pediatric Radiology. Pediatr Radiol. 2010;40(2): 237–50.
36. Fiumara K, Kucker N, Fanikos J, et al. Predictors of major hemorrhage following fibrinolysis for acute pulmonary embolism. Am J Cardiol. 2006;97:127–9.
37. Cannizzaro V, Berger F, Kretschmar O, Saurenmann R, Knirsch W, Albisetti M. Thrombolysis of venous and arterial thrombosis by catheter-directed low-dose infusion of tissue plasminogen activator in children. J Pediatr Hematol Oncol. 2005;27(12):688–91.
38. Beitzke A, Zobel G, Zenz W, Gamillscheg A, Stein JI. Catheter-directed thrombolysis with recombinant tissue plasminogen activator for acute pulmonary embolism after fontan operation. Pediatr Cardiol. 1996; 17(6):410–2.
39. Babyn PS, Gahunia HK, Massicotte P. Pulmonary thromboembolism in children. Pediatr Radiol. 2005; 35:258–74.
40. Gelfand MJ, Gruppo RA, Nasser MP. Ventilation-perfusion scintigraphy in children and adolescents is associated with a low rate of indeterminate studies. Clin Nucl Med. 2008;33(9):606–9.
41. Remy J, Remy-Jardin M, Giraud F, et al. Angioarchitecture of pulmonary arteriovenous malformations: clinical utility of three dimensional helical CT. Radiology. 1994;191:657–64.
42. White Jr RI. Pulmonary arteriovenous malformations: how do I embolize? Tech Vasc Interv Radiol. 2007; 10(4):283–90.
43. Fairfax AJ, Ball J, Batten JC, Heard BE. A pathological study following bronchial artery embolization for haemoptysis in cystic fibrosis. Br J Dis Chest. 1980; 74(4):345–52.
44. Yovichevich S. Commentary on bronchial artery embolization for hemoptysis in young patients with cystic fibrosis. Radiology. 2003;228(3):903; author reply 903–4.
45. Zuckerman DA, Sterling KM, Oser RF. Safety of pulmonary angiography in the 1990's. J Vasc Interv Radiol. 1996;7(2):199–205.

Arterial Interventions: Gastrointestinal

8

John M. Racadio

Introduction

In children, arterial interventions involving the gastrointestinal (GI) tract and liver are performed primarily for diagnosis and therapy for GI bleeding, liver trauma, and complications of liver transplantation. GI bleeding in infants and children is a fairly common problem in the practice of general pediatrics and accounts for about 10–15 % of referrals to pediatric gastroenterologists [1]. Intervention for liver trauma and complications of liver transplant are limited to Level I trauma centers and transplant centers, respectively. Therefore, this chapter will focus on GI bleeding.

Gastrointestinal Bleeding

The upper GI tract extends from the esophagus to the ligament of Treitz, while the lower GI tract includes the small bowel, colon, and rectum. The distinction is important because some characteristics are relatively unique to each location, and these may affect the therapeutic strategy. Common causes of upper GI bleeding in children include gastritis/esophagitis, Mallory-Weiss tear, trauma secondary to gastrostomy tubes, and eosinophilic gastroenteropathy. Common causes of lower GI bleeding include infectious diarrhea, eosinophilic gastroenteropathy, anal fissure, nodular lymphoid hyperplasia, inflammatory bowel disease, and Henoch-Schonlein purpura [1]. Less common causes of GI bleeding include Meckel's diverticulum, typhlitis (especially in neutropenic patients), angiodysplasia, and esophageal varices secondary to portal hypertension. Iatrogenic causes include posttraumatic hemobilia following percutaneous liver biopsy.

In most children, GI bleeding ceases on its own early in the child's hospital course, and if bleeding persists, the majority respond to conservative medical management including fluid resuscitation, correction of coagulopathy, and administration of blood products. When more invasive investigation is needed, endoscopy is the procedure of choice for both upper and lower GI hemorrhage. Unfortunately, particularly in lower GI bleeding, precise endoscopic detection and treatment may be difficult if rapid bleeding is present. In general, arteriography and transcatheter intervention are reserved for those patients with massive acute GI bleeding requiring frequent blood transfusions to maintain an adequate hemoglobin/hematocrit level.

Although arteriographic diagnosis and therapy have been reviewed extensively in the adult literature, little experience has been reported in children. In one published pediatric study that

J.M. Racadio, M.D. (✉)
Department of Radiology, Cincinnati Children's Hospital and Medical Center, 3333 Burnett Avenue, Cincinnati, OH 45229, USA
e-mail: john.racadio@cchmc.org

M. Temple and F.E. Marshalleck (eds.), *Pediatric Interventional Radiology: Handbook of Vascular and Non-Vascular Interventions*, DOI 10.1007/978-1-4419-5856-3_8,

evaluated 27 children who underwent arteriography for GI bleeding, arteriography had an overall positive diagnostic rate of 64 %. In acute GI bleeding, arteriography provided a correct diagnosis in 71 % of patients, while in chronic or recurrent GI bleeding, arteriography was correct in 55 % of patients [2]. These success rates are comparable to several adult series [3–5].

Indications and Contraindications for Arterial Intervention

Indications for arteriography include bleeding that is not responsive to conservative medical management and requires continued blood replacement (>500 mL in 8 h for adults), and endoscopy failed, inconclusive, or unavailable. Although persistent melena, hematemesis, or hematochezia may indicate active hemorrhage, hemodynamic instability despite aggressive resuscitation is the best indicator of active bleeding that may be angiographically detectable [6]. Even in life-threatening bleeding, diagnosis of the precise anatomic source can be difficult due to the intermittent nature of GI bleeding. In general, more severe bleeding is best evaluated by angiography and less severe bleeding is best evaluated by endoscopy. The strength of endoscopy is in its ability to provide diagnostic information in the absence of active bleeding, but it may be severely limited in bowel that is poorly prepped or filled with a large amount of blood during severe acute bleeding. On very rare occasions, bleeding may be too brisk for the time required for transcatheter intervention and immediate surgical exploration may be preferable.

Relative contraindications are rare but include patients with a history of severe allergic reaction (anaphylaxis) to iodinated contrast and patients with considerable residual retained barium within their bowel from recent contrast barium enema or upper GI examination.

Preprocedure Evaluation

Imaging studies may be useful if a bleeding source cannot be identified by endoscopy or if transcatheter intervention is being considered. Because GI hemorrhage is typically intermittent, detection by angiography is only possible during active bleeding at the time of examination; in adults, bleeding rates of 0.5–1.0 mL/min are necessary to visualize contrast extravasation angiographically [7]. Radionuclide technetium-99m (Tc-99m)-tagged red blood cell (RBC) scans are more sensitive and can detect active GI bleeding at rates as low as 0.1 mL/min [8]. However, due to the intermittent nature of GI bleeding, it can be difficult in practice to determine whether or not bleeding rates have reached these thresholds.

Previous studies, primarily in adults, have reported positive detection rates of 22–96 % for Tc-99m RBC scans [9]. In a recent pediatric series of 22 patients undergoing Tc-99m RBC scintigraphy for acute massive GI bleeding, the diagnostic sensitivity was 39 % [9]. In the absence of massive ongoing hemorrhage and hemodynamic instability, a Tc-99m RBC scan may be performed first to confirm active bleeding and help localize the source of bleeding prior to angiography. In an adult study, a positive nuclear bleeding scan prior to angiography increased the likelihood of a positive angiogram from 22 to 53 % [6–10]. Others argue that because of the time it takes to obtain the tagged RBC scan, the patient may stop bleeding prior to arriving in the angiography suite. A potentially useful algorithm is to take hemodynamically unstable patients directly to angiography and to obtain initial nuclear medicine imaging in hemodynamically stable patients. Although the sensitivity and specificity of multidetector row helical CT in localizing the source of acute massive GI bleeding have been reported to be as high as 90 % in adults [11], the role of CT in the overall work-up of GI bleeding has yet to be clearly defined.

Before beginning angiographic intervention, the patient should be stabilized as much as possible and supportive therapy, including correction of coagulopathy and blood transfusion, initiated. Additional blood products should be immediately available in the angiography suite if needed during the procedure. Standard pre-angiographic work-up and patient monitoring should be performed and informed consent obtained. If endoscopy has been performed, the findings should be discussed with the gastroenterologist. The treatment plan should also be discussed with the referring physician and surgeon.

Equipment

Depending on patient size, a 4 F or 5 F arterial sheath should be placed in the common femoral artery. Catheter configurations that have an angled hook, such as the Cobra, Sos Omni, and Simmons, are useful in selecting the celiac and superior mesenteric artery (SMA) origins, while selective catheterization of a cephalad coursing vessel, such as the left gastric artery, may require the formation of a Waltman loop. For accessing the inferior mesenteric artery (IMA), catheters such as the Simmons, Sos Omni, or RIM are useful. If coaxial microcatheter techniques are anticipated, it is important to size the microcatheter appropriately to fit through the selective catheter. Injection and image acquisition parameters should allow not only for visualization of the arterial phase but also for the parenchymal and venous phases. Proper collimation and practice of ALARA principles should be followed, but the field of view must include the entire vascular territory of the artery that is being investigated.

Procedure Technique

Diagnostic Arteriography

Selective catheter angiography has been shown to be able to detect GI bleeding when the bleeding rate is as low as 0.5 mL/min [12]. However, the intermittent nature of bleeding in many patients can result in a false-negative angiographic study. Provocative angiography, including the use of anticoagulants, vasodilators, and fibrinolytic agents to prolong, augment, or reactivate the bleeding, has been shown to complement conventional angiography and increase the diagnostic efficacy in the detection of lower GI bleeding in adults [13, 14]. However, these provocative measures are not routinely used in adults, and their use in pediatric patients has not been described. Prior to angiography, brief fluoroscopy of the abdomen may be performed to evaluate the amount of bowel peristalsis, which may lead to motion artifact on digital subtraction angiography (DSA). If peristalsis is substantial, intravenous glucagon may be given to inhibit peristalsis.

Although aortography provides a general overview of the visceral anatomy, selective angiography is almost always necessary to identify the source of bleeding. If contrast or volume overload is a concern, aortography can be bypassed, and selective catheterization can be performed directly, beginning with the artery supplying the most likely site of bleeding as determined by the available clinical, endoscopic, and imaging data. For suspected upper GI hemorrhage, the celiac artery should initially be evaluated. The SMA must also be evaluated, since it too may contribute to a site of upper GI hemorrhage through the pancreaticoduodenal arcade.

Similar to the upper GI tract, a series of interconnected arcades provide collateralized supply throughout the lower GI tract. Therefore, for suspected lower GI hemorrhage, both the SMA and the IMA must be selectively catheterized. The primary territories within the distribution of the SMA are the small bowel and the ascending and transverse colon. The IMA supplies the splenic flexure, the descending and sigmoid colon, and the rectum and anus. There is additional arterial supply to the rectosigmoid and anus that arises from the internal iliac arteries. Congenital variant vascular anatomy must also be considered. For example, the entire middle colic artery may originate from the dorsal pancreatic artery in up to 2 % of patients, and an anomalous ileocolic artery or middle mesenteric artery may rarely arise directly from the abdominal aorta [6]. Although angiographic evaluation should begin with the most likely bleeding source vessel, because of the rich collateral vascular supply of the entire GI tract, selective catheterization and angiography of the celiac, SMA, and IMA should be included in all GI bleeding evaluations.

The classic angiographic finding that confirms active GI bleeding is extravasation of contrast material. Other entities that can mimic extravasation include hypervascular bowel mucosa, adrenal gland vascular blush, and DSA misregistration artifact from bowel peristalsis or respiratory motion. Other angiographic findings of GI bleeding besides intraluminal contrast extravasation may be seen in certain pathologic conditions and are suggestive of the cause and/or source of the GI bleeding. For example, in ulcer disease small, persistent contrast collections may be seen within the ulcer crater. Occasionally, contrast may pool within gastric folds or haustra mimicking the appearance of a vein. This may be differentiated from a true venous structure by the unusual location and appearance as well as by the persistence beyond the venous phase of the contrast injection. Rarely, arterial pseudoaneurysm formation is another angiographic abnormality that may be a manifestation of GI hemorrhage and may serve to localize the site of bleeding. This occurs most frequently in patients (usually adults) with chronic pancreatitis.

Arteriography of a Meckel's diverticulum may show clusters of small tortuous irregular arteries representing persistent vitelline arteries that originate from the distal SMA [15], a dense capillary stain caused by ectopic gastric mucosa [16], and/or a mesodiverticular band artery (an abnormal ileal artery passing to the antimesenteric border of the ileum) [17]. The combination of these angiographic findings should suggest the diagnosis and direct surgical intervention.

Typhlitis can be identified by arteriographic signs such as hypervascularity of the cecum with intense blush, contrast-filled superficial ulcers, and dilated ileal arteries and veins [18]. Neutropenic patients also have a high incidence of enteritis (including cytomegalovirus infection, pseudomembranous colitis, graft-versus-host disease, and chemotherapy-induced mucositis), which can involve necrosis and ulceration of the epithelium leading to vascular injury in the lamina propria and resulting in GI bleeding [19]. This is often complicated by thrombocytopenia or dysfunctional platelets. Angiography in these patients typically shows diffuse hypervascular blush of the affected colon. A point source of hemorrhage is not always identified.

Unlike adults, in whom angiodysplasia of the colon represents 40 % of lower GI bleeding [20], the incidence in children is unknown but certainly less frequent than in adults [21]. Angiographic criteria of angiodysplasia include abnormal vascular tufts in the intestinal wall, early-filling veins (4–5 s after injection), and dense, persistent, slowly emptying veins in the late phase of the injection [22]. Although angiography is the most valuable method for diagnosing angiodysplasia, occasionally, no angiographic abnormality is detected, especially when the lesions are very small and the blood flow is sluggish [2]. In contrast to the adult population in whom angiodysplasia tends to occur in the right colon and cecum, occurrence in the small bowel and left hemicolon is more common in children [2, 21].

Intervention

One of the main advantages of angiographic diagnosis of GI bleeding is the ability to perform transcatheter treatment after localization of the bleeding site. The two main transcatheter therapies are intra-arterial vasopressin infusion and embolization. In addition, initial clinical experience with the creation of a transjugular intrahepatic portosystemic shunt (TIPS) in children suggests that this process is technically feasible and as safe in children as in adults [23]. Although a full discussion of TIPS in children is beyond the scope of this review, TIPS can aid in management of complications of portal hypertension in children (including variceal hemorrhage), especially in those patients needing temporary relief as a bridge to liver transplantation [23]. As a general rule, no matter what strategy is used to treat GI bleeding, correction of any underlying coagulopathy is important. In adults, embolization has been shown to be 2.9 times more likely to fail in patients with coagulopathy [24].

Vasopressin

Vasopressin, a naturally occurring hormone produced by the neurohypophysis of the pituitary gland, causes constriction of very small arteries, arterioles, and capillaries. Since the initial report of selective intra-arterial infusion of a pharmaceutical preparation of vasopressin to control acute lower GI hemorrhage [7], transcatheter therapy has gained wider acceptance as a first-line means of management. This is in part because of a significant perioperative mortality rate reported with emergent surgery in adults with acute gastrointestinal bleeding [25, 26]. However, with continued advancements in microcatheter technology and embolization techniques, the use of intra-arterial vasopressin infusion to treat GI bleeding has decreased. Vasopressin remains a useful alternative to embolization when microcatheter arterial sub-selection is not possible due to technical or anatomic reasons. In general, vasopressin is more successful in controlling lower GI bleeding than upper GI bleeding and is most successful in cases of diffuse mucosal hemorrhage or bleeding from small vessels [27]. Profuse bleeding from larger vessels is less likely to be controlled by intra-arterial vasopressin infusion, and embolotherapy is preferable [28–31]. In the adult literature, vasopressin infusion is reported to achieve hemostasis in 70–90 % of cases [27, 32–34], and rebleeding rates upon discontinuation of therapy are reported to be approximately 20 % [27, 34]. In general, the devices needed for vasopressin infusion are cheaper and less complex than those used for embolization. A typical vasopressin infusion technique established in the adult population consists of placing a standard 4 F or 5 F catheter proximally into the bleeding artery (e.g., proximal SMA or IMA) and beginning vasopressin infusion at 0.2 U/min for 20–30 min. A repeat angiogram is then performed to evaluate the vasoconstrictive efficacy of this vasopressin infusion rate. If the repeat angiogram shows continued bleeding, the infusion rate is increased incrementally first to 0.3 U/min and then to 0.4 U/min. Each incremental increase is followed by an additional waiting period of 20–30 min to assess the vasoconstrictive effects of that rate. If bleeding is not controlled after an infusion rate of 0.4 U/min, further increase in dose rate is not beneficial, and embolization or surgery should be considered [28]. If vasopressin therapy is successful in controlling bleeding, infusion is continued for up to 48 h. For children, an appropriate vasopressin dosage has not been defined, although one investigator has suggested that a dose of 0.1–0.4 U/min/1.73 m^2 body surface area be used [35].

The patient should remain in the intensive care unit during vasopressin infusion. Potential serious complications of vasopressin infusion that have been described in adults include cardiovascular side effects (4 %), such as myocardial infarction, severe arrhythmia, or hypertension; bowel ischemia-infarction (0.8 %); peripheral vascular ischemia manifested by mottling and pain (0.5 %); antidiuretic hormone effect of vasopressin (1 %); and catheter-related thrombosis, false aneurysm, or sepsis (2 %) [32]. The antidiuretic side effects of vasopressin may appear within 6–8 h after initial infusion causing decreased urine output and electrolyte imbalance. Water retention may be treated with furosemide. Additional complications related to prolonged arterial access include hematoma, pseudoaneurysm, arterial spasm, arterial dissection, catheter dislodgement, and infection. It may not be prudent to perform intra-arterial vasopressin infusion after unsuccessful embolization because an increased rate of bowel necrosis has been described [27, 36, 37].

Embolization

Transcatheter embolization for both upper and lower GI bleeding has been shown to be safe and effective in several adult reports [6, 24, 38–40]. With the exception of treatment for diffuse mucosal hemorrhage, vasopressin infusion has for the most part been replaced by transcatheter embolization. Embolotherapy produces more rapid control of hemorrhage and helps avoid problems of long-term catheter placement and the cardiovascular and antidiuretic side effects of vasopressin. However, in the setting of prior failed vasopressin infusion, one should wait at least 30 min after vasopressin infusion before attempting transcatheter embolization to avoid an increased risk of bowel ischemia [28, 29]. Waiting 30 min for the vasoconstrictive effects to resolve will also minimize false-positive results after embolization. Indications for transcatheter embolization that were initially described in adult populations were upper GI bleeding or bleeding from large vessels eroded by gastric or duodenal ulcers. However, with improved technology and smaller microcatheters, embolization has also now been proven successful and safe in adults with lower GI bleeding [38, 39, 41].

The most common temporary embolic agent is Gelfoam (Pfizer Pharmaceuticals, New York, NY). Gelfoam is a sterile gelatin sponge that may be applied to bleeding surfaces to aid in hemostasis.

It is insoluble in water, porous, and malleable. It is considered a temporary embolic because it allows vessel recanalization in several days to several weeks. The most commonly used permanent embolic agents are standard and microcoils and polyvinyl alcohol (PVA) particles. PVA is a permanent embolic agent that incites intraluminal thrombosis with an associated inflammatory reaction. It is supplied in a small vial and has a gross appearance similar to sand, with particles ranging in size from 100 to 1,000 μm. Microcoils are made of stainless steel or platinum and, when deployed, function in a similar manner to a surgical ligation. They are biocompatible but highly thrombogenic due to the addition of synthetic fibers attached to the coil. Microcoils decrease perfusion pressure and induce local vasospasm. This enables the patient to more effectively form clot, leading to hemostasis. Trisacryl gelatin microspheres (Embospheres, Biosphere Medical, Inc., Rockland, MA) and detachable balloons are additional permanent solid embolic agents that have been successfully used in adults. Liquid embolic materials include *N*-butyl cyanoacrylate (NBCA) and Onyx, an ethylene vinyl alcohol copolymer (ev3 Endovascular, Inc., Plymouth, MN).

Embolization should ideally decrease perfusion pressure enough to arrest hemorrhage, but not to the extent of total devascularization. Due to the limited collateral blood flow in the colon, overly aggressive embolization must be avoided. Superselective embolization limits the segment of bowel at risk for ischemia. In some patients, asymptomatic submucosal ischemia may develop but typically resolves over a short time. Late ischemic complications such as bowel stricture have been reported but appear to be quite sporadic.

Upper GI Embolization

Due to the extensive collateral blood supply to the upper GI tract, it is important, if technically possible, to "bridge" the site of bleeding (to embolize both proximally and distally) so that collateral flow does not cause rebleeding. Embolization of the left gastric artery is effective in gastric mucosal bleeding with little risk of gastric ischemia, because of multiple sources of blood supply and a rich submucosal plexus interconnecting major arteries. Successful embolic control of gastric hemorrhage has been described by multiple investigators in the adult literature, and complications are rare [30]. In a recent adult synopsis of outcomes from 15 published series of upper GI bleeding refractory to endoscopic treatment, transcatheter embolization was technically successful in 69–100 % of patients and clinically successful in 63–97 % [24]. From the analysis, the authors concluded that superselective catheterization of the culprit vessel, "sandwich" occlusion (both proximal and distal to the bleeding source), and even "blind embolization" (no evidence of active bleeding on pre-embolization arteriography but guided by endoscopic information regarding the location of the bleeding vessel) should be considered as first-line therapy for massive upper GI bleeding refractory to endoscopic treatment.

Lower GI Embolization

Historically, the most significant risks of transcatheter lower GI embolization have been ischemia and infarction, the latter of which has been reported to occur in up to 20 % of cases [36]. However, as catheter technology has improved, newer and smaller caliber catheters and microcatheters have enabled more sub-selective catheterization of distal vessels. Microcoil deployment at the level of the vasa recta in the large bowel has been shown to be effective in achieving hemostasis while minimizing ischemic complications [39]. Particle embolization has also been shown to be safe and effective in treating lower GI bleeding [41]. It is important to avoid very small particles or gelatin sponge powder, which may reach the intramural circulation distal to the collaterals, increasing the risk for infarction. Initially, the role of embolization in small bowel hemorrhage was unclear because of reports of a significant incidence of small intestine infarction induced by embolization. However, many of these cases were in patients in whom embolotherapy was performed shortly after vasopressin infusion, which may have had lingering vasoconstrictive effects on collateral circulation [42]. From an anatomic viewpoint, the level of small bowel embolization in the mesenteric artery is quite critical [42]. To avoid bowel infarction, the ideal embolization site is that which occludes only one of the nearest

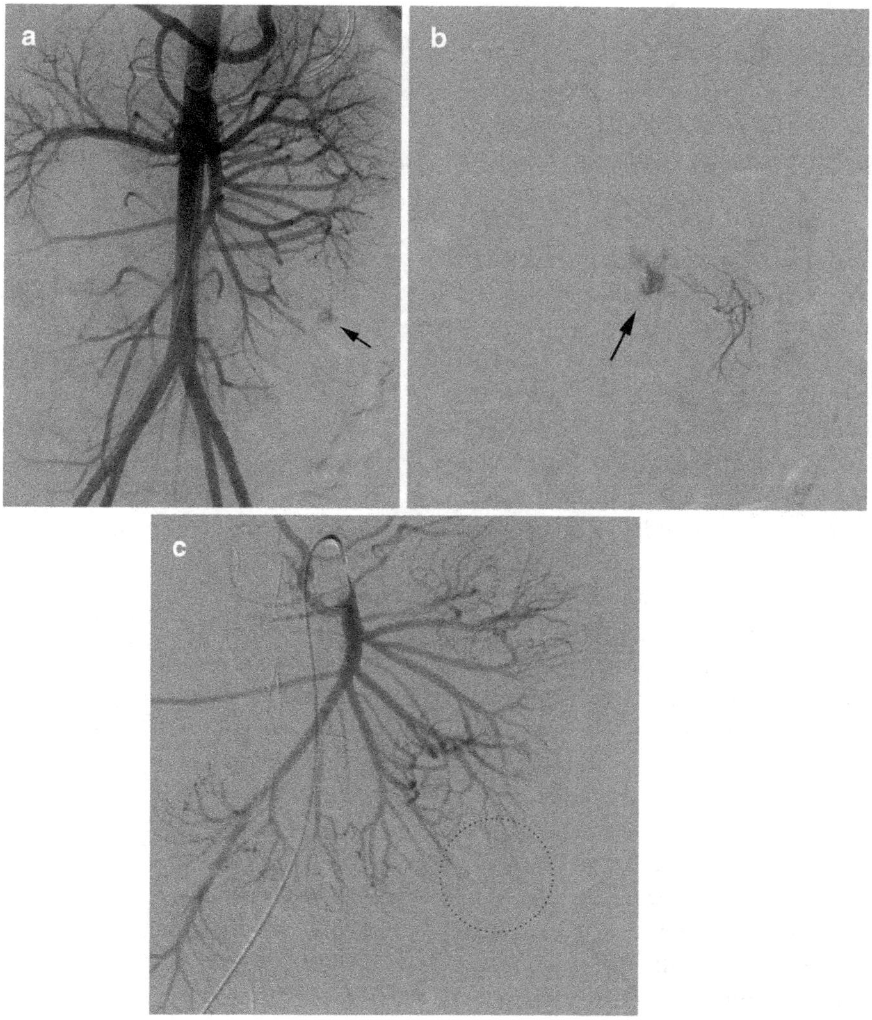

Fig. 8.1 A 16-year-old boy with hemophagocytic lymphohistiocytosis (HLH) presented with melena, abdominal pain, anemia (hemoglobin 7.9 g/dL, previously 11.5 g/dL), and tachycardia. He was admitted to the PICU and an esophagogastroduodenoscopy was performed. No bleeding site was identified. After becoming hemodynamically unstable and requiring aggressive resuscitation, he was transferred urgently to the interventional suite. (**a**) Although visualization of GI bleeding usually requires selective catheterization and angiography, in this patient flush aortography demonstrated active intraluminal contrast extravasation (*arrow*) from a distal jejunal branch. (**b**) After selection of the SMA with a 4 F cobra catheter, coaxial microcatheter sub-selection confirmed active extravasation (*arrow*) and localized the culprit vessel. The microcatheter was advanced slightly more distally into the culprit vessel, and 500–700 μm polyvinyl alcohol (PVA) particle embolization was performed. (**c**) Post-embolization SMA angiography shows cessation of active bleeding in the region of prior extravasation (*dotted circle*). The patient stabilized following embolization and had no episodes of rebleeding and no signs of bowel ischemia

arcade of the vasa recta of the segmental branch such that the vasa recta itself are not occluded [42]. After embolization, collateral circulation develops via arterial arcades distal to the occlusion and longitudinal communications between mural branches of vasa recta within the wall of the small intestine, which decreases the risk of infarction. The goal of embolization in small intestinal hemorrhage is to reduce pulse pressure, allowing spontaneous hemostasis. Embolization of lower GI bleeding has been shown to be safe and effective, with recently reported success rates of 90–100 % and ischemic complication rates of 0–5 % [39, 41, 42]. An example of a successful lower GI (jejunal) embolization is shown in Fig. 8.1.

Postprocedure Care

All patients should be watched for signs of rebleeding. The patient may still pass melanotic stools long after the bleeding has been stopped; therefore, stability of vital signs and hematocrit are more important to monitor. Any coagulopathy should also continue to be monitored and corrected. Although not reported in the literature, since femoral arterial access may be significantly more technically challenging and time-consuming in small children than in adults, if the initial diagnostic arteriography is negative, one may consider leaving the femoral arterial sheath in place for a short time (<24 h) in order to expedite any additional arteriography for recurrent bleeding. Of course, the risk of complications from extended femoral artery catheterization, including femoral artery thrombosis, should be considered.

For patients who have received vasopressin therapy, once an initial dose rate has been established and control of bleeding has been confirmed, the dose rate should be tapered over 24–48 h. After vasopressin has been tapered, normal saline should be infused for an additional 6–12 h, so that if bleeding recurs, the catheter is still in place and vasopressin can be restarted. The patient must remain in the ICU during vasopressin infusion with careful monitoring for antidiuretic or cardiovascular side effects.

Chapter Summary

Background

- Etiology
  - Liver: trauma, transplantation
  - Gut:
    - Gastritis/espophagitis
    - Esophageal varices (portal hypertension)
    - Mallory-Weiss tear
    - Gastrostomy tubes
    - Eosinophilic gastroenteropathy
    - Infectious diarrhea
    - Anal fissure
    - Nodular lymphoid hyperplasia
    - Inflammatory bowel disease
    - Henoch-Schonlein purpura
    - Meckel's diverticulum
    - Typhlitis (neutropenic patients)

Indications and Contraindications

- No response to conservative management
- Continued blood requirements (>500 mL in adult sized patients)
- Endoscopy failed, inconclusive or unavailable
- No absolute contraindications

Pre-procedure Evaluation

- Coagulation and hemoglobin optimized as possible
- Blood products in room
- Workup as for other forms of angiography

Equipment

- 4/5 F vascular sheath
- Selection of angiographic catheters
  - Cobra
  - Sos Omni
  - Simmons
  - RIM
  - Microcatheters

Procedure Technique

- Diagnostic arteriography
- Intervention
  - Embolization
    - Particles
    - Microcoils
    - Glue
  - Drugs
    - Vasopressin

Post-procedure Care

- Wean vasopressin
- Monitor for signs of recurrent bleeding

References

1. Arain Z, Rossi TM. Gastrointestinal bleeding in children: an overview of conditions requiring nonoperative management. Semin Pediatr Surg. 1999;8(4):172–80.
2. Meyerovitz MF, Fellows KE. Angiography in gastrointestinal bleeding in children. AJR Am J Roentgenol. 1984;143(4):837–40.

3. Whitaker SC, Gregson RH. The role of angiography in the investigation of acute or chronic gastrointestinal haemorrhage. Clin Radiol. 1993;47(6):382–8.
4. Rollins ES, et al. Angiography is useful in detecting the source of chronic gastrointestinal bleeding of obscure origin. AJR Am J Roentgenol. 1991;156(2):385–8.
5. Rahn III NH, et al. Diagnostic and interventional angiography in acute gastrointestinal hemorrhage. Radiology. 1982;143(2):361–6.
6. Walker TG, Salazar GM, Waltman AC. Angiographic evaluation and management of acute gastrointestinal hemorrhage. World J Gastroenterol. 2012;18(11):1191–201.
7. Nusbaum M, Baum S. Radiographic demonstration of unknown sites of gastrointestinal bleeding. Surg Forum. 1963;14:374–5.
8. Orellana P, et al. [99mTc red blood cell scintigraphy for the assessment of active gastrointestinal bleeding]. Rev Med Chil. 1998;126(4):413–8.
9. Lee J, et al. Red blood cell scintigraphy in children with acute massive gastrointestinal bleeding. Pediatr Int. 2008;50(2):199–203.
10. Gunderman R, et al. Scintigraphic screening prior to visceral arteriography in acute lower gastrointestinal bleeding. J Nucl Med. 1998;39(6):1081–3.
11. Yoon W, et al. Acute massive gastrointestinal bleeding: detection and localization with arterial phase multi-detector row helical CT. Radiology. 2006;239(1):160–7.
12. Baum S. Arteriographic diagnosis and treatment of gastrointestinal bleeding. In: Baum S, Pentecost M, editors. Abram's angiography interventional radiology. Philadelphia: Lippincott Williams & Wilkins; 2006. p. 488.
13. Johnston C, et al. Use of provocative angiography to localize site in recurrent gastrointestinal bleeding. Cardiovasc Intervent Radiol. 2007;30(5):1042–6.
14. Rosch J, et al. Interventional angiography in the diagnosis of acute lower gastrointestinal bleeding. Eur J Radiol. 1986;6(2):136–41.
15. Routh WD, et al. Meckel's diverticula: angiographic diagnosis in patients with non-acute hemorrhage and negative scintigraphy. Pediatr Radiol. 1990;20(3):152–6.
16. Faris HC, Whitley JE. Angiographic demonstration of Meckel's diverticulum. Case report and review of the literature. Radiology. 1973;108(2):285–6.
17. Takeda I, et al. A bleeding Meckel's diverticulum diagnosed by arteriography. Gastroenterol Jpn. 1977;12(1):76–9.
18. Meyerovitz MF, Fellows KE. Typhlitis: a cause of gastrointestinal hemorrhage in children. AJR Am J Roentgenol. 1984;143(4):833–5.
19. Donnelly LF, et al. CT appearance of clinically occult abdominal hemorrhage in children. AJR Am J Roentgenol. 1998;170(4):1073–6.
20. Hemingway AP. Angiodysplasia as a cause of iron deficiency anaemia. Blood Rev. 1989;3(3):147–51.
21. de la Torre Mondragon L, et al. Angiodysplasia of the colon in children. J Pediatr Surg. 1995;30(1):72–5.
22. Phillips J, Yao J. Congenital vascular malformations. In: Neiman H, editor. Angiography of vascular disease. New York: Churchill Livingston; 1985. p. 393–419.
23. Hackworth CA, et al. Transjugular intrahepatic portosystemic shunt creation in children: initial clinical experience. Radiology. 1998;206(1):109–14.
24. Loffroy R, et al. Embolization of acute nonvariceal upper gastrointestinal hemorrhage resistant to endoscopic treatment: results and predictors of recurrent bleeding. Cardiovasc Intervent Radiol. 2010;33(6):1088–100.
25. Behringer GE, Albright NL. Diverticular disease of the colon. A frequent cause of massive rectal bleeding. Am J Surg. 1973;125(4):419–23.
26. Olsen WR. Hemorrhage from diverticular disease of the colon. The role of emergency subtotal colectomy. Am J Surg. 1968;115(2):247–63.
27. Athanasoulis CA, et al. Mesenteric arterial infusions of vasopressin for hemorrhage from colonic diverticulosis. Am J Surg. 1975;129(2):212–6.
28. Kadir S. Principles of management of gastrointestinal bleeding. In: Kadir S, editor. Current practice of interventional radiology. Philadelphia: BC Decker; 1991. p. 408–14.
29. Kadir S. Treatment of pyloroduodenal bleeding. In: Kadir S, editor. Current practice of interventional radiology. Philadelphia: BC Decker; 1991. p. 418–24.
30. Gomes AS, Lois JF, McCoy RD. Angiographic treatment of gastrointestinal hemorrhage: comparison of vasopressin infusion and embolization. AJR Am J Roentgenol. 1986;146(5):1031–7.
31. Eckstein MR, et al. Gastric bleeding: therapy with intraarterial vasopressin and transcatheter embolization. Radiology. 1984;152(3):643–6.
32. Kandarpa K. Acute gastrointestinal bleeding. In: Aruny K, Machan L, editors. Handbook of interventional radiologic procedures. Boston: Little, Brown and Company; 1996. p. 130–8.
33. Browder W, Cerise EJ, Litwin MS. Impact of emergency angiography in massive lower gastrointestinal bleeding. Ann Surg. 1986;204(5):530–6.
34. Athanasoulis CA, et al. Angiography: its contribution to the emergency management of gastrointestinal hemorrhage. Radiol Clin North Am. 1976;14(2):265–80.
35. Roy CC, Morin CL, Weber AM. Gastrointestinal emergency problems in paediatric practice. Clin Gastroenterol. 1981;10(1):225–54.
36. Guy GE, et al. Acute lower gastrointestinal hemorrhage: treatment by superselective embolization with polyvinyl alcohol particles. AJR Am J Roentgenol. 1992;159(3):521–6.
37. Prochaska JM, Flye MW, Johnsrude IS. Left gastric artery embolization for control of gastric bleeding: a complication. Radiology. 1973;107(3):521–2.

38. Cherian MP, et al. Arterial interventions in gastrointestinal bleeding. Semin Intervent Radiol. 2009;26(3):184–96.
39. Kwak HS, Han YM, Lee ST. The clinical outcomes of transcatheter microcoil embolization in patients with active lower gastrointestinal bleeding in the small bowel. Korean J Radiol. 2009;10(4):391–7.
40. Sudheendra D, et al. Radiologic techniques and effectiveness of angiography to diagnose and treat acute upper gastrointestinal bleeding. Gastrointest Endosc Clin N Am. 2011;21(4):697–705.
41. Kickuth R, et al. Acute lower gastrointestinal hemorrhage: minimally invasive management with microcatheter embolization. J Vasc Interv Radiol. 2008; 19(9):1289–96.e2.
42. Okazaki M, et al. Emergent embolotherapy of small intestine hemorrhage. Gastrointest Radiol. 1992; 17(3):223–8.

Section III

Vascular Interventions: Venous

9 Central Venous Access and Related Interventions

Kevin M. Baskin

Background/Overview

As both a clinician and a proceduralist, the interventional radiologist can have a tremendous impact on central venous access (CVA) services. The ubiquitous nature of CVA in modern medical practice has a tremendous impact both positive and negative. CVA allows administration of transvenous therapies and blood sampling but can also result in infections and other complications. A significant portion of healthcare costs relate to CVA and its complications.

Most CVA devices are placed for short-term indications such as a single course of antibiotic therapy and are unlikely to result in significant patient risk. However, patients who require recurrent or lifelong venous access are more likely to see complications such as recurrent bloodstream infections or venous injury leading to thrombosis, stenosis, and occlusion.

While attention to stringent technique helps produce desirable outcomes when performing venous access, decisions regarding the approach to complex patients are best made in association with all disciplines involved in the clinical care of the patient. For patients whose underlying diagnosis predicts long-term reliance on CVA, or whose venous history is already marked by difficult access or significant central stenosis, venous access procedures should be performed at a center with expertise in advanced access and salvage techniques.

Indications/Contraindications

Common indications are summarized in Table 9.1. Relative contraindications are included in the risk factors summarized in Table 9.2.

Preprocedure Workup

The clinical history and requirements for venous access should be evaluated with special regard to venous access history and factors that may predispose to related complications.

Communication

After referral for venous access, the choice of device and route is determined after discussion of the urgency, indications, and expected duration of treatment with the patient's primary care team. Children should be referred to interventional radiology for the medical indication for CVA, not merely for the procedure. It should be the judgment and experience of the interventional radiologist that determines the appropriate

K.M. Baskin, M.D. (✉)
Advanced Interventional Institute,
5427 Wilkins Avenue, Pittsburgh, PA 15217, USA
e-mail: kevinbaskin@comcast.net

M. Temple and F.E. Marshalleck (eds.), *Pediatric Interventional Radiology: Handbook of Vascular and Non-Vascular Interventions*, DOI 10.1007/978-1-4419-5856-3_9,

Table 9.1 Common indications for central venous access

- Therapeutic indications
  - Blood products
  - Parenteral nutrition/lipids
  - Antibiotics
  - Dialysis/apheresis
  - Chemotherapy
  - Chelation therapy
  - Fluids/electrolytes
  - Systemic anticoagulation/thrombolysis
  - Delivery of caustic agents (e.g., Ca^{2+})
  - Other medications
- Diagnostic indications
  - Phlebotomy
  - Pressure transduction
  - Cardiac function evaluation

Table 9.2 Risk factors for central venous access complications

- Known medical allergies
- Immune status
- Evidence of current infection with systemic signs and symptoms
- Concurrent antibiotic administration
- Coagulopathy
- History of active infection or prior central venous access related infections
- History of difficult access or known venous anomalies/abnormalities
- Coexisting central venous access or implanted medical devices (e.g., pacemaker, shunt)
- History of major surgery or trauma
- Admission to an intensive care unit
- High risk group
  - Severe burns
  - Intestinal failure
  - Renal failure
  - Diabetes mellitus
  - Solid organ transplant, small bowel transplant, or multivisceral transplant
  - Functional or quantitative neutropenia
  - Severe malnutrition
  - Chronic respiratory disease
  - Complex congenital heart disease
  - Morbid obesity

device and route. This philosophy should be consistently represented to referring clinicians, families, and patients, so that no child leaves the interventional suite without safe and durable access, with preservation of essential venous capital, when access is indicated and achievable.

Indication and Expected Duration

For acute indications with a brief expected duration (hours to days), a temporary device via a groin or neck vein may be best. When temporary devices are deployed as an interim measure, replacement with a permanent device should occur within 5–10 days when possible (Fig. 9.1). For indications requiring longer-term continuous access, either a peripherally or tunneled, centrally inserted device with a centrally located tip is best. Intermittent access may best be served with an indwelling subcutaneous venous port, while special indications may require purpose-driven devices, such as apheresis and hemodialysis catheters.

Diagnosis and Comorbidities

It is helpful to prospectively clarify the specific diagnosis or diagnoses being treated using venous access, using the International Classification of Diseases (currently ICD-10). Risk stratification also depends on accurate understanding of risk factors and comorbidities (Table 9.2). There are certain referrals to the interventional suite that should provoke anticipatory consideration for concurrent CVA device insertion if one is not already in place, such as biopsy of suspected malignancy, drainage of an abscess with systemic symptoms of sepsis, and thoracostomy tube insertion for parapneumonic effusion.

Venous History

Prior to selection and insertion of a CVA device, the patient's pertinent history should be reviewed, including prior insertions and their outcomes. Potential venous anomalies, thromboses, stenosis, or occlusions should be assessed by reviewing any previous venography, vascular ultrasound, contrast-enhanced CT venography, or

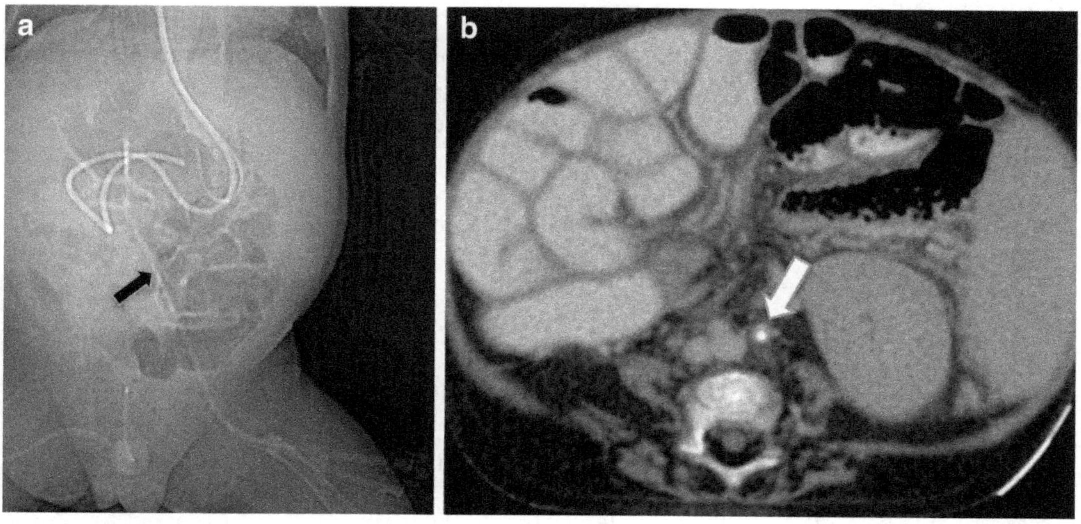

Fig. 9.1 (**a**) A left groin temporary catheter was placed in an infant in PICU without image guidance. The catheter tip (*arrow*) projects just left of the spine on a post-insertion portable radiograph. (**b**) CT 3 weeks later shows the catheter tip (*arrow*) within the left common iliac artery. Fortunately, no complications occurred with this prolonged inadvertent arterial malposition

MR venography. When collateral vessels are prominently visualized, the point of stenosis or occlusion should be identified and this information encompassed in the venous access plan.

Cardiac arrhythmias can be precipitated by electrolyte abnormalities such as hyperkalemia and hypocalcaemia. Electrolyte levels should be determined in at-risk patients.

Premedication, Laboratory Analysis, and Antibiotic Prophylaxis

Other than p.r.n. anxiolysis, there is seldom a need for preprocedure medication or antibiotic administration. At this time, there is no good evidence to support the practice of administering prophylactic antibiotics prior to a CVA procedure or for patients with indwelling central venous catheters. Practices vary by institution.

For placement of a peripherally inserted central catheter (PICC), virtually no preprocedure labs are necessary as, even in the face of uncorrectable coagulopathy, the entry site is easily accessible for compression. For other central catheter insertions, preprocedure platelet count and coagulation studies are routinely obtained. If possible, platelets should be above 50,000/μL, and the INR should be below 1.5 for elective procedures. If there is a more urgent need for access, the potential benefits must be weighed against the potential risks before proceeding.

Equipment

Innumerable CVA catheters are available. These include temporary and long-term devices, PICC (cuffed, uncuffed), port (single, double), tunneled central venous lines (CVLs) (cuffed, uncuffed; single, dual, or triple lumen; apheresis, dialysis), and special-purpose catheters such as CT-compatible catheters and antibiotic catheters. CT-compatible catheters (PICC, port, and CVL) are constructed of thin-walled, strong material that permits much higher flow rates, up to 7 mL/s in some catheters, which can be used for rapid bolus studies such as CT angiography and cardiac studies. Antibiotic-treated or antibiotic-impregnated catheters may provide increased protection against catheter-related bloodstream infections (CRBSIs) for 60 days or longer. In select high-risk patients, including those with renal failure and complex congenital heart disease; patients in the intensive care unit; children after liver, small bowel, or multivisceral

Table 9.3 Common sizes of central venous devices used in children

Weight	<5 kg	5–15 kg	15–30 kg	>30 kg
PICC				
Single lumen	1.9–3 or †	1.9–3	3–4	4–6
Double lumen	2.6–4 or †	2.6–4	4–5	5–7
Tunneled central catheter				
Single lumen	3	3–4	3–4	4–6
Double lumen	4	4–5	4–5	5–7
Port[1]				
Single lumen	5[2]	5	5–6	5–9
Hemodialysis/apheresis (DL)				
Acute (non-tunneled)	6.5	8	10	11.5
Maintenance (tunneled)	8	10	12	14
Bone marrow transplant/stem cell collection (DL)				
Donor (non-tunneled)[3]	6.5	8	10	10
Recipient (tunneled)	4	4–7	7	12[4]

This table compiles the French sizes of catheters by patient weight and device type. These represent the preferences of the author and editors and should be considered advisory rather than prescriptive
DL double-lumen catheter
† Consider a tunneled central catheter
[1]Low-profile devices commonly used in children
[2]Small-diameter "mini" port chamber available for infants
[3]For all allogeneic donors and autologous collection
[4]Can be used for autologous stem cell collection

transplant; and children dependent upon chronic IV nutritional support such as those with short bowel syndrome, there may be as much as a 15 times reduction in risk of infection with use of antibiotic-impregnated catheters [1]. Selective use of these catheters in stratified populations may yield significantly improved outcomes.

Device Selection

A catheter with the smallest diameter and the least number of lumens that meet the treatment requirements should be used to minimize the risks of infection and thrombosis. Table 9.3 provides examples of catheter sizes for various weights and indications. Features like catheter taper, material properties, and inner diameter necessitate different procedural considerations for catheters with the same nominal French size, so these recommendations should be interpreted with respect to the operator's experience, the institution's preferences, and the patient's individual needs.

For expected treatment lengths of 5 days to 6 months, a PICC is usually the best choice. Currently, the smallest PICC that can be manipulated with a guide wire is 1.9 Fr. The author prefers a 3-Fr PICC in children less than 10 kg, or where the length is less than 20 cm, and a 4-Fr PICC in larger children, or where a longer catheter is required. In infants less than 5 kg, a tunneled, cuffed catheter placed in a central vein may be easier to place than a PICC, but positive pressure ventilation during insertion is recommended.

For long-term continuous venous access, a tunneled, cuffed catheter placed via a central vein works well. When more than two lumens are required, there are a number of options available. A second temporary or permanent single- or dual-lumen catheter can be inserted in lieu of a triple-lumen device.

For chronic intermittent access, an indwelling subcutaneous venous port provides reliable access with the lowest risk of infection or other complications. Varying chamber sizes allow placement in patients ranging in size from adults to premature infants. "Mini" ports have been placed in infants as small as 1.4 kg with good outcomes. Dual-lumen ports are used for only a few indications such as osteosarcoma or recurrent red blood cell exchange in sickle cell disease. CT-compatible ports that allow the use of power injectors have recently become available in a wide variety of sizes and profiles. Low-profile ports may also be used in peripheral locations, such as the arm, without increasing risk.

Apheresis and hemodialysis catheters are usually placed via the jugular or femoral veins. Kidney Disease Outcomes Quality Initiative (KDOQI) guidelines indicate jugular access is preferred. For short-term use, temporary catheters

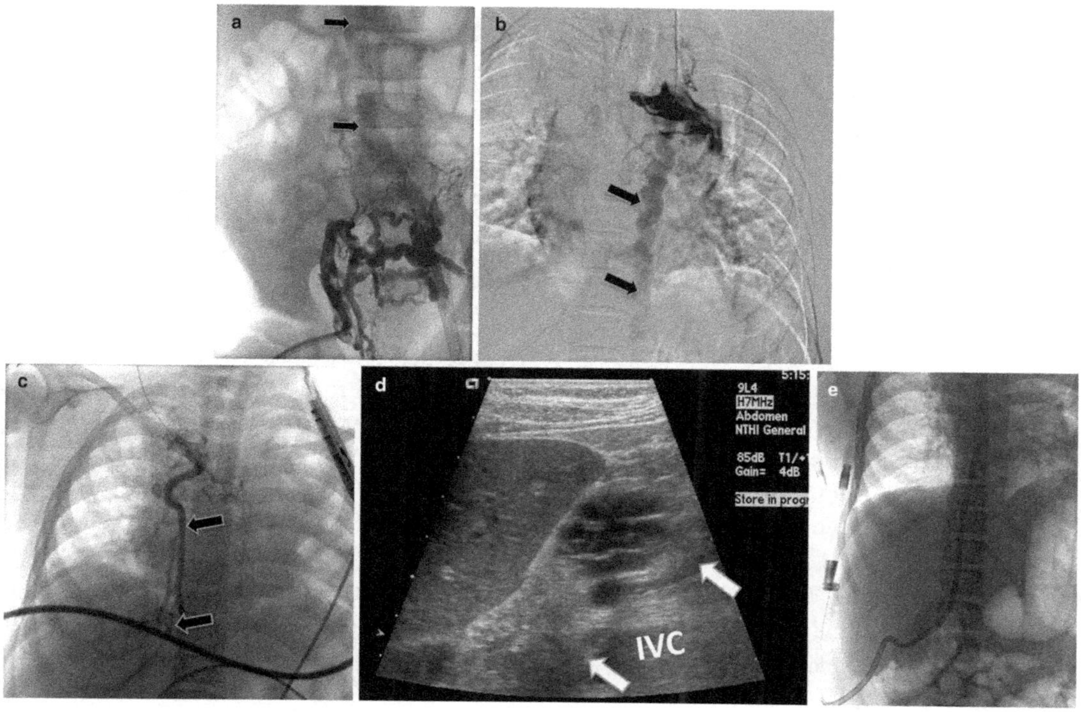

Fig. 9.2 A 12-year-old male with dysfunctional right femoral hemodialysis access. (**a**) Contrast study through the existing catheter (*arrows*) shows complete occlusion of the right common iliac vein and indwelling stents. (**b**) The left and (**c**) right upper extremities and neck veins are completely occluded centrally. (**d**) A percutaneous translumbar access to the IVC was obtained with ultrasound guidance and a 21-gauge echogenic needle (*arrows*) just inferior to the dysplastic kidney. (**e**) A tunneled, cuffed hemodialysis catheter was inserted

may be placed, while for chronic use, tunneled catheters are preferred. The catheter diameter should be selected based on the flow rates required, in consultation with the referring clinician and the apheresis/dialysis staff. In the younger age groups, device selection is limited as catheters with a diameter of 6–14 Fr are required to achieve satisfactory flow rates in most cases. Patients with chronic renal failure are at high risk for mechanical and infectious complications related to their central venous catheters and often accumulate venous injuries that may result in loss of all conventional routes of access (Fig. 9.2). Minimizing risk of venous injury in this patient group is essential. This can be facilitated by close communication between multiple disciplines and referral of all venous access-related procedures in these patients to the lowest-risk provider available. Early creation of arteriovenous fistulae to avoid or delay hemodialysis is advocated by some groups.

Procedure Technique

Comfort, Sedation, Anesthesia, Analgesia

Pediatric anesthesia and sedation are covered in Chap. 3. However, the following are some considerations related to venous access procedures. Safe and effective percutaneous venous access and secure guide wire access to the atrium should be the goal of sedation. In many cases, adequate local anesthesia and brief immobilization of the access site will be sufficient. In some cases, the inherent hazards of a procedure, elevated anxiety, or sensitivity to pain may require general anesthesia and even paralysis.

Numerous resources can be utilized to facilitate desirable outcomes and improve the experience of the patient and family. These include involvement of parents, child life specialists and play therapists, patient liaisons, sedation specialists, and anesthesiologists. Use of distraction techniques, sedation, or general anesthesia is based on patient need, procedure complexity, and resource availability.

Venous Access

Positioning

The patient should be positioned so that the potential access site is freely accessible and immobile. During real-time ultrasound guidance, which is recommended for all venous access procedures, the ultrasound monitor should be placed so that it is in line with the entry site and with the operator's natural line of sight. A small roll placed directly under the intended venous entry site can often make the site more easily accessible.

Skin Preparation and Draping

In order to minimize the potential for CRBSI, strict sterile technique should be used for venous access procedures. Proper hand washing technique and surgical gowns, gloves, and masks should be employed. A large area should be cleansed with a suitable agent such as 2 % chlorhexidine. To avoid a chemical skin burn, lower concentrations of chlorhexidine (1 %) or Betadine should be considered for use in premature infants. Adhesive drapes help to isolate the sterile field.

Site Selection

In selecting a site for venous access safety, comfort, avoidance of complications, and accommodation to venous abnormalities should be considered. Access should be performed through intact skin without evidence of local infection.

Placing a catheter from the right side provides a straighter course to the atrium from the right arm or neck and is less likely to be malpositioned in a lumbar vein from the right groin. For tunneled, cuffed central catheters, the internal jugular and common femoral veins are equally useful with a similar rate of complications, except that placement of long-term (tunneled) catheters from the groin has a higher rate of accidental dislodgement in the author's experience. The subclavian vein should be avoided except as a last recourse for most applications, as the rate of both mechanical and infectious complications is highest for these catheters. If it must be used, image-guided puncture lateral to the costoclavicular ligament will avoid catheter pinch-off syndrome (Fig. 9.3).

Alternative Access Sites

When the usual sites for venous access are not available, a variety of less commonly used routes can be employed. These include peripheral systemic veins such as scalp veins, forearm, hand, thigh, and leg veins. All of these are accessible using ultrasound. If a tunneled catheter is required, a tunnel may be formed once access is secured. In most of these locations, a low-profile port could be placed if needed.

If the pathways proximal to the usual access sites are obstructed and cannot be salvaged, then collateral pathways can be used. These include the external jugular and internal mammary veins, as well as paravertebral and intercostal collaterals above the diaphragm (Fig. 9.4) and occasionally pelvic and paraspinal collaterals below the diaphragm. Collateral pathways tend to be tortuous and constricted at branch points that can often make insertion of a guide wire and catheter challenging or impossible. When using a collateral pathway, it is important to advance the catheter tip to the lower SVC beyond the azygos arch, as these collateral pathways often communicate with spinal and epidural vessels and could transmit caustic medications to the spinal cord resulting in transverse myelitis and potential paralysis.

When subclavian and jugular veins are occluded, retroclavicular transmediastinal access to the brachiocephalic veins or even to the distal SVC may be possible (due to inflow from the azygos system). In this case, the patent pathway

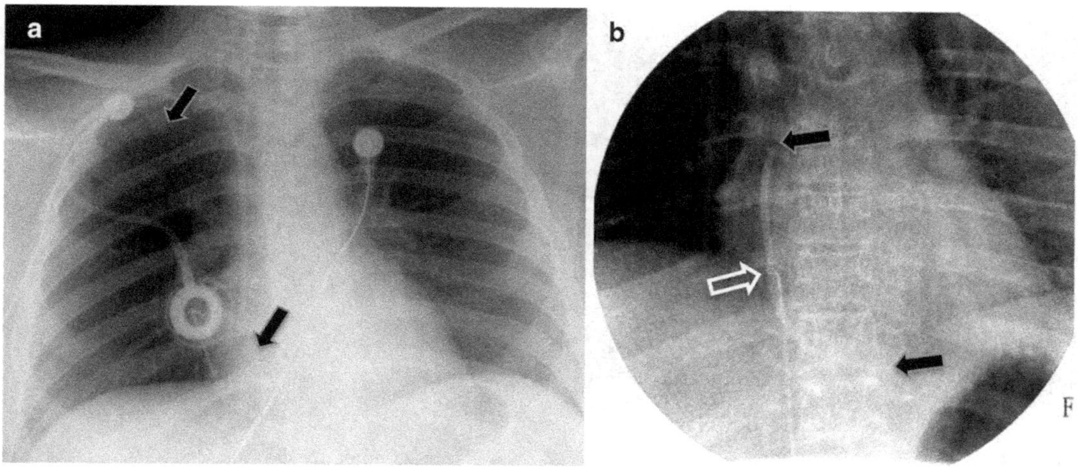

Fig. 9.3 A 12-year-old female underwent removal of a right subclavian port. (**a**) The distance from costoclavicular ligament to its tip measures 11.5 cm (between *arrows*). (**b**) This is the same length as the catheter fragment (*arrows*) that was retrieved with a transfemoral loop snare (*open arrow*) after port explantation. Catheter pinch-off syndrome is a common cause of complication for catheters inserted by this route

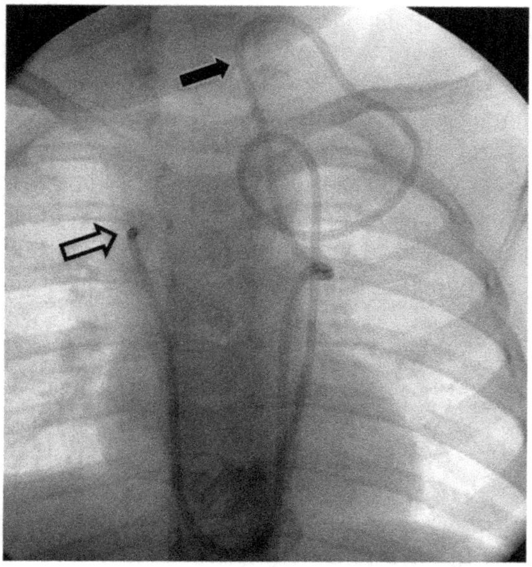

Fig. 9.4 A 7-year-old on chronic parenteral nutrition with extensive systemic venous occlusions. A dual-lumen cuffed, tunneled catheter enters a paravertebral collateral vein in the neck (*arrow*), descends through tortuous hemizygos collaterals and crosses below the diaphragm into the azygos veins, and ascends to the azygos arch (*open arrow*). This was achieved by snaring the guide wire from a transfemoral approach (the so-called body-floss technique of guide wire stabilization)

to the right atrium may be visualized by directing a paracoronal ultrasound beam toward the atrium from a supraclavicular approach (Fig. 9.5). In this view, the cupola of the lung and the brachiocephalic or subclavian artery may also be visualized so that pneumothorax and inadvertent arterial puncture can be avoided. Similarly, from below the diaphragm, it is possible to gain access to the IVC by a translumbar or a transhepatic approach. Ultrasound and fluoroscopy can be used in combination to guide such access. Three-dimensional imaging, using cone-beam CT on the angiography table or conventional CT, can be a helpful adjunct for route planning or guidance. It is worth noting that the transhepatic route especially is associated with very high rates of infection, infusate extravasation, and accidental catheter dislodgment and should be reserved as a last resort.

Principles of Image Guidance

Before ultrasound became the mainstay for guidance during venipuncture, venous access was obtained using visual guidance (under direct visualization, transillumination, or use of topographical landmarks) or using venography. Visual access attempts favor selection of more fragile superficial veins that are more prone to rupture and thrombophlebitis and are also more likely to result in inadvertent puncture of

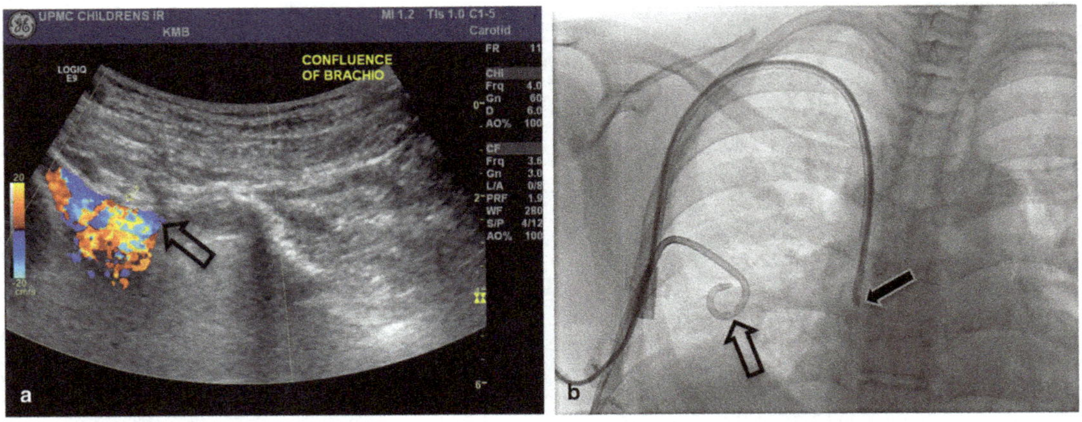

Fig. 9.5 A 22-year-old male on hemodialysis. Pelvic, neck, and upper extremity veins are chronically occluded. (**a**) The brachiocephalic confluence is visualized with color Doppler imaging using a right retroclavicular, coronal approach. The access route (between *open arrows*) was chosen to minimize the path length. (**b**) This access was used to deliver the 14 Fr dual-lumen cuffed, tunneled hemodialysis catheter shown here (*black arrow*). The right pigtail thoracostomy drainage tube (*open arrow*) was preexisting

nontarget structures such as the pleurae and arteries (Fig. 9.6). Venography is more reliable for deep vein puncture, but requires use of contrast and ionizing radiation (Fig. 9.7). As a planar modality, it also increases risk of transgression of nontarget structures like arteries and nerves.

Minimizing vessel trauma during access is important, as repeated trauma (such as from multiple punctures) promotes intimal injury and platelet aggregation and ultimately may progress to thrombosis, fibrosis, stenosis, and occlusion. With exquisite high-resolution near-field imaging, ultrasound can enable navigation into even tortuous or very small caliber vessels while avoiding vital structures such as arteries, nerves, and pleurae. The target vessel can be interrogated along its length to assure patency and to define a safe pathway for access.

Initial Access

While either longitudinal or transverse imaging can be useful, most venous access is performed in transverse section (Fig. 9.8). Tilting the transducer slightly away from the needle can help make the beveled tip more conspicuous. If the imaging plane is maintained just ahead of the needle tip, then the bright tip artifact will always be entering the image as the needle is advanced, making it easier to keep control of the position of the needle tip and avoiding inadvertent puncture through the back wall of the vein. A short sharp darting motion will allow inertia to help stabilize the wall while the bevel (and, importantly, the cannula if an angiocatheter (i.v. catheter) is used) pierces the wall and fully enters the lumen. While controlling the tip position with ultrasound, the needle and cannula can be advanced well within the lumen, so that guide wire access can be achieved with decreased risk of dislodgement. In infants with small veins, double-wall puncture may be required.

Guide Wire Advancement

Soft, gently curved guide wires facilitate advancement through the venous system. The earlier in the procedure that the guide wire is advanced to or beyond the right atrium, the fewer events can occur which lead to loss of access. Imaging confirmation of its central progress is helpful to assure the wire is properly placed to guide the catheter tip to its desired location.

Inability to pass a guide wire into the central circulation may be due to (1) extravascular position of the access needle tip, (2) malposition,

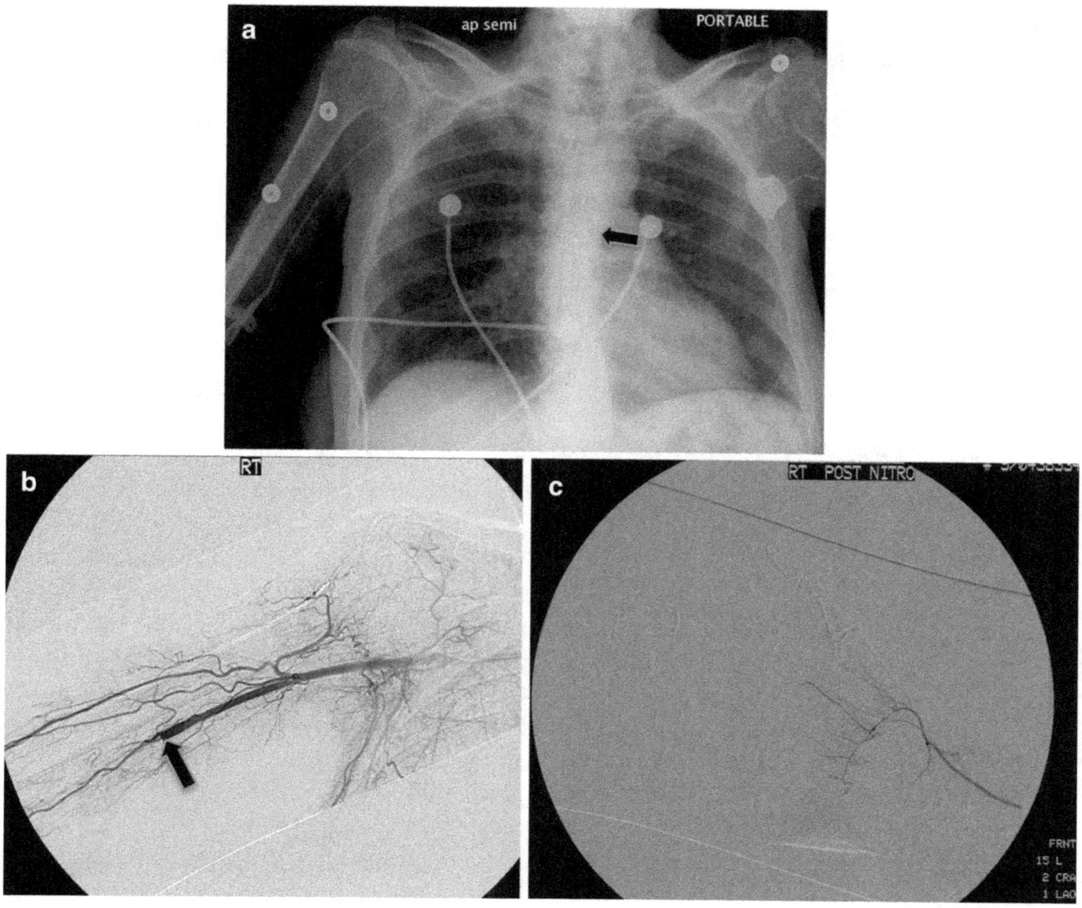

Fig. 9.6 Pain and ischemic symptoms following PICC insertion. (**a**) On the immediate post-insertion radiograph, the catheter tip is located at the level of the carina to the left of the spine, suggesting inadvertent arterial malposition. (**b**) Although the catheter was promptly removed, an arteriogram shows the "meniscus" sign (*arrow*) of thrombotic occlusion at the insertion site with distal reconstitution but (**c**) very poor flow to the hand despite nitroglycerin administration. This case emphasizes the hazards associated with venous access performed without adequate real-time image control

(3) spasm, or (4) stenosis or occlusion. If not within the vein, the wire can coil outside the vessel or travel along the neurovascular connective tissue sheath until it reaches a transition point, such as the axilla. If the guide wire advances into a difficult accessory or collateral pathway, recognition and reposition is essential to successful central placement.

When venospasm occurs, the guide wire or the PICC catheter cannot be advanced, usually beyond the upper arm or axilla. It can be provoked by any manipulation of the vein. The appearance on venography is often equivocal, and one may simply see extravasation of contrast distal to the access point or near the tip of the catheter or dilator. Calming the child, warming the affected region, or simply allowing time to pass are usually the most successful treatment strategies. Pharmacologic measures (e.g., nitroglycerin, papaverine) may be attempted but are often not helpful. In some cases, a peel-away sheath or metal stiffener inserted over a mandril wire from a micropuncture set can be used to gently bypass the area of stenosis. It may be most useful to simply select an alternative access point that does not involve the spastic segment.

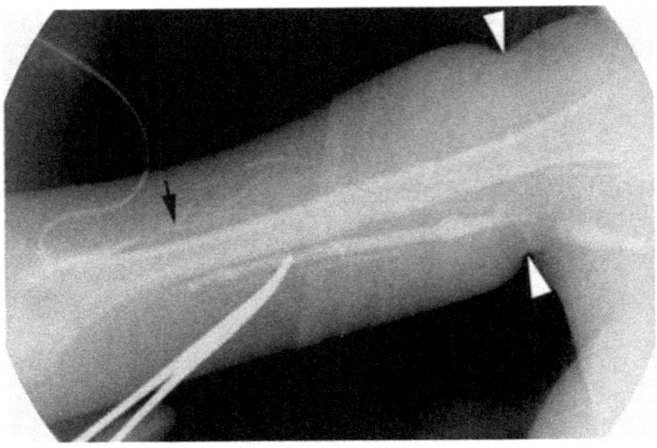

Fig. 9.7 Through a 22-gauge angiocatheter (*arrow*) in a right cephalic branch, intravenous contrast is administered during fluoroscopic imaging to plan a route for percutaneous venous access for a PICC insertion. A tourniquet (*arrowheads*) improves reflux of contrast into arm veins. The tip of a hemostat is being used to identify a route of access to the brachial vein in the mid-arm. Effacement of contrast (not shown here) by the tip of the needle during attempted access is a sign that the tip is compressing the target vein wall

In distinction to venospasm, stenosis and occlusion are fixed or progressive. Once injury has progressed to fibrosis, tight stenosis, or occlusion, it may be impossible to provide access through the affected venous pathway without specific intervention. Again, it is easiest and quickest when such issues are encountered to simply move on to another vessel and write off the affected pathway. However, unlike self-limited spasm, failure to address the issue of stenosis or occlusion when it is encountered may be equivalent to reducing the patient's venous reserve. When all the access routes are spent, the access-dependent patient will die. It is not the last vessel standing that should command our attention so much as the first vessel at risk. Guide wire and related techniques to salvage stenotic or occluded venous pathways are addressed in "Recanalization and Venoplasty."

Tract and Pocket Preparation

Local and Regional Anesthesia

Topical anesthetic agents are a great aid in children as they will decrease the pain associated with venipuncture and local anesthetic injection. Care must be taken when local anesthetic is injected prior to venipuncture as it can result in compression of the vein and loss of visualization. Use of epinephrine (1:200,000) in the local anesthetic and longer-acting local agents (e.g., 0.25 % bupivacaine) and regional blockade (e.g., of intercostal nerves in port pocket preparation) can be useful adjuncts for greater and more durable patient comfort.

PICC and Peripheral Port Sites

Basilic, brachial, and cephalic veins can be used. The basilic has the lowest incidence of thrombosis. The cephalic vein is often problematic because of its narrow caliber and tortuous course. It is best to select an insertion site just high enough above the antecubitum that the patient can easily bend and use the arm after the catheter has been placed and dressed. When accessing the brachial vein, the relationship of the vein to the artery and nerve (Fig. 9.8) is variable and should be carefully noted. Transgression of the nerve causes pain and paresthesia.

Port pockets for peripheral ports may be formed distal to the venous entry site, or the tract may be curved so that the port can be placed more proximally, taking care that the tract is not sharply curved to avoid catheter kinking.

Catheter Insertion

Peel-Away Sheath

In most cases, a catheter is introduced to the venous system through a peel-away sheath, either directly, as for a PICC or temporary catheter, or after having been drawn through a subcutaneous tunnel, as for a tunneled central line or indwelling port.

In the thorax, sheath insertion should be monitored under fluoroscopy to stay properly aligned and avoid perforation of the vein or atrium wall. The sheath should never be advanced without its dilator, as the unprotected tip is relatively sharp.

As air embolism is possible, many peel-away sheaths are now manufactured with a valve that prevents ingress of air after the dilator has been

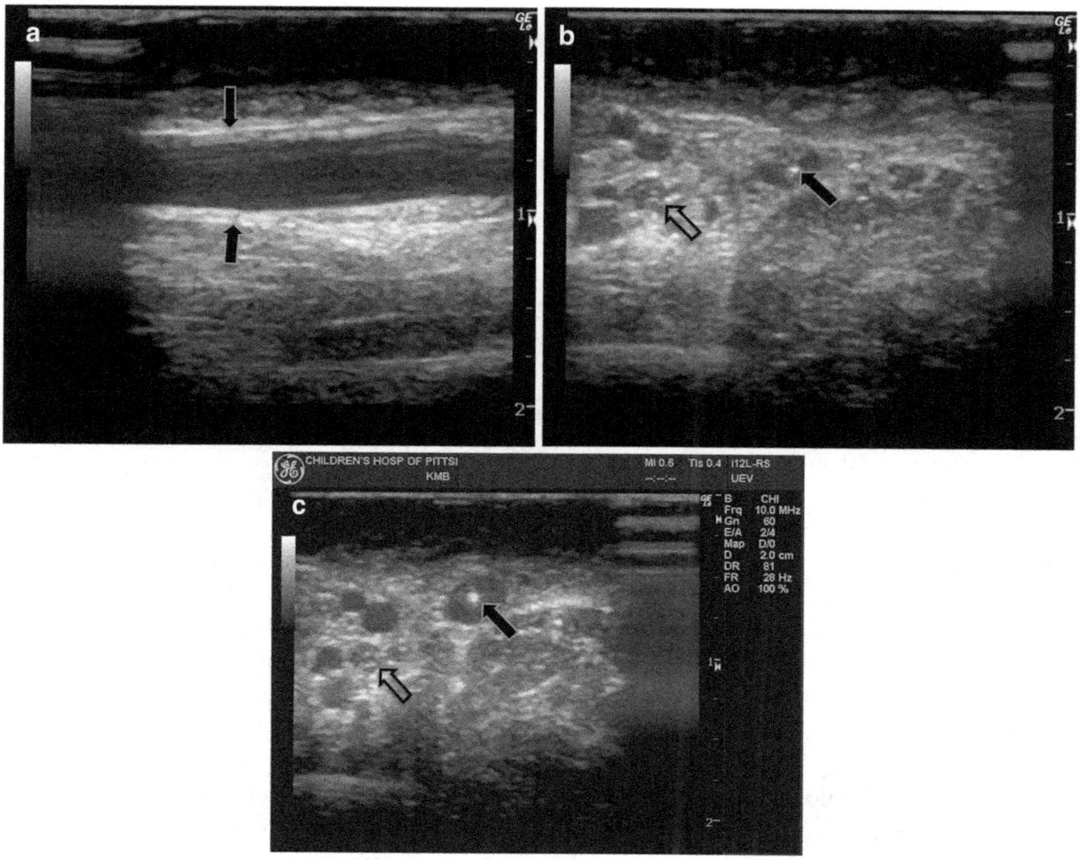

Fig. 9.8 (**a**) The basilic vein is visualized with longitudinal ultrasound in the mid-arm of a 6-month-old infant. The anterior and posterior walls of the vessel (*arrows*) are most echogenic when the vein is centered in the beam. (**b**) The same vein is visualized in transverse section. Slight caudal angulation of the transducer enhances conspicuity of the tip (*arrow*). In this image, although the tip appears to be within the lumen, the vein has not yet been punctured. Note also the brachial nerve (*open arrow*) adjacent to the brachial artery characterized on ultrasound as a noncompressible structure filled with small echogenic circles that represent the perineurium of the nerve fascicles. (**c**) Note the increased echogenicity of the beveled tip of the angiocatheter stylet when it is completely within the vessel lumen compared with the extraluminal tip seen in (**b**) above

removed. Placing the patient in Trendelenburg position helps assure a positive pressure gradient. It is also possible to clamp the sheath outside the skin until the catheter tip has been introduced, although this may cause damage to the sheath.

After the catheter has been advanced through the sheath, it must be controlled during sheath removal to prevent inadvertent malposition or dislodgement. It may be helpful to confirm with fluoroscopy that the catheter has been adequately advanced before peeling the sheath away and to observe with fluoroscopy while removing the sheath if there is any uncertainty.

Catheter Measurement

Hemodialysis and apheresis catheters, and those with specialized tips, such as Groshong-type valved catheters, are inserted without modifying the catheter length. However, most catheters are trimmed to length so as to position the tip at a desired location (*see* "Tip Position"). There are several methods that can be used to determine the proper length such as pre-marked guide wires, the modified bent guide wire technique, and cutting to length from surface measurement. Each involves placing the wire or catheter tip at the target point and then measuring the distance to the skin entry point.

Catheter Advancement

Once a peel-away sheath is in place and the catheter has been measured and trimmed, the catheter is advanced through the sheath. The sheath is removed and the final position is evaluated under fluoroscopic control.

Tip Position

The actual goal is to position the catheter tip at the safest place with the lowest risk of infectious or mechanical complications. We do not have very reliable data about where this point might be for each catheter type, each patient size and age, and each medical indication. For most situations, experience suggests this is at or near the cavoatrial junction, at the superior limit of the right atrium from above the diaphragm, and at the inferior limit of the atrium from below the diaphragm. Since the venous anatomy cannot be seen without contrast or cross-sectional imaging, this point can best be approximated as a point 2 vertebral bodies below the carina for the superior cavoatrial junction (Fig. 9.9e) and a point just above the diaphragmatic margin for the inferior cavoatrial junction.

Recommendations of the KDOQI of the National Kidney Foundation state that the distal catheter tip of hemodialysis catheters should be located within the right atrium (Fig. 9.10).

Apheresis and temporary catheters are usually not constructed to reach the cavoatrial junction and are not trimmable to length, so they must be positioned so as to optimize function and minimize complications. They may also be more tapered and stiffer than permanent catheters. From above the diaphragm, they should be placed with their tip well into the SVC if possible, that is, below the carina and, better, below the inferior margin of the right mainstem bronchus. When placed from the left, they should be advanced so as to hang freely within the SVC lumen and not project against the lateral vein wall. From below the diaphragm, the tip should be within the IVC if possible and not obstruct either the renal or the hepatic venous outflow.

For catheters in a persistent left superior vena cava (Fig. 9.11), there is no consensus on tip position.

Catheter Fixation, Wound Closure, and Dressing

Where possible, it is best to avoid retention sutures in children. PICCs, for example, can be reliably fixed to the skin with an adhesive device that "locks in" the PICC hub to help prevent its accidental dislodgement.

A sterile dressing that is self-wicking and does not require gauze underneath the occlusive dressing can usually remain in place for a week before it needs to be changed. Dressings that include a gauze covering should be changed much more often, while blood-soaked dressings, dirty dressings, and dressings that are no longer occlusive should be changed immediately on recognition.

Ingrowth of subcutaneous fibrous tissue provides stability in cuffed catheters. However, during the first 7–10 days, the stability of the catheter must be protected by some other means. Tunneled, cuffed catheters as well as temporary catheters are often fixed to the skin with interrupted sutures through suture tabs or around suture points. Form a suture loop in the skin and then fix the tab to the loop, rather than passing the skin loop through the suture tab. This decreases risk of the suture cutting the skin or causing necrosis. Alternatively, these catheters as well as catheters without suture tabs can be fixed to the skin with an adhesive device similar to that described above. The skin entry wound should be closed around the exiting catheter with an interrupted suture, taking care not to kink the catheter! Similarly, the skin entry wound at the venous entry site can be closed with a single interrupted suture, taking care not to perforate the catheter in the process. Both wounds should be covered with a sterile occlusive dressing until primary healing has occurred. The sutures may usually be removed after 10–14 days.

The hub of an indwelling venous port can be fixed to the superficial muscle fascia with interrupted sutures. The incision is usually closed in layers, with interrupted sutures deeply and either a running subcuticular suture or tissue adhesive to close the superficial layer. If tissue adhesive is not used, Steri-Strips are often applied as a final protection against early dehiscence of the wound.

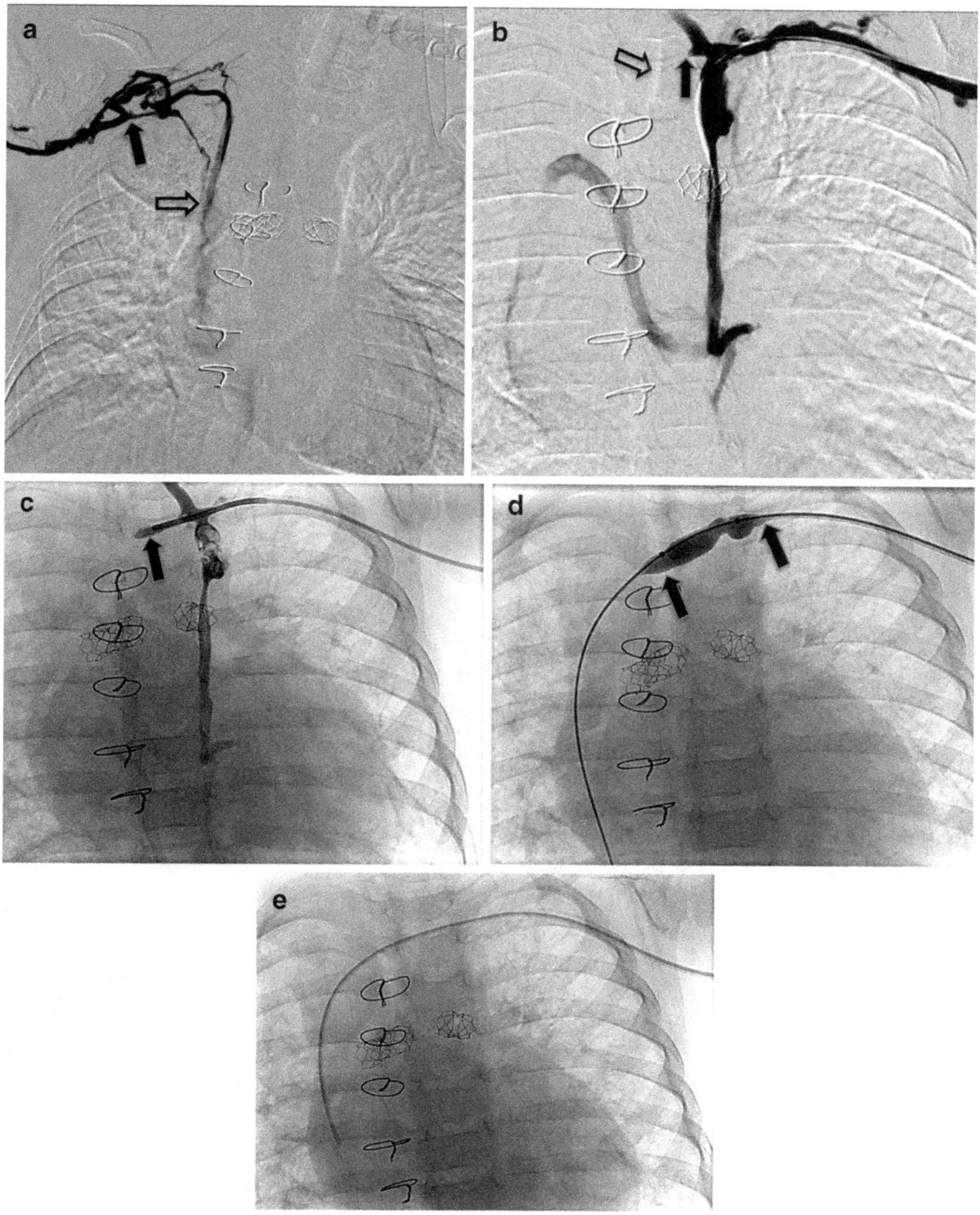

Fig. 9.9 A 1-year-old female with truncus arteriosus post repair presented for PICC insertion. (**a**) Venography from the right shows complete occlusion of the axillary vein (*black arrow*) with prominent collaterals that drain to the right atrium via the azygos (*open arrow*). (**b**) Left extremity venogram shows occlusion of the left brachiocephalic vein, with preferential decompression via the hemiazygos to azygos, returning through the arch (*asterisk*) to the right atrium. (**c**, **d**) Wire recanalization and serial angioplasty to 5 mm was performed to allow for restoration of flow (**e**) and line insertion. The tip of the catheter projects 2 vertebral bodies below the carina, a close approximation of the cavoatrial junction

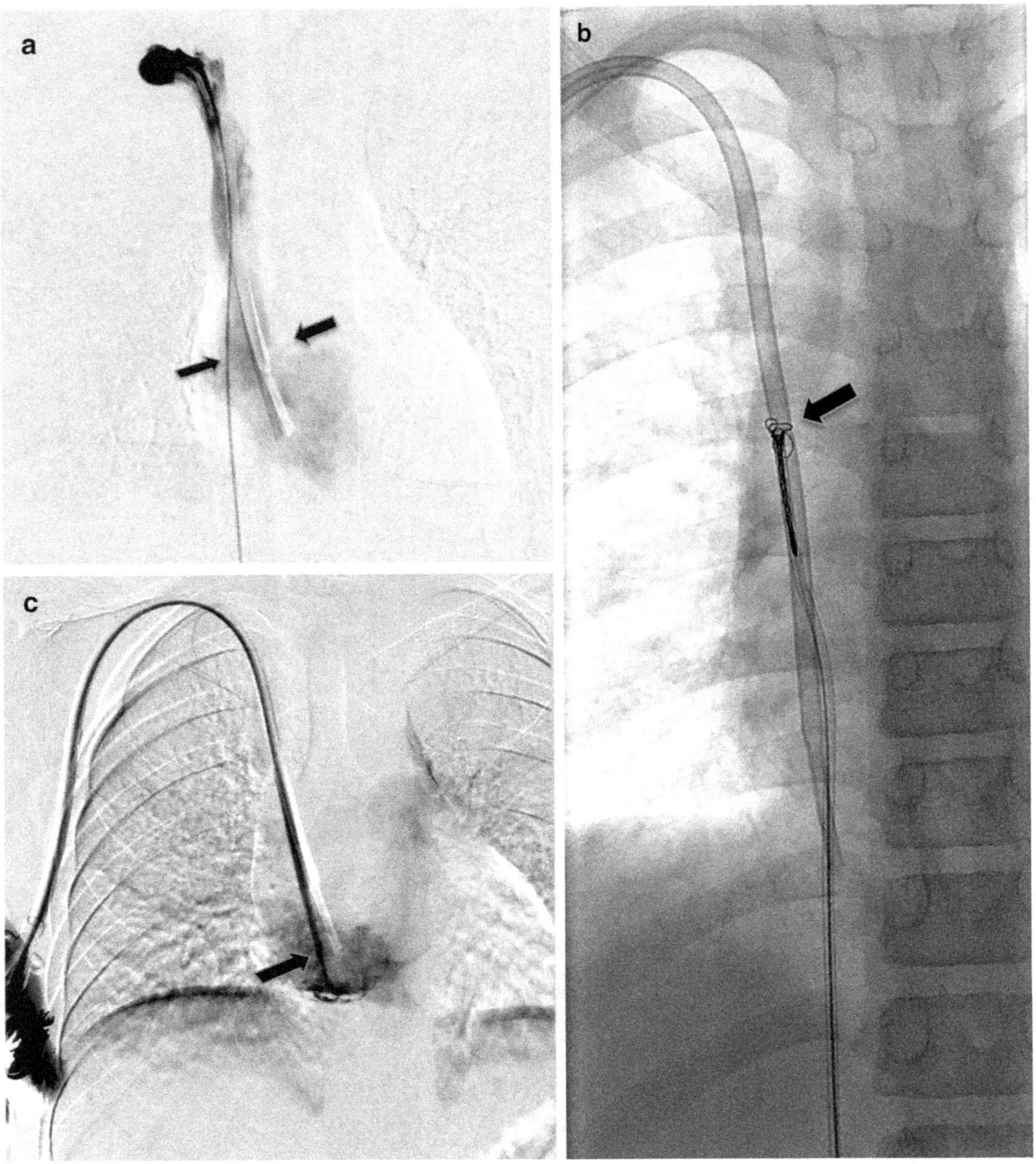

Fig. 9.10 (**a**) Dysfunctional hemodialysis catheter in an 11-year-old male with chronic renal failure. A catheter contrast study showed that both channels were positioned below the cavoatrial junction, as recommended by KDOQI guidelines. (**b**) Neither port would flush or withdraw properly. A snare was advanced from the femoral vein over the intravascular portion of the catheter, and after snugging it against the catheter (*arrow*), it was pulled down off the tip. (**c**) Repeat contrast injection demonstrated unimpaired flow. This type of salvage procedure can usually be accomplished much more quickly than placing a new catheter and at significantly lower risk to the patient

If the port will not be used immediately after insertion, then the wound can be covered with a sterile dressing after heparin administration. If it will be used, then it should be accessed with the appropriate non-coring needle. The needle-hub access device can be supported with a split gauze dressing, fixed to the skin with Steri-Strips, and then covered with a sterile dressing. Once the wound heals, no dressing is required when the port is not accessed.

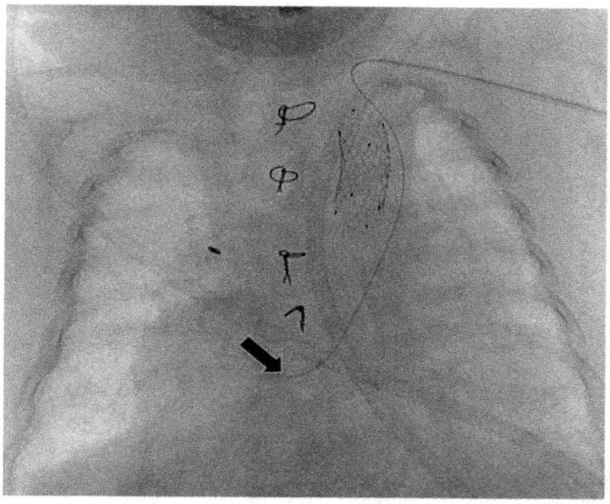

Fig. 9.11 This 4-month-old male required central venous access but had marked right upper extremity edema. During the procedure for insertion of a left arm PICC, the guide wire was noted to advance into a persistent left superior vena cava. Catheters can be situated in a left SVC, but the safest tip position has not been determined

Managing Complications and Catheter Salvage

Procedural Complications

Immediate major complications encountered during the access procedure include cardiorespiratory compromise (perhaps related to sedation, airway compression, or a cardiac rhythm disturbance), perforation or arterial puncture with cardiac tamponade or hemothorax, air embolism, and pneumothorax. Although a discussion of treatment for these conditions is outside the scope of this chapter, such events signal the end of the elective procedure and the beginning of resuscitation: the transition must be made without delay.

Mechanical Complications

Device Dysfunction

Catheter dysfunction may be the result of a number of factors. Inability to draw from or flush through the catheter may be secondary to kinking or suture occlusion of the catheter, a flipped or disconnected port chamber, improperly accessed port, malposition of the tip, occlusion with medication, or thrombus/fibrin sheath. Careful evaluation of the external portions of the catheter and a chest radiograph will often reveal the underlying cause of dysfunction. If not, fluoroscopy with contrast is helpful.

Comparison with imaging obtained at the time of insertion can help discern more subtle evidence of catheter tip migration or embolization after fracture. Contrast outside the catheter may relate to a connection failure (at the port hub, Fig. 9.12) or catheter fracture or perforation. Fracture or perforation is most commonly seen in "subclavian" catheters that pass through the costoclavicular ligament on their way to the anterolateral wall of the brachiocephalic vein: the so-called catheter pinch-off syndrome (Fig. 9.3). If the catheter appears shortened compared to earlier images or measurement at the time of insertion, the thorax should be searched for an embolized fragment (Fig. 9.13). Deviation of the contrast stream at the catheter tip suggests either adherence to the vessel wall, a fibrin sheath, or a tip thrombus (Fig. 9.14).

A flipped port can sometimes be manipulated through the skin into its normal position, but if it is recurrent or cannot be restored in this way, the port pocket may have to be opened in order to suture the hub more securely to the muscle fascia. A fibrin sheath or tip thrombus may respond to thrombolytics at dose volumes just large enough to fill the catheter.

For devices that remain dysfunctional and are difficult to replace, like ports and hemodialysis catheters, it may be worthwhile attempting to strip the tip of the catheter with a snare (Fig. 9.10). If this does not work, there is little choice but to replace the catheter or place a new one at a new location.

Dehiscence

Rarely, if the port hub or subcutaneous catheter is too shallow or there is pressure on the overlying skin, it may erode through the skin or result in wound dehiscence. There is little that can be done about these complications other than to administer appropriate antibiotics and re-site the device.

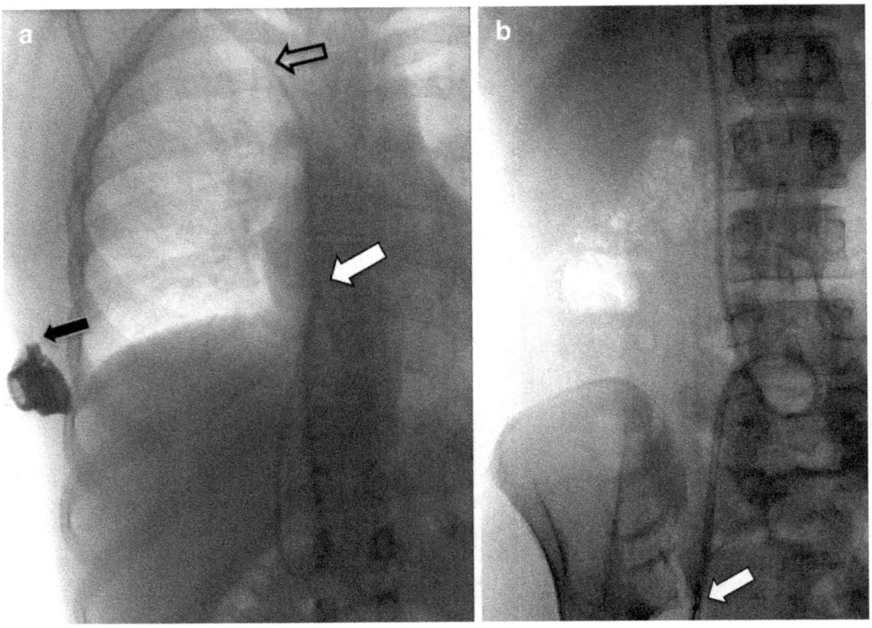

Fig. 9.12 A 18-year-old female with sickle cell disease experiencing pain and swelling of the port pocket during drug administration. (**a**) This chest radiograph shows that the port hub (*black arrow*) has separated from the catheter (*open arrow*). The catheter tip (*white arrow*) has embolized to the suprahepatic IVC after coiling in the ostium of the left hepatic vein. (**b**) A snare was used to capture the superior end of the catheter, which was withdrawn safely through the groin sheath. The port hub had to be removed from the port pocket and a new port was inserted

Swelling

Swelling near the insertion site or port pocket is usually infectious or inflammatory, but may be mechanical in origin. If the swelling and any associated discomfort worsen during infusion, it may represent infusate infiltration, signifying discontinuity somewhere between the hub and the venous entry site. If there is a pulsatile swelling or if the swelling continues to increase in size without relation to use, this may signify an inadvertent arterial injury, such as arteriovenous fistula or pseudoaneurysm.

Infectious Complications

Central venous catheters in children are removed far more often due to misdiagnosis of infection than to proven infection. Reasonable efforts should be made to exclude common noninfectious reasons for catheter-related symptoms and common reasons for non-catheter-related symptoms of infection, before removing an otherwise functioning catheter.

Pain, erythema, and swelling overlying the access vein with or without fever, especially in close proximity to the access procedure, usually represent self-limited phlebitis or phlegmasia. A warm compress, elevation of the affected extremity, and time will usually see these findings pass without further incident, although many catheters are removed under such conditions in the mistaken belief that the underlying cause is infectious.

Erythema, tenderness, and a purulent discharge without bacteremia are prima facie evidence of a soft tissue infection and may be seen at the catheter exit site, at the venous entry site wound, along the subcutaneous tunnel, or in the port pocket. A swab of the purulent discharge should be submitted for microbiologic analysis. Antibiotics should be administered and the catheter or port should be removed.

Unequivocal evidence of a CRBSI includes catheter tip and blood cultures with a single organism known to cause such infections, without another source, and with clinical signs and symptoms of sepsis. Differential time to positivity of

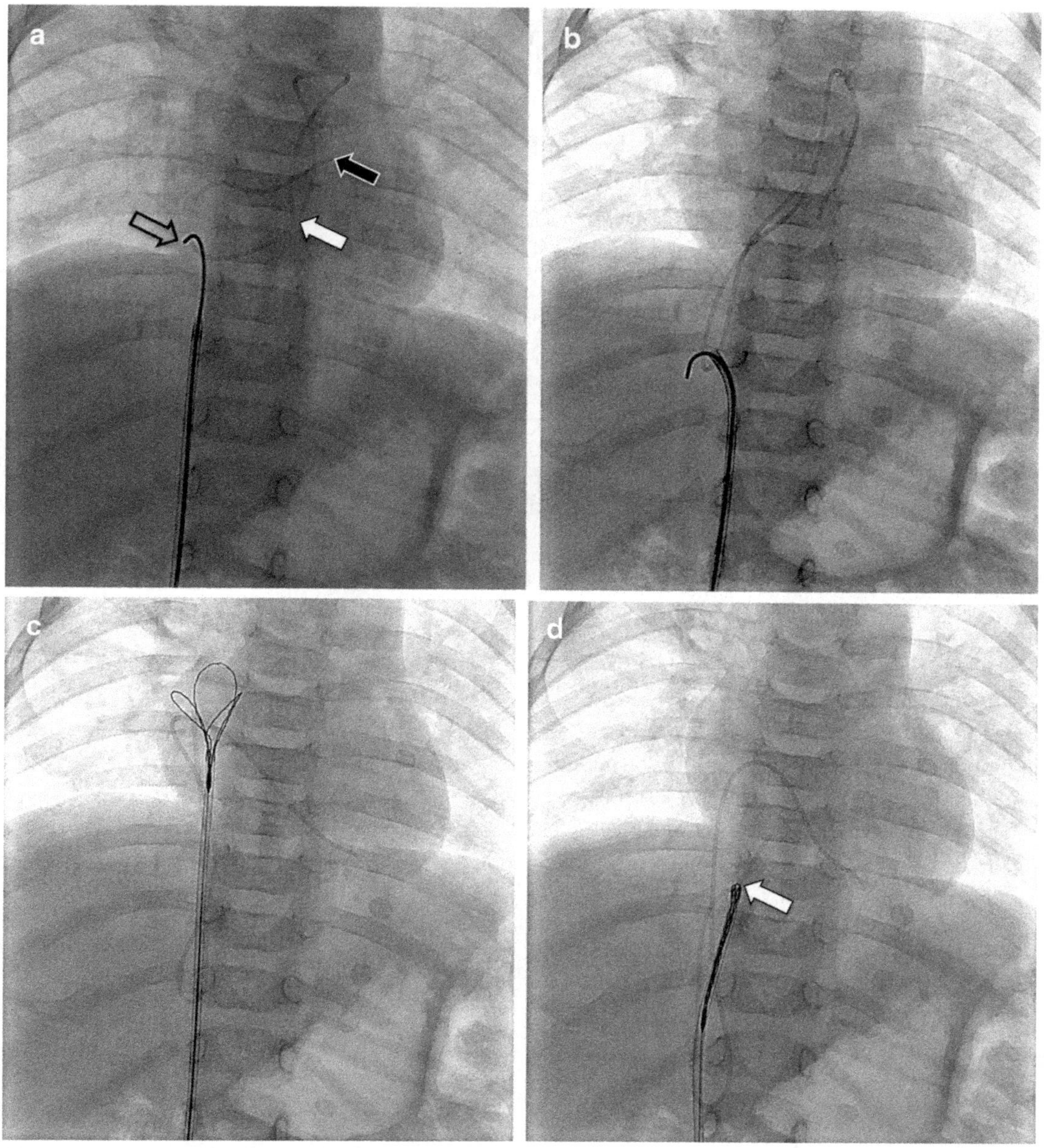

Fig. 9.13 Two days following PICC removal in a 10 month old, an unsuspected fragment was discovered. (**a**) Tips of the embolized fragment project over the inflow (*black arrow*) and outflow (*white arrow*) portions of the right ventricle. Rather than advancing a device across the tricuspid valve, a tip-deflecting wire (*open arrow*) was passed transfemorally and activated within the right atrium to capture the loop of catheter. (**b**) The loop was then drawn down into the IVC in order to bring one tip of the catheter in range of a snare loop. (**c**) A snare (*arrow*) was then advanced superior to the intra-atrial catheter tip and retracted until the tip was captured. (**d**) The captured tip (*white arrow*) was then withdrawn through the transfemoral sheath to complete the foreign body retrieval

catheter and peripheral cultures are strongly predictive of catheter-related infection. The samples should be of equal volume and drawn simultaneously, and the transcatheter culture should be positive 2 h or more before the peripheral culture. Such evidence should be sought especially in patients at high risk for catheter-related infections, because they are subject to severe complications related to multiple venous interventions and cannot afford to have functioning

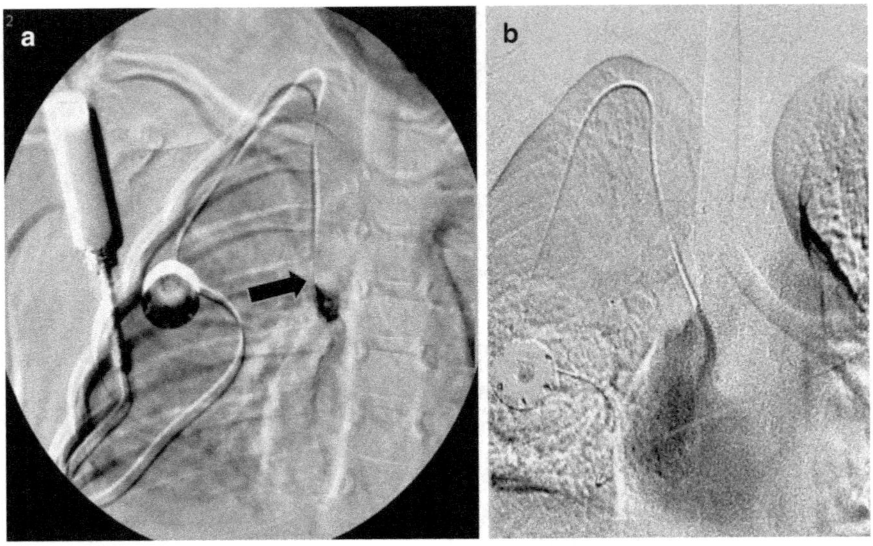

Fig. 9.14 (**a**) A 3-year-old boy with nephrotic syndrome and port dysfunction. Medial deviation of contrast indicates a tip thrombus or fibrin sheath. Relative immobility of the catheter tip (*arrow*) also suggests catheter adherence to the vessel wall. (**b**) A tip-deflecting wire placed transfemorally was used to strip the catheter tip free from the vessel wall. Contrast in this subtracted image now shows the stream to be directed straight from the tip, as normally expected. This salvage procedure added more than 300 days to the life of this catheter

noninfected catheters removed. A positive blood culture with resolution of signs and symptoms within 24 h of catheter removal is also presumptive evidence of a CRBSI, but presumes removal of the catheter before diagnosis. The most common organisms associated with CRBSI include *Staphylococcus aureus* and coagulase-negative staphylococci, *Enterococcus faecalis*, *Escherichia coli*, *Pseudomonas aeruginosa*, and *Candida albicans*. Of course, this is a retrospective diagnosis made after removal of the catheter. Fever without a positive culture is not evidence of a CRBSI.

It is difficult to make a definitive diagnosis while the catheter is still in place and to preserve the catheter in cases where it is not involved. If another source can be identified and successfully treated, the catheter usually does not need to be removed. Some CRBSI can be treated with antibiotics without removing the catheter. This should be undertaken through consultation with a specialist in treatment of pediatric infectious diseases. It is important to understanding outcomes, identifying risks and sources of infection, and improving practice to correctly differentiate CRBSI and catheter-related soft tissue infections from non-catheter-related events. Each institution should collect data on each central venous catheter from the first use of an access site to the final removal of a catheter from that site, as part of the procedural and outcomes data summarized in Appendix. The calculation of this data according to events per catheter day provides information that can usefully be compared across experiences and locations.

Venography

Although MRI or CT can be used, venography is the common method to diagnose significant venous stenosis or occlusion. The most common etiologies in children are related to previous venous access for causes such as hemodialysis, dependence on parenteral nutrition, and complex congenital heart disease. A venogram can delineate the level of obstruction, demonstrate evidence of accessibility of central systemic veins (Fig. 9.15), or suggest an alternative pathway to the right atrium. The author's preference is to perform simultaneous bilateral injections of distal peripheral veins in the upper or lower extremities, as indicated. Imaging should focus on

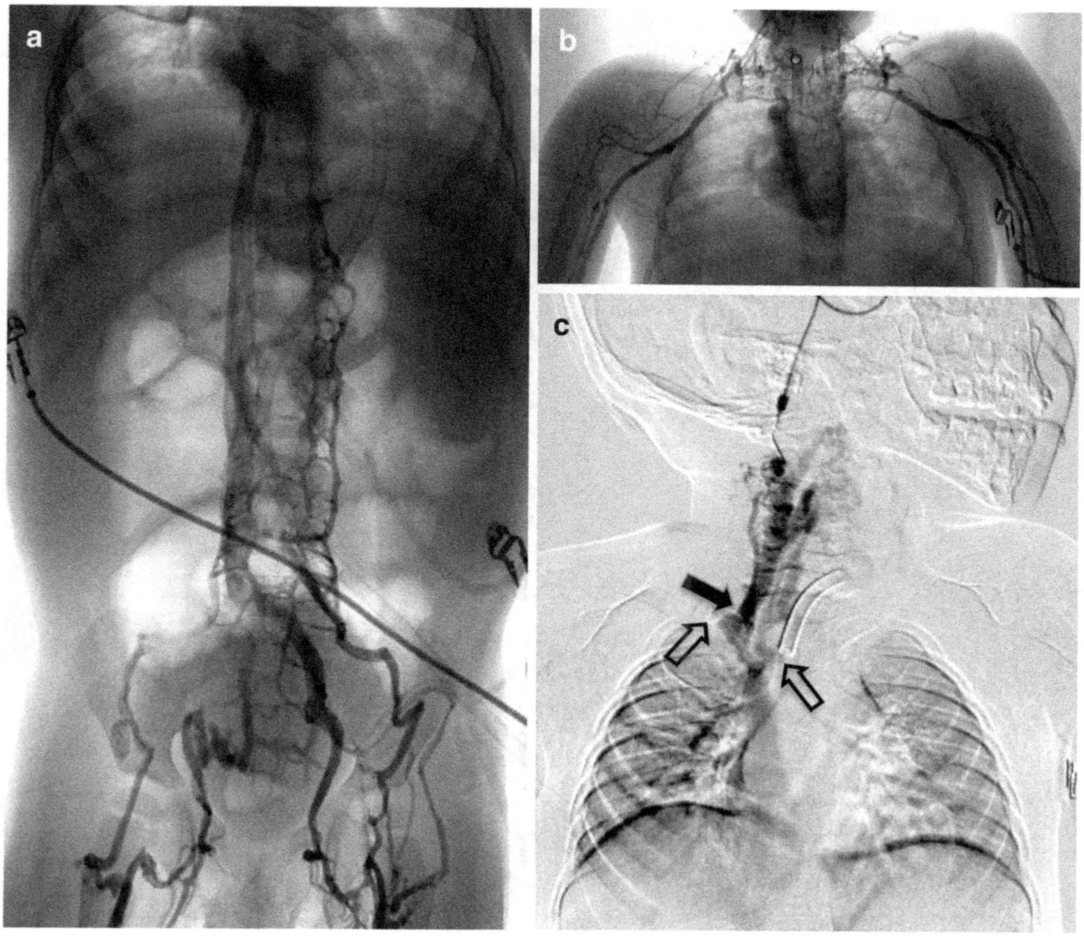

Fig. 9.15 A 5-year-old male with biliary atresia following multivisceral transplant. (**a**) Bilateral lower extremity venography shows occlusion of both common femoral veins with numerous pelvic collaterals reconstituting the IVC. (**b**) Simultaneous upper extremity venography shows bilateral axillary occlusions with extensive collateralization to the hemizygos/azygos system. (**c**) It shows severe narrowing of the proximal jugular vein, right brachiocephalic vein, and distal SVC. (**d**) Dilation of the severe stenosis with a 7-mm noncompliant balloon (*arrow*) was incomplete. (**e**) Completion venography showed improved flow through the region with little filling of collaterals. (**f**) Catheter retraction post initial placement requiring guide wire placement into the IVC and subsequent reinsertion with the use of a longer peel-away sheath (**g**, **h**)

central vessels, from the upper arm to the diaphragm for upper extremity venography and from the groin to the atrium for lower extremity venography. Additional veins can be interrogated individually.

Ultrasound evaluation of the veins can often complement contrast venography, using the two modalities to piece together an answer on a task-oriented basis. If a contrast-enhanced CT study of the area of interest is available, it can add considerably to understanding the anatomy and dissecting a complex array of overlapping vessels that characterize the planar images of the venogram.

Recanalization and Venoplasty

In patients with temporary CVA requirements, if a venous stenosis or occlusion is present, it is usually best to move the catheter to another vessel. In contrast, a more aggressive approach may

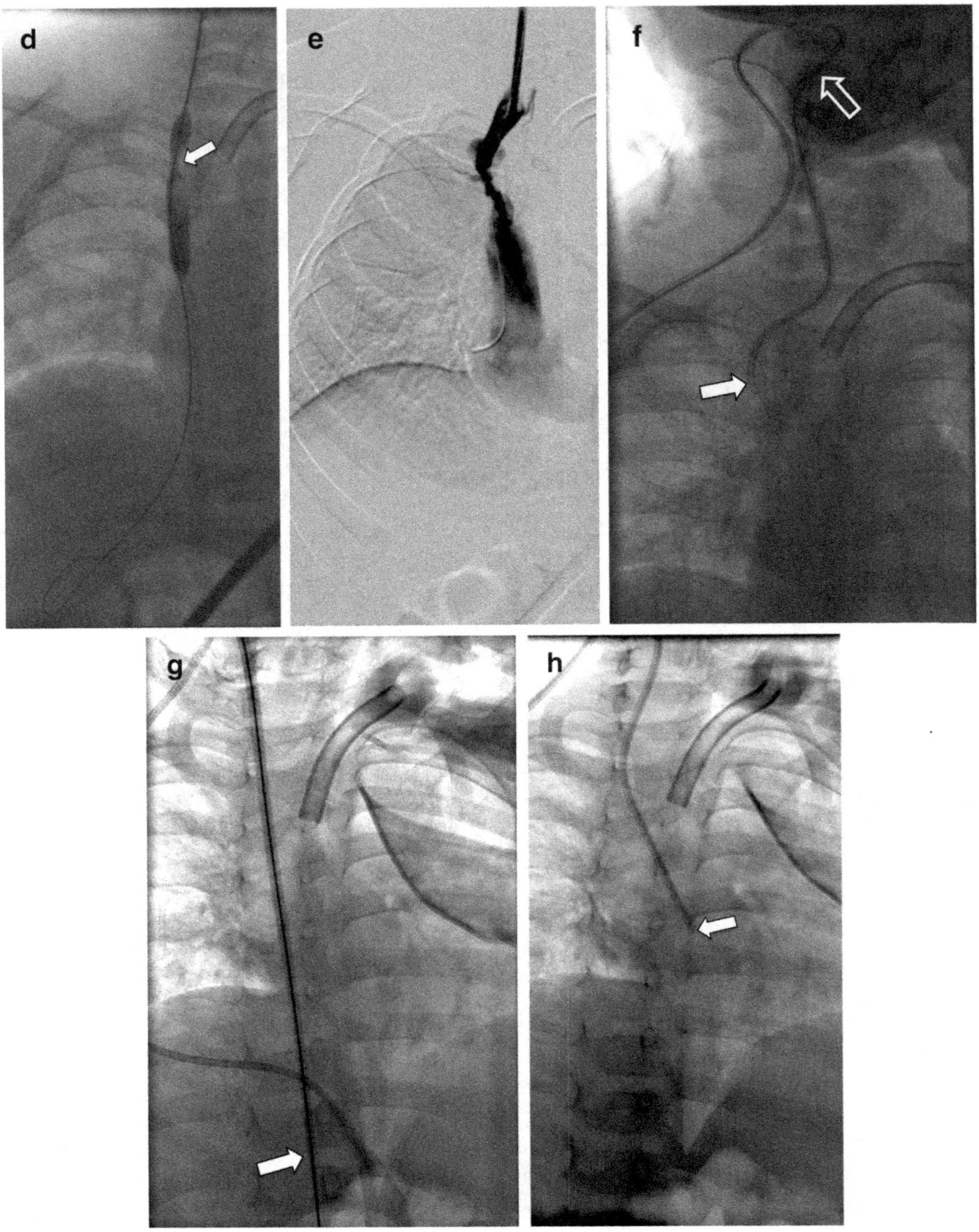

Fig. 9.15 (continued)

be warranted in patients who are reliant upon long-term venous access. Reutilizing or recanalization of an obstructed vein will maintain easier access routes for later in life and could even improve life expectancy. For example, absence of durable access above the diaphragm may preclude transplantation in some patients. Patients with superior vena cava syndrome (Fig. 9.16) have a significant risk of mortality if nothing is done to correct their restricted venous drainage.

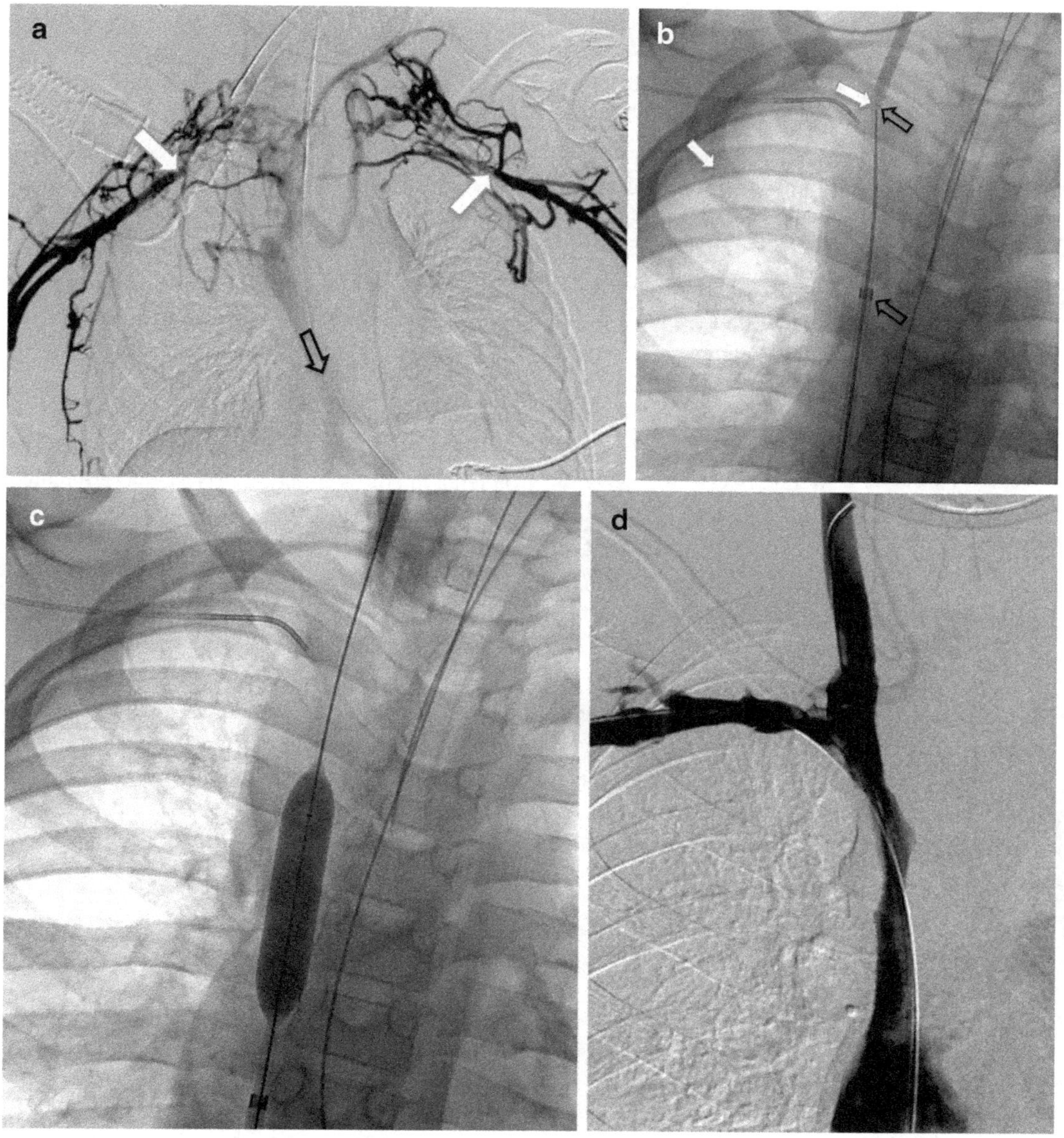

Fig. 9.16 A 12-year-old boy with nephrotic syndrome presenting with symptomatic SVC syndrome. (**a**) Simultaneous bilateral upper extremity venography shows complete occlusion of the upper extremity drainage (*white arrows*) with collateral flow ultimately to the azygos system. (**b**–**d**) Central line insertion ultimately obtained using a combination of sharp recanalization (trans-septal needle), body-floss technique (jugular and femoral access), and venoplasty

Venous stenosis or occlusion should be treated with the least intensive intervention possible. Guide wire access beyond the occlusion is an essential first step. If stiff or hydrophilic wires are unsuccessful, an endovascular sheath can be used in combination with a directional catheter and a stiff hydrophilic wire for microdissection through the occluded region. In some situations, an endovascular sheath/dilator combination or even a noncompliant balloon can replace the directional catheter (Fig. 9.9). If an occlusion cannot be crossed, a retrograde "rendezvous" approach (from the opposite side) can be attempted. Venous recanalization using a needle or radiofrequency wire has been described.

Augmentation of the recanalized lumen may be necessary to insert the desired catheter. Initial venoplasty may be performed with low-profile balloons over a 0.018-in. wire or using slightly larger caliber balloons over a 0.035-in. wire. In children, very high-pressure balloons are almost never required. Conventional noncompliant balloons of 8–16 atmospheres burst pressure are usually adequate. The final balloon diameter can be oversized by 1–2 mm compared to the normal diameter of the vein. If more aggressive interventions or larger caliber balloons are planned, it is prudent to consult surgical backup in the event of venous perforation or rupture.

Catheter Removal and Replacement

PICC and Tunneled Catheters

While non-tunneled catheters are simply removed by gentle traction, removal of a cuffed catheter requires blunt dissection. When a cuff is very deep, a cutdown may be required in order to remove the catheter. The explanted catheter should be measured to assure that catheter fracture or embolization has not occurred.

Ports

Indwelling ports are explanted by making an incision wide enough to remove the port hub and then using a combination of blunt and sharp dissection to clear away the fibrous tissue that normally envelops the hub. The sharp tip of a towel clamp can be used to grasp one of the suture holes in the base of the hub, making it much easier to pull the hub free. The wound is then closed in the same manner as when the port was inserted.

Catheter Exchange

Exchange over a wire can be performed if the insertion site is uncomplicated. A peel-away sheath can be inserted over the wire prior to insertion of the catheter if desired.

When replacing ports or tunneled hemodialysis catheters, it is possible to remove the old catheter over one or even two guide wires (one through each lumen) through the original subcutaneous tunnel, although it can be problematic advancing the new catheter through the venotomy site, especially if the tract is sharply angled. In some cases a peel-away sheath can be placed over the wire(s) in such a manner that the tip of the sheath is intravascular when the dilator is removed. Again, if the tract is sharply angled, this may be difficult and uncomfortable for the patient, and the angulation may lead to premature splitting of the tip of the sheath.

If the catheter is replaced over a wire, a contrast study can be performed through the existing catheter after pulling the catheter back so that it remains intravascular. This may show that a fibrin sheath remains like a cast of the catheter. Replacement with a new catheter may simply slip into the old fibrin sheath. If a residual sheath is demonstrated, it can be disrupted with inflation of a relatively low-pressure balloon.

Documentation and Communication

After initial consultation with the referring physician, the interventional radiologist is responsible for providing a recommendation based on the patient or treatment need. Informed consent and treatment undertaken is then documented. It is important to communicate any significant deviations from standard technique, adverse events, or unexpected findings.

If unexpected complications occur during the procedure, it is helpful to discuss the findings with the referring clinician prior to progressing to non-emergent salvage procedures. Emergent salvage procedures should be undertaken without delay as in any other circumstance. If further discussion or informed consent issues require, elective procedures can be delayed until these important details are completed.

Research reporting standards for CVA have been established for adults. Pediatric reporting standards are under development and should soon be available from the Society of Interventional Radiology.

Appendix: Central Venous Access Procedure and Outcome Measures

Guidelines are available in the literature for quality improvement [2] prevention of catheter-related infections [3] and reporting standards [4] for CVC placement. To improve outcome and quality assurance analysis, it may be helpful to record the following information for each CVA device referral or deployment:

1. Demographic information (patient name, unique identification number, date and time of procedure, age, sex, weight, date of birth, etc.)
2. Underlying disease, patient acuity, comorbid illness, ASA class, competence of patient, or primary caregiver
3. Any contraindicating or complicating factors
   (a) Coagulopathy
   (b) Fever, sepsis, known infection, immunodeficiency, nutritional status
   (c) Venous stenosis
   (d) Acute thrombosis
   (e) Local skin infection
4. Referring service provider, inpatient or outpatient status
5. Provider or patient preference for CVC device or position
6. Indication(s) for venous access placement or replacement, intended function (e.g., dialysis, plasmapheresis, phlebotomy, simultaneous delivery of medications that cannot be mixed)
7. Anticipated endpoint for venous access
8. Provider responsible for access (interventionalist, surgeon, nurse, etc.)
9. Procedure location (interventional suite, operating room, bedside, etc.)
10. Provider responsible for anesthesia/sedation (anesthesiologist, nurse, etc.)
11. Preprocedural interventions (e.g., antibiotics, blood products, imaging)
12. Initial access
    (a) Entry side and site (e.g., basilic vein, internal jugular vein, common femoral vein)
    (b) Method (e.g., visual, fluoroscopic venography, ultrasound)
    (c) Device (e.g., angiocatheter, single-wall needle)
    (d) Number and location of unsuccessful and successful attempts
    (e) Complications (e.g., arterial puncture, pneumothorax)
    (f) Reason for deferral, discontinuation, or failure, if insertion not completed
13. Access device and position
    (a) Catheter manufacturer, description, lumen number and diameter, final length, composition, coating or impregnation, etc.
    (b) Implanted, tunneled, or direct? (if tunneled, length and exit site)
    (c) Cuffed or uncuffed? (if cuffed, material and position)
    (d) Tip position and catheter function (satisfactory position? How were position and function confirmed?)
    (e) Method of catheter fixation, wound closure, and dressing
14. Equipment and supplies used, cost
15. Procedure time, fluoroscopy time, or estimated radiation dose
16. Type, duration, and adequacy of anesthesia/sedation/analgesia
17. Procedural complications (e.g., venospasm, extravasation) and management
18. Adjunctive therapies required (e.g., papaverine, nitroglycerine, tPA, hot packs)
19. Complications, including
    (a) Catheter-related infection (include dates)
    - Type (phlebitis, catheter-related sepsis, bacteremia, colonization, exit site, tunnel or pocket infection, etc.)
    - Suspected (basis) or proven (method and results)
    - Management (e.g., antibiotics, catheter removal, repeat cultures)

    - Result of catheter tip and blood cultures
    - Outcome
  (b) Catheter dysfunction (include dates)
    - Type (e.g., phlegmasia, extravasation or infiltration, fracture, fragment embolization, etc.)
    - Management
    - Outcome
  (c) Occlusion, fibrin sheath formation, or thrombosis (include dates)
    - Method of diagnosis or documentation
    - Location and extent
    - Management
    - Outcome
  (d) Dislodgment, migration, or malposition (include dates)
    - Method of diagnosis or documentation
    - Management
    - Outcome
20. Other catheter-related complications or interventions
21. Complications, additional details
  (a) Major
    - Admission to hospital for therapy
    - Unplanned increase in level of care
    - Prolonged hospitalization
    - Permanent adverse sequelae
    - Death
  (b) Minor
    - No sequelae
    - Nominal therapy
    - Short hospital stay (for observation)
  (c) Procedurally related (within 24 h of insertion)
  (d) Early (within 30 days of placement)
  (e) Late
22. Removal or replacement (reason and date; endpoint achieved?)

Chapter Summary

Indications
- See Table 9.1

Contraindications
- Active infection
- Coagulopathy

Preprocedure Workup
- Venous access referral
- Review history for complication risks (Table 9.2)
- Review venous history and applicable imaging
- Choose access route and device
- Consider CBC, PT/INR, PTT, and electrolytes:
  - Platelets >50,000 U and INR ≤1.5 for CVL/port
  - Assess K^+ and Ca^{2+} in at-risk patients
- No scientific support for antibiotic prophylaxis at this time

Equipment
- Innumerable catheter choices based on need:
  - Temporary vs. permanent
  - Number of lumens
  - Flow rates required
  - Specific needs: CT compatible, antibiotic coated
- See Table 9.3 for size ranges.
- PICC:
  - Sizes available that allow IR intervention as small as 1.9 Fr single lumen and 2.6 Fr double lumen
  - 3–4 Fr average size for pediatric patients
- CVL (tunneled catheters):
  - Single, double, and triple lumen
  - Apheresis/dialysis
    - 6–14 Fr
- Ports:
  - Single, double, CT compatible

Procedure Technique

CVA Insertion
- Local, sedation, or GA based on device and patient requirements
- Position to allow access
- Prep and drape skin:
  - 2 % chlorhexidine
  - Consider 1 % chlorhexidine or Betadine in premature infant
- Obtain access:
  - Ultrasound, occasionally venography
- Insert guide wire
- Prepare pocket (port), tunnel catheter if required
- Place peel-away sheath
- Measure catheter:
  - Surface measurement or wire techniques

- Advance catheter
- Assure adequate tip position and function:
  - Reposition if necessary
- Fix, heparinize, and dress catheter

Catheter Removal/Replacement

- Blunt dissection for cuffed catheters:
  - Cutdown may be required if very deep
  - Measure catheter
- Sharp and blunt dissection for port removal
- Can often be exchanged over a wire:
  - May require dilation at venotomy site
  - Consider balloon disruption of fibrin sheath

Recanalization

- Wire, sheath, needle, or RF wire could be used to cross occlusion:
  - Use least-invasive method possible
- Noncompliant usually adequate:
  - Can oversize balloon by 1–2 mm
  - High-pressure balloons not often required
- Consider surgical backup and have stents available for higher-risk procedures

Postprocedure Care

- No specific requirements
- Consider analgesia for CVLs/ports

Complications

- Procedural:
  - Air embolism
  - Pneumothorax
  - Arterial puncture
  - Catheter perforation/cardiac tamponade (early or late)
- Mechanical:
  - Device dysfunction
    - Catheter "kink"
    - Tip malposition
    - Disconnection/catheter breakage
  - Wound dehiscence
  - Tissue swelling
- Infectious

Follow-Up

- None specific

References

1. Kevin MB, Christopher H, Megan EB, Elan DC, John JC, Charles RF. Long-term central venous access in pediatric patients at high risk: conventional versus antibiotic agent–impregnated catheters. JVIR. 2014;25(2).
2. Lewis CA, Allen TE, Burke DR, et al. Quality improvement guidelines for central venous access. J Vasc Interv Radiol. 2003;14:S231–5.
3. Miller DL, O'Grady NP. Guidelines for the prevention of intravascular catheter-related infections: recommendations relevant to interventional radiology. J Vasc Interv Radiol. 2003;14:S355–8.
4. Silberzweig JE, Sacks D, Khorsandi AS, Bakal CW. Reporting standards for central venous access. J Vasc Interv Radiol. 2003;14:S443–52.

Suggested Reading

Dubois J, et al. Incidence of deep vein thrombosis related to peripherally inserted central catheters in children and adolescents. CMAJ. 2007;177(10):1185–90.

Baskin KM, et al. Cavoatrial junction and central venous anatomy: implications for central venous access tip position. J Vasc Interv Radiol. 2008;19(3):359–65.

Management of Varicocele in Pediatrics

10

Josée Dubois and Laurent Garel

Introduction

Varicocele is an abnormal dilatation of the pampiniform plexus. The incidence in the general population is between 15 and 17 %. In young boys, below 10 years of age, the incidence is approximately 1 % and in late adolescence increases to 15 % [1]. Ninety percent of varicoceles are unilateral and on the left side. Ten percent are bilateral. Isolated right-sided varicoceles are reported in only 0.4 %. The diagnosis of an isolated right-sided varicocele necessitates further investigation to rule out retroperitoneal and abdominal tumors.

Causes

Varicoceles occur for a number of reasons:

1. Compression of the left renal vein between the aorta and superior mesenteric artery creating renal vein hypertension (nutcracker phenomenon).
2. Modification and remodeling of the venous system during the embryonic stage.
3. Absence of valves in the gonadal vein with progressive functional impairment (controversial cause because it was demonstrated at autopsy in men without varicocele).
4. Right angle entry of the left spermatic vein within the high-pressure system left renal vein [2].

Infertility

Varicocele is the most frequent cause of male infertility. The thermal effects of stagnant venous blood and reflux of adrenal metabolites and prostaglandins cause testicular alterations that result in sperm dysfunction. The diminished semen quality is a result of lower semen density with less mobility and abnormal form.

Barwell et al. [3] first demonstrated varicocele-related infertility and estimated the rate to be between 9 and 15 %. However, controversy remains regarding the relationship between varicocele and infertility. While varicocele is seen in approximately 40 % of males seeking evaluation for infertility, 85 % of men with varicoceles are fertile [1, 4–6]. Still, significant evidence in the literature supports the hypothesis that varicocele has a significant negative effect on the testis and fertility and that varicocele repair can reverse or prevent this effect [7–10].

The treatment of varicoceles associated with sperm parameter alterations in adulthood may result in normal fertility in only half of patients [11, 12].

J. Dubois, M.D., F.R.C.P.(C.), M.Sc. (✉)
L. Garel, M.D.
Department of Medical Imaging, Sainte-Justine Mother and Child University Hospital Center, 3175 Cote Ste-Catherine Road, Montreal, QC, Canada H3T 1C5
e-mail: josee-dubois@ssss.gouv.qc.ca; laurent_garel@ssss.gouv.qc.ca

M. Temple and F.E. Marshalleck (eds.), *Pediatric Interventional Radiology: Handbook of Vascular and Non-Vascular Interventions*, DOI 10.1007/978-1-4419-5856-3_10,

Diagnosis

The patients are referred to the imaging department mostly for scrotal pain or discomfort. The diagnosis is made by physical examination. Dubin and Amelar [13] described a grading system for the clinical diagnosis of varicocele:

Grade 0 = not palpable

Grade 1 = palpable only with the patient standing and performing a Valsalva maneuver

Grade 2 = a moderate varicocele palpable without Valsalva

Grade 3 = a large varicocele that is visible without the need for palpation

To confirm the diagnosis, an abdominal ultrasound will rule out renal or abdominal pathology, and high-resolution, real-time ultrasound with color Doppler flow is used to assess the testicles. Ultrasonography can determine the testes volume and detect subclinical varicoceles. The grading system for Doppler ultrasonography is:

Grade 1 = the absence of varicose veins but venous reflux with Valsalva

Grade 2 = the presence of varicose veins >3 mm in diameter with the presence of venous reflux during a Valsalva maneuver

Grade 3 = the presence of varicose veins >3 mm with the presence of venous reflux without Valsalva maneuver

Anatomy

The left internal spermatic vein (ISV) joins the left renal vein. At the level of the femoral head, the ISV divides in multiple venous channels called the pampiniform plexus, draining the venous blood from the testicle. The right ISV joins directly into the inferior vena cava (IVC) on the anterolateral wall just below the right renal vein.

Variations of the classic pattern have to be recognized. On the right, the ISV can drain in the right renal vein in 8 % and by multiple terminating veins in the IVC and the renal vein in 16 %. On the left side, multiple terminating veins in the left renal vein can be seen in 20 % of cases. Rarely, one of multiple branches may terminate in the infrarenal IVC [14, 15].

Multiple collateral communications exist between the retroperitoneal, peritoneal, adrenal, and portal veins. Cross-communication between the left and right ISVs at the level of L3 can be seen. The prevalence of the circumaortic left renal vein is 8.7 % and the retroaortic left renal vein 2.1 % [16]. The prevalence of left inferior vena cava is 0.2–0.5 % and double inferior vena cava is 0.2–3 % [16].

Bähren Classification (Fig. 10.1)

Bähren et al. [17] developed the following anatomic classification system:

- *Type 0* = no evidence of venous reflux on venography
- *Type I* = reflux into a single gonadal vein without duplication (Fig. 10.2)
- *Type II* = reflux into a single gonadal vein that communicates with accessory gonadal, lumbar, and/or iliac veins, or the vena cava (Fig. 10.3)
- *Type III* = reflux into a gonadal vein duplicated caudally, coalescing into a single trunk at the renal vein junction (Fig. 10.4)
- *Type IV* = competent valves at the renal/gonadal junction but reflux into a renal hilar and capsular collateral vessel that communicates with the gonadal vein (Fig. 10.5)
- *Type V* = reflux into a gonadal vein that drains into a circumaortic renal vein (Fig. 10.6) [18]

In our series of 93 pediatric varicoceles, we encountered 54 % type 1, 10 % type II, 17 % type III, 14 % type IV, and 5 % type V [19].

Indications for Treatment

The main indications for varicocele treatment in adolescents are pain, discomfort, testicular atrophy, and recurrence after surgical ligation. The timing of treatment is controversial in the literature. The Best Practice Policy Committee of the American Urological Association and the Practice Committee of the American Society for Reproductive Medicine recommend that adolescents and young men with a varicocele but a normal-size ipsilateral testicle or normal semen analysis, or both, should be offered annual follow-up monitoring [20].

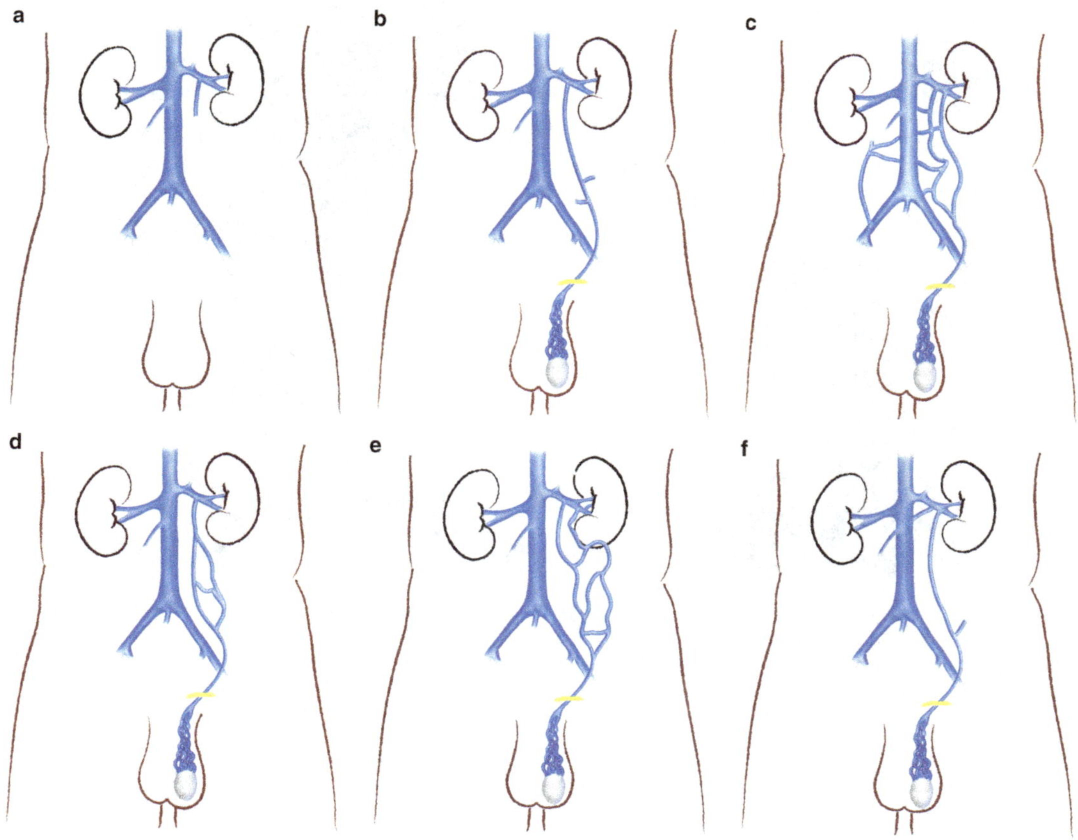

Fig. 10.1 Bähren classification. (**a**) Type 0 (normal), no venous reflux. (**b**) Type I, single gonadal vein without duplication. (**c**) Type II, single gonadal vein with accessory veins (gonadal, lumbar, iliac veins, IVC). (**d**) Type III, duplicated gonadal vein with a single trunk. (**e**) Type IV, competent renal/gonadal junction with reflux to collateral vessel(s). (**f**) Type V, gonadal vein that drains into a circumaortic renal vein

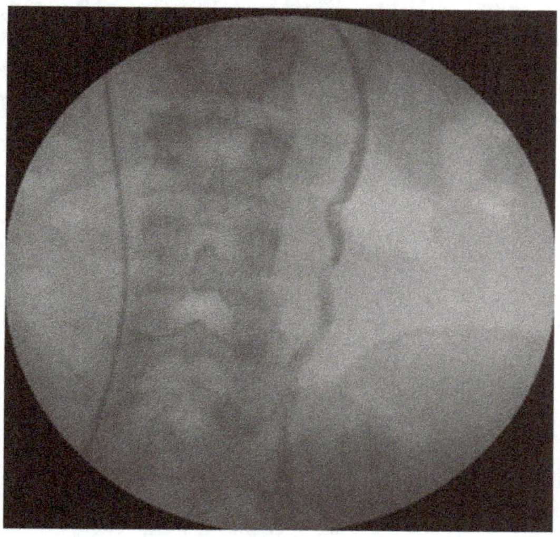

Fig. 10.2 A 12-year-old boy with left varicocele. Type I was demonstrated with a single gonadal vein

Equipment: Occluding Agents

Many agents have been used to occlude the ISV. The most frequently used agents are Sotradecol (STS), foam, and coils [2]. Some authors also reported varicocele treatment with glue, detachable balloons, particles, and hot contrast material [2, 12, 14, 16, 21]. Selected embolic materials are described below.

Sotradecol

1 % or 3 % sodium tetradecyl sulfate creates an endothelial surface damage-induced inflammatory reaction. STS has a low risk of extravasation, systemic dispersion, and adverse reactions.

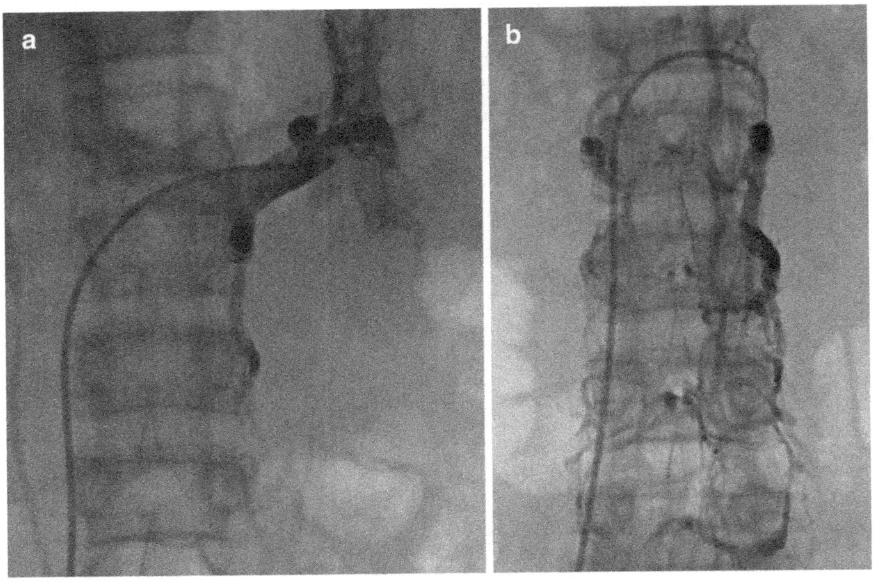

Fig. 10.3 A 14-year-old boy with left-sided varicocele. (**a**) Selective catheterization of the left renal vein shows the anastomosis of the internal spermatic vein (ISV) with the left renal vein. (**b**) ISV catheterization shows multiple collaterals with lumbar veins (type II)

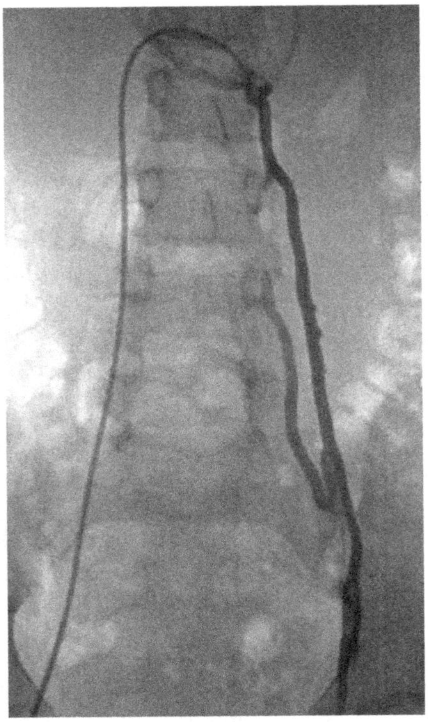

Fig. 10.4 A 13-year-old boy with type III varicocele with duplicated veins coalescing into a single trunk

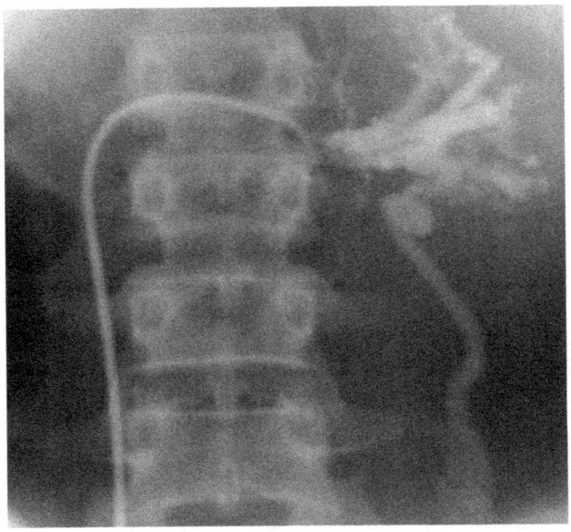

Fig. 10.5 A 14-year-old boy with renal hilar collateral vessels (type IV)

STS Foam

STS foam is a mixture of 2 mL STS, 1 mL Lipiodol, and 3 mL of air. It improves the distribution of the sclerosing agent and its contact with the endothelial wall. Gandini uses two 10 mL Luer-Lock syringes containing 1 mL of 3 % STS and 4 mL air connected through a three-way stopcock that is vigorously mixed to form the foam prior to injection.

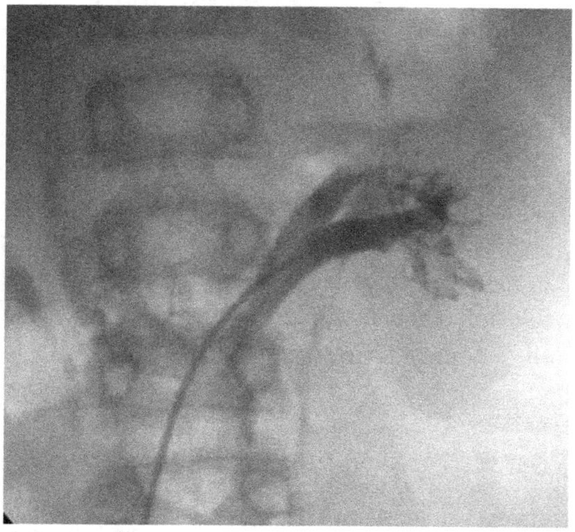

Fig. 10.6 A 15-year-old boy with a circumaortic renal vein (type V)

Coils

Some authors have reported good results with coils alone. However, early recurrence will take place with the endogenous lysis of the thrombus. We suggest the use of coils in association with a sclerosing agent. Also, late recurrence is frequently related to coil erosion. In Shlansky-Goldberg et al.'s study, the technical failure was 12 % and recurrence 4 % with coils in 173 varicoceles [22].

Glue (*n*-Butyl Cyanoacrylate)

Glue (*n*-butyl cyanoacrylate) is a tissue adhesive agent. This agent is permanent; however, recanalization can be observed. Sze et al. reported no recurrence in 17 patients who had undergone embolization for postsurgical recurrence [18].

Absolute Ethanol

Absolute ethanol is a permanent agent that induces thrombosis by denaturing blood proteins, dehydrating vascular endothelial cells, and precipitating their protoplasm; the agent denudes the vascular wall.

Treatment

Surgery

Surgery is performed by high retroperitoneal or transinguinal ligation of the ISV. The problem is the high frequency of venous collaterals, with either recurrence or persistence of the varicocele. Surgical recurrence rate or persistence of venous reflux in the pampiniform plexus ranges between 0 and 28 % [22]. Following a laparoscopic approach, the recurrence rate reported is 7–9 % [20], and for microsurgical technique, the recurrence rate is 0–3 % of cases [23, 24].

Percutaneous Embolization of Varicocele

Patients are treated on an outpatient basis under sedation or general anesthesia. See Chap. 3 for sedation information. Intraprocedural monitoring includes heart rate, blood pressure, and pulse oximetry.

When performing varicocele embolization, careful collimation, pulsed fluoroscopic acquisition, and appropriate gonadal shielding are important to minimize the patient dose. Videocapture is used rather than exposures.

Traditional technique involves the use of a sclerosing agent in the lower ISV and placement of coils in the proximal portion. Sandwich technique was described by Goffette et al. (Fig. 10.7) [25]. Distal occlusion is performed with a nest of coils just above the pubic ramus. Thereafter, sclerosing agent is injected to reach all potential collaterals. Finally, coil occlusion is performed proximally. This approach avoids the reflux of the sclerosing agent to the scrotum and prevents phlebitis of the pampiniform plexus. Success rate of this technique is 91 % and lack of recurrence is reported in 73 % of cases. Mazzoni et al. [21] reported no recurrence in 79.4 % and Feneley et al. in 81 % [26].

Access is usually performed through the femoral veins, although, when accessing the right ISV, a jugular or antecubital puncture may be helpful. Infiltration of the right groin with 1 % lidocaine without epinephrine (max: 5 mg/kg) is

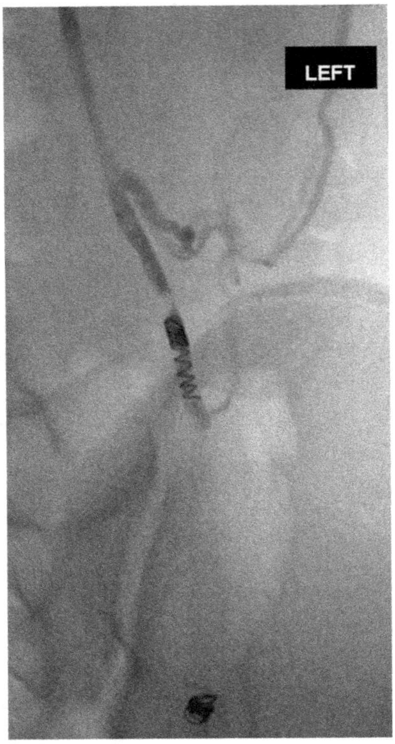

Fig. 10.7 Sandwich technique: distal occlusion is performed with coils (stainless steel: 25–5 mm –5 cm) just above the pubic ramus. Sclerosing agent (5 cc of Sotradecol) is injected. Finally, proximal coils (stainless steel: 25–5 mm –5 cm) occlusion is performed

performed at the site of the puncture. Under ultrasonography, the puncture of the right common femoral vein is performed with an 18G needle followed by placement of a long or short 7 Fr vascular sheath depending on operator preference. A 4 Fr catheter such as a C2 or C3 cobra is used to selectively catheterize the left renal vein and then the orifice of the left ISV. In problematic cases, a 4 Fr hydrophilic catheter or a microcatheter may be helpful. The ISV is injected with 10–15 mL of contrast material with Valsalva maneuver when possible. When the ISV is incompetent, the catheter is advanced to the distal ISV just above the pubic symphysis. Retrograde phlebography is performed in order to identify the presence of any collaterals. Embolization (with coils) is started below the origin of the lowest collateral, usually between the level of the acetabulum and the lower half of the sacroiliac joint, assuring complete thrombosis of the ISV while carefully avoiding coiling within the inguinal canal and distal embolization of coils/sclerosant into the pampiniform plexus. At our institution, we then inject 3–6 mL of plain or foamed 3 % sodium tetradecyl sulfate selectively into the gonadal vein. A few minutes later, some authors advocate gentle injection of contrast medium for the evaluation of the occlusion of the gonadal vein. In our opinion, delayed opacification is not necessary in most instances. The occlusion is then completed with proximal insertion of coils or a vascular occlusion plug.

Postprocedural and Follow-up Care

The sheath and catheter are removed and manual inguinal compression is applied to control hemostasis. Postprocedure bed rest is recommended for 4 h. The patient is discharged 6 h postprocedure. The patient is advised to limit their activity for 2 days. Any heavy lifting and sports should be avoided for 2 weeks. Pain is controlled with anti-inflammatory drugs if necessary. No antibiotic is needed. The assessment of results is based upon the follow-up clinical examinations and Doppler ultrasonography at 3 and 12 months.

Complications

The complications related to percutaneous varicocele sclerosing treatment are uncommon.

Fever, nausea, groin hematoma, reaction to contrast material, and femoral vein thrombosis (<1 %) are seen in less than 5 % of cases [2, 27]. Thrombosis of the pampiniform plexus can occur in 1–4 %. The symptoms are significant pain, swelling, or both. It is treated with anti-inflammatory medication and antibiotics.

Outcomes

Technical success rates range from 90 to 97 % with all agents described. The recurrence rate is between 4 and 27 % [2, 27]. Technical failure occurs in 1–12 % [19, 22, 28]. Recurrences are related to dilation of collaterals not seen at the time of the procedure. Recurrence after surgical failure is more easily managed with percutaneous sclerotherapy treatment.

In our series of pediatric patients, technical failure was more frequent with types II, IV, and V, respectively (22 %, 15 %, and 60 %) [19]. No technical failure was seen with types I and III. We did not assess the semen parameters. However, some adult studies report improvement of semen parameters in 27–78 % of patients after embolotherapy, comparable with the surgical correction.

Conclusion

Anatomic variants of the ISV are frequent in children. Types II, IV, and V represent a technical challenge. Transcatheter embolization of varicocele is a feasible, safe, quick, and cost-effective procedure with minimal morbidity in children. The preventive value of the treatment of varicocele in this age group remains an issue because there is no consensus about the endpoints of intervention.

Chapter Summary

General/Background Information

- Abnormal dilatation of pampiniform plexus
- 90 % left side, 10 % bilateral, 0.4 % right side
- Isolated right varicoceles require investigation for cause
- Most frequent cause of male fertility

Indications/Contraindications

- Pain, discomfort, testicular atrophy, recurrence postsurgery
- No contraindications

Preprocedure Work-up

- Ultrasound
- Blood work, antibiotic prophylaxis not required

Equipment

- 7 Fr vascular sheath—long or short
- Angiographic catheter
  - C2 or C3 cobra
  - 4 Fr hydrophilic catheter
  - Microcatheter
- Contrast
- Sclerosing agent
  - Sodium tetradecyl sulfate—plain or foam
  - Glue
  - Ethanol
  - Boiling contrast
- Coils/vascular plug

Procedure Technique

- GA or sedate
- Right femoral access for left varicocele
- Consider jugular/brachial access for right varicocele
- Define anatomy
- Embolize
  - Traditional technique: embolization, coils
  - Sandwich technique: coils, embolization, coil

Pearls

- Vein access: right antecubital vein and jugular vein approach aid in cannulation of a right-sided varicocele. Femoral access is the authors' first choice for treatment of left-sided varicoceles.
- Valsalva maneuver is useful to facilitate catheterization and allows an optimal distribution of the sclerosing agent through the gonadal vein avoiding proximal migration.
- To improve opacification of the gonadal veins, the spermatic cord can be compressed between the thumb and index finger with the ipsilateral hand during Valsalva maneuver at the time of contrast injection according to Gandini [2].
- Failure can occur due to the presence of unopacified collateral vessels (e.g., internal iliac supply).

Postprocedure Care

- Bed rest × 4 h
- Limit activity 2 days
- No contact sports 2 weeks
- Anti-inflammatory medications for symptomatic relief

Complications

- Pampiniform plexus thrombosis
- Fever
- Nausea
- Hematoma

Follow-up

- Ultrasound at 3 and 12 months
- Sperm count

References

1. Diamond DA. Adolescent varicocele: emerging understanding. BJU Int. 2003;92 Suppl 1:48–51.
2. Gandini R et al. Male varicocele: transcatheter foam sclerotherapy with sodium tetradecyl sulfate–outcome in 244 patients. Radiology. 2008;246(2):612–8.
3. Barwell R. One hundred cases of varicocele treated by the subcutaneous wire loop. Lancet. 1885;125(3222): 978.
4. Evers JL, Collins JA. Assessment of efficacy of varicocele repair for male subfertility: a systematic review. Lancet. 2003;361(9372):1849–52.
5. Redmon JB, Carey P, Pryor JL. Varicocele–the most common cause of male factor infertility? Hum Reprod Update. 2002;8(1):53–8.
6. Salzhauer EW, Sokol A, Glassberg KI. Paternity after adolescent varicocele repair. Pediatrics. 2004;114(6): 1631–3.
7. Gat Y et al. Induction of spermatogenesis in azoospermic men after internal spermatic vein embolization for the treatment of varicocele. Hum Reprod. 2005; 20(4):1013–7.
8. Gat Y et al. Varicocele: a bilateral disease. Fertil Steril. 2004;81(2):424–9.
9. Gat Y, Gornish M. Re: varicocele. Where, why and, if so, how? J Urol 2005;173(6):2208; author reply 2208–9.
10. Greenfield SP, Seville P, Wan J. Experience with varicoceles in children and young adults. J Urol. 2002; 168(4 Pt 2):1684–8. discussion 1688.
11. Onozawa M et al. Clinical study of varicocele: statistical analysis and the results of long-term follow-up. Int J Urol. 2002;9(8):455–61.
12. Schlesinger MH, Wilets IF, Nagler HM. Treatment outcome after varicocelectomy. A critical analysis. Urol Clin North Am. 1994;21(3):517–29.
13. Dubin L, Amelar RD. Varicocele. Urol Clin North Am. 1978;5(3):563–72.
14. Grieme B, Venbrux A. Management of male varicocele. In: Mauro MA et al., editors. Image-guided interventions. Philadelphia: Saunders/Elsevier; 2008. p. 887–92.
15. Lechter A et al. Anatomy of the gonadal veins: a reappraisal. Surgery. 1991;109(6):735–9.
16. Bass JE et al. Spectrum of congenital anomalies of the inferior vena cava: cross-sectional imaging findings. Radiographics. 2000;20(3):639–52.
17. Bähren W et al. [Side effects, complications and contraindications for percutaneous sclerotherapy of the internal spermatic vein in the treatment of idiopathic varicocele]. Rofo. 1983;138(2):172–9.
18. Sze DY et al. Persistent and recurrent postsurgical varicoceles: venographic anatomy and treatment with N-butyl cyanoacrylate embolization. J Vasc Interv Radiol. 2008;19(4):539–45.
19. Alqahtani A et al. Percutaneous embolization of varicocele in children: a Canadian experience. J Pediatr Surg. 2002;37(5):783–5.
20. Report on varicocele and infertility. Fertil Steril. 2004;82 Suppl 1:S142–5.
21. Mazzoni G et al. Varicocele: a multidisciplinary approach in children and adolescents. J Urol. 1999;162(5):1755–7. Discussion 1757-8.
22. Shlansky-Goldberg RD et al. Percutaneous varicocele embolization versus surgical ligation for the treatment of infertility: changes in seminal parameters and pregnancy outcomes. J Vasc Interv Radiol. 1997;8(5):759–67.
23. Kocvara R et al. Lymphatic sparing laparoscopic varicocelectomy: a microsurgical repair. J Urol. 2005;173(5):1751–4.
24. Orhan I et al. Comparison of two different microsurgical methods in the treatment of varicocele. Arch Androl. 2005;51(3):213–20.
25. Goffette P et al. Recurrence of varicocele after spermatic vein embolization in young patients: radiological aspect. Acta Urol Belg. 1995;63(2):55–6.
26. Feneley MR et al. Retrograde embolization and causes of failure in the primary treatment of varicocele. Br J Urol. 1997;80(4):642–6.
27. Reyes BL et al. Percutaneous embolotherapy of adolescent varicocele: results and long-term follow-up. J Vasc Interv Radiol. 1994;5(1):131–4.
28. Rivilla F et al. Percutaneous venography and embolization of the internal spermatic vein by spring coil for treatment of the left varicocele in children. J Pediatr Surg. 1995;30(4):523–7.

11 Venous Interventions: IVC Filters

Kamlesh Kukreja and Joao Amaral

Background

Deep venous thrombosis (DVT) is a significant cause of morbidity and mortality in North America. The incidence of DVT is estimated to be 0.07–0.14/10,000 children [1, 2] and 5.3/10,000 admissions. However, due to the increased complexity of medical conditions in children and the advent of new therapies, this incidence may be underestimated. In a recent multicenter retrospective review in the United States (2001–2007), it was noted that the number of pediatric admissions due to DVT increased by 70 % during the 7-year study period [3]. Pulmonary embolism (PE) is the most feared complication related to DVT. It occurs rarely in children with an incidence of 0.014–0.09/10,000 children [2] and 0.86–5.7/10,000 hospital admissions [1, 4].

The standard therapy for DVT is anticoagulation [5]. Vena cava filters are not recommended for systematic use. However, there are cases when children are at an increased risk of PE, and prophylaxis with anticoagulants have failed or might be contraindicated and undesirable. Anticoagulation carries a 3.75 % risk of acute major bleeding complication after 10 days of use and 10.3 % risk of late major bleeding after 2 years of use in adults [6, 7]. In children, the risk of major bleed related to anticoagulation for PE may reach up to 21.8 % as previously reported [4]. In such cases, a possible alternative is the placement of a vena cava filter to reduce the chance of a life-threatening PE. Vena cava filters are not intended to prevent formation of new clot or to promote lysis of existing clot.

The idea of caval filtration/PE prevention is not new. In 1874 John Hunter described femoral vein ligation [8] and in 1944 Homans suggested inferior vena cava (IVC) ligation to prevent recurrent PE [9]. Although effective, the side effects of these procedures (chronic venous stasis) were significant. In 1967, an umbrella filter (Mobin-Uddin) was developed, but the rate of vena cava thrombosis was still high (60 %) [10]. In 1973, Greenfield developed the first permanent stainless steel filter [11]. Since then, filter technology has significantly evolved and new retrievable filters are now available in the market.

The only randomized trial comparing anticoagulation alone vs. anticoagulation and vena cava filter in adults showed a lower rate of PE on the filter group vs. the anticoagulation alone at 2

K. Kukreja, M.D.
Department of Radiology, Cincinnati Children's Hospital Medical Center, 3333 Burnet Ave, ML 5031 Cincinnati, OH 45229, USA
e-mail: kamlesh.kukreja@cchmc.org

J. Amaral, M.D. (✉)
Department of Medical Imaging, University of Toronto, Toronto, ON, Canada

Department of Diagnostic Imaging - Image Guided Therapy Centre, The Hospital for Sick Children, 555 University Ave Room 2172B Toronto, ON, Canada M5G 1X8
e-mail: joao.amaral@sickkids.ca

M. Temple and F.E. Marshalleck (eds.), *Pediatric Interventional Radiology: Handbook of Vascular and Non-Vascular Interventions*, DOI 10.1007/978-1-4419-5856-3_11,

years' (3.4 % vs. 6.3 %) and at 8 years' follow-up (6.2 % vs. 15.1 %). However, the incidence of long-term DVT was higher in the filter group at 2 years' (20.8 % vs. 11.6 %) and at 8 years' (35.7 % vs. 27.5 %) follow-up [6, 7].

Indications

According to the Guidelines for the use of Retrievable or Convertible Vena Cava Filters from the Society for Interventional Radiology [12], some indications include:

1. Absolute
   (a) Recurrent venous thromboembolism (VTE) despite adequate anticoagulation
   (b) Documented DVT with a contraindication to anticoagulation
   - Head trauma
   - Intracranial hemorrhage, hemorrhagic stroke
   - Brain tumors
   - Severe bleeding diathesis
   - Acute or active internal hemorrhage (e.g., gastrointestinal bleeding)
   - Recent major surgery

   (c) Inability to achieve/maintain therapeutic anticoagulation
   (d) Complication of anticoagulation
   - Retroperitoneal bleed
   - Intracranial hemorrhage
2. Relative
   (a) Iliocaval DVT
   (b) Large, free-floating thrombus; large residual thrombus
   (c) Thrombolysis or mechanical thrombectomy of DVT with risk of PE
   (d) DVT or PE in patient with limited cardiopulmonary reserve
   (e) Poor patient compliance with anticoagulants
   (f) High risk of complication with anticoagulation
3. Prophylaxis
   (a) Major surgery in patient with high risk of postoperative DVT or PE
   (b) Trauma in patient with high risk of DVT or PE
   (c) Medical condition with high risk of VTE (e.g., Klippel-Trenaunay patient during sclerotherapy)

Contraindications

Some of the contraindications for vena cava filter insertion include [12]:

1. Absolute
   (a) Occlusion (total thrombosis) or the absence of vena cava
   (b) Lack of venous access (occlusion of jugular, subclavian, and femoral veins)
   (c) Infection at access site
2. Relative
   (a) Maximum diameter of vena cava (2.8 cm for some devices)
   (b) Minimum diameter of vena cava (1 cm) [13]

Filter Types

Multiple vena cava filters are available in the market (Table 11.1). These filters are not designed specifically for children. Therefore, pediatric interventional radiologists have to adapt and use vena cava filters available for adults. Besides the indication and expected length of use, filter diameter and filter length (pre- and post-deployment) are important elements to consider when choosing the device for caval filtration. Some filters will not open or work properly if they are not fully deployed. Vena cava diameter and infrarenal length of IVC are also important parameters to assess before and during vena cava filter insertion. In some cases, suprarenal deployment will be the only alternative.

Vena cava filters are classified as temporary, optional/retrievable/recoverable, or permanent:

- Temporary filters: these are filters that must be removed or repositioned after a certain time. They are usually tethered devices with a segment (catheter/wire) exiting through the skin at the insertion site.
- Optional or retrievable/recoverable filters: these are permanent filters with the option to be removed if caval filtration is no longer

Table 11.1 Vena cava filters currently available

Name	Manufacturer	Retrievable (R)/ permanent (P)	Access (delivery size, French ID)	Material	Maximal IVC filter (mm)	MRI compatibility[+]	Minimum IVC diameter (mm)	Retrieval set	Pediatric use
Celect	Cook	R/P	Femoral, jugular (8.5 Fr)	Conichrome	30	Y (1.5, 3 T)*	15	Jugular (11 Fr)	Y
Gunther tulip	Cook	R/P	Femoral, jugular (8.5 Fr)	Conichrome	30	Y (1.5, 3 T)*	N/A	Jugular (11 Fr)	Y
Gianturco-Roehm Bird's Nest	Cook	P	Femoral, jugular (12 Fr)	Stainless steel	40	Y (6 weeks delay)*	N/A	N/A	
Tempofilter II	B Brawn	P	Jugular (6 Fr)	Phynox	28	N/A	N/A	N/A	
Trapease	Cordis	P	Femoral, jugular, brachial (6 Fr)	Nitinol	30	Y (1.5 T)	N/A	N/A	
Optease	Cordis	R/P	Femoral, jugular (6 Fr)	Nitinol	30	Y (3 T)*	N/A	N/A	
Vena Tech LP	B Brawn	P	Femoral, jugular (7 Fr)	Phynox	35	Y	N/A	N/A	
G2	Bard	R/P	Femoral (7 Fr), jugular (10 Fr)	Nitinol	28	Y (1.5 T)	N/A	Recovery Cone system (10 Fr)	Y
G2X	Bard	R/P	Femoral (7 Fr), jugular (10 Fr)	Nitinol	28	Y (3 T)*	N/A	Snare (7 Fr), Recovery Cone system (10 Fr)	
Option	Rex Medical	R/P	Femoral, jugular (5 Fr)	Nitinol	30	Y (3 T)*	N/A	Snare and sheath combination	
Safeflow	Rafael Medical	P	Femoral, jugular (6 Fr)	Nitinol	27	N/A	N/A		
ALN	ALN	R/P	Femoral, jugular, brachial (7 Fr)	316 L amagnetic stainless steel	32	Y	N/A		
Vena Tech LGM	B Brawn	P	Femoral, jugular (10 Fr)	Phynox	28	Y	N/A	N/A	
Eclipse	Bard	R/P	Femoral (7 Fr), jugular (10 Fr)	Nitinol Electropolished G2X	28	Y (3 T)*	N/A	Snare (7 Fr), Recovery Cone system (10 Fr)	
Simon Nitinol	Bard	P	Femoral, jugular, brachial (7 Fr)	Nitinol	28	Y	N/A	N/A	
Meridian	Bard	R/P	Femoral (8 Fr), jugular, subclavian (10 Fr)	Nitinol-titanium alloy	28	Y (1.5, 3 T)*	N/A	Snare and 10 Fr sheath	N

[+]Information available at each company's website at the time of publication
*MR conditional

needed up to a predetermined time limit. They are excellent devices for prophylaxis (duration of PE risk is short) or as a bridge to anticoagulation. They are the preferred filters in children as there is an option to remove the filter and avoid a permanent device in a child with long life expectancy. They can also be left as a permanent device if the clinical status of the patient requires or if large thrombus burden is trapped in the filter.

- Permanent filters: these devices should not be removed or repositioned.

Pre-procedure Assessment

D-dimer levels help to detect recent thrombus formation or prothrombotic states. Patients with an elevated D-dimer [D-dimer normal levels <0.51 μg/mL FEU (fibrinogen equivalent unit)] and clinical signs/symptoms suggestive of DVT have a high probability of venous thromboembolic events. These patients should be further investigated with imaging.

Ultrasound is the best imaging modality to assess the venous system and to determine the extent of thrombosis. Compressibility on ultrasound of deep veins on the lower limbs (common femoral veins, superficial femoral veins, or popliteal veins), upper limbs, and neck (jugular veins) is considered the gold standard exam to detect DVT. Other sonographic signs include lack of augmentation in the vessel lumen, lack of respiratory variability, or absent flow on pulsed and color Doppler.

The anatomy and patency of the IVC are confirmed with US, CT, or MRI. Vena cava anatomy and size is further evaluated during the procedure with a venogram.

Computed tomography angiography (CTA) of the chest/pulmonary arteries is required in cases of PE suspicion.

If a decision is made to insert a vena cava filter, the rationale to insert a vena cava filter in a child is slightly different from an adult (Fig. 11.1). Children have a long life expectancy and the indication for filter insertion generally is not permanent. Therefore, retrievable/recoverable or optional filters are preferred.

Insertion Technique

Percutaneous approach is preferred as new lower profile delivery systems are available.

1. Obtain informed consent including potential risks [14] of:
   (a) Recurrent PE (3–5 %)
   (b) Complete occlusion of vena cava (5 %)
   (c) Filter migration, fracture, malposition, vena cava perforation (1 %)
   (d) Development of (new) symptomatic DVT if prophylactic filter is placed (3–20 %) [7]
2. Local anesthesia/sedation or general anesthesia according to the patient age.
3. Sterile technique.
4. Venous access: the vast majority of filters have a jugular or femoral delivery system. The most commonly used access sites are the right femoral vein and the right jugular vein. Alternative accesses such as the basilic vein, subclavian vein, and external jugular vein may be used in some patients. Access is obtained under real-time US guidance to reduce procedure length and potential complications such as arterial puncture [11] or arteriovenous fistula creation.
5. Place a ruler on the angiographic table parallel to the IVC to determine the IVC diameter and to help mark the location of the renal veins. Alternatively, modern angiography equipment may isocenter the patient and estimate the size of objects quite accurately. Measurements from pre-procedure noninvasive imaging methods (US, CT, or MRI) may also be used. Measuring the IVC is critical in children.
6. Perform A cavogram using a catheter (such as a pigtail catheter) positioned at the confluence of the common iliac veins (jugular or femoral approach) or through an angiocatheter placed in the non-involved femoral vein. Contrast volume injected depends on patient age/size. In general, 10–20 mL of contrast is needed to opacify the IVC. The maximum volume of contrast should not exceed 6–8 mL/kg [15]. Diluted nonionic iodinate contrast (50 %) can

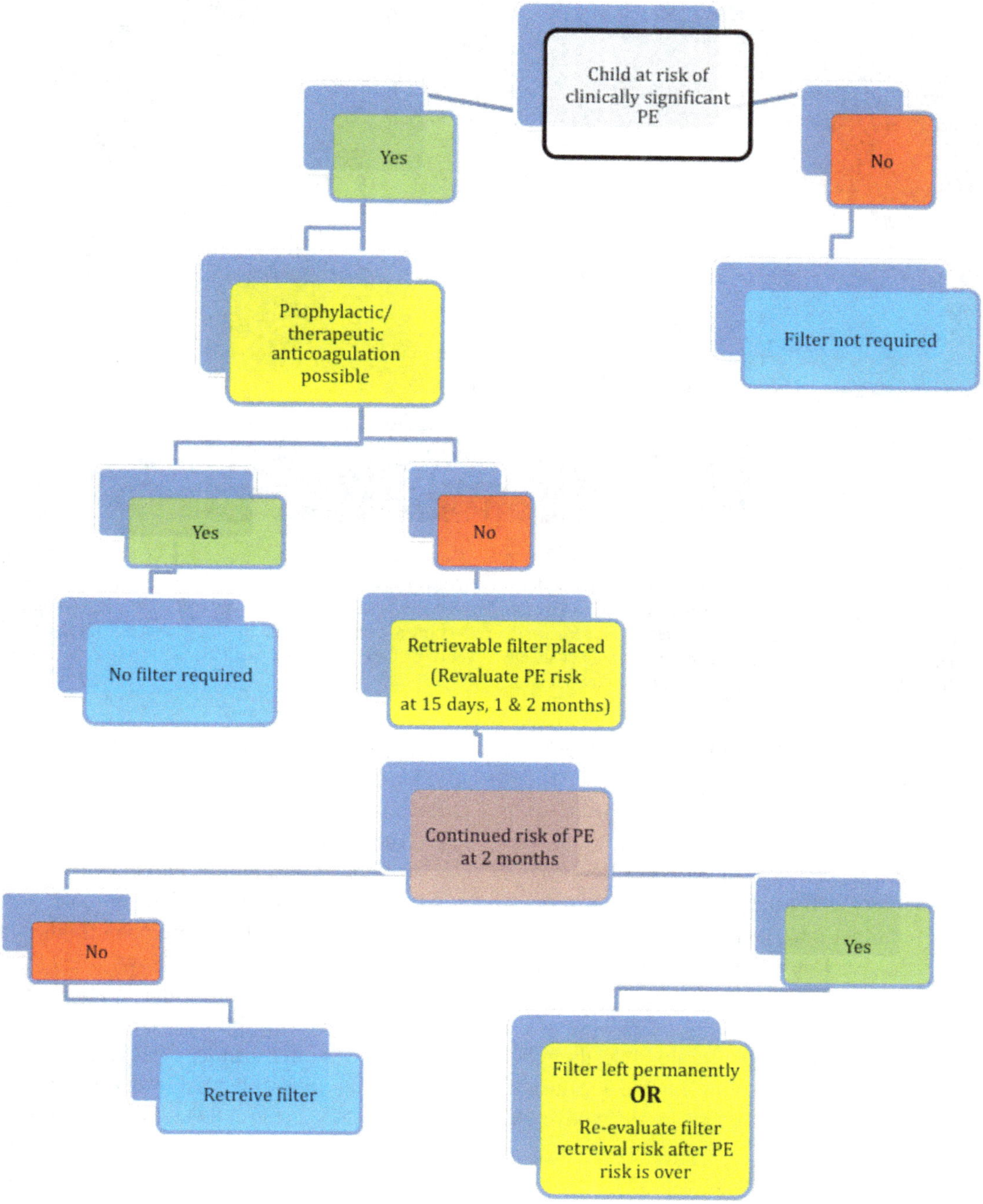

Fig. 11.1 Rationale algorithm to insert a vena cava filter in a child

be used to minimize contrast exposure. Digital subtraction angiography (DSA) with suspended respiration, filming at 2–6 frames/s, is ideal (Fig. 11.2a).

(a) The cavogram defines the vena cava anatomy, its patency and its size. Absent IVC with azygos continuation occurs in 0.15 % of patients [16]. Drainage occurs through the azygos venous system precluding IVC filter placement. Megacava (IVC with a diameter >28 mm) is found in 1 % of patients and may be a contraindication for

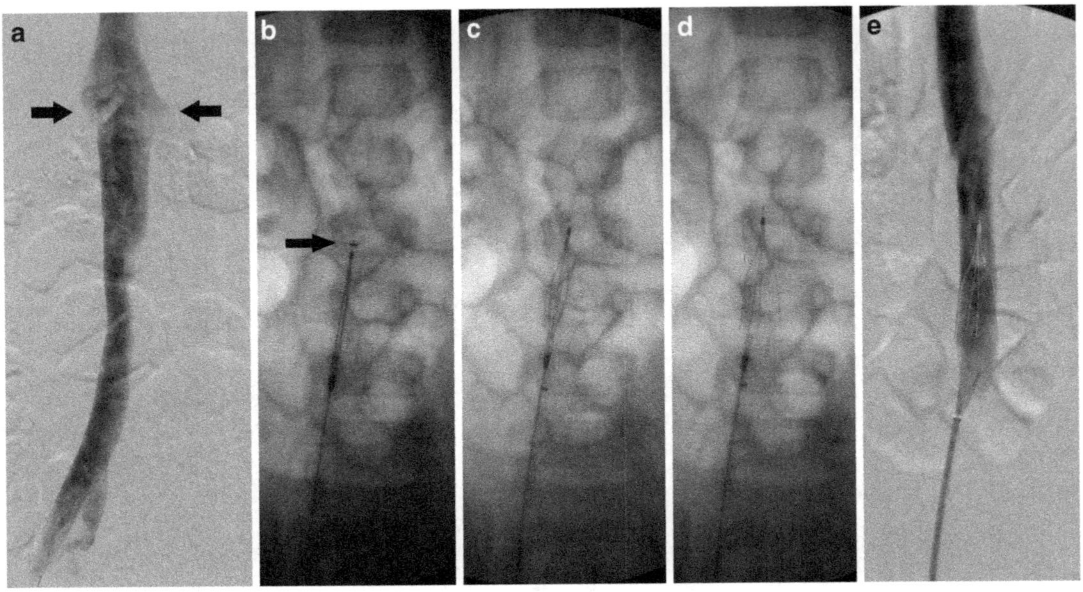

Fig. 11.2 Vena cava filter insertion technique (femoral approach): (**a**) Cavogram through the right common femoral vein delineating the inferior vena cava (IVC), its contours and diameter, the position of the renal veins (*arrows*), and the absence of clot in the lumen. (**b**) Introducer sheath with marker (*arrow*) positioned at the level that the hook of the filter (seen inside the sheath) will be deployed. (**c**) Introducer sheath pulled back exposing filter. (**d**) Vena cava filter released and deployed in the IVC. (**e**) Venogram to confirm position of the filter, clearance from the renal veins' ostium, and patency of IVC

some filters due to the potential risks of filter migration.

(b) The cavogram also determines the position of the renal veins, seen as a faint non-opacified inflow of blood in the pool of contrast in the IVC or by reflux of contrast into their orifices. Alternatively, the renal veins may be selectively catheterized with a guidewire to determine their locations.

(c) The cavogram detects possible thrombus in the IVC, assisting on the location to place the IVC filter (always above the thrombus).

7. Insert a stiff guidewire in the IVC, and advance a guiding/delivery sheath over the wire to the position where the filter will be deployed. The ruler and anatomical landmarks help determine the proper position. Serial dilation of the venous entry point may be necessary to allow insertion of large guiding/delivery sheaths.
8. Remove the guidewire (unless you are using an over the wire filter), check the correct orientation of the filter, and advance the filter to the end of the delivery sheath (Fig. 11.2b).
9. Recheck filter position.

(a) The majority of filters are placed in an infrarenal position (1 cm below the renal veins) to reduce the risk of renal vein thrombosis and filter migration (higher in suprarenal filters—27.5 % vs. 3 %) [17]. These may be challenging in small children where the infrarenal portion of the IVC is shorter than the filter length and in patients with scoliosis due to acute angulation of IVC (Fig. 11.3). Filter arms or legs should not be placed at the level of the renal veins due to the risks of filter dislodgement, filter tilting, filter fracture, and renal vein thrombosis.

(b) Suprarenal filters are reserved for situations where the thrombus originates from the renal veins, the thrombus extends above an indwelling vena cava filter, or the infrarenal IVC is too short (some children) and cannot accommodate the vena cava filter.

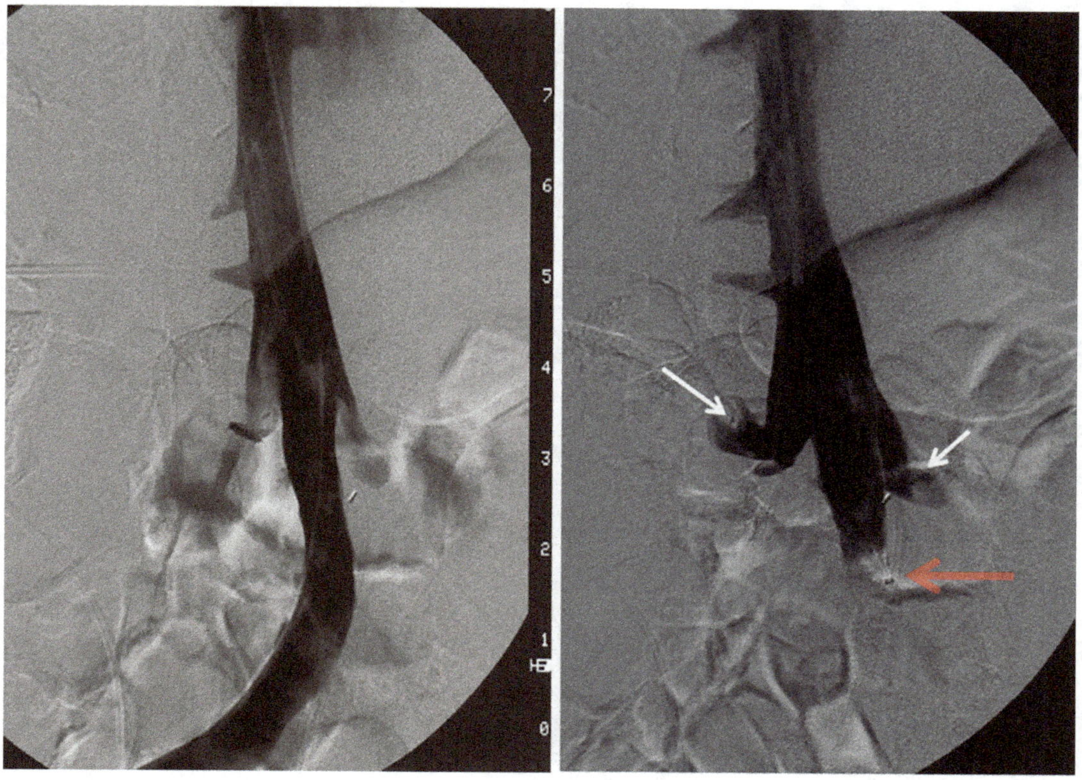

Fig. 11.3 Digital subtraction venography shows tortuous course of IVC due to severe scoliosis requiring partial placement of Trapease filter (*red arrow*) at the level of renal veins (*white arrows*)

(c) The most common anatomical variant is a circumaortic renal vein present in 4–5.5 % of patients [18]. The filter should be placed below the circumaortic left renal vein to prevent inadvertent clot bypassing the filter through the circumaortic left renal vein and main renal vein.

(d) Persistent left IVC occurs in 2 % of patients [19] and presents either as a single left IVC (1 %) or as duplicated IVCs (1 %). Typically the left IVC drains into the left renal vein. A suprarenal filter or two IVC filters should be inserted to protect the patient.

10. Deploy the filter (follow the manufacturer's recommendation) withdrawing the delivery sheath (Fig. 11.2) and allowing the filter to expand in the IVC (majority of filters) (Fig. 11.2d).
11. Pull back the delivery sheath into distal IVC and repeat the cavogram. Check the position of the filter and its orientation/degree of tilting (Fig. 11.2e).

Cava filter delivery through a jugular approach is slightly different as shown in Fig. 11.4.

Troubleshooting Insertion Procedural Problems

1. Filter is not deployed properly (legs do not open or filter is tilted): usually it has no consequences and no action is required. If significant asymmetry or tilting, consider retrieval and redeployment of the filter.
2. Filter completely in the wrong location: retrieve and redeploy filter through a jugular approach (for IVC filters) or deliver another filter above it.
3. Sheath kinks during filter delivery: advance sheath and filter as a unit and then try to advance filter; if no success, remove filter and exchange sheath [20].

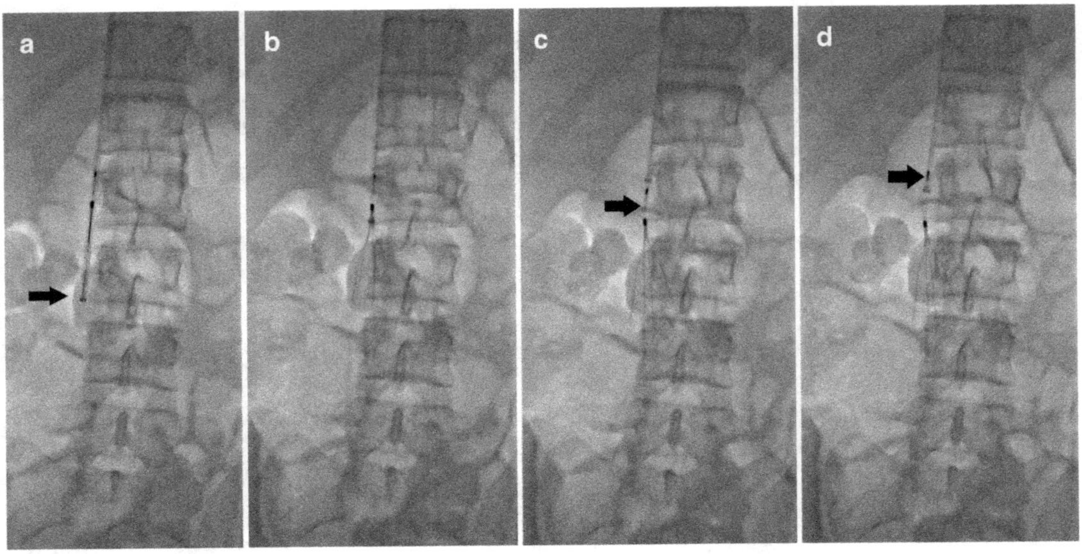

Fig. 11.4 Vena cava filter insertion technique (jugular approach): (**a**) Introducer sheath with marker (*arrow*) positioned at the level that the legs of the filter (seen inside the sheath) will be deployed. (**b**) Introducer sheath pulled back deploying filter's legs in the IVC. (**c**) Filter hook still connected to the delivery system (*arrow*). (**d**) Filter released (*arrow*) in the IVC

Special Considerations

- SVC filters lead to a higher major complication rate in comparison to IVC filters (3.8 % vs. 0.3 %). Its use is controversial as the real rate of PE related to upper limb DVT is not known [21].
- SVC filters utilize the same filter systems as IVC except that through jugular approach, the femoral delivery system should be used to avoid an upside-down filter.
- Duplicate SVC occurs in less than 1 % of patients and the left SVC generally drains into the coronary sinus. If needed, two SVC filters have to be placed.
- Transabdominal ultrasound alone has been used to guide IVC filter placement outside the angiography suite, but visualization of the IVC and renal veins is limited and post-deployment filter configuration cannot be determined [14].

Indications to Retrieve a Vena Cava Filter

1. The indication for caval filtration no longer exists.
2. The risk of significant or life-threatening PE is acceptably low (e.g., effective anticoagulation; post-prophylactic use—surgery, trauma).

Retrieval Technique

IVC filters can be retrieved by the commercially available retrieval kits (Cook, Bloomington IN; Bard Peripheral Vascular, Tempe, AZ) or by a combination of gooseneck snare and 6/11 Fr sheath [13].

1. Obtain venous access with ultrasound guidance (IJV or femoral vein depending on type of filter).
2. Place a 5 Fr vascular sheath. Use a 5 Fr catheter (like a JB 1) with a wire (0.035 angled

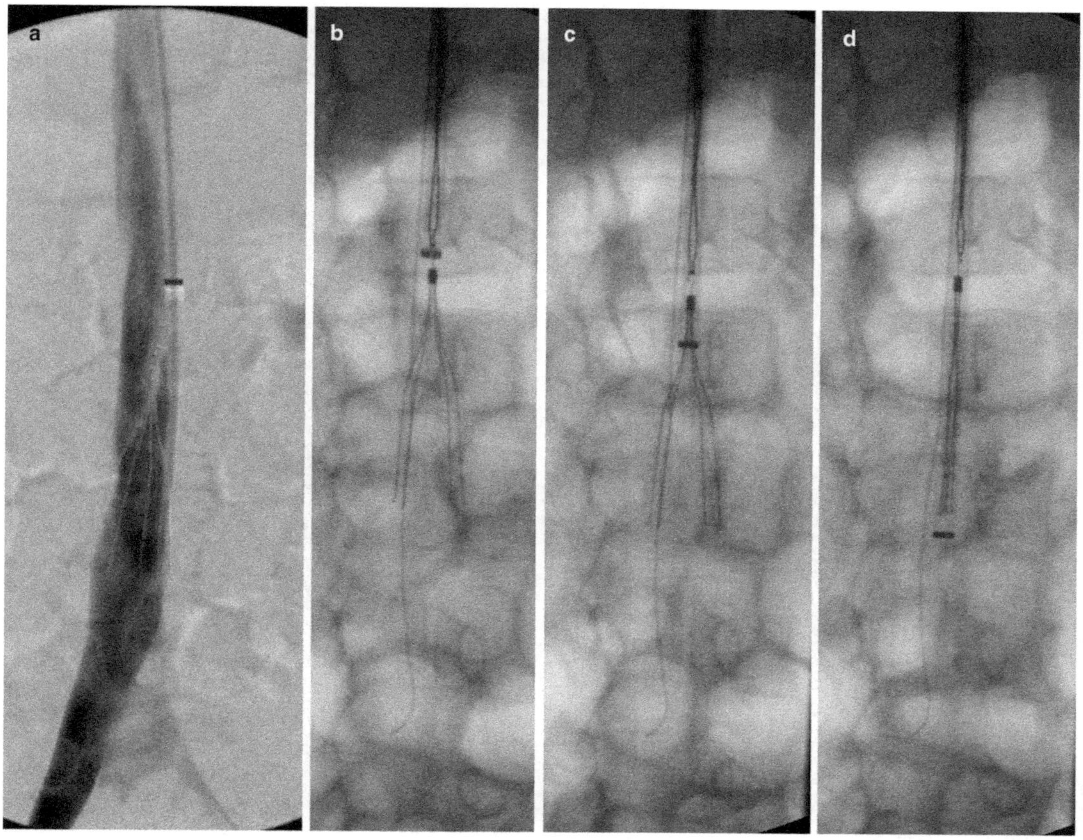

Fig. 11.5 Vena cava filter removal technique (jugular approach): (**a**) Venogram to confirm the absence of large clots in the IVC or entrapped in the filter. (**b**) Vascular sheath inserted and proximal hook of the filter snared (*arrow*). (**c**) Vascular sheath advanced over the filter, closing its legs. (**d**) Filter completely covered by vascular sheath, allowing filter removal

glide wire/straight Benson wire) to navigate distal to the filter.

3. Exchange directional catheter for a 5 Fr pigtail catheter. Perform pre-retrieval cavogram (Fig. 11.5a).
4. Assess for filter thrombus, hook and filter leg position, and any variations from placement venogram.
5. If more than 25 % of the filter has thrombus, reschedule filter retrieval after a month of anticoagulation therapy. If less than 25 % thrombus burden, the filter may be retrieved.
6. Exchange the sheath and the pigtail catheter for a snare and sheath combination or cone retrieval system (Bard Peripheral Vascular, Tempe, AZ). The wire is removed and the loop of the snare is utilized to snare the hook of the filter (Fig. 11.5b). A cone (Bard Peripheral Vascular, Tempe, AZ) can be used to grab the hook of the filter.
7. Once the snare/cone is snug, the sheath is slowly advanced (Fig. 11.5c) over the snare/cone to capture the filter within the sheath (Fig. 11.5d).
8. Remove filter or filter/sheath combination.
9. Perform a post procedure cavogram if removal is difficult.
   - With a Cook (Bloomington, IN) filter retrieval kit, three sheaths are present. The innermost sheath is a non-radiopaque black sheath which fixes the snare loop to the hook. The middle radiopaque sheath is primarily used to retrieve the filter. The outer blue sheath can be left in place after filter retrieval for post-retrieval cavogram.

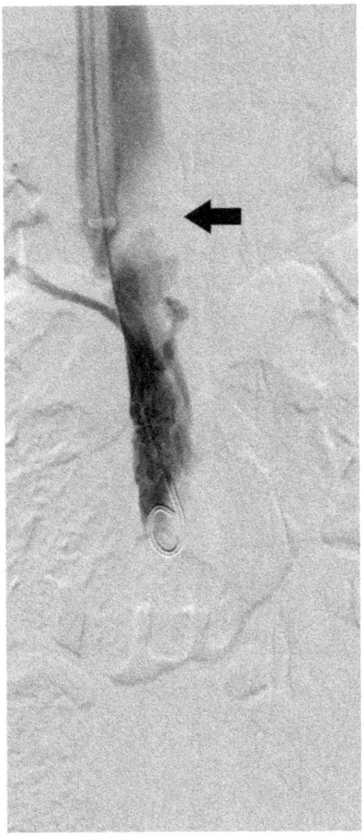

Fig. 11.6 IVC endothelial tear (*arrow*) following difficult filter removal

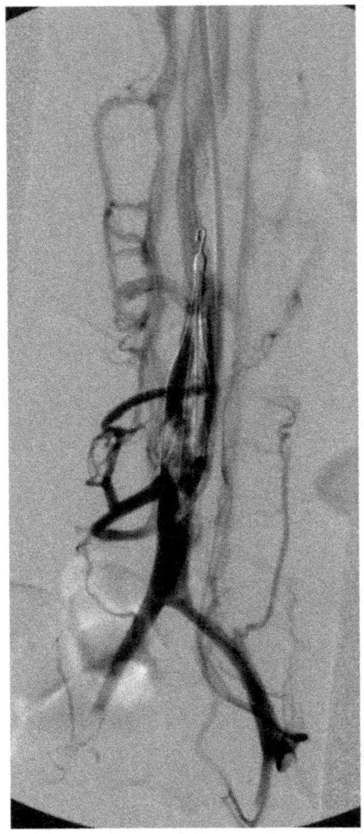

Fig. 11.7 Large clot (more than 25 %) entrapped in the IVC filter

- Post-retrieval cavogram is optional and usually not performed unless there was significant difficulty during filter retrieval. Cavogram may show damage to the IVC wall (Fig. 11.6).
- Filter retrieval by using endobronchial forceps, laser, and several other advanced techniques have been used in adults but have not been reported in children [22–24].

Troubleshooting Retrieval Procedural Problems

1. Filter hook cannot be snared: the hook may be close to or embedded in the IVC wall. Perform lateral venogram or CT (Conebeam or multislice CT) to assess position. Access femoral vein and a balloon can be used to correct filter tilt and snare the filter from the jugular access [22].
2. More than 25 % of thrombus in the filter (Fig. 11.7): mechanical thrombectomy can be performed and retrieval may be attempted if there is significant thrombus clearance.
3. Filters in place for prolonged periods may require significant force to remove the legs due to significant endothelialization.
4. Snare stuck to the filter hook: wire of snare can be cut from femoral approach and left in place.

Postprocedure Care

Immediate

1. Head of bed elevated to 20°, if jugular access.
2. Keep neck or leg still for 4 h.
3. Watch for bleeding at access site.

Mid- and Long Term

1. Watch for infection of access site.
2. Assess for limb edema, which may indicate DVT, post-thrombotic syndrome, or caval thrombosis.
3. If the filter is left permanently, filter position can be observed on future studies or scheduled yearly radiographs may be performed.

Follow-up

Follow-up is very crucial in children. Almost all children can receive retrievable filters as most of the currently available retrievable filters are approved for permanent use. Retrieval in children can be assured by scheduling follow-up appointments at 2 weeks, 1 and 2 months after filter placement to assess the continued need for the filter. The responsibility of retrieval is shared by the pediatric interventional radiologist and the referring clinician. IVC filter clinics [25] may be impractical in children since many institutions place 0–10 filters a year in children. Filters may be repositioned if prolonged protection is required [26]. Alternatively filters with long retrieval time like Celect (Cook, Bloomington, IN) and Meridian (Bard Peripheral Vascular, Tempe, AZ) can be used to reduce risks related to repositioning and anesthesia.

Outcomes and Complications

The limited numbers of studies in children is a major limitation to properly assess outcomes of IVC filters in children. The role of IVC filters in children in thrombosis prophylaxis has been assessed in small studies, which have shown that placement and removal of IVC filters is technically feasible in children with acceptable complications rate [3, 27]. Complications like symptomatic IVC penetration [28], IVC stenosis, and recurrent DVT [27] have been described in children. Other complications such as filter embolism or breakthrough PE, have not been described in children. The role of IVC filters in prophylaxis against PE in trauma patients is yet to be fully evaluated; however, the incidence of VTE and vena cava filters is uncommon in pediatric trauma [29].

In adults, complications include:

- Recurrent pulmonary embolism: 5 %
- Symptomatic complete IVC occlusion: 5 %
- Symptomatic insertion site thrombosis: 2 %
- Major filter migration (heart, lungs, iliac veins): <1 %
- Filter fracture (Fig. 11.8) with clinical consequences: <1 %
- Symptomatic perforation of major structures: <1 %

Postprocedural Problems and Management

In most postprocedural problems, if the patient is asymptomatic, no intervention is performed. Asymptomatic filter/filter fragment migration to the heart however, requires percutaneous or surgical removal. Specific situations are discussed below:

1. Suspected recurrent PE:
   (a) Confirm PE by imaging (pulmonary CTA).
   (b) Anticoagulation. If anticoagulation is contraindicated:
      - Abdominal X-ray for assessment of present filter:
        – If filter is malpositioned/migrated, place new filter.
        – If filter is in normal position, assess source of PE (new lower extremity DVT, renal vein thrombosis, filter thrombus, or no source found?): place filter above existing filter.
      - Upper extremity DVT: consider SVC filter (controversial).
2. Suspected filter/IVC occlusion:
   (a) Confirm diagnosis and level of occlusion by imaging.
   (b) Anticoagulation.
   (c) Consider mechanical thrombolysis, especially if anticoagulation is contraindicated: the goal is to restore the flow and not clear filter of thrombus.
   (d) Continued risk of PE: place filter above the thrombus.

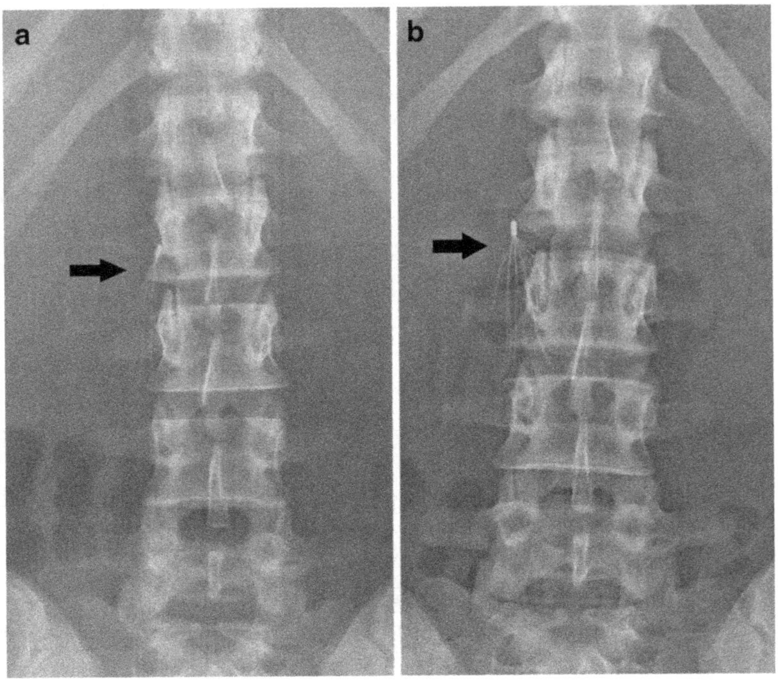

Fig. 11.8 (**a**) Upper legs of the filter bent (*arrow*). (**b**) Upper legs of the filter missing (*arrow*) due to breakage and migration to chest

3. Suspected filter migration:
   (a) Confirm by comparison to prior imaging.
   - If continued PE risk or if filter function is compromised, place new filter.

   (b) Migration to iliac veins: place new filter.
   (c) Migration to the heart: surgical or percutaneous removal even if asymptomatic.
   (d) Migration to pulmonary arteries: can be left alone.
4. Suspected filter fragment fracture:
   (a) Confirm by comparison to prior imaging.
   - If continued PE risk or filter function is compromised, place new filter.

   (b) Symptomatic due to fragment: CT to assess location.
   (c) Endovascular or surgical removal, if possible.
5. Suspected IVC wall penetration
   (a) Majority are asymptomatic and observed (Fig. 11.9).

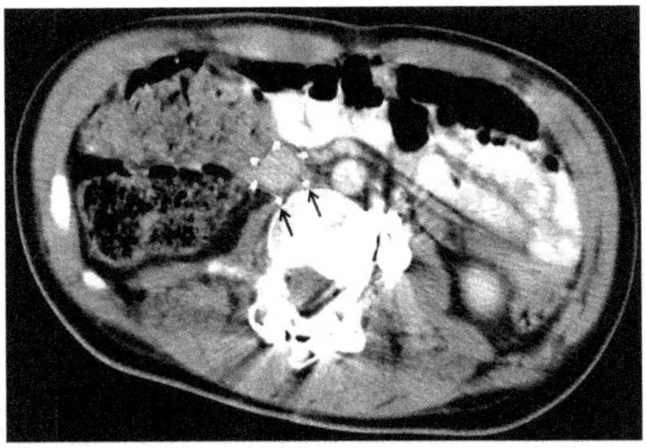

Fig. 11.9 A 16-year-old with asymptomatic IVC wall penetration. Axial CT image demonstrates filter struts outside the IVC lumen (*black arrows*)

   (b) Symptomatic: assess position.
   - Consider alternative diagnosis of symptoms.
   - Manage by analgesics or endovascular or surgical removal.

Chapter Summary

Background

- IVC filters are used to reduce chance of life-threatening PE
- Placed when anticoagulation failed or contraindicated

Indications

- See Page 142
- *Absolute*: recurrent VTE in anticoagulated patient, contraindication/complication/inadequate anticoagulation
- *Relative*: iliocaval DVT, free-floating thrombus, undergoing thrombosis intervention, poor cardiorespiratory reserve, poor compliance, or high-risk anticoagulation
- *Prophylaxis*: surgery, trauma, and medical treatment risk (e.g., Klippel–Trenaunay sclerotherapy)

Contraindications

- *Absolute*: Occlusion or the absence of IVC
- Lack of access or infected access site
- *Relative*: cava >2.8 cm (some devices) or <1 cm [13]

Equipment

- Temporary filters: must be removed/repositioned
- Optional/retrievable/recoverable filters: permanent filters that can be removed
  - Preferred option in children
- Permanent filters: should not be removed or repositioned

Pre-procedure Assessment

- Elevated D-dimer levels with DVT have high probability of PE
- Ultrasound: Doppler, compression, augmentation, respiratory variability
- CTA chest for suspected PE

Procedure Technique

IVC Filter Insertion

- Informed consent.
- Local anesthesia, sedation, GA based on age and availability.
- Venous access—jugular or femoral
- Localization:
  - Consider placement of ruler on table or isocenter patient
- Cavogram, DSA, 2–6 frames/s:
  - Anatomy, patency, size, thrombus distribution
- Insert delivery sheath over guidewire
- Place filter in position and withdraw sheath
- Deploy filter in appropriate position:
  - Usually ~1 cm below renal veins
  - Suprarenal deployment if infrarenal IVC is too short, thrombus is above indwelling IVC filter, or renal vein thrombus
  - Below circumaortic renal vein
- Repeat cavogram
- Assess filter legs, tilt, and location—revise if necessary

IVC Filter Removal

- Remove when placement indication no longer exists and <25 % thrombus burden in filter
- Consent, sedation, and venous access as above
- Cavogram (below filter)
  - Assess for thrombus burden and filter position
- Insert retrieval device (snare, cone, etc.) to capture filter
  - Hook can be endothelialized—lateral cavogram ± CT may be helpful
- Advance sheath over filter; remove filter
- Perform cavogram if removal is difficult
- Advanced techniques (laser, forceps, balloons, etc.) are not described in children

Postprocedure Care

- Bed rest 4 h
- Elevate head of bed 20° if jugular access
- Monitor for bleeding, site infection, and leg edema

Follow-up

- Remove filters in timely manner
  - Assess in the clinic at 2 weeks, 1 and 2 months

Complications

- Recurrent PE
- Filter/IVC occlusion
- Filter migration
- Filter fracture
- IVC penetration

References

1. Andrew M, David M, Adams M, et al. Venous thromboembolic complications (VTE) in children: first analyses of the Canadian Registry of VTE. Blood. 1994;83:1251–7.
2. van Ommen CH, Heijboer H, Buller HR, Hirasing RA, Heijmans HS, Peters M. Venous thromboembolism in childhood: a prospective two-year registry in The Netherlands. J Pediatr. 2001;139:676–81.
3. Raffini L, Huang YS, Witmer C, Feudtner C. Dramatic increase in venous thromboembolism in children's hospitals in the United States from 2001 to 2007. Pediatrics. 2009;124:1001–8.
4. Biss TT, Brandao LR, Kahr WH, Chan AK, Williams S. Clinical features and outcome of pulmonary embolism in children. Br J Haematol. 2008;142: 808–18.
5. Monagle P, Chalmers E, Chan A, et al. Antithrombotic therapy in neonates and children: American College of Chest Physicians Evidence-Based Clinical Practice Guidelines (8th Edition). Chest. 2008;133: 887S–968.
6. Eight-year follow-up of patients with permanent vena cava filters in the prevention of pulmonary embolism: the PREPIC (Prevention du Risque d'Embolie Pulmonaire par Interruption Cave) randomized study. Circulation. 2005;112:416–22.
7. Decousus H, Leizorovicz A, Parent F, et al. A clinical trial of vena caval filters in the prevention of pulmonary embolism in patients with proximal deep-vein thrombosis. Prevention du Risque d'Embolie Pulmonaire par Interruption Cave Study Group. N Engl J Med. 1998;338:409–15.
8. Mauro M, Murphy KPJ, Thomson KR, Venbrux AC, Zollikofer CL, editors. Image-guided interventions. 1st ed. Philadelphia, PA: Saunders Elsevier; 2008.
9. Neuerburg JM, Gunther RW, Vorwerk D, et al. Results of a multicenter study of the retrievable Tulip Vena Cava Filter: early clinical experience. Cardiovasc Intervent Radiol. 1997;20:10–6.
10. Kinney TB. Update on inferior vena cava filters. J Vasc Interv Radiol. 2003;14:425–40.
11. Athanasoulis CA, Kaufman JA, Halpern EF, Waltman AC, Geller SC, Fan CM. Inferior vena caval filters: review of a 26-year single-center clinical experience. Radiology. 2000;216:54–66.
12. Kaufman JA, Kinney TB, Streiff MB, et al. Guidelines for the use of retrievable and convertible vena cava filters: report from the Society of Interventional Radiology multidisciplinary consensus conference. J Vasc Interv Radiol. 2006;17:449–59.
13. Chaudry G, Padua HM, Alomari AI. The use of inferior vena cava filters in young children. J Vasc Interv Radiol. 2008;19:1103–6.
14. Kandarpa K, Aruny JE. Handbook of interventional radiologic procedures. 3rd ed. Philadelphia: Lippincott Williams & Wilkins; 2002.
15. Heran MK, Marshalleck F, Temple M, et al. Joint quality improvement guidelines for pediatric arterial access and arteriography: from the Societies of Interventional Radiology and Pediatric Radiology. J Vasc Interv Radiol. 2010;21:32–43.
16. Koc Z, Oguzkurt L. Interruption or congenital stenosis of the inferior vena cava: prevalence, imaging, and clinical findings. Eur J Radiol. 2007;62: 257–66.
17. Matchett WJ, Jones MP, McFarland DR, Ferris EJ. Suprarenal vena caval filter placement: follow-up of four filter types in 22 patients. J Vasc Interv Radiol. 1998;9:588–93.
18. Koc Z, Ulusan S, Oguzkurt L, Tokmak N. Venous variants and anomalies on routine abdominal multidetector row CT. Eur J Radiol. 2007;61:267–78.
19. Bass JE, Redwine MD, Kramer LA, Huynh PT, Harris Jr JH. Spectrum of congenital anomalies of the inferior vena cava: cross-sectional imaging findings. Radiographics. 2000;20:639–52.
20. Kaufman J, Lee MJ. Vascular and interventional radiology. Philadelphia: Mosby; 2004.
21. Owens CA, Bui JT, Knuttinen MG, Gaba RC, Carrillo TC. Pulmonary embolism from upper extremity deep vein thrombosis and the role of superior vena cava filters: a review of the literature. J Vasc Interv Radiol. 2010;21:779–87.
22. Iliescu B, Haskal ZJ. Advanced techniques for removal of retrievable inferior vena cava filters. Cardiovasc Intervent Radiol. 2012;35:741–50.
23. Kuo WT, Cupp JS. The excimer laser sheath technique for embedded inferior vena cava filter removal. J Vasc Interv Radiol. 2010;21:1896–9.
24. Stavropoulos SW, Dixon RG, Burke CT, et al. Embedded inferior vena cava filter removal: use of endobronchial forceps. J Vasc Interv Radiol. 2008;19:1297–301.
25. Minocha J, Idakoji I, Riaz A, et al. Improving inferior vena cava filter retrieval rates: impact of a dedicated inferior vena cava filter clinic. J Vasc Interv Radiol. 2010;21:1847–51.
26. Haider EA, Rosen JC, Torres C, Valenti DA. Serial repositioning of a Gunther tulip retrievable inferior vena cava filter in a pediatric patient. Pediatr Radiol. 2005;35:1135–8.
27. Kukreja KU, Gollamudi J, Patel MN, Johnson ND, Racadio JM. Inferior vena cava filters in children: our experience and suggested guidelines. J Pediatr Hematol Oncol. 2011;33:334–8.
28. Bogue CO, John PR, Connolly BL, Rea DJ, Amaral JG. Symptomatic caval penetration by a Celect inferior vena cava filter. Pediatr Radiol. 2009;39:1110–3.
29. Cook A, Shackford S, Osler T, Rogers F, Sartorelli K, Littenberg B. Use of vena cava filters in pediatric trauma patients: data from the National Trauma Data Bank. J Trauma. 2005;59:1114–20.

12 Hemodialysis Graft and Fistula Access and Intervention

Francis E. Marshalleck

Background/General Information

The incidence of renal failure in children is 1–2/100,000 as compared to 30/100,000 in adults. Although the method of dialysis depends on many factors, in some European countries, hemodialysis is preferred in children older than 5 years with peritoneal dialysis used in younger children and those less than 10 kg in weight [1]. The National Kidney Foundation (NKF) has developed the Kidney Disease Outcomes Quality Initiative (K/DOQI) guidelines that serve as the standards of hemodialysis access management. Methods of dialysis access that are used in patients requiring hemodialysis include (1) hemodialysis catheters, (2) arteriovenous grafts (AVGs), and (3) arteriovenous fistulae (AVFs). One of the current goals of the DOQI guidelines is to have an AVF placed in at least 50 % of patients with new onset renal failure and in at least 40 % of patients requiring hemodialysis. The DOQI guidelines also recommend that catheters should be used in less than 10 % of patients requiring hemodialysis [2]. This chapter will focus on the management of dysfunctional AVGs and AVFs.

F.E. Marshalleck, M.D. (✉)
Interventional Radiology, Indiana University School of Medicine, Riley Hospital for Children, 705 Riley Hospital Drive, Room 1053, Indianapolis, IN 46202, USA
e-mail: frmarsha@iupui.edu

In 1966, Brescia and Cimino successfully created a fistula between the radial artery and cephalic vein for hemodialysis. The fistula can be created using a side-to-side, end-to-side, or end-to-end anastomosis (Fig. 12.1). Similarly, an AVF can be created between the brachial artery and cephalic vein. In addition, the basilic vein can be transposed to a more superficial location and subsequently anastomosed to the ulnar or brachial artery. AVFs, once mature, have long durability; however, AVFs can fail due to surgical factors, competing collaterals, and inadequate size of the cephalic vein. In adults, a higher rate of maturity is seen when the cephalic vein is greater than 2 mm in size.

AVGs are synthetic grafts made of Dacron or polytetrafluoroethylene (PTFE) usually 6–8 mm in diameter. Nonsynthetic grafts include bovine carotid artery or venous grafts (cadaveric or noncadaveric). Loop grafts are usually placed within the forearm and anastomosed to the brachial artery and to the basilic or brachial vein (Fig. 12.2). Grafts in the upper arm are usually straight connecting the brachial artery to either the antecubital, cephalic, basilic, or axillary vein. Generally, the venous limb of a forearm loop graft is placed within the medial aspect of the forearm with the exception of reversed grafts where the arterial limb is located medially. AVGs can be placed within the groin to anastomose the femoral artery to the femoral vein or to the greater saphenous vein. AVGs are easier to cannulate and mature quicker but are

M. Temple and F.E. Marshalleck (eds.), *Pediatric Interventional Radiology: Handbook of Vascular and Non-Vascular Interventions*, DOI 10.1007/978-1-4419-5856-3_12,

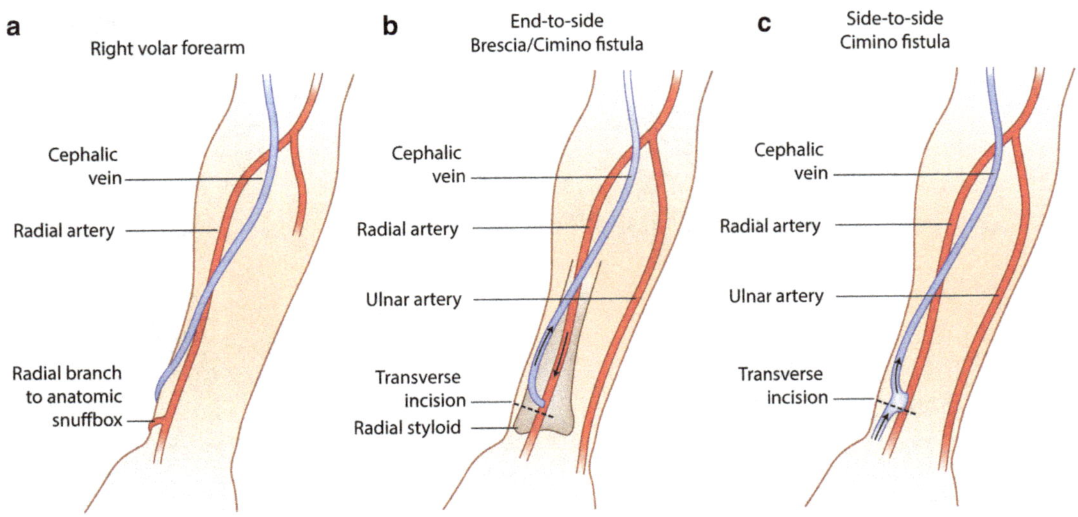

Fig. 12.1 Types of anastomoses seen in Brescia–Cimino fistulae. (**a**) Normal anatomy. (**b**) End-to-end anastomosis. (**c**) End-to-side anastomosis

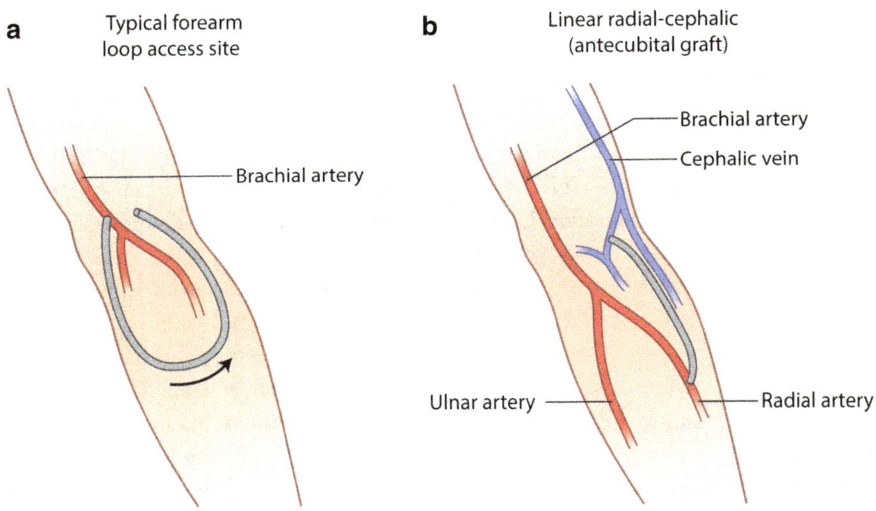

Fig. 12.2 Typical types of upper extremity grafts. (**a**) Loop graft. (**b**) Straight graft

less durable than AVFs [3]. It is generally recommended that AVGs be placed only if AVFs cannot be created.

Indications/Contraindications

A hemodialysis access is deemed dysfunctional if there is a hemodynamically significant stenosis, if the access (AVF) has failed to mature, if the access cannot be cannulated for hemodialysis, or if the access has thrombosed. A hemodynamically significant stenosis occurs when there is a greater than 50 % reduction in normal vessel diameter [2]. The most common cause of hemodialysis access dysfunction is venous outflow stenosis in greater than 80 % of cases. In AVGs, venous stenoses typically occur at the venous anastomosis but can also occur in a more central location. Subclavian and brachiocephalic vein

Table 12.1 Causes of hemodialysis access failure

1. Thrombosis
2. Stenosis
(a) Venous (80 % in AVGs, 25 % in AVFs)
(b) Arterial anastomotic (10 % in AVGs, 52 % in AVFs)
(c) Central (27 %)
3. Pseudoaneurysm formation (5 % in AVGs and 15 % in AVFs)
4. Arterial steal

Table 12.2 Measured flow rate parameters indicating access dysfunction (DOQI)

1. Direct intra-access flow measurement (Transonics) of less than 600 mL/min (AVGs) or less than 1000 mL/min (AVFs) or a decrease by more than 25 % over 4 months
2. Elevated static (venous limb pressure>40 % systemic pressure) or dynamic venous pressure (>150 mmHg at 200–250 mL/min)
3. Non-urea recirculation of >5 % indicating retrograde flow. Urea-based (two-needle method) recirculation of >10–20 % (AVFs)
4. Unexplained decreases in the amount of hemodialysis delivered (decreased Kt/V)
5. Elevated negative arterial pressure resulting in decreased blood flow

stenoses are typically result from prior placement of central venous catheters. In AVFs, the area of stenosis is typically within 3 cm of the anastomosis [3]. Arterial stenosis occurs in less than 5 % of cases (Table 12.1).

Hemodialysis access dysfunction requiring fistulography can be detected with various surveillance modalities (Table 12.2). Physical examination is an important monitoring tool [4, 5]. The loss of a continuous thrill indicates flow rates <450 mL/min and that an intervention is necessary. Other clinical indicators include prolonged bleeding after decannulation; extremity swelling; a rigid, enlarging, or abnormally flat pseudoaneurysm; a loss of a continuous bruit on auscultation; palpable outflow stenosis (AVFs); the presence of prominent skin veins; or a decompressed outflow vein (AVFs). Evaluation of central venous stenosis after surgical thrombectomy and evaluation of vascular steal are additional indicators for fistulography. The main indication for thrombectomy is to restore patency of a thrombosed graft.

The only absolute contraindication to intervention is infection within a thrombosed access. Relative contraindications include significant metabolic disturbance, right to left shunts, severe pulmonary compromise, significant contrast allergy, and severe right heart failure.

Central venous angioplasty is not advised in patients who are coagulopathic since venous rupture would be life threatening. In the treatment of thrombosed grafts, the use of tissue plasminogen activator is contraindicated in patients with recent cerebrovascular accident, active internal bleeding, recent surgical procedures, and the presence of an intracranial aneurysm. In those cases, mechanical thrombectomy rather than thrombolysis would be performed. Severe contrast allergy can be pretreated prior to the procedure.

Preprocedure Workup

A clinical examination of the AVF or AVG is important to confirm a thrombosed graft, absence of a thrill, to evaluate pseudoaneurysms, to evaluate for superficial collateral veins, and to evaluate location of the arterial and venous limb of the AVG. Ultrasound is a great tool for use in AVFs to evaluate patency of the anastomosis as well as location of thrombus and/or stenoses which will aid in determining the point of access prior to intervention. Cardiorespiratory examination is important to evaluate for fluid overload. If the patient has missed more than two dialysis sessions, it is important to rule out hyperkalemia. An ill patient with an elevated serum concentration of potassium greater than 5 mEq/L who has not been dialyzed may be better served with a temporary dialysis catheter. Emergent therapy of hyperkalemia is indicated especially with the presence of ECG changes if the serum concentration of potassium is greater than 6.5 mEq/L [6]. Obtaining coagulation values is recommended prior to central venous intervention.

Sedation

All children will require some degree of sedation during fistulography. Younger children under the age of 12 will likely require general anesthesia.

Older children greater than 12 years of age may respond well to moderate sedation. The majority will require general anesthesia for percutaneous thrombectomy.

Fistulography

The goal of fistulography is to image the arterial inflow, the entire fistula or graft, and the entire venous outflow including the central veins.

Fistulography: Arteriovenous Grafts

If the interventionalist is unsure which limb of the graft is venous or arterial, manually compressing the apex of the graft will result in absence of pulsatility within the venous limb with continued pulsatility of the arterial limb. The venous limb is typically punctured in an antegrade fashion pointing toward the venous outflow with subsequent contrast injection since venous outflow stenosis is the main cause of hemodialysis access dysfunction (Fig. 12.3). A second retrograde puncture of the venous limb may be required if the arterial inflow or intragraft stenosis of the arterial limb needs to be treated (Fig. 12.4). Alternatively, the apex of the graft can be punctured to allow access to both the venous and arterial limb. Once the venous outflow has been treated, the access can be reversed to allow intervention on the arterial limb [7]. A 6 Fr high-flow sheath is typically sufficient to allow placement of up to a 10 Fr balloon. Upsizing to a larger sheath will be needed for placement of a covered stent. In order to visualize the arterial anastomosis and the arterial limb, reflux fistulography is performed. This can be accomplished during balloon inflation when treating the venous outflow, by manual compression of the venous limb or by venous outflow compression using a blood pressure cuff with simultaneous injection of contrast. Alternatively, direct fistulography can be performed by catheterization of the arterial inflow through the retrograde venous limb access in order to visualize the entire AVG and arterial anastomosis.

Fistulography: Arteriovenous Fistulae

Ultrasound-guided puncture of the outflow vein will allow for easier access in veins that are prone to vasospasm. This is particularly important in AVFs that are not well matured resulting in a small outflow vein. Ultrasound evaluation of the outflow vein can also be extremely helpful in determining where to access the outflow vein by evaluating for the presence of stenoses and thrombus. A retrograde venous puncture (within the forearm or arm) will allow access to majority of stenoses as well as to the anastomosis thereby limiting the number of punctures (Fig. 12.5). Alternatively, the inflow brachial artery can be punctured in a retrograde fashion above the elbow using ultrasound guidance with subsequent

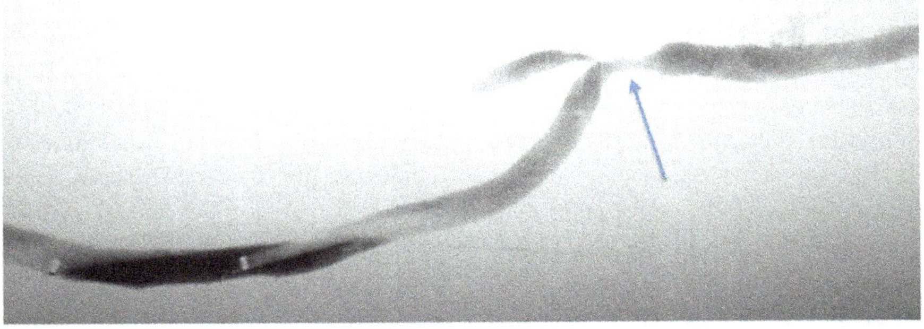

Fig. 12.3 Forearm loop fistulography post declotting procedure demonstrating a significant venous anastomotic stenosis

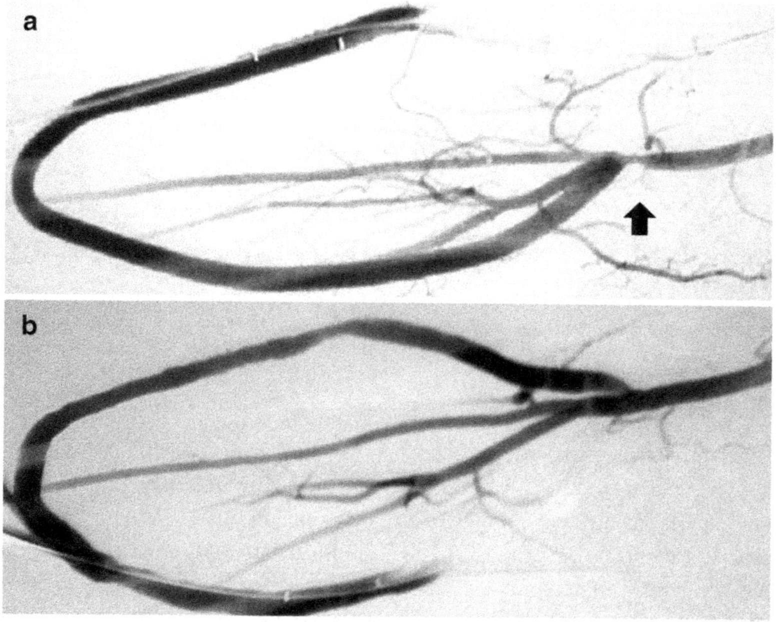

Fig. 12.4 (**a**) Forearm loop fistulography post-declot procedure demonstrating a significant arterial anastomotic stenosis (*arrow*). (**b**) Fistulogram demonstrates an arterial limb stenosis

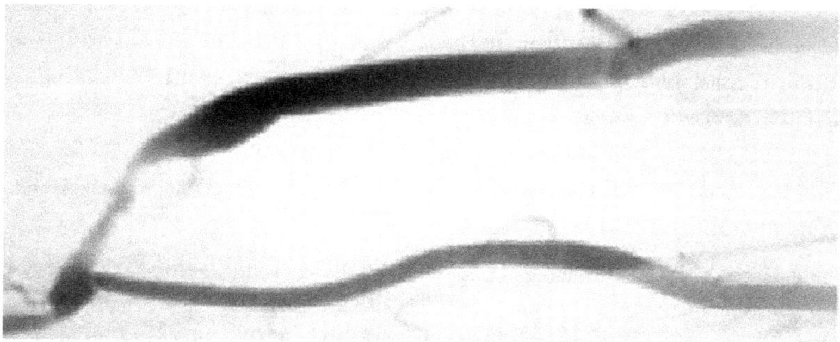

Fig. 12.5 Native wrist fistulography demonstrating a severe juxta-anastomotic venous outflow stenosis

contrast injection through a small (3 Fr) dilator to evaluate the anastomosis. This is done in situations where venous puncture is not possible (not well matured) or if the anastomosis is not well visualized despite venous puncture (Fig. 12.6). An antegrade puncture is necessary for treatment of central stenoses.

Angioplasty/Endoluminal Stent Insertion

Once a stenosis is encountered, an appropriately sized high-pressure balloon is used for angioplasty [8]. It is important to avoid balloon

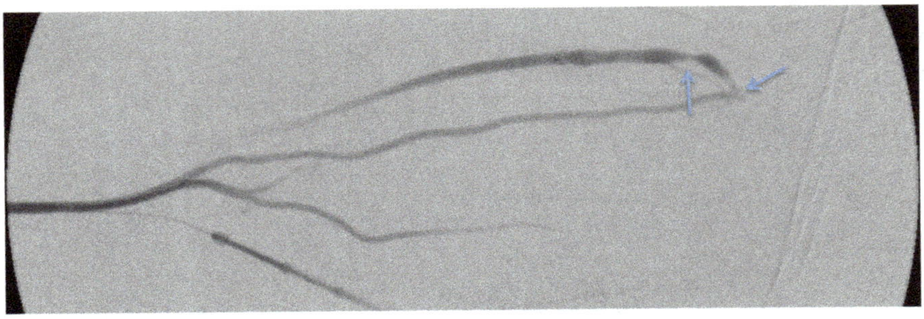

Fig. 12.6 Retrograde brachial arteriogram demonstrating a patent radial artery–cephalic vein arteriovenous fistula with multiple venous stenosis (*arrows*)

oversizing in children where the veins are already of small caliber. This is also true for the cephalic arch and native fistula anastomosis which are prone to rupture. Intravenous heparin (50–100 units/kg) can be given to prevent thrombosis especially in children with smaller-size veins or if prolonged inflations (greater than 2 min) are required. A typical inflation time is 1–2 min. Repeat or prolonged angioplasty (up to 5 min) may be needed if there is a suboptimal result or significant elastic recoil. Injection of perivenous lidocaine at the site of angioplasty can help with pain control. If the angioplasty balloon cannot be effaced due to an underlying resistant stenosis, consider using a cutting balloon [9]. Alternatively, a guidewire can be placed alongside an existing balloon to create a cutting effect during angioplasty (parallel wire technique) [10]. A good outcome of angioplasty is indicated by palpation of a continuous thrill (clinical), less than 30 % residual stenosis, absence of a flow-limiting dissection flap (anatomic), and venous pressure less than 30 % of the measured systolic arterial blood pressure (hemodynamic). DOQI guidelines dictate that angioplasty should result in a primary patency rate of at least 50 % at 6 months [2]. Recurrent stenosis after two angioplasties within a 3-month period is considered failure. Failure of angioplasty should result in surgical revision or stent insertion in patients who are not surgical candidates.

Percutaneous insertion of an intravascular stent is generally recommended to treat venous rupture not responding to prolonged inflation, to treat an elastic stenosis, and for failure of angioplasty or recurrent central stenosis within 3 months of previous angioplasty [2]. It has been shown that for peripheral veins, stents do not increase the patency rate when compared to angioplasty [11]. When placing a stent, it is important to only cover the lesion and avoid as much normal vein as possible. Typically, flexible self-expandable nitinol stents are used and ideally should only be placed within a vessel that is not surgically accessible. Covered stents may have a role to treat a stenosis at the venous anastomosis of AVGs, to treat focal graft or venous rupture and to exclude AVG pseudoaneurysms [12–15]. Stents are generally avoided in the pediatric population due to the smaller caliber of veins.

Thrombectomy Technique

The principle of thrombectomy centers on the removal of existing clot, the removal of the arterial plug, and the treatment of an underlying stenosis. In addition to a similar workup as for fistulography, intravenous antibiotics are typically administered due to the risk of existing silent infected thrombus [15]. Intravenous heparin (50–100 units/kg) is also administered to decrease rethrombosis risk/rate.

Ultrasound surveillance of AVFs immediately prior to the procedure will facilitate detection of the offending stenosis and the extent of thrombus burden and can limit access to a single puncture. Two puncture sites may be necessary to treat concurrent juxta-anastomotic and more central stenoses. In order to facilitate access to the venous and arterial anastomoses of AVGs, the venous limb may be punctured in an antegrade and retrograde fashion with placements of high-flow sheaths. Alternatively, an antegrade access within the arterial limb with retrograde access within the venous limb would achieve the same objective.

Thrombus removal techniques include the following:

(a) Lyse and wait: 2–4 mg t-PA is injected into the access 30 min prior to the procedure. Thrombus is removed with balloon maceration.
(b) Pulse spray: 3–5 mg t-PA can be administered though the entire length of the thrombus through crossing infusion catheters over a few minutes followed by balloon maceration.
(c) Thromboaspiration: using removable hub sheaths to aspirate clots within each limb of the graft.
(d) Mechanical thrombectomy: using a mechanical device to macerate existing clot. The type of device used will be dependent on patient size.

Using a mechanical thrombectomy device is the preferred method used at the author's institution to declot AVGs. The device is initially activated within the venous limb through an antegrade sheath and subsequently placed through a retrograde sheath within the venous limb to declot the arterial limb and remove the arterial plug as the device is retracted and activated at the arterial anastomosis. The plug can also be removed using an over-the-wire Fogarty balloon catheter, adherent clot catheter, or an angioplasty balloon. Once flow has been established within the access, fistulography is performed and the stenosis is then treated with angioplasty as described earlier. A single retrograde puncture technique usually suffices to declot an AVF when the stenosis is juxta-anastomotic. A mechanical thrombectomy device is used to remove the plug at the anastomosis and thrombus within the outflow vein. A second puncture (antegrade) will be necessary to treat more central stenoses.

The Nonmaturing AVF

In order for an AVF to be functional for dialysis, the venous outflow needs to increase in size to become easily palpable, possess adequate flow, and be large enough to allow cannulation during dialysis. The development of adequate flow depends upon the presence of competing flow and venous resistance. Angioplasty can be used to assist maturation by treating an underlying stenosis. Competing venous collaterals result in decreased flow within the main outflow vein and can be treated with surgical ligation or coil embolization. If competing collaterals coexist with an underlying stenosis, angioplasty alone may suffice [3].

Complications

The most common complication that occurs during hemodialysis access intervention is focal venous rupture due to angioplasty. This occurs in 2–3 % of cases. Manual compression and balloon tamponade are both effective to control bleeding. If these maneuvers fail, then stent insertion becomes necessary. Embolization of thrombus to the inflow artery can occur in up to 9 % of cases. The back-bleeding technique is used to treat clinically significant arterial emboli that may occur during thrombectomy. In this technique, a Fogarty balloon is placed within the inflow brachial artery above the anastomosis and inflated while the patient opens and closes the hand repeatedly for about a minute. The balloon is subsequently deflated with repeat fistulography. If this technique fails, the embolus may be removed using thromboaspiration, thrombolysis, or a pullback technique to dislodge the embolus back into the graft. Allergic contrast reactions may occur; therefore, appropriate preprocedure therapy is indicated in patients with known contrast allergy. Severe complications such as symptomatic pulmonary embolism or death occur in less than 1 % of patients [16].

Postprocedure Care

Adequate hemostasis is usually achieved with manual compression using Gelfoam or a hemostasis patch. A purse-string suture can be used for AVGs and should be removed within 48 h to prevent infection. Various devices exist to aid in compression of AVGs. The goal is to avoid too much compression resulting in graft occlusion with rethrombosis. Once hemostasis is achieved, dialysis can be performed immediately. Access surveillance as discussed in the indications section is then continued to determine the need for repeat intervention as necessary.

Chapter Summary

Indications for Treatment

- Hemodynamically significant stenosis; >50 % decrease in vessel diameter
- Failure of maturation
- Inability to cannulate
- Thrombosis
- Loss of thrill
- Prolonged bleeding
- Abnormal pseudoaneurysm

Contraindications

- Venoplasty/angioplasty in coagulopathic patients
- Infected, thrombosed fistula or graft
- Relative:
  - Metabolic disturbances (e.g., hyperkalemia)
  - Right to left shunt
  - Severe pulmonary compromise
  - Right-sided heart failure
  - Contrast allergy
  - Recent surgery, active bleeding, or recent cerebrovascular event (thrombolysis)

Workup

- Clinical evaluation
  - Thrill
  - Veins
- Ultrasound
- Coagulation values (prior to central venous intervention)

Equipment

- Vascular sheath
- Balloons—angioplasty, high pressure for venoplasty, cutting occasionally
- Stent—occasionally
- Thrombectomy device
- Multi-side hole infusion catheters
- Aspiration catheters
- TPA
- Heparin
- Lidocaine

Complications

- Venous rupture
- Arterial embolization
- Pulmonary embolism
- Death

Postprocedure Care

- Purse-string suture removed after 48 h
- Surveillance monitoring

References

1. Fischbach M, Terzic J, Menouer S, Provot E, Bergere V. Hemodialysis in children: principles and practice. Semin Nephrol. 2001;21:470–9.
2. NKF-K/DOQI Clinical practice guidelines for vascular access: update 2000. Am J Kidney Dis. 2001;37 (1 Suppl 1):S137–81.
3. Altman SD, Clark T, Dolmatch, Bien-Soo T. Society of Interventional Radiology annual meeting's workshop text. Creation and management of hemodialysis access. 2008;259–85.
4. Treotola SO, Scheel Jr PJ, Powe NR, Prescott C, Freely N, He J, et al. Screening for dialysis access graft malfunction: comparison of physical examination with US. J Vasc Interv Radiol. 1996;7(1):15–20.
5. Safa AA, Valji K, Roberts AC, Ziegler TW, Hye RJ, Ogelvie SB. Detection and treatment of dysfunctional hemodialysis access grafts: effect of a surveillance program on graft patency and the incidence of thrombosis. Radiology. 1996;199(3):653–7.
6. Waybill PN, Brown DB. Patient care in vascular and interventional radiology. Periprocedural Management of Fluids, Electrolytes and Acid-base Disturbances 2nd ed. SIR syllabus series. p. 156–7.
7. Hathaway PB, Vesely TM. The apex puncture technique for mechanical thrombolysis of loop hemodialysis grafts. J Vasc Interv Radiol. 1999;10(6):775–9.
8. Trerotola SO, Kwak A, Clark TW, et al. Prospective study of balloon inflation pressures and other technical aspects of hemodialysis access angioplasty. J Vasc Interv Radiol. 2005;16(12):1613–8.
9. Vesely TM, Siegel JB. Use of the peripheral cutting balloon to treat hemodialysis related stenoses. J Vasc Interv Radiol. 2005;16(12):1593–603.
10. Fukasawa M, Matsushita K, Araki I, et al. Self-reversed parallel wire balloon technique for dilating unyielding strictures in native dialysis fistulas. J Vasc Interv Radiol. 2002;13(9 Pt 1):943–5.

11. Quinn SF, Schuman ES, Demlow TA, et al. Percutaneous transluminal angioplasty versus endovascular stent insertion in the treatment of venous stenoses in patients undergoing hemodialysis: intermediate results. J Vasc Interv Radiol. 1995;6(6):851–5.
12. Vesely TM. Use of stent grafts to repair hemodialysis graft-related pseudoaneurysms. J Vasc Interv Radiol. 2005;16:1301–7.
13. Dale JD, Dolmatch BL, Duch JM, et al. Expanded polytetrafluoroethylene-covered stent treatment of angioplasty-related extravasation during hemodialysis access intervention: technical and 180-day patency. J Vasc Interv Radiol. 2010;21:22–6.
14. Bent CL, Rahan DK, Tan K, et al. Effectiveness of stent-graft placement for salvage of dysfunctional arteriovenous hemodialysis fistulas. J Vasc Interv Radiol. 2010;21:496–502.
15. Ayus JC, Sheikh-Hamad D. Silent infection in clotted hemodialysis access grafts. J Am Soc Nephrol. 1998;9(7):1314–7.
16. Aruny JE, Lewis CA, Cardella JF, et al. Quality improvement guidelines for percutaneous management of the thrombosed or dysfunctional dialysis access. J Vasc Interv Radiol. 1999;10:491–8.

13 Congenital Portosystemic Shunts: Diagnosis and Percutaneous Management

Francis E. Marshalleck and Paul Haste

Background/General Information

Congenital portosystemic shunts (CPSS), first described in 1793 by London surgeon John Abernethy, are rare congenital communications between the portal and the systemic venous system. These shunts are caused by the anomalous development of the hepatic vasculature during the embryologic period. During normal embryonic development, the right and left vitelline veins emerge from the yolk sac to enter the primitive liver (septum transversum). Around the fourth week of development, cross-communicating veins develop between the vitelline veins. These crossing veins anastomose with each other in a figure-eight arrangement around the developing duodenum. The left vitelline vein ultimately involutes and the remaining right vitelline vein forms a portion of the inferior vena cava, the hepatic veins, and the portal vein. The left and right umbilical veins, likewise, course through the primitive liver. The network of veins formed from the umbilical and vitelline veins drains into the ductus venosus and ultimately into the inferior vena cava. The entire right umbilical and a portion of the left umbilical vein involute. The remaining portion of the left umbilical vein carries oxygenated blood from the placenta to the fetal liver and drains into the IVC via the ductus venosus.

Congenital absence of the portal vein is thought to arise due to an early involution of the periduodenal vitelline veins. Shunts between the right portal vein and systemic systems are thought to arise due to persistence of the right vitelline vein [1]. Shunts between the left portal vein and systemic circulation are thought to be due to persistence of the left vitelline vein.

Classification

These congenital shunts can be classified into different types depending on the specific anatomy of the shunt. Congenital extrahepatic portosystemic shunts (CEPSS) were first studied by Abernethy in 1793 and a formal classification was proposed by Morgan and Superina in 1994 (Table 13.1, Fig. 13.1) [2]. Park proposed a classification for congenital intrahepatic portosystemic shunts (CIPSS) in 1990 (Table 13.2, Fig. 13.2) [1, 3].

F.E. Marshalleck, M.D.
Interventional Radiology, Indiana University School of Medicine, Riley Hospital for Children, 705 Riley Hospital Drive, Room 1053, Indianapolis, IN 46202, USA
e-mail: frmarsha@iupui.edu

P. Haste, B.S., M.D. (✉)
Department of Radiology, Indiana University School of Medicine, 5260 Carrollton Avenue, Indianapolis, IN 46220, USA
e-mail: phaste@inpui.edu

M. Temple and F.E. Marshalleck (eds.), *Pediatric Interventional Radiology: Handbook of Vascular and Non-Vascular Interventions*, DOI 10.1007/978-1-4419-5856-3_13,

Table 13.1 Congenital extrahepatic portosystemic shunts (Morgan and Superina classification)

Type I (Abernethy malformation): end-to-side communication with the portal system to the IVC (most common), azygous vein, renal vein, right atrium, or iliac veins (Fig. 13.1a)
Type Ia: the splenic vein (SV) and superior mesenteric vein (SMV) each drains separately into the systemic circulation
Type Ib: the SV and SMV join to form a common trunk and directly drain into the systemic circulation bypassing the liver
Type II: side-to-side anastomosis of the portal with the IVC (Fig. 13.1b)
Type IIa: congenital type II shunts
Type IIb: acquired type II shunts

Patient Presentation

Regardless of which type of shunt occurs, the presenting symptoms constitute a wide spectrum. CPSS may be asymptomatic or associated with varying degrees of encephalopathy. In fact, the majority of shunts are discovered during screening for metabolic diseases. Due to portal blood bypassing the liver, these patients often have hypergalactosemia, elevated ammonia levels, and sometimes hyperbilirubinemia.

In type I CEPSS, there is a congenital absence of the portal vein with complete diversion of portal blood into the systemic circulation. Intrahepatic portal radicles may be hypoplastic and undetectable [4]. Type 1 shunts are more commonly seen in females and are associated with other anomalies including biliary atresia, polysplenia, malrotation, situs inversus, multicystic dysplastic kidneys, Goldenhar syndrome (oculoauriculovertebral dysplasia), choledochal cyst, skeletal anomalies, and cutaneous hemangiomas.

Type II CEPSS are more common in boys with less association with congenital anomalies but can be seen in patients with pulmonary valve atresia, patent ductus arteriosus, Goldenhar syndrome, polysplenia, and IVC anomalies.

Associated congenital anomalies are much less common with CIPSS but can still occur, e.g., biliary atresia, cutaneous hemangiomas, and congenital heart disease.

Excessive shunting results in accumulation of toxic metabolites such as bile acids, cholylglycine, galactose, and ammonia resulting in varying degrees of hepatic encephalopathy. Signs of portal hypertension such as varices, ascites, and splenomegaly may occur but are infrequent. Features of portal hypertension usually indicate that the existing shunt is compensatory and not congenital. Patients with CIPSS can present with postprandial hyperglycemia seen especially in diabetic patients. Both CEPSS and CIPSS may be associated with the development of intrahepatic lesions (fatty liver, focal nodular hyperplasia, adenoma, nodular regenerative hyperplasia, hepatoblastoma, and hepatocellular carcinoma) which may regress after treatment. Any remaining nodules are generally evaluated with follow-up imaging and do not typically require percutaneous biopsy since the occurrence of hepatocellular carcinoma is rare. It is thought that hepatic tumors occur as a compensatory response to the decrease in intrahepatic flow of blood, but the exact mechanism of hepatic nodule formation is unknown. Hepatopulmonary syndrome (hepatic dysfunction, lung vascular alteration, and hypoxemia) may occur with either type of shunt and can result in significant pulmonary hypertension [5–8].

Preprocedure Workup

Abdominal ultrasound with hepatic Doppler evaluation is the initial radiologic workup when a malformation is suspected. US evaluation is inexpensive, is noninvasive, and does not expose the patient to radiation. The vast majority of shunts can be visualized with US alone (Fig. 13.3). After the malformation has been recognized, the next step is to utilize cross-sectional imaging (CT or MR) to demonstrate the exact course of the shunt and visualize the remainder of the portal system in order to plan subsequent management. Cross-sectional imaging more accurately demonstrates the extrahepatic venous anatomy, features of portal hypertension (ascites, splenomegaly, varices), and the presence of intrahepatic masses (Fig. 13.4). The advantage

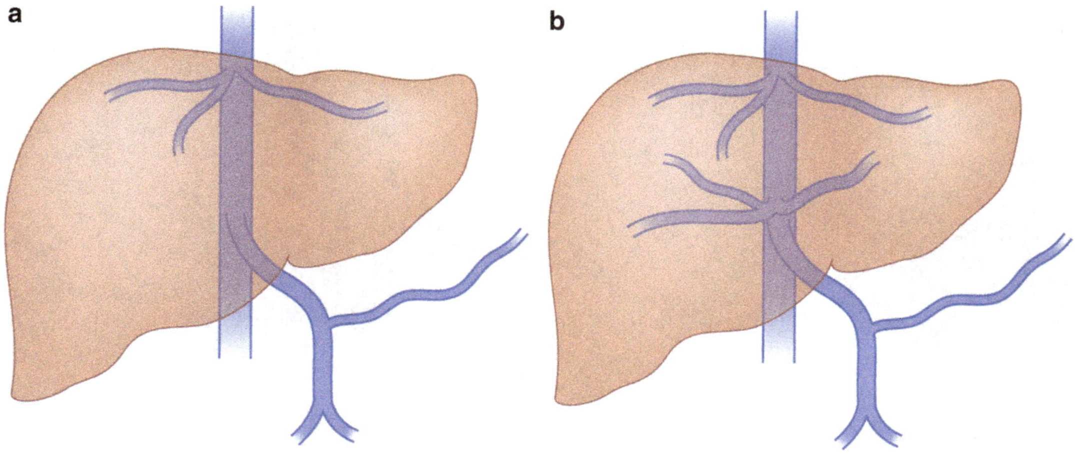

Fig. 13.1 Congenital extrahepatic portosystemic shunts. (**a**) Type I—end-to-side communication of portal vein to IVC. (**b**) Type II—side-to-side anastomosis of portal vein with IVC

Table 13.2 Congenital intrahepatic portosystemic shunts (Park classification)

Type I—a single large vessel connecting the right portal vein to the intrahepatic IVC (Fig. 13.2a)
Type II—one or more communications between the peripheral portal and hepatic vein branches within a *single* hepatic segment (Fig. 13.2b)
Type III—type II shunt with an intervening venous aneurysm (Fig. 13.2c)
Type IV—multiple portosystemic communications between portal and hepatic veins within *multiple* hepatic segments (Fig. 13.2d)
Type V—the fifth type of intrahepatic shunt is a patent ductus venosus. This type of shunt is an abnormal persistence of the embryologic vascular connection between the proximal left portal vein and the IVC (Fig. 13.2e)

of MR imaging is the lack of ionizing radiation. Nuclear medicine studies such as iodine 123 iodoamphetamine administered rectally have been used to calculate shunt ratios between the liver and the lung primarily for type II CEPSS. A shunt ratio of greater than 30 % indicates an increased risk of encephalopathy [9]. Catheter-directed angiography is usually reserved for use during percutaneous intervention. Additional laboratory evaluation such as platelet count and coagulation parameters may also be obtained if a transhepatic intervention is contemplated. Urea and creatinine levels are important to obtain prior to contrast administration. Percutaneous liver biopsy is useful primarily in suspected type I CEPSS to evaluate for hypoplasia or absence of intrahepatic portal radicles.

Indications for Treatment

Depending on the degree of shunting, CPSS can significantly affect neurocognitive function especially if associated with elevated ammonia levels, galactose levels, and encephalopathy. This is an important consideration in children since neurological effects can decrease productivity in adulthood. It is generally recommended that early shunt closure be performed to restore hepatic blood flow to prevent possible long-term neurological and pulmonary effects [7, 9] especially if the patient is already encephalopathic.

For CEPPS, an elevated iodine 123 iodoamphetamine shunt ratio of greater than 30 % indicates that encephalopathy can be precipitated and a shunt ratio of greater than 60 % indicates that encephalopathy will occur spontaneously and that treatment is mandatory [10]. In the past, patients with type I CEPSS underwent liver transplantation, but successful outcomes have been reported following surgical banding [4]. Type II CEPSS can be treated with percutaneous embolization or surgical ligation depending on the anatomy of the shunt.

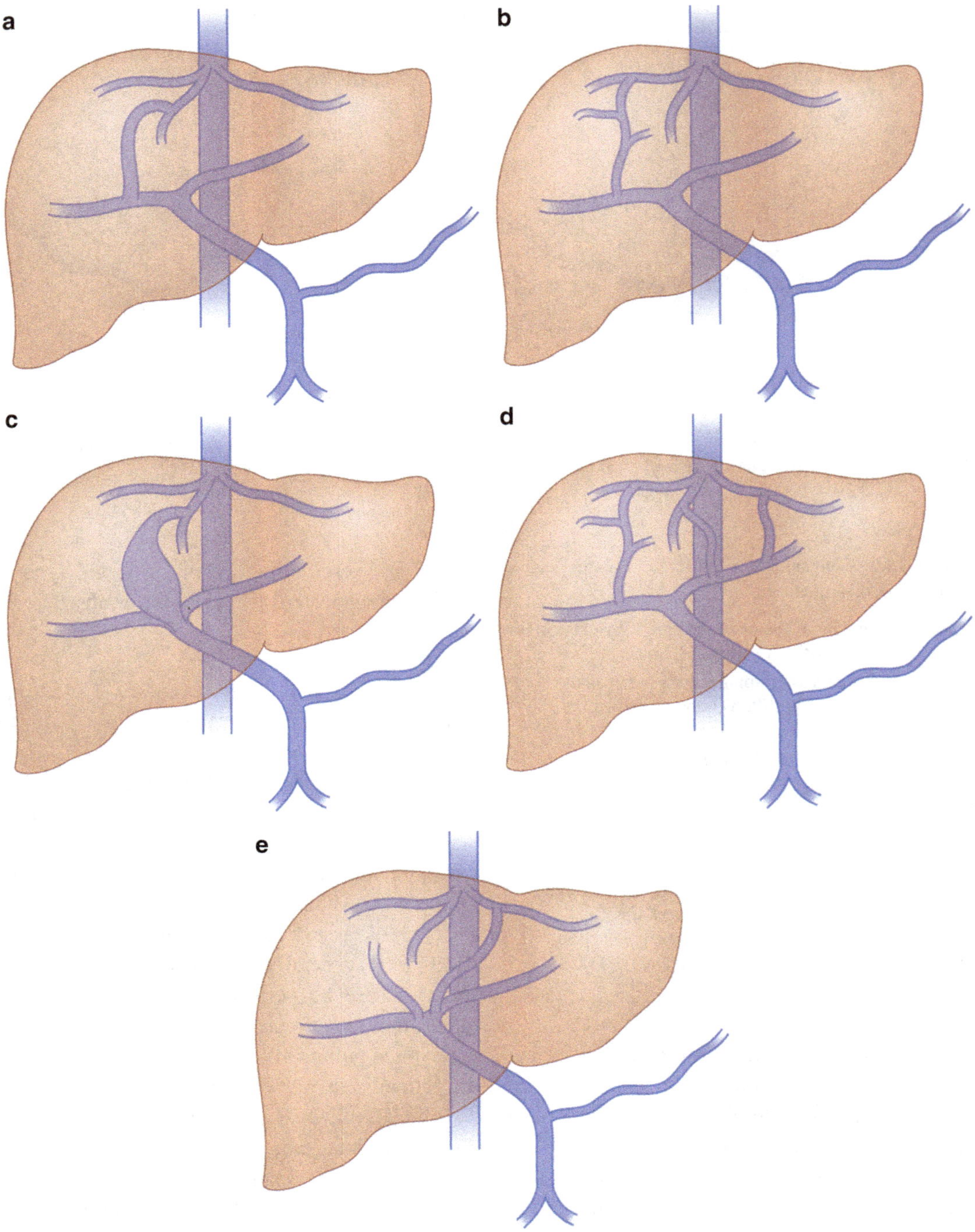

Fig. 13.2 Congenital intrahepatic portosystemic shunts. (**a**) Type 1—right portal vein to intrahepatic IVC. (**b**) Type II—peripheral portal to hepatic vein connection, single segment. (**c**) Type III—type II with aneurysm. (**d**) Type IV—multiple portal hepatic connections, multiple segments. (**e**) Type V—patent ductus venosus

Unlike CEPSS, cases of spontaneous regression of CIPSS have been reported during the first year or 2 of life. Asymptomatic patients can be followed for the first 2 years of life and treated only if symptoms develop or if ammonia or galactose levels begin to rise [4, 8]. Symptomatic patients and those over 2 years of age should be treated with percutaneous embolization.

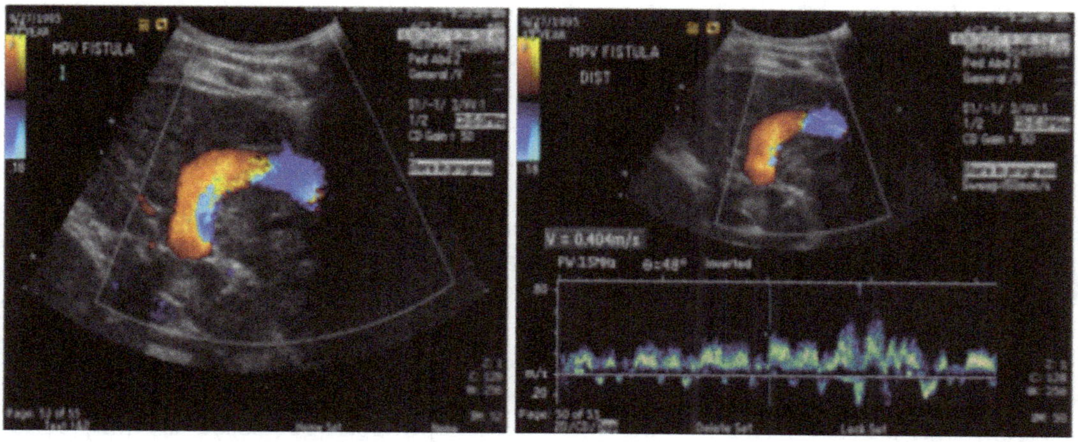

Fig. 13.3 Doppler ultrasound images demonstrating a large congenital shunt from the left portal vein to the IVC (patent ductus venosus)

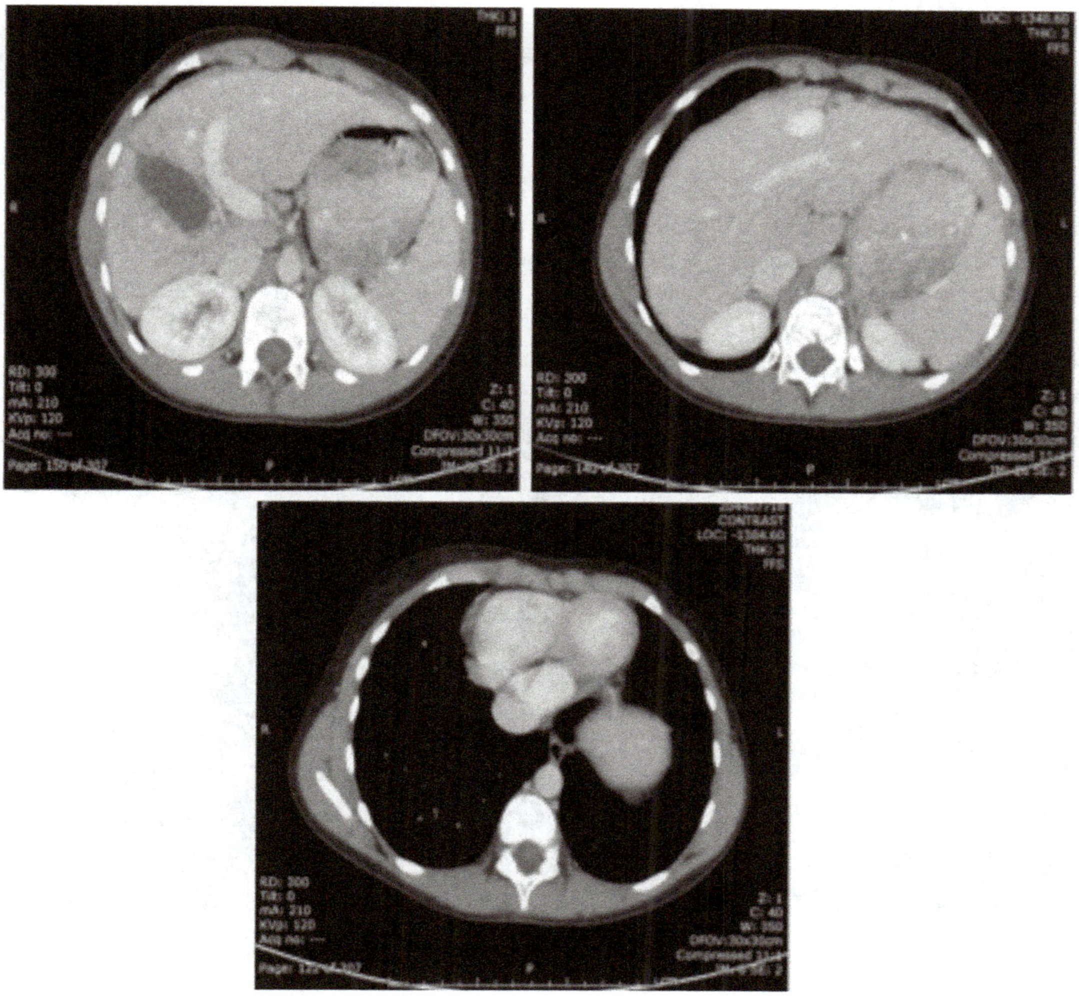

Fig. 13.4 Axial CT images demonstrating a patent ductus venosus. Cross-sectional imaging has the advantage of also illustrating abnormalities within the solid organs

Asymptomatic patients are treated with medical therapy and dietary management.

Contraindications

It is important to note that only primary congenital shunts should be treated. Shunt closure should not be performed in cases where the shunt occurs as a compensatory mechanism to portal hypertension as seen in neonatal hemochromatosis. Shunt closure in the presence of portal hypertension due to intrinsic liver disease can result in fatality due to mesenteric venous congestion and bowel ischemia [11]. Coagulopathy would be a contraindication only if a transhepatic route was contemplated to percutaneously treat intrahepatic shunts.

Technique

The procedure is typically performed with general anesthesia. The treatment of CPSS is variable depending on shunt anatomy. The indicated treatment for a type I extrahepatic shunt is liver transplantation due to the lack of a suitable vessel for embolization. The other types of shunts are best managed with endovascular therapy when feasible. Surgical ligation is an option for patients with an unfavorable shunt anatomy for endovascular closure. Embolization of these shunts can be performed using transjugular, transfemoral, transhepatic, mesenteric, umbilical venous, or transcaval routes [8].

Catheterization of congenital shunts is often successful using a transjugular route. Once access is gained into the portal vein, manometric assessment is performed to obtain a baseline pressure measurement. Direct portography is also performed to determine shunt anatomy in order to decide whether embolization can be performed safely. An occlusion balloon is subsequently inflated within the portal vein with repeat portography and manometric assessment. Occlusion portography is performed to confirm the presence of intrahepatic portal radicles and to determine the effect of shunt closure on portal venous pressure (Fig. 13.5). Opinion varies regarding the pressure gradient that warrants staged closure (avoiding abrupt closure that could lead to significant acute portal hypertension). Authors have

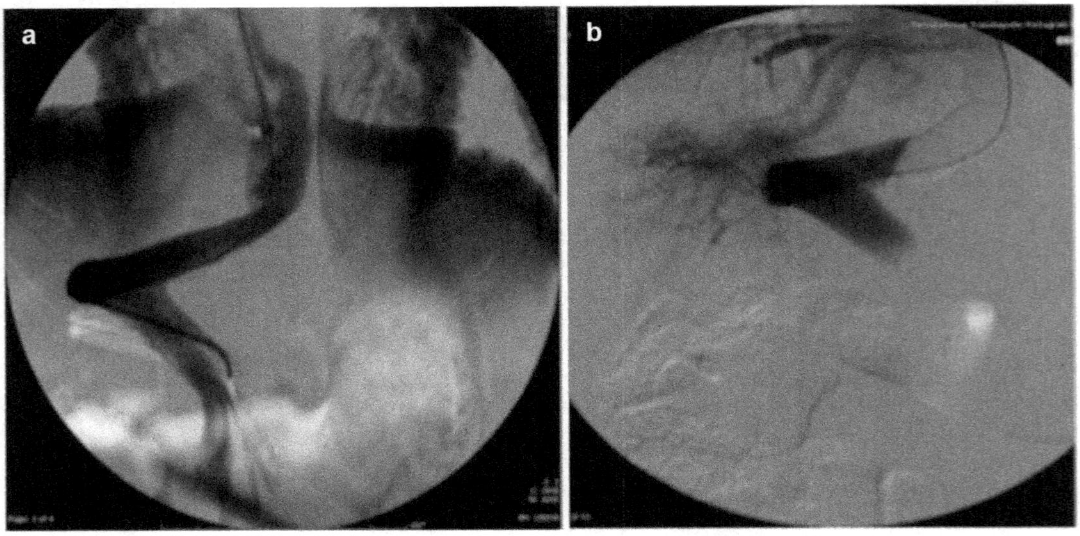

Fig. 13.5 Occlusion portogram. (**a**) Angiographic image demonstrating catheterization of a congenital ductus venosus from a jugular approach. Intrahepatic radicles are not clearly seen. (**b**) Occlusion portography obtained by injection of contrast during balloon inflation within the shunt demonstrates that intrahepatic portal venous radicles exist. Multiple small shunts between the portal vein and hepatic veins are also seen

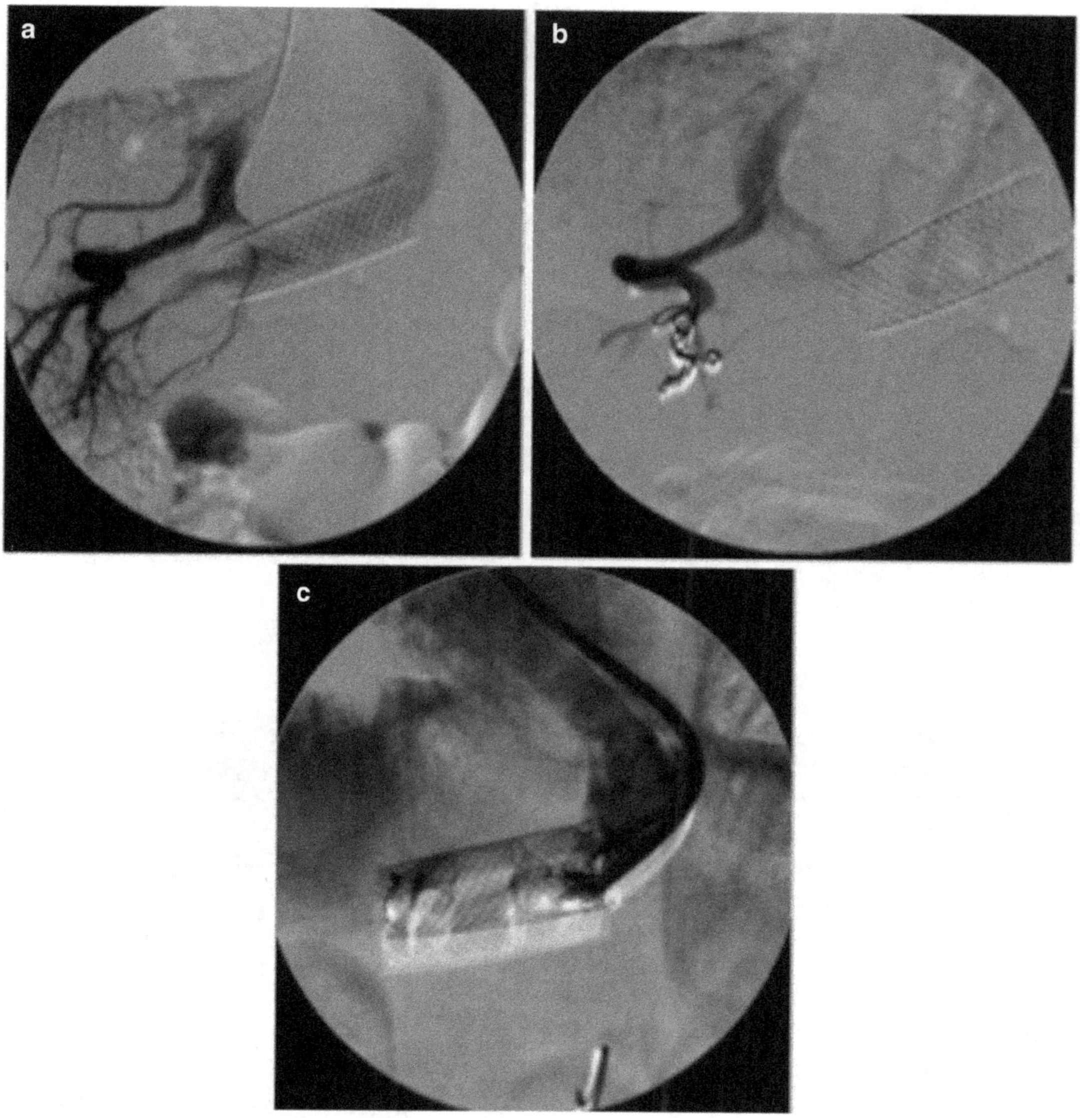

Fig. 13.6 Staged shunt closure. (**a**) Patent ductus venosus with a wall stent placed to induce intimal hyperplasia. Occlusion portography had demonstrated a portal pressure of >20 mmHg indicating unfavorable conditions for immediate shunt closure. (**b**) Coil embolization of portal vein to hepatic vein shunt in the same patient. (**c**) Final shunt closure with an Amplatzer plug device placed within the existing stent after occlusion portography demonstrated a portal pressure of <20 mmHg

suggested pressure gradients ranging from 20 to 32 mmHg as the indicator for staged closure [4]. If the gradient is favorable, i.e., <20–32 mmHg, then primary closure can be performed using metallic coils (large coils up to 20 mm in diameter are available). Likewise, the Amplatzer occlusion device (AGA Medical Corporation, MN) can be used especially for larger-diameter fast flow fistulae. Detachable coils play a vital role in smaller-diameter shunts where precise deployment is necessary [9, 12]. In the case of a short-length, large-diameter shunt, endovascular exclusion of the shunt by placement of a covered stent within the IVC has been reported (Fig. 13.6) [13]. If staged closure is warranted, this can be achieved using a reducing stent technique (Fig. 13.7). A self-expanding Wallstent (Boston Scientific, USA) is initially placed within the

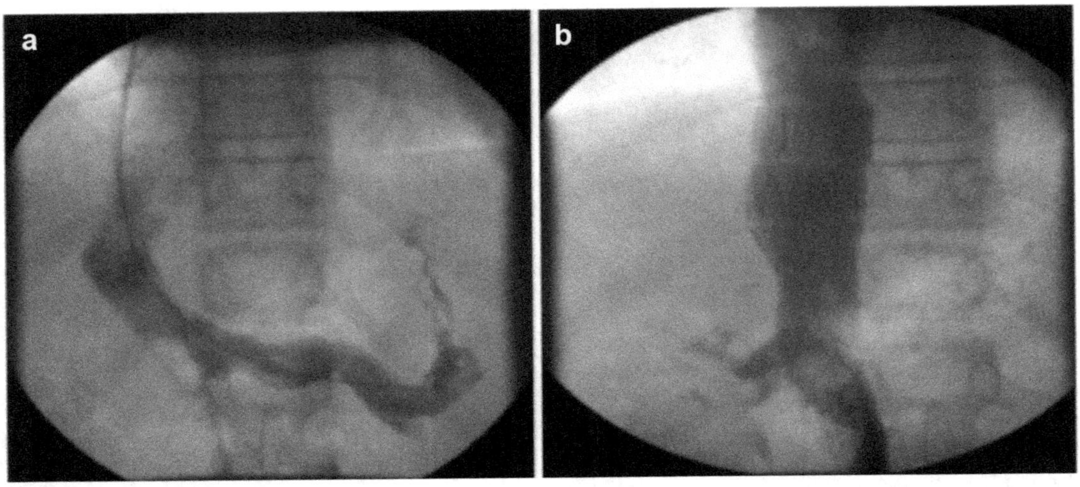

Fig. 13.7 Covered IVC stent; femoral Swan-Ganz. (**a**) Angiographic image demonstrating catheterization of a congenital extrahepatic shunt short in length but with a wide diameter precluding adequate embolization. (**b**) Exclusion of the shunt by placement of covered stents within the IVC after occlusion portography demonstrated portal pressure <20 mmHg

shunt to incite intimal hyperplasia followed by coaxial placement of a reducing stent to further close the shunt after a 2-month interval [8]. If there are multiple shunts, staged embolization of the various shunts may be employed. Concomitant arterial access (visceral angiography) is necessary not only to visualize the shunt on delayed imaging but also to evaluate for shunt closure after embolization (Fig. 13.8). In cases where there is significant hepatopulmonary syndrome, pulmonary arterial pressure can be monitored during the procedure with the placement of a Swan-Ganz catheter (Fig. 13.7a).

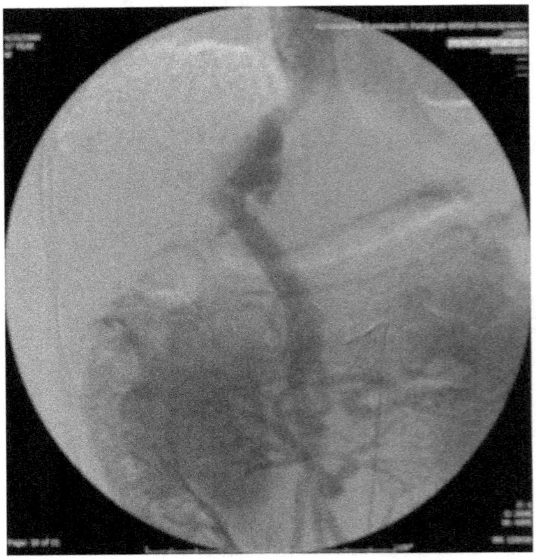

Fig. 13.8 Arterial access. Venous phase of SMA angiography delineating a type III congenital intrahepatic shunt. Arteriography is needed before and after intervention to assess for adequate shunt closure

Complications

As with any embolization procedure, nontarget embolization can occur but could be avoided with proper sizing of coils, the use of detachable coils, or the use of the Amplatzer occlusion device especially to treat larger-diameter shunts. Due to the risk of portal vein thrombosis, it is advised that intravenous heparin is administered during the procedure at a dose of 50–100 units/kg. Significant portal hypertension can be avoided with staged closure. As previously stated, shunt closure should be avoided when a portacaval shunt is secondary to portal hypertension caused by intrinsic liver disease. Complications related to arteriography as well as contrast reactions can also occur.

Follow-up Care

Doppler sonography at routine intervals (1, 3, 6 months, and annually) is recommended to assess shunt closure and development of intrahepatic portal branches. Follow-up blood work is also done to confirm decreasing ammonia and galactose levels. Repeat clinical assessment is also recommended to follow improvement in encephalopathy and to monitor cognitive function.

Chapter Summary

Presentation

- Variable presentation
- Encephalopathy
- Hypergalactosemia
- Hyperammonemia
- Hyperbilirubinemia
- Portal hypertension
- Hepatic nodules/masses
- Hepatopulmonary syndrome

Preprocedure Workup

- Ultrasound liver with Doppler evaluation
- CT/MR
  - Define shunt anatomy
  - Portal hypertension sequelae
  - Intrahepatic masses
- Iodine 123 iodoamphetamine (type II CEPSS)
- Blood work: platelet count, INR/PTT, BUN, creatinine
- Liver biopsy (type I CEPSS)

Indications for Treatment

- Type II CEPSS
- ^{123}I shunt ratio >30 %; >60 %
- CIPPS: may involute in the first year—consider surveillance if ammonia stable and no encephalopathy

Contraindications

- Secondary portosystemic shunt (e.g., hemochromatosis)
- Intrinsic liver disease
- Coagulopathy

Equipment

- Angiographic catheters, wires, sheaths
- Occlusion balloon
- Pressure monitoring equipment
- Coils, occlusion devices
- Heparin

Complications

- Nontarget embolization
- Portal vein thrombosis
- Portal hypertension—mesenteric venous congestion, bowel ischemia

Follow-up

- Doppler ultrasound
  - 1, 3, 6, and 12 months then yearly
- Clinical follow-up to assess for encephalopathy
- Ammonia, galactose levels

References

1. Gallego C, Miralles M, Marin C, Muyor P, Gonzalez G, Garcia-Hidalgo E. Congenital hepatic shunts. Radiographics. 2004;24(3):755–72.
2. Morgan G, Superina R. Congenital absence of the portal vein: two cases and a proposed classification system for portasystemic vascular anomalies. J Pediatr Surg. 1994;29(9):1239–41.
3. Senocak E, Oguz B, Edguer T, Cila A. Congenital intrahepatic portosystemic shunt with variant inferior right hepatic vein. Diagn Interv Radiol. 2008;14(2):97–9.
4. Franchi-Abella S, Branchereau S, Lambert V, Fabre M, Steimberg C, Losay J, et al. Complications of congenital portosystemic shunts in children: therapeutic options and outcomes. J Pediatr Gastroenterol Nutr. 2010;51(3):322–30.
5. Howard ER, Davenport M. Congenital extrahepatic portocaval shunts—the Abernethy malformation. J Pediatr Surg. 1997;32(3):494–7.
6. Murray CP, Yoo SJ, Babyn PS. Congenital extrahepatic portosystemic shunts. Pediatr Radiol. 2003;33(9):614–20.
7. Ohno T, Muneuchi J, Ihara K, Yuge T, Kanaya Y, Yamaki S, et al. Pulmonary hypertension in patients with congenital portosystemic venous shunt: a previously unrecognized association. Pediatrics. 2008;121(4):e892–9.
8. Stringer MD. The clinical anatomy of congenital portosystemic venous shunts. Clin Anat. 2008;21(2):147–57.
9. Eroglu Y, Donaldson J, Sorensen LG, Vogelzang RL, Melin-Aldana H, Andersen J, et al. Improved

neurocognitive function after radiologic closure of congenital portosystemic shunts. J Pediatr Gastroenterol Nutr. 2004;39(4):410–7.
10. Alonso-Gamarra E, Parron M, Perez A, Prieto C, Hierro L, Lopez-Santamaria M. Clinical and radiologic manifestations of congenital extrahepatic portosystemic shunts: a comprehensive review. Radiographics. 2011;31(3):707–22.
11. Tsai A, Paltiel HJ, Sena LM, Kim HB, Fishman SJ, Alomari AI. Neonatal hemochromatosis and patent ductus venosus: clinical course and diagnostic pitfalls. Pediatr Radiol. 2009;39(8):823–7.
12. Alonso J, Sierre S, Lipsich J, Questa H, Faella H, Moguillansky S. Endovascular treatment of congenital portal vein fistulas with the Amplatzer occlusion device. J Vasc Interv Radiol. 2004;15(9):989–93.
13. Hoover W, Ackerman V, Schamberger M, Kumar M, Marshalleck F, Hoyer M. The congenital porto-caval fistula: a unique presentation and novel intervention. Pediatr Pulmonol. 2008;43(2):196–9.

Section IV

Vascular Interventions: Other

14 Vascular Anomalies

Philip John

Overview of Vascular Anomalies

The International Society for the Study of Vascular Anomalies (ISSVA) classifies vascular anomalies into vascular tumors and vascular malformations (Table 14.1). This division is based on the biological and clinical behavior of these anomalies (including physical characteristics, natural history, and cellular features) [1]. Its usage provides a common language for most diagnoses.

Infantile hemangioma is the commonest vascular tumor, initially presenting a few weeks after birth. Fetal hypoxic stress is considered a likely trigger for the development of these tumors; however, placental emboli have previously been implicated as they share pathological features in common. Although most vascular tumors are not associated with vascular malformations, the so-called "segmental" type of infantile hemangioma may be associated with developmental vascular and other anomalies, as in PHACES syndrome [2].

Vascular malformations are different to infantile hemangiomas as they are present at birth (although not always evident), show commensurate growth with the patient, and persist throughout life. They are due to errors of vascular morphogenesis affecting vascular channels exhibiting low flow (capillaries, veins, and lymphatics) or high flow (arteries). A vascular anomaly is characterized as high flow when arteriovenous shunting occurs. Gene mutations are now recognized in many patients with vascular malformations, e.g., somatic mutations of the TIE2 gene are seen in 50 % of sporadic venous malformations (VM).

Establishing an accurate diagnosis allows for appropriate treatments to be undertaken and prevents inappropriate treatments. Most postnatal diagnoses can be made from history and physical examination and supplemented by diagnostic imaging (and occasionally other investigations) when diagnoses are unclear or lesions are deeply located.

Interventional radiology has a major role in providing treatment options for many of these patients. The interventionalist should have knowledge of these anomalies and their imaging findings. Skills are needed for endovascular techniques (particularly sclerotherapy, transcatheter embolization, and endovenous laser) and other relevant therapies (compartmentalizing lesions and laser therapies). Participation in a specialist multiprofessional team providing patient care is essential.

Before the interventionalist undertakes radiological treatments, it is important to review up-to-date imaging of the lesions and understand the aim and expected outcomes of the planned treatment.

P. John, M.B.Ch.B., D.C.H., F.R.C.R., F.R.C.P.C. (✉)
Department of Diagnostic Imaging, The Hospital for Sick Children, 555 University Avenue, Toronto, ON, Canada
e-mail: Philip.john@sickkids.ca

M. Temple and F.E. Marshalleck (eds.), *Pediatric Interventional Radiology: Handbook of Vascular and Non-Vascular Interventions*, DOI 10.1007/978-1-4419-5856-3_14,

Table 14.1 Classification of vascular anomalies

Vascular tumors	Vascular malformations
Hemangiomas	*Low flow (single channel)*
– Infantile (superficial/deep)	– Capillary malformation (CM)
– Congenital (RICH/NICH)	– Venous malformation (VM)
Kaposiform hemangioendothelioma (KHE)	– Lymphatic malformation (LM)
Tufted angioma (TA)	*Low flow (combined channels)*
	– CLM/CVM/VLM
	High flow
	– Arteriovenous malformation (AVM)
	– Arteriovenous fistula (AVF)
	Complex combined
	– Klippel–Trenaunay syndrome (CLVM)
	– Parkes Weber syndrome (CLAVF)

Most interventional treatments in pediatrics require general anesthesia as this provides a safe, controlled pain-free environment enabling procedures to be done efficiently and effectively. Chapter 3 covers pediatric sedation and includes a section describing anesthesia for vascular anomaly interventions.

Sclerotherapy is done for low-flow vascular malformations by injecting a sclerosant directly into the lesion. It is usually performed as a day-case procedure with patients discharged after 4–6 h. Embolization for high-flow vascular anomalies is performed by injecting embolic agents via an angiographic catheter or by direct needle puncture into the lesion and usually requires a 24-h stay in hospital. If significant swelling is likely post treatment in lesions located in the oral cavity (including tongue) or airway, then planned admission to intensive care may be needed for airway support and management. If multiple treatments are required over a long period for large anomalies affecting the oral cavity and airway (particularly in infancy), gastrostomy and tracheostomy may be required for feeding and airway support, respectively. It is important to be aware of post-procedure requirements, which are dependent on patient age, patient well-being (including psychosocial), and disease type and location. For example, large pelvic or urogenital malformations may need a Foley catheter for several days until post-procedure swelling resolves.

Imaging of Vascular Anomalies

Not all patients with vascular anomalies require imaging to confirm the diagnosis. Most (between 80 and 90 %) can be diagnosed from clinical history and physical examination [3]. For example, most babies with infantile hemangiomas do not need imaging; however, close clinical follow-up is needed.

Imaging is undertaken to aid diagnosis and when full evaluation of the anomaly is required (including its full extent and tissue involvement). Ultrasound (US) and magnetic resonance (MR) are the most useful modalities due to their high tissue specificity [4]. For most patients, MR angiographic (MRA) sequences are not needed to establish the diagnosis. In patients with high-flow lesions, MRA is useful for mapping the affected vascular anatomy. US has limitations when lesions are extensive or deeply located.

Vascular tumors on MR and US demonstrate a hypervascular parenchymal tumor in which vascular shunting may be seen (Figs. 14.1 and 14.2). In infantile hemangiomas, the vascularity and shunts decrease and fibrofatty tissue increases over time.

Vascular malformations show no parenchymal tumor with VMs showing dysplastic venous spaces, thrombi, and phleboliths (Figs. 14.3 and 14.4).

Lymphatic malformations (LM) show cysts, some containing hemorrhagic fluid or thrombi

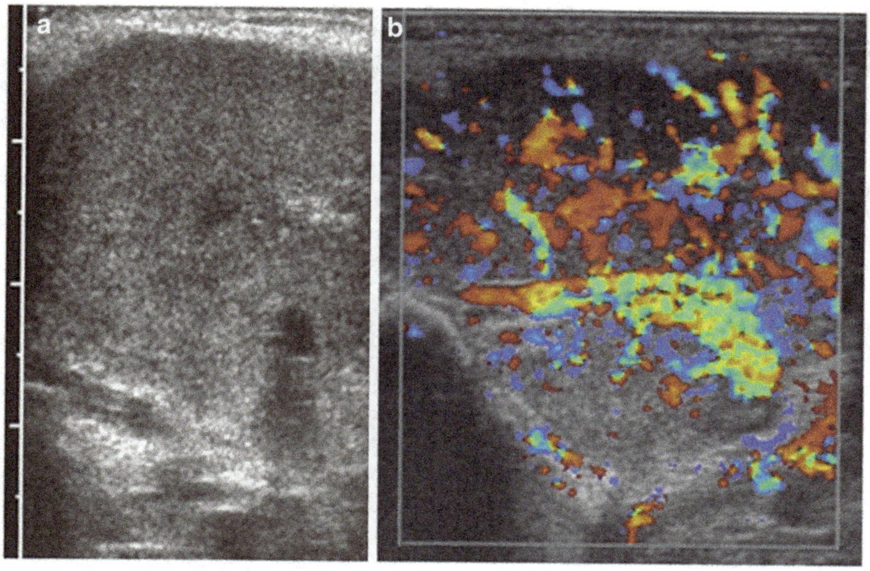

Fig. 14.1 Ultrasound parotid hemangioma. Solid, densely hypervascular lesion. The solid component (**a**) represents the parenchymal component of the vascular tumor (**b**), distinguishing this lesion from an arteriovenous malformation

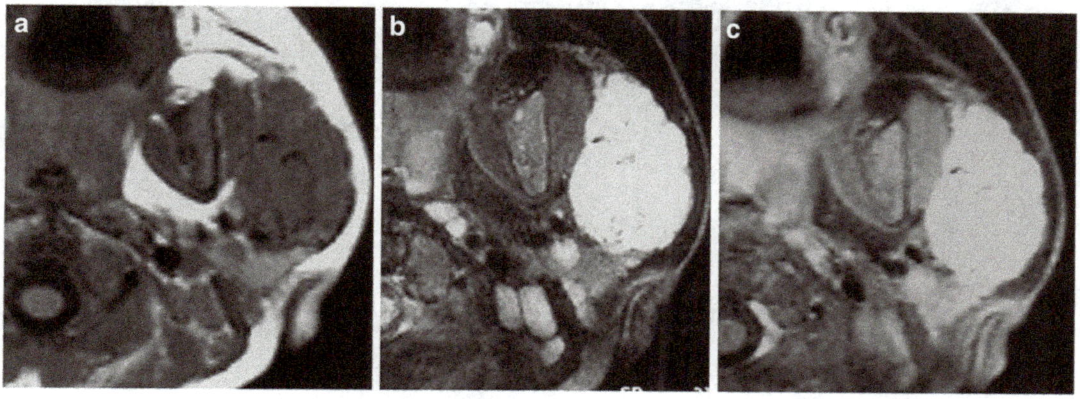

Fig. 14.2 MR parotid hemangioma. Parotid gland proliferative phase infantile hemangioma. Tumor parenchyma is isointense on T1 (**a**) and hyperintense on T2 (**b**), showing avid uniform contrast enhancement (**c**). Flow voids present

adjacent to the cyst walls (Figs. 14.5 and 14.6). The microcystic type of LMs which have no identifiable cysts on imaging appears as areas of solid echogenic tissue. VMs and LMs can have fluid-fluid levels.

Arteriovenous malformations (AVM) show lesional hypervascularity and vascular shunting, with perilesional soft tissue edema. Localized increased fatty areas can be seen around some soft tissue VMs and AVMs. Enlargement of inflow arteries and outflow veins with AV shunting can be seen in both vascular tumors and high-flow vascular malformations.

"Bedside" US is extremely useful in vascular anomalies, providing a rapid diagnosis in the clinic when lesions may have little or no visible abnormality on the skin surface. US can demonstrate local complications such as superficial blood clots in venous malformations when patients present with pain. During interventional, radiology US is essential and provides image guidance for endovascular procedures.

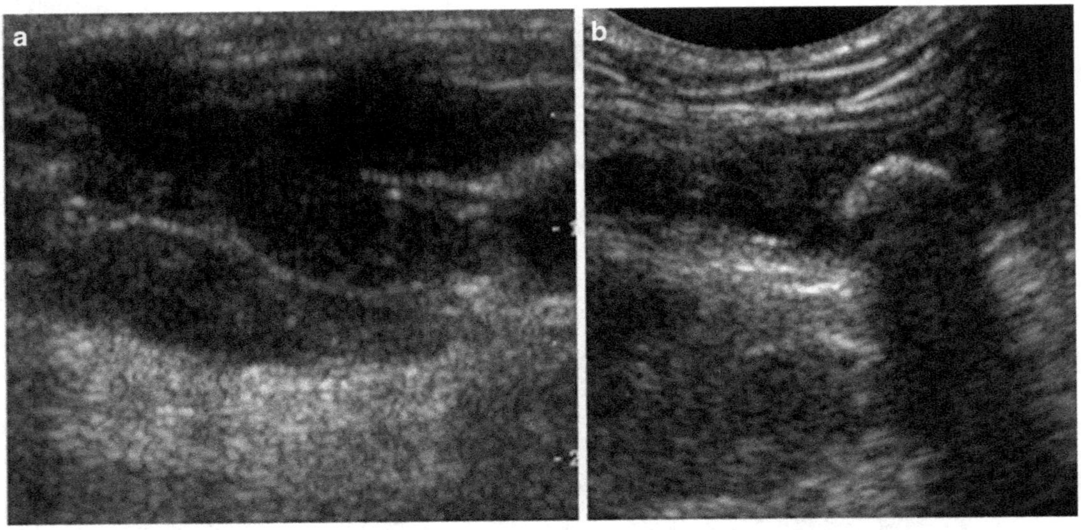

Fig. 14.3 Ultrasound venous malformation (VM). VM shows anechoic channels within soft tissue mass (**a**). Intralesional phlebolith present in anechoic channel (**b**)

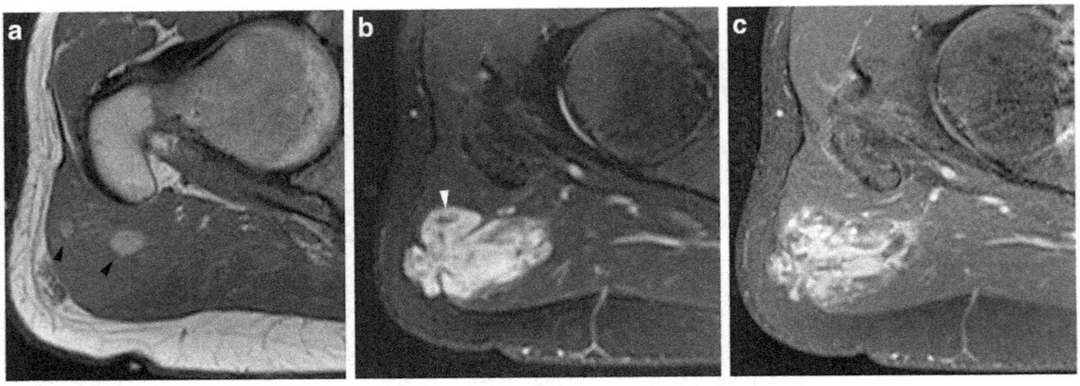

Fig. 14.4 MR venous malformation (VM). VM is isointense on T1 (**a**), hyperintense on T2 (**b**), and nonuniform lesion enhancement with contrast (**c**). Small hyperintense focal thrombus present on T1 (*black arrowheads*). Focal signal void phlebolith present on T2 (*white arrowhead*)

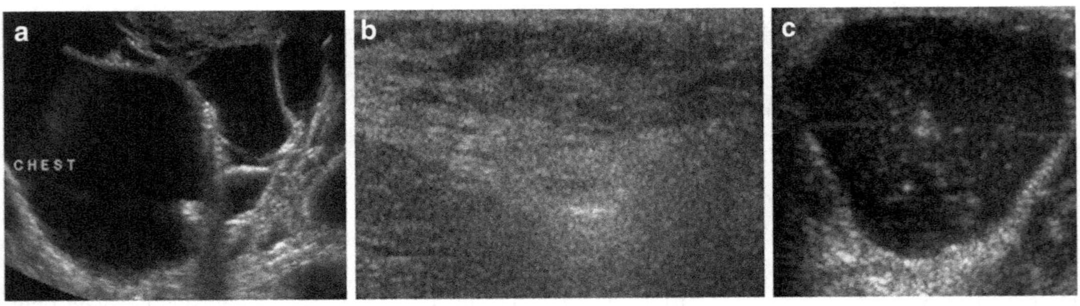

Fig. 14.5 Ultrasound lymphatic malformation (LM). Mixed LM (macro- and microcysts) (**a**). Microcystic LM as "solid echogenic tissue" with no ultrasound visible cysts (**b**). Macrocystic hemorrhage containing echogenic fluid (**c**)

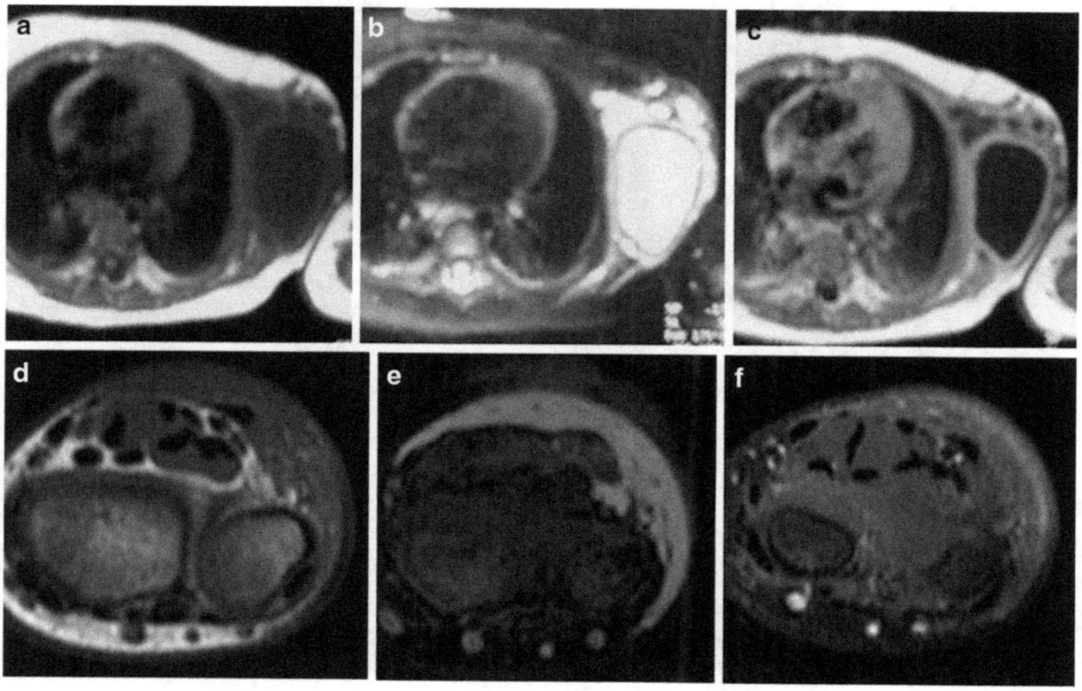

Fig. 14.6 MR of lymphatic malformation (LM). Macrocystic (**a–c**) and microcystic (**d–f**) LMs show similar T1 and T2 signal intensity (isointense on T1 (**a**, **d**), hyperintense on T2 (**b**, **e**)). Morphologically however these lesions differ. Cyst rim enhancement occurs in macrocystic LM (**c**). Microcystic LM rarely shows contrast enhancement and if so appears as a slight diffuse enhancement throughout the lesion (**f**)

Plain X-ray and CT scan are not required in most for diagnosis (they have a low tissue specificity). They may be required to assess abnormalities of skeletal growth associated with vascular malformations, to assess extremity overgrowth in Klippel–Trenaunay syndrome (KTS), and to evaluate challenging vascular anomalies involving the skeleton.

Conventional venography and catheter angiography are not required in the majority of patients. Venography is occasionally undertaken in VMs with significant phlebectasia to assess potential closure methods and in some patients to delineate communications between the VM and normal functioning veins. This can be done at the time of sclerotherapy. In KTS, venography to assess anomalous veins and the deep venous system prior to endovascular therapy is required as MR venography (MRV) is often inadequate (Fig. 14.7). Routine direct percutaneous puncture venography of VMs is only required during injection sclerotherapy Catheter arteriography is done during embolization in selected high-flow vascular anomalies (Fig. 14.8). Nuclear medicine has no role in imaging these disorders.

Equipment/Drugs

The array of equipment, embolic agents, and sclerotherapy agents is vast. Suggestions for materials for specific indications are listed in each section below.

Prophylactic Medications

Steroids, antibiotics, and nonsteroidal anti-inflammatory medication may be required as single intravenous doses for selected sclerotherapy and embolization procedures.

Dexamethasone (0.1 mg/kg, maximum 8 mg) is given if the lesion is in a confined space such as the orbit or airway.

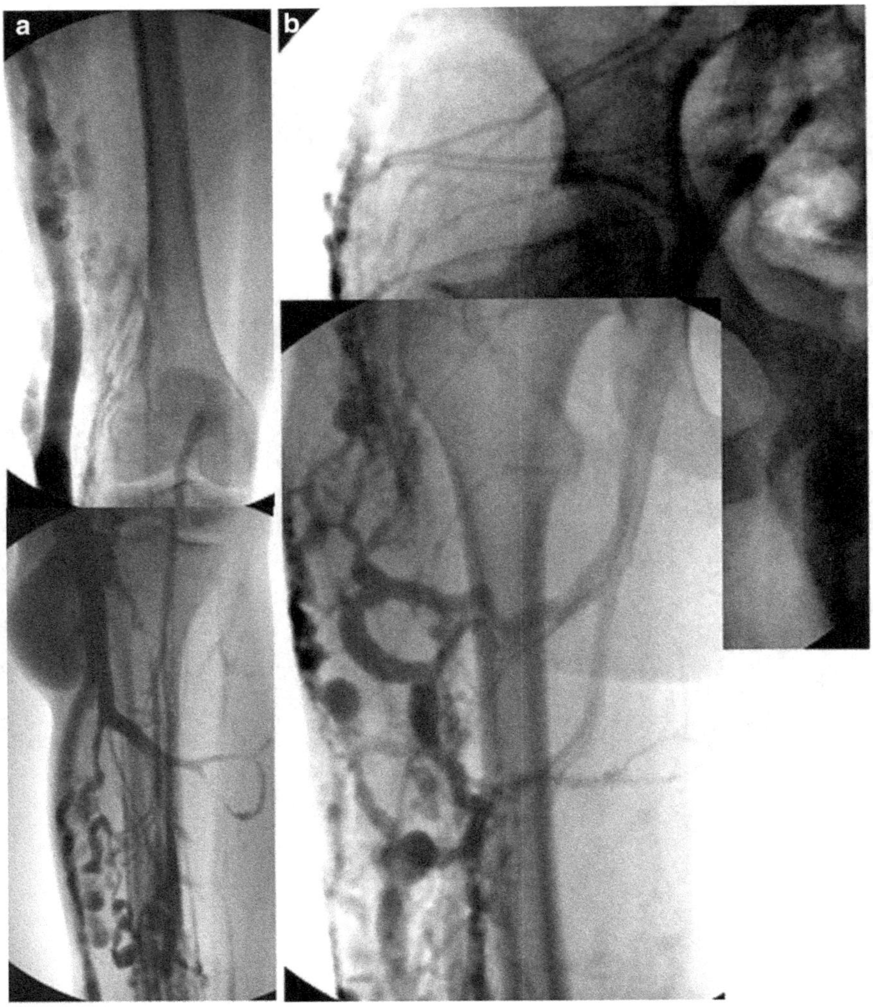

Fig. 14.7 Venogram of lateral marginal embryonic vein in Klippel–Trenaunay Syndrome. Performed by direct lower calf injection. In this patient, the lateral marginal vein is a single large channel, associated with a large superficial venous aneurysm below the knee (**a**). The embryonic vein drains via posterior channels in the upper thigh to the femoral vein and via gluteal channels to the iliac vein (**b**). The embryonic vein may also be composed of multiple intercommunicating channels

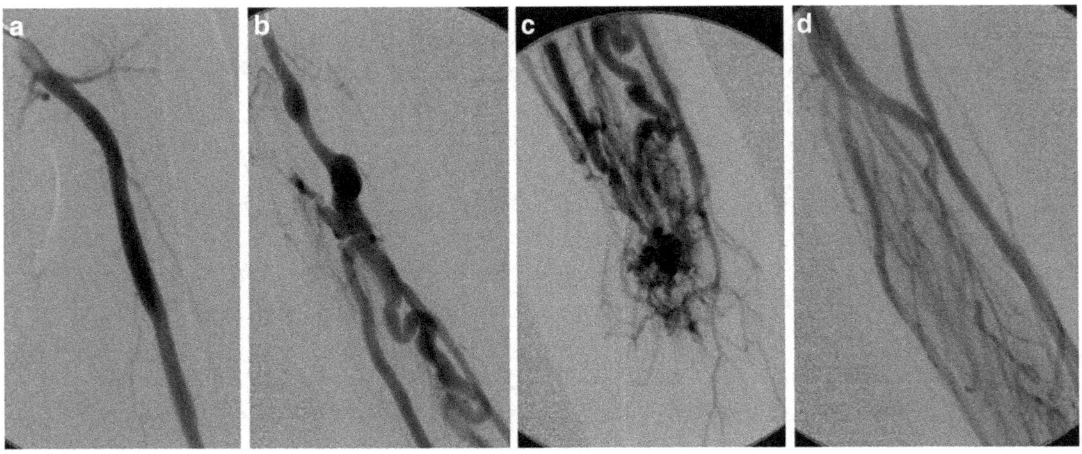

Fig. 14.8 Global catheter angiogram of upper extremity arteriovenous malformation (AVM). Typical finding with enlarged brachial artery (**a**); runoff into enlarged tortuous radial, ulnar, and interosseous arteries; arterial aneurysms at the elbow (**b**); shunts (nidi) in the distal forearm and palm (**c**); and early drainage into enlarged veins (**d**)

Cefazolin (30 mg/kg, maximum 1 g) should be given when treating oral, orbital, or perineal/perianal lesions.

Ketorolac (0.5 mg/kg, maximum 15 mg in those <16 years) is good at providing post-procedural pain (and can be repeated every 6 h if needed).

Vascular Tumors

The ISSVA classification of vascular tumors includes hemangiomas, kaposiform hemangioendotheliomas (KHEs), and tufted angioma. A description of vascular tumor types and associated treatments (including treatment of Kasabach–Merritt phenomenon [KMP]) follows.

Infantile Hemangiomas (IH)

IHs are the most common tumor of infancy, appearing a few weeks after birth. These flat red lesions are commonly cutaneous and present in the head and neck area [5]. 20 % have multiple lesions. Visceral hemangiomas occur in the liver, gastrointestinal tract, and brain. When more than five cutaneous lesions are present, liver ultrasound is performed to exclude hepatic involvement.

Infantile hemangiomas have a characteristic three-phase life cycle (Fig. 14.9). The first phase, the "proliferative phase," occurs within the first 9–12 months of postnatal life with rapid tumor growth and tumor angiogenesis. During this phase, tumor hypervascularity and high flow vascular shunting can be seen. The second phase, the slow "involuting phase," occurs over the next 5–7 years, with reduced vascularity, reduction in overall size. Reduced vascular flow and some fibrofatty replacement. The third or "involuted phase" occurs after 5–7 years with resultant fibrofatty residue. After involution, lesions do not recur, and approximately half of all patients will have e lesion.

When involving the superficial dermis, the flat, red lesions become raised during proliferation. Ulceration and bleeding can be seen in rapidly growing, large superficial tumors. Tumors in the lower dermis and subcutaneous tissue appear bluish or have no alteration in color to the overlying skin. During involution, the color of the tumor fades.

IH can be mistaken for other skin stains such as capillary malformations. Deep (i.e., subcutaneous) IH can be mistaken for VMs or LMs because of the bluish discoloration through the skin. IH showing high flow can be mistaken for AVMs, but the age at onset, growth pattern, and presence of tumor parenchyma in IH distinguish these two lesions.

The location of the IH may be associated with specific problems during the proliferative phase

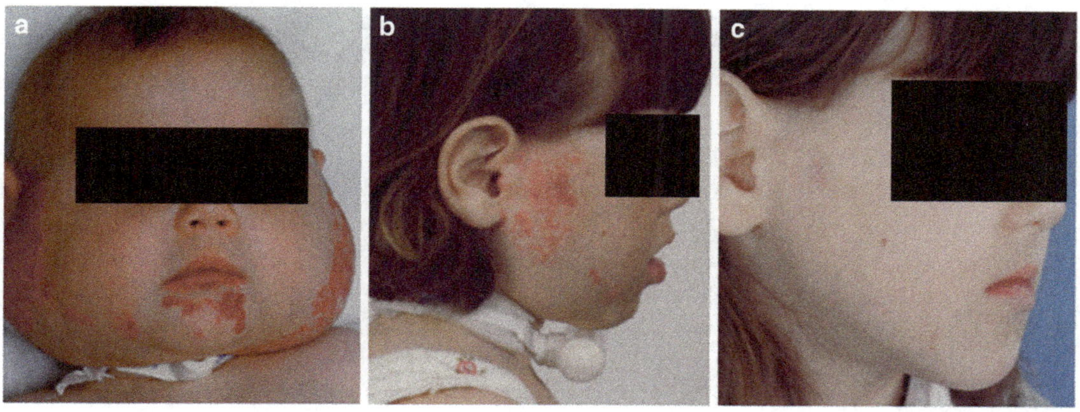

Fig. 14.9 3-phase life cycle of infantile hemangioma (IH). The progression of a patient with a "beard area" IH, is shown over time. IH also affected the airway (explaining the tracheostomy which was taken down when airway tumors involuted). (**a**) Phase 1: proliferative. (**b**) Phase 2: involuting. (**c**) Phase 3: involuted

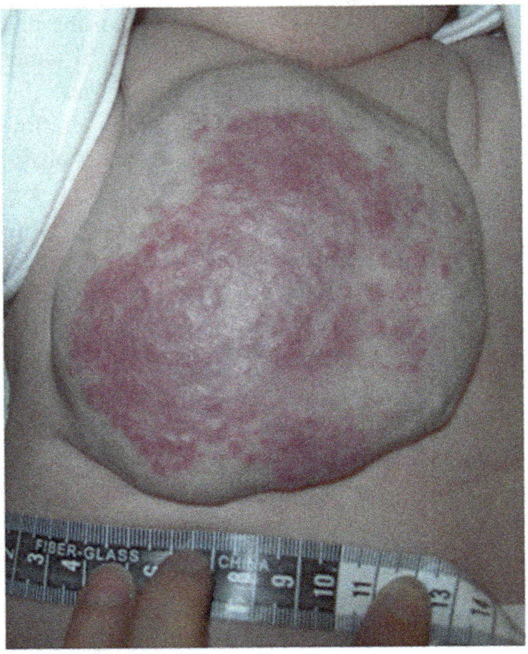

Fig. 14.10 Rapidly involuting congenital hemangioma (RICH). Large raised tumor extending across the posterior chest and abdominal wall of a baby. The blue periphery is due to large draining veins from AV shunting; however, infant was not in cardiac failure

when the tumor is rapidly increasing in size. Airway obstruction, visual impairment, gastrointestinal bleeding, high-output congestive heart failure from vascular shunting within large or multiple hemangiomas (particularly in the liver), and tissue necrosis can potentially occur.

Congenital Hemangiomas (CH)

CHs are rare and are distinct from IH [6, 7]. They arise antenatally and are fully developed at birth. They do not usually exhibit postnatal growth unless infants are preterm when they will continue to grow for some time. There are two types: the rapidly involuting congenital hemangioma (RICH) and the non-involuting congenital hemangioma (NICH) (Figs. 14.10, 14.11, 14.12, and 14.13). Clinically, they are quite different. RICHs are often impressive protuberant masses, whereas a NICH tends to be a flat to a slightly raised rounded skin lesion with telangiectasias and a pale surrounding halo. RICHs regress spontaneously usually by 12–14 months of postnatal life, whereas NICHs persist throughout life. Both are hypervascular tumors. Significant arteriovenous shunting can occur in the RICH before tumor regression which can potentially lead to cardiac failure. CHs can potentially be confused with vascular malformations; however, their clinical features and presence of tumor parenchyma provide clues to the antenatal and postnatal diagnosis. These tumors, although called hemangiomas, are quite distinct from IH. Interestingly, "hemangiomas" infrequently have features in common with both tumor types (IH and CH) in the same lesion.

Infantile Hepatic Hemangioma

There are three recognized types of infantile hepatic hemangioma (IHH): focal, multifocal, and diffuse (Fig. 14.14) [7]. The classical presentation with heart failure, anemia, and hepatomegaly is rare, and certainly not all hepatic hemangiomas are life-threatening.

Focal lesions are single, often large, and present antenatally. They do not grow after birth with regression usually seen in the first 12–14 months of postnatal life (similar to a RICH).

Multifocal hepatic hemangiomas have a three-phase life cycle, similar to typical cutaneous his. Small lesions, even when numerous, can be completely asymptomatic. Macrovascular shunts, if present in the focal and multifocal IHHs, can lead to high-output cardiac failure and require emergent catheter embolization, sometimes done as staged procedures [8–10].

In focal IHH, the onset of cardiac failure usually occurs at, or soon after, birth. In multifocal IHHs, the onset of cardiac failure may not occur for several months after birth. Embolization (Figs. 14.15, 14.16, and 14.17) should be performed in conjunction with other intensive medical support and medical therapy (including steroids and beta-blockers to promote tumor involution).

In the diffuse type, most of the liver parenchyma is replaced by tumor, typically causing

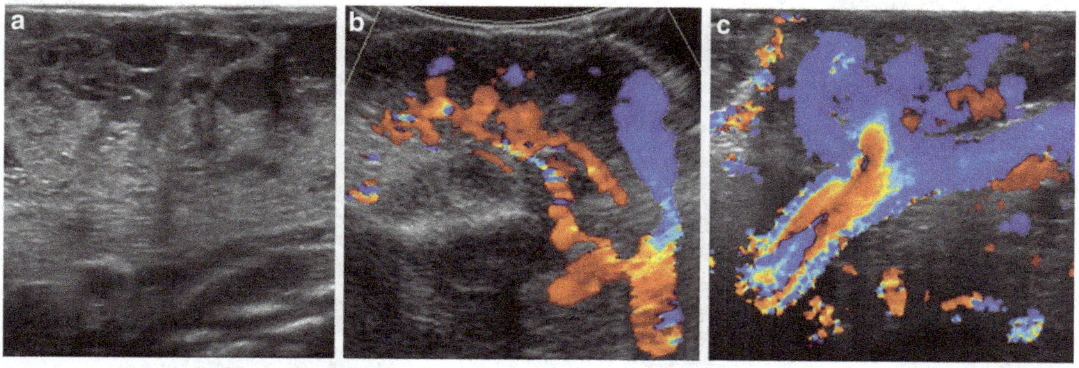

Fig. 14.11 Ultrasound RICH. Typical soft tissue tumor containing vascular spaces (**a**). Prominent arterial inflow (**b**) and venous outflow (**c**) on Doppler

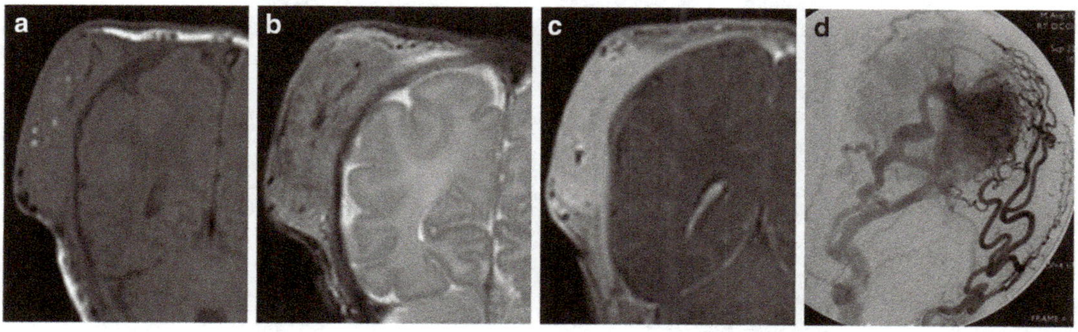

Fig. 14.12 MR and catheter angiogram of cephalic RICH. Typical appearances of RICH on MR showing T1 hypointensity (**a**), T2 hyperintensity (**b**), and diffuse contrast enhancement (**c**). Small intralesional hyperintense thrombi present on T1. Catheter angiogram shows prominent and tortuous feeding arteries and draining veins with staining of tumor parenchyma (**d**). Catheter angiography is not required in most RICH tumors unless embolization is required

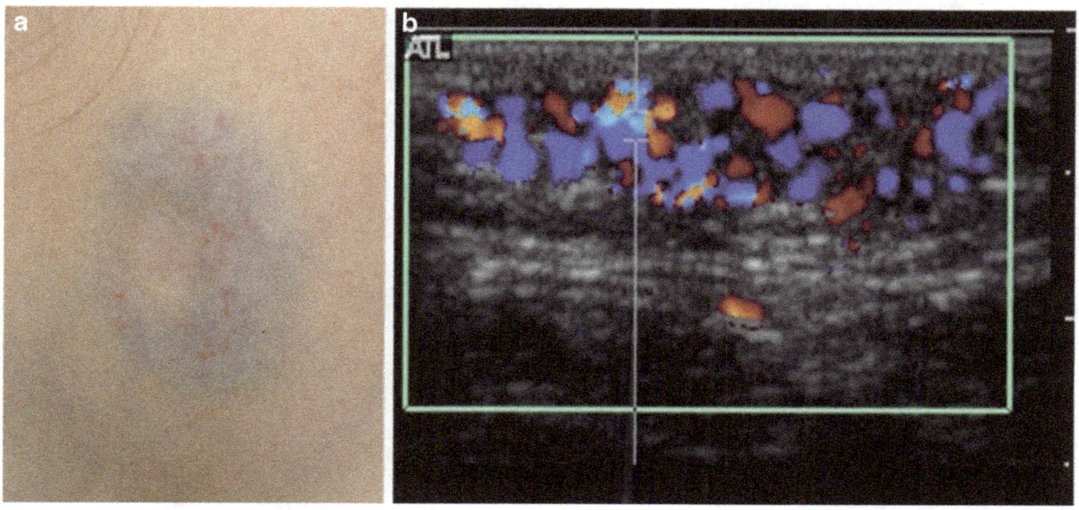

Fig. 14.13 Non-involuting congenital hemangioma (NICH). Typical appearance of NICH. Flat skin lesion with telangiectasias surrounded by a blue/pale "halo" (**a**). Ultrasound shows expected subcutaneous hypervascularity of NICH (**b**)

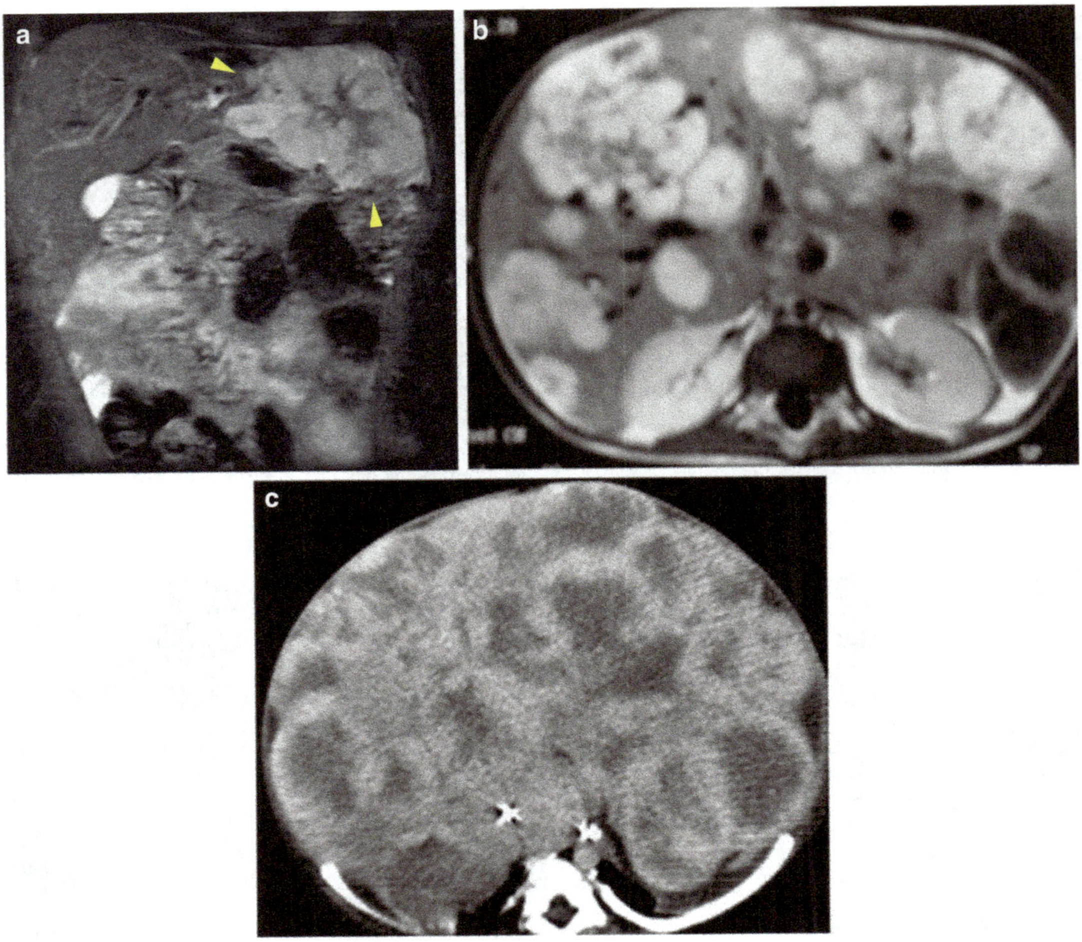

Fig. 14.14 Infantile hepatic hemangioma (IHH). The three types of IHH. Focal IHH (*yellow arrowheads*) (**a**) and multifocal IHH (**b**) are shown on T2W MR. Post-contrast CT demonstrates diffuse IHH (**c**)

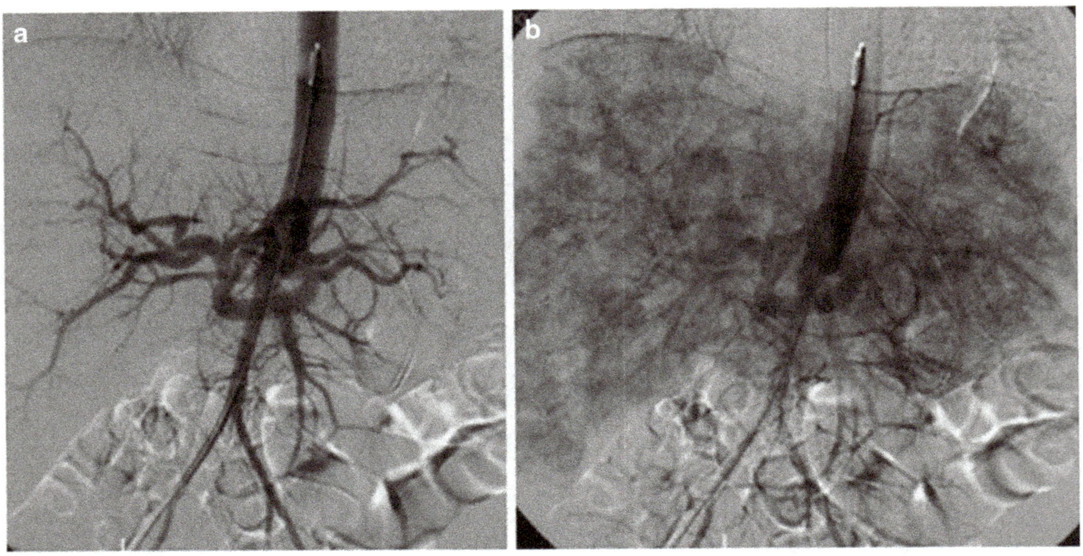

Fig. 14.15 Catheter angiography in infantile hepatic hemangioma (IHH). (**a**) and (**b**) Typical findings in multifocal IHH with enlarged aorta above the celiac trunk, enlarged hepatic artery, and multifocal hypervascular tumors. A femoral approach for catheterization may be difficult as aortoiliac vessels below the celiac trunk can be small especially with significant shunts. In this infant, no shunting was evident

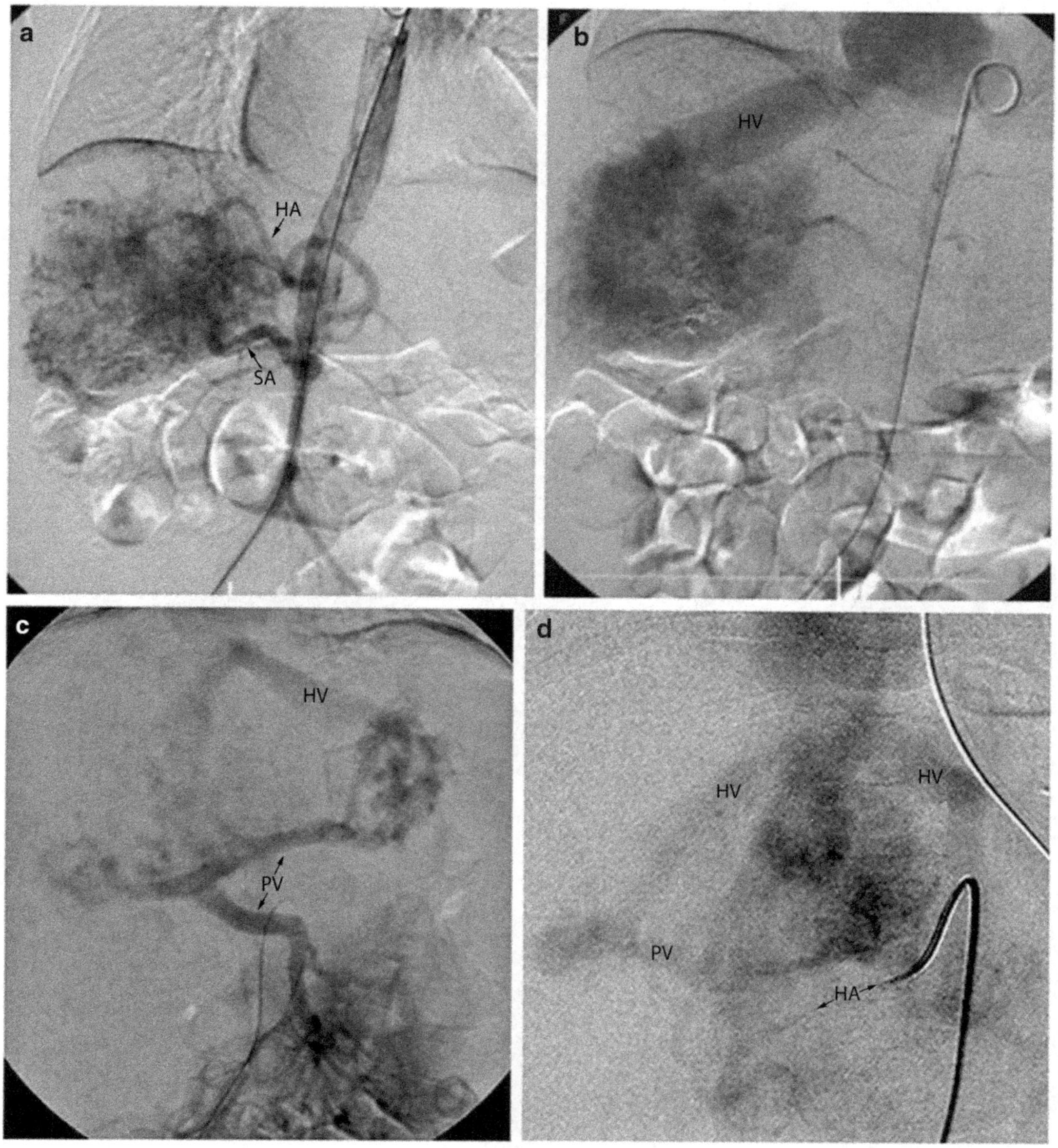

Fig. 14.16 Angiography of vascular shunts in infantile hepatic hemangioma. Arteriovenous shunts (hepatic artery/other systemic arteries to hepatic veins) (**a**, **b**), portovenous shunts (portal vein to hepatic vein) (**c**), and arterioportovenous shunts (hepatic artery/other systemic artery to portal vein to hepatic vein) (**d**) can occur within the tumors. *HA* hepatic artery, *SA* systemic artery, *HV* hepatic vein, *PV* portal vein

massive hepatomegaly, abdominal compartment syndrome, and respiratory compromise. The diffuse type can lead to severe hypothyroidism until there is tumor involution as the tumor produces type 3 iodothyronine deiodinase which inactivates circulating thyroid hormones. Large thyroxine doses are required by these infants. Diffuse IHH carries the highest mortality rates, and liver transplantation may be required for survival.

Tufted Angioma (TA) and Kaposiform Hemangioendothelioma

These sometimes aggressive and invasive vascular tumors are often present at birth, but they can present later. KHE is usually more extensive than TA. The tumors are often located on the trunk, shoulder, thigh, or retroperitoneum [11]. TA appears as a red skin plaque and KHE as

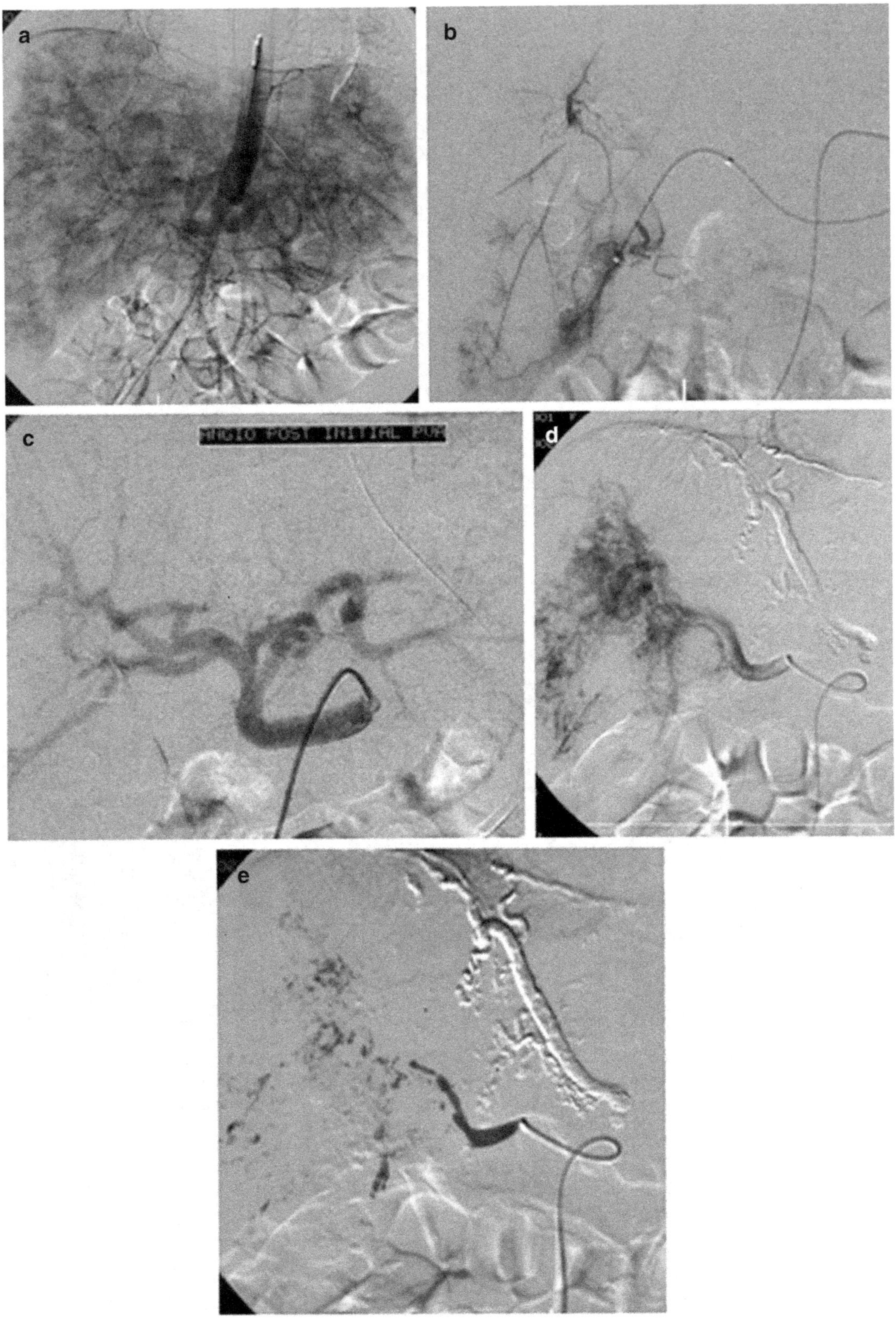

Fig. 14.17 Catheter embolization in infantile hepatic hemangioma. Coaxial technique with microcatheters will improve safety. Particles (e.g., PVA) can be used if there are no macroshunts (**a**). Particles can devascularize tumor reducing tumor staining (**b**) and preserve main vessels (**c**). When IHH macroshunts are present, proximal embolization of feeding vessels with glue (**d**)/other agents is effective (**e**)

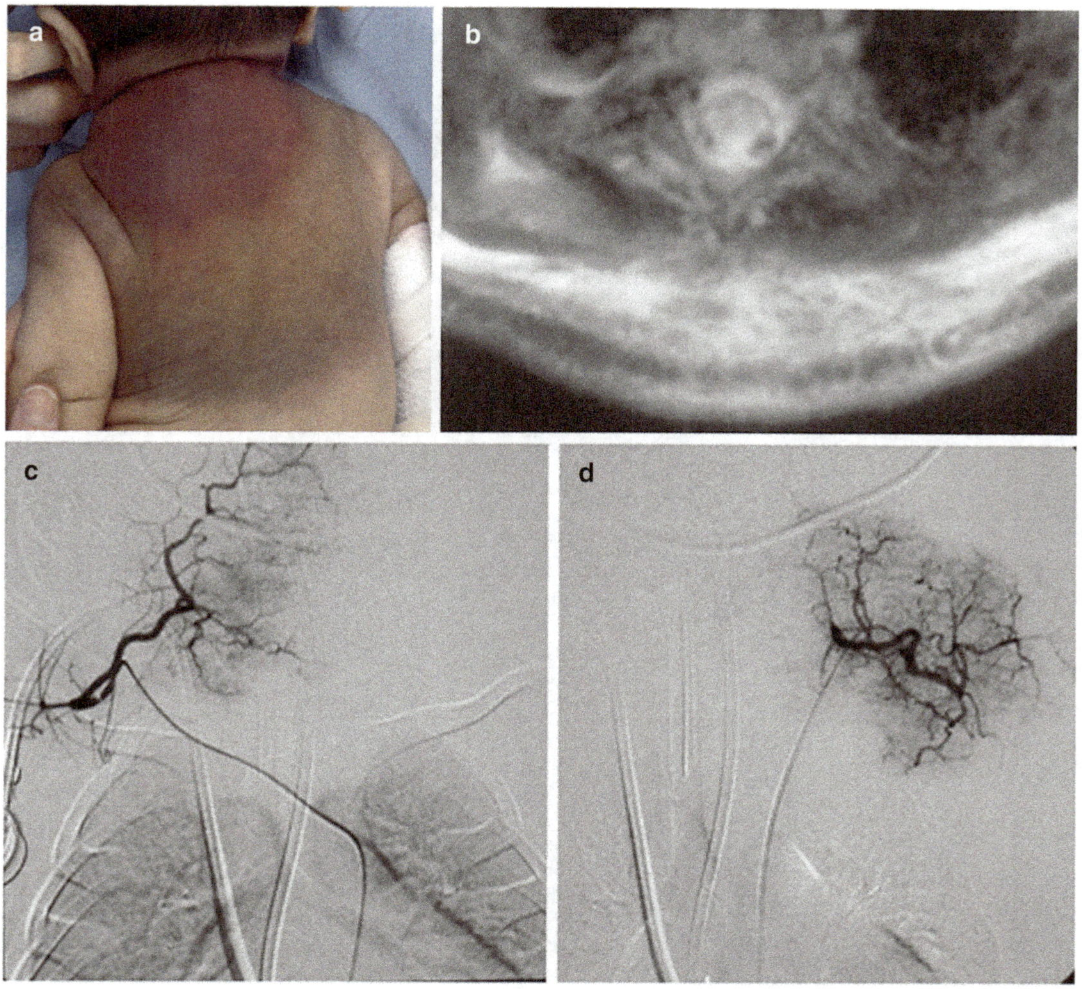

Fig. 14.18 Kaposiform hemangioendothelioma (KHE). Typical physical appearance of KHE with violaceous tumor (**a**). MR (T2) shows hyperintense soft tissue tumor with typical subcutaneous stranding from dilated subdermal lymphatics (**b**). Selective microcatheter angiography shows typical hypervascular tumor with no shunting (**c, d**)

violaceous skin lesion (Fig. 14.18). MR is excellent at evaluating these rare vascular tumors (Fig. 14.18). MR typically demonstrates stranding in the subcutaneous tissue in KHE (Fig. 14.18).

Tissue biopsy is not always required; however, a percutaneous image-guided needle biopsy can occasionally be helpful. Histology reveals infiltrating sheets of slender endothelial cells with positive staining for lymphatic elements.

Kasabach–Merritt Phenomenon

KMP refers to thrombocytopenia from platelet consumption associated with a coagulopathy and occurs in KHE and TA only. It does not occur in other vascular tumors or any vascular malformation.

Typically, the thrombocytopenia is severe with a platelet count <10,000 × 10/μL (10 × 10^9/L in SI units). A coagulopathy occurs with reduced fibrinogen levels are elevated prothrombin and partial thromboplastic times. Bleeding is can be seen. Treatment for most is medical, as tumors may be large and extensive [12, 13]. Supportive measures in critical care may be needed. Low-dose weekly intravenous vincristine and oral corticosteroids are usually given. In KMP, the mortality is between 20 and 30 %, and tumors

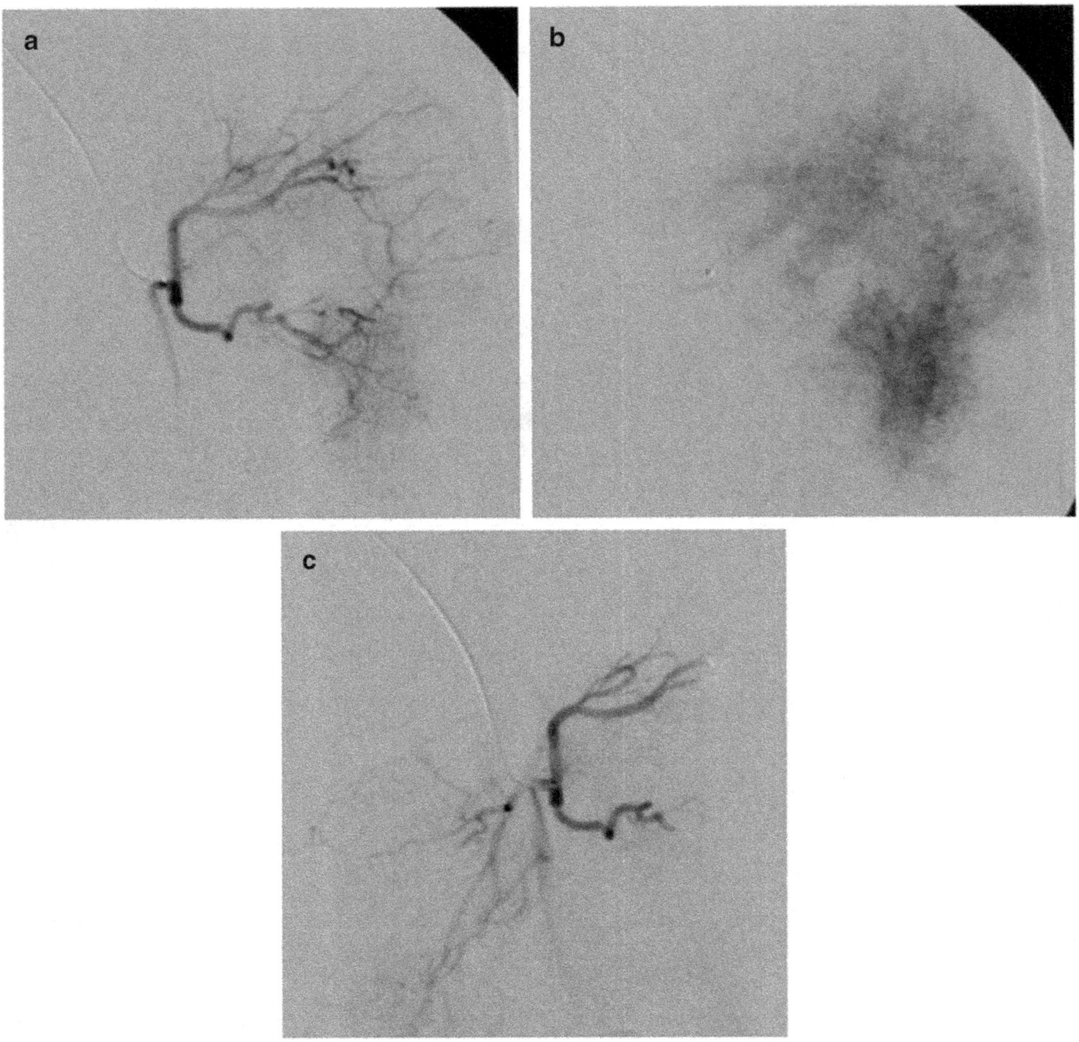

Fig. 14.19 Catheter embolization of kaposiform hemangioendothelioma (KHE). Typical angiographic appearance of KHE with tumor staining (**a**, **b**). For embolization, particles (e.g., PVA) are used to devascularize the tumor parenchyma, reduce tumor staining, and preserve main arterial trunks (**c**)

show proliferation into early childhood with eventual incomplete regression despite being otherwise asymptomatic. Platelet transfusions are usually reserved for patients with platelet counts <10,000 × 10/μL where there is a risk of spontaneous intracranial hemorrhage. Routine platelet transfusion is not recommended as this can lead to increase in tumor size.

Transcatheter arterial embolization using polyvinyl alcohol particles (size range 250–350 μm) can improve the thrombocytopenia (Figs. 14.18 and 14.19) and may need to be repeated. Most patients nowadays, as mentioned above, receive low-dose weekly vincristine, and catheter embolization is not required. Particle embolization should be considered as adjunctive therapy if the thrombocytopenia is refractory to vincristine and angiogenesis inhibitors (steroids).

Treatment of Vascular Tumors

The majority of IHs do not require specific treatment other than observation and reassurance for the family. Previously, approximately 10 % of IHs were treated as they were "endangering" by virtue of their location or functional risks, e.g., airway compromise or heart failure. Nowadays, more infants with cutaneous IHs are treated medically, usually with oral beta-blockers (propranolol) or angiogenesis inhibitors, mainly corticosteroids (prednisone), often up until 10–12 months of age. Intralesional corticosteroid injection can be undertaken for IHs that cause local deformity or ulceration. Ultrasound guidance can help target the injection into the solid tumor component. Systemic low-dose chemotherapy with vincristine (via a central venous catheter or PICC) may be considered in challenging cases.

In selected patients, surgical excision may be considered. Surgical resection is sometimes undertaken for IHs during/after the involuting phase and also for NICHs. Nd:YAG lasing with epidermal ice cooling has been recommended as an option to treat the deeper subcutaneous component of IHs. It is important to wait for completion of regression of RICHs and completed involution in IHs before plastic surgery is considered to deal with cosmetic issues.

Catheter angiography and embolization is rarely needed for infants with vascular tumors. It can be extremely useful and sometimes lifesaving when endovascular closure of macroshunts (Figs. 14.16–14.18) or devascularization of the tumor bed is required (Figs. 14.19 and 14.20) (Table 14.2).

Practical Tips for Catheter Angiography and Embolization in Infants with Vascular Tumors

1. Avoid "routine" catheter angiography unless combined with embolization (preservation of vascular access is vital for repeat procedures).
2. Staged embolization may be needed (complex lesions, limited contrast volume).
3. Limit contrast volume to a maximum of 6 mL/kg/procedure (300 mg/mL iodinated contrast). Selective angiography, dilute contrast, and minimizing unnecessary nonselective injections (including aortography) can maximize usable contrast.
4. Use the smallest sized vascular introducer sheaths and catheters for the procedure (e.g., 4F sheath, 4F outer coaxial catheter, and microcatheter systems).
5. Use US-guided arterial access. For femoral and left brachial artery catheterization in neonates, use a 24G angiocatheter, a short 0.014″ wire, and 3 Fr dilator. Then upsize the guidewire to a short 0.018″, and then place a 4 Fr vascular introducer sheath. For brachial arteries, pass a 0.0014″ or a 0.018″ wire into the descending thoracic aorta advancing over it a 4 Fr angiographic catheter preloaded with the microcatheter.
6. For IHH, evaluate shunt type(s). If the arteriovenous shunts are supplied solely by the hepatic artery (with no portal vein shunting), perform nonselective embolization of the hepatic artery. Portovenous shunts can be closed by transjugular access of the hepatic veins to access the portal vein. Alternatively, direct transhepatic puncture of the portal vein and shunts can be performed.
7. Small femoral arteries and a small infra-celiac aorta are challenging for catheterization when significant arteriovenous shunts exist in IHH. Consider brachial artery approach.
8. Pump inject contrast via a high-flow microcatheter for abdominal aortography (1 mL/kg over 2 s) with DSA 6 frames/s and for arterioportography via SMA (0.8 mL/kg over 4 s) with DSA 4 frames/s.
9. For selective angiography into aortic branches and portal vein, use hand injections.
10. Use a coaxial technique (with a maximum 4 Fr outer catheter) for delivery of embolics.
11. Be familiar with suitable embolic agents. Glue, particles, and microcoils should be delivered via suitable microcatheters.
12. Do not use ethanol or sodium tetradecyl sulfate (STS) for vascular tumor embolization as they will cause tissue necrosis. Do not use particles for macroshunts.
13. Glue (Histoacryl, B Braun, Aesculap AG, Tuttlingen, Germany) should be mixed with Lipiodol Ultra Fluid (Guerbert, EZEM, Montreal, QC, Canada). See section on AVM.
14. If Amplatzer Vascular Plugs are used (AGA Medical Corporation, Plymouth, MN, USA),

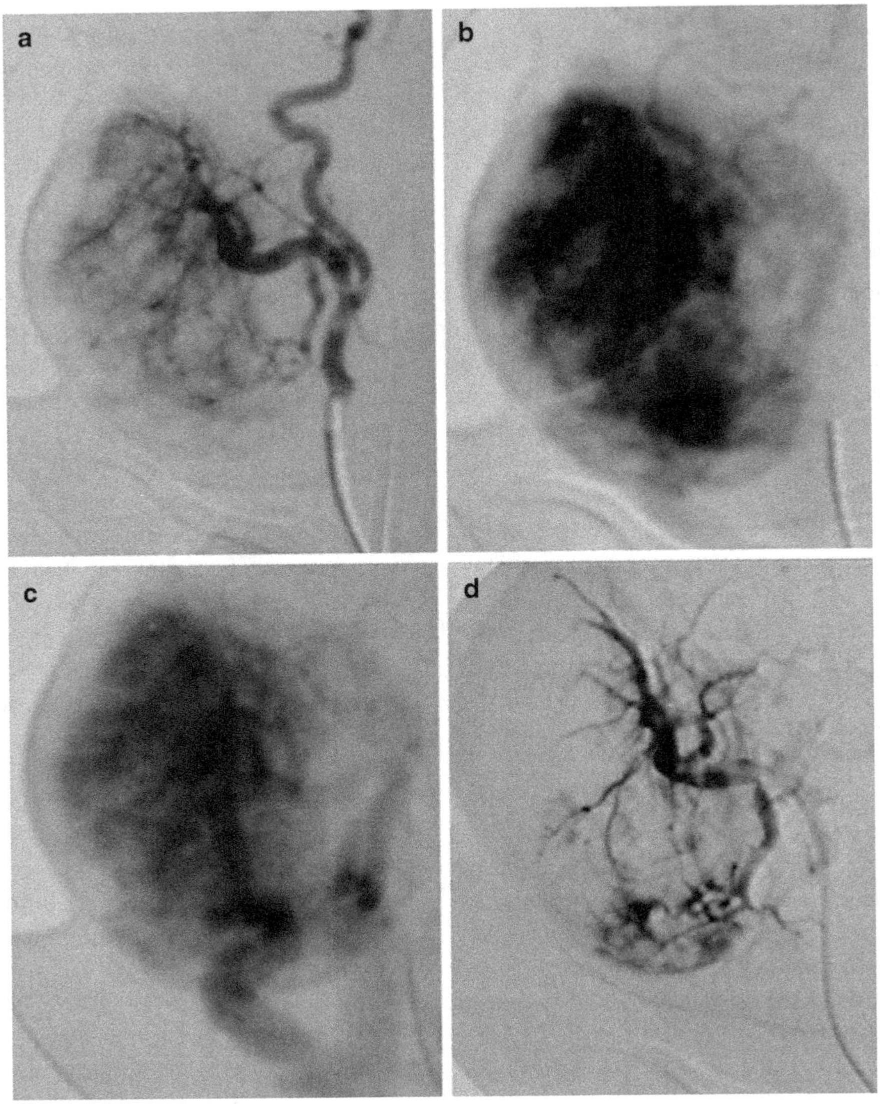

Fig. 14.20 Catheter angiography and embolization in proliferative phase infantile hemangioma (IH). Infant with large parotid IH. Enlarged inflow facial artery (**a**), intense tumor parenchymal staining (**b**), and enlarged draining veins (**c**) typify proliferative IH. Particle embolization results in significant devascularization (**d**). N.B. most infants with IH do not require catheter angiography/embolization

an AVP 4 is useful as this can be delivered via a 4 Fr catheter.

15. In the absence of bleeding, give systemic heparin for the procedure (initial 100 units/kg, repeating every 2 h depending on activated clotting time).
16. Small arteries can spasm. Use nitroglycerine via vascular sheaths prior to removal and if needed during the case via the vascular sheath/angiographic catheter (bolus dose = 3 μg/kg). Consider application of topical nitroglycerine gel at the brachial artery puncture site after the sheath is withdrawn (spread gel using a 4 mm length of gel/kg).

Vascular Malformations

The ISSVA classification of vascular malformations (Table 14.1) is based on the flow characteristics of the lesion and the vascular channel type involved. Lesions are subtyped/secondarily

Table 14.2 Vascular tumor embolization

Vascular tumor	Clinical problem	Procedure urgency	Embolic agent	Aim of embolization
IHH	Cardiac failure 2°	Emergent	Glue	Selectively close shunts in IHH. General tumor devascularization in RICH
RICH	Vascular shunting within the tumor		Coils Particles Vascular plugs	N.B. IHH shunts can be arteriovenous (hepatic artery and or other systemic arteries to hepatic veins), portovenous (portal to hepatic veins), arterioportovenous, or combinations of these
KHE	KMP, platelets $<10\times10^9$/L	Emergent	Particles, e.g., PVA	Selectively devascularize small peripheral arterial branches within the tumor. Maintain patency of main feeding vessels
All	Refractory bleeding, e.g., from skin, intra-abdominal/hepatic, and airway lesions	Emergent/semi-elective	Glue Coils Vascular plugs Particles	General tumor devascularization
	Prior to surgical excision of tumor	Elective		

classified based on the tissue of origin and anatomy. The most commonly encountered vascular malformations are discussed below.

Low-Flow Vascular Malformations

Capillary Malformation (CM)

CM is the most common vascular malformation. They are commonly called "port-wine stains" and are frequently located as focal skin stains in the head and neck area (Fig. 14.21). The low-flow, cutaneous lesions are flat and pink-red in color and are present at birth. They can be localized or extensive. CMs do not fade and are permanent throughout life.

Syndromic CMs, such as Sturge–Weber syndrome (SWS), occur more rarely. In SWS, the CM is located on the face and affects the first and second trigeminal dermatomes. It is associated with ipsilateral leptomeningeal vascular malformations and cerebral atrophy. In the complex combined low-flow vascular malformation, KTS, the CM commonly affects a lower extremity.

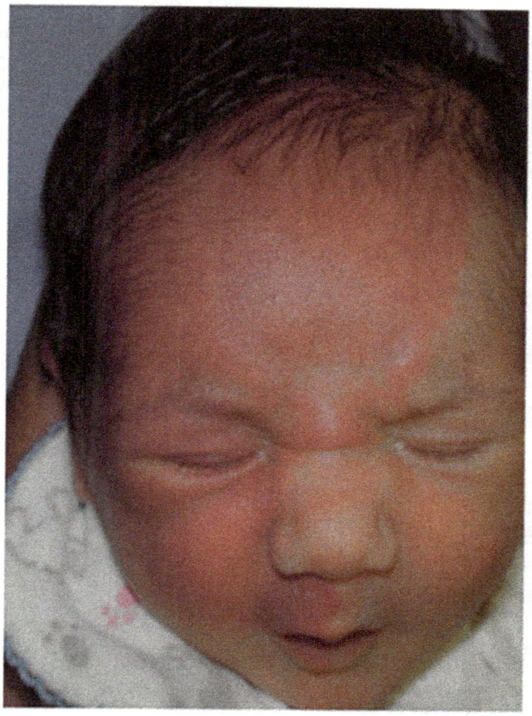

Fig. 14.21 Capillary malformation (CM). Typical physical appearance of CM with flat red skin stain or "port-wine stain" affecting first and second trigeminal dermatomes

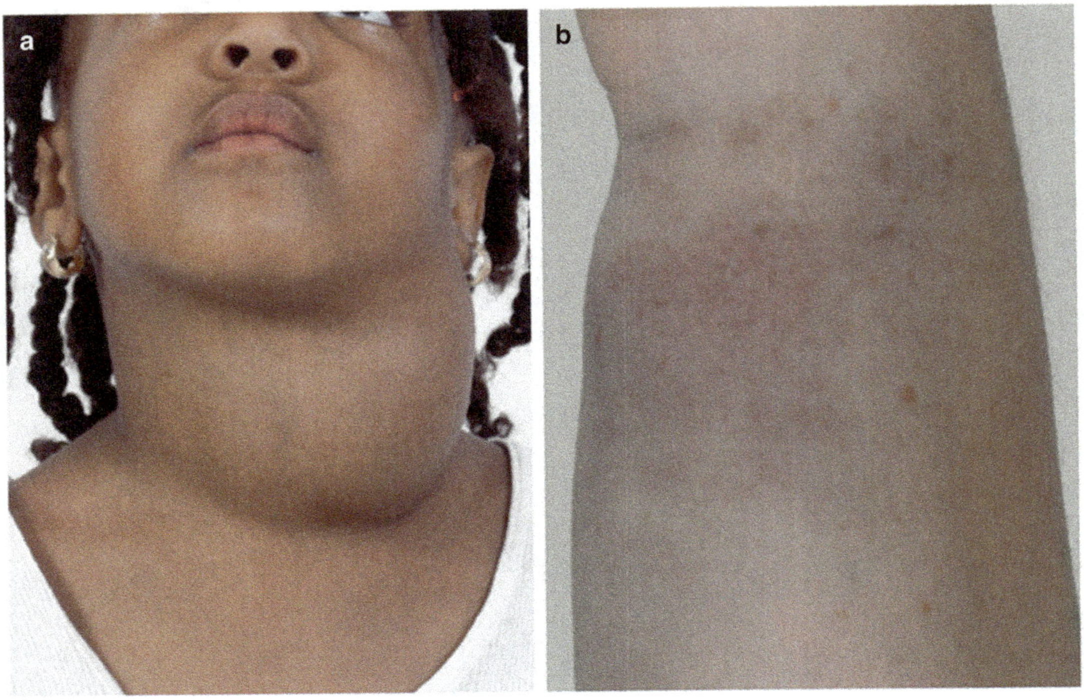

Fig. 14.22 Lymphatic malformation (LM). Typical physical findings in 2 patients. Soft, partly compressible swelling of the neck caused by a large macrocystic LM (**a**). Firm expansion of the wrist with bruising (from spontaneous intralesional hemorrhage) in a microcystic LM (**b**)

The diagnosis of a CM is clinical. No imaging is required for diagnosis (unless brain imaging is undertaken for those with SWS). Treatment of CMs is for cosmesis with flash-lamp pulsed-dye laser therapy being the treatment of choice [14].

There is no role for interventional radiology in the treatment of CMs.

Lymphatic Malformation (LM)

LMs are made up of cysts containing lymphatic fluid which exhibit low-flow characteristics and are classified as macrocystic, microcystic, or mixed LMs [15]. Outdated terminology such as "cystic hygromas" and "lymphangiomas" should no longer be used.

The definition of macro- and microcysts has been inconsistent. Some consider macrocysts to be those with cyst cavities visible on imaging, whereas microcysts have no visible cyst on imaging and are evident only on histopathology. However, many consider macrocysts to be those with cyst diameters >1 cm and microcysts with cyst diameters <1 cm. Mixed LMs are those with both macro- and microcystic elements.

LMs often present as localized masses, but infiltrative lesions can be seen. Fluid leakage (chylous fluid in body cavities or weeping from skin vesicles) can occur (Fig. 14.22). LMs are usually noted at birth; however, they can be seen at any age including prenatally on imaging. Although skin and soft tissues (subcutaneous and fascial planes in muscle) are most commonly affected, LMs can involve bone and more rarely viscera such as the GI tract and lungs. The axillary, thoracic, cervicofacial, mediastinal, retroperitoneal, buttock, and anogenital regions are commonly affected. Soft tissue and skeletal hypertrophy can occur with LMs. Macrocystic LMs appear as soft partially compressible masses. These can be differentiated from VMs as macrocystic LMs show no increase in size on dependency and no refilling after release of compression. Lymphedema can occur if there is diffuse infiltration of subcutaneous tissues. Interestingly, infection and intralesional bleeding can occur in all types of LMs, leading sometimes to alarming expansion of the lesion with pain and a red/blue skin discoloration (appearing like a bruise). With infection, a clinical presentation of cellulitis can be seen. Sepsis has been reported when infection occurs in extensive LMs.

The problems associated with LMs can often be related to their location, e.g., proptosis from periorbital LMs, airway obstruction in cervicofacial LMs, clear fluid and bleeding from tongue surface LM vesicles, and protein-losing enteropathy in GI tract disease. LMs of the extremities can be associated with overgrowth and limb length discrepancy. In Gorham's syndrome soft tissue and skeletal LMs with progressive osteolysis, pathological fractures and vertebral instability can occur.

LM Imaging

LMs are best imaged by US and MRI (Figs. 14.5 and 14.6) [4]. MR better documents the full extent of deeper, larger, and more complex LMs. Macrocystic structures on US and MR are easily seen when cysts are larger than 1 cm in diameter. Microcystic LMs may only have cysts seen on histopathology and often appear as predominantly solid lesions with no identifiable cysts on imaging. LMs on MRI appear hypointense on T1 and hyperintense on T2 (because of high water content). Macrocystic LMs show septal contrast enhancement. Microcystic LMs may not show contrast enhancement or ill-defined enhancement of the entire lesion. Fluid-fluid levels in cysts are due to layering of protein or blood. Enlarged or anomalous venous channels can sometimes be seen in close proximity to LMs. Contrast lymphangiography can identify abnormal lymphatic channels and leaks in those lymphatic anomalies of the thoracic duct and in patients with chylous effusions.

LM Treatment

The indications for treatment of LMs include troublesome symptoms with recurrent swelling, pain, infections, functional impairment, leakage of fluid from the LM into body cavities/skin, and cosmesis. Treatment options include injection sclerotherapy, surgical interventions, laser techniques, conservative measures, and combinations of these [16, 17]. Recently, medical therapy with rapamycin and sildenafil has been suggested for selected patients [18, 19]. Focal and macrocystic lesions can be treated by both sclerotherapy and resection with excellent results [17, 20]. The advantages of sclerotherapy for macrocystic LMs include avoidance of surgical scars, reduced risk of neurovascular injury, and uneventful recoveries in most (Fig. 14.23). Diffuse and predominantly microcystic LMs are difficult to eradicate although sclerotherapy can offer some reduction in lesion size, depending on the number of cysts that can be injected [17]. Surgical resection of complex and microcystic LM can be beneficial and usually needs to be well planned and staged. The recurrence rate however post surgery for this type of LM is approximately 40 % and is due to regrowth and or re-expansion of residual disease. Scars from multiple surgeries are not uncommon and themselves can lead to problems including disease developing along scar edges. It has been suggested that sclerotherapy of the resection cavity may help reduce disease "recurrence."

It has been difficult to compare treatment outcomes from surgery and injection sclerotherapy. Invariably, surgical results are based on cosmetic appearances with no postsurgical imaging to assess deep residual disease.

Intralesional bleeding causing sudden enlargement of LMs and pain can be treated conservatively with analgesics. LM enlargement occurring with systemic viral/bacterial infections usually resolves without specific treatment. Bacterial infections occurring in the LM resulting in a "cellulitis-like" presentation with reddening, enlargement, hardening, and pain require appropriate antibiotics, often intravenous. Rarely are long-term prophylactic antibiotics required. Good pain management may be required for those with extensive disease suffering troublesome pain.

LM Sclerotherapy

Pre-procedure Work-Up

No special pre-procedure work-up is needed. Most injection sclerotherapy procedures are done

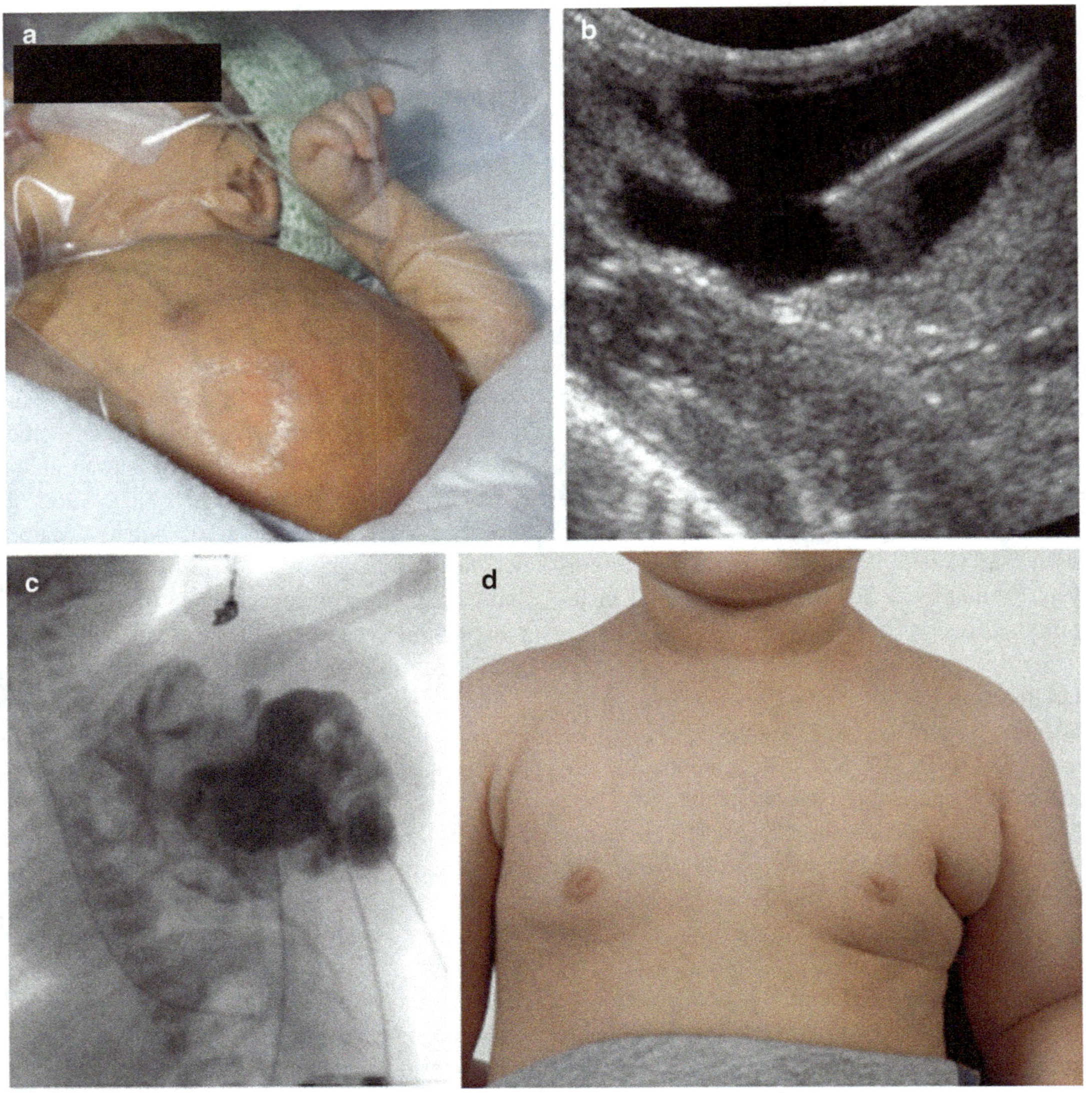

Fig. 14.23 Lymphatic malformation (LM) sclerotherapy. Large macrocystic chest wall LM present at birth (**a**). Ultrasound-guided needle puncture (**b**) and drain placement for doxycycline sclerotherapy (**c**). Three treatment sessions performed with excellent sclerotherapy result. No residual LM was seen on 18-month follow-up US scan. Significant tissue expansion caused by the large LM results in excess skin folds at 18 months (**d**)

with ultrasound guidance. Fluoroscopic or CT guidance is rarely needed for LM sclerotherapy unless drains are placed/challenging locations are treated (as with mediastinal/intrathoracic/intraosseous disease).

Procedure

Cysts to be treated are evaluated with US, the patient is placed in an optimum position to access the cysts, and the skin is prepped. Cysts are then punctured with a 21 or 22 gauge needle (sheathed or non-sheathed) using US guidance. Fluid is aspirated and sclerosant injected. Small drains can be placed into one or more of the larger macrocysts with ultrasound guidance, and cyst fluid aspirated before sclerosant is injected (Fig. 14.23). Sclerosant agents used for LM sclerotherapy include doxycycline (APP Pharmaceuticals LLC, Schaumburg, IL, USA), 3 % STS (Omega, Montreal, QC, Canada), ethanol or dehydrated alcohol 100 % (Sandoz Canada, Boucherville, QC, Canada), and bleomycin (Hospira, Saint-Laurent, QC, Canada).

Doxycycline solution is used at a concentration of 10 mg/mL. Approximate maximum doses of doxycycline for one treatment session are 300 mg in babies and 1,200 mg for children 12 years and older. When using doxycycline, half the volume of the aspirated fluid is replaced with the doxycycline solution. Some cysts visible on ultrasound are too small to be aspirated, and therefore a small volume of doxycycline is injected into each cyst. When drains are placed into larger macrocysts (>5 cm diameter), a 4 Fr micropuncture access is useful. Over the 0.0018″ wire, exchange the 4 Fr dilator for a short 5 Fr drain (e.g., 5 Fr Duan drain (COOK Medical, Bloomington, IN, USA)). Larger and longer drains may be required. All cyst fluid is aspirated, and again half the volume is replaced with doxycycline. Irrigation of those cysts with a drain, initially with 3 % STS liquid, may add to the effectiveness of the doxycycline. Drains should be closed for 6 h post sclerosant injection and then opened. Repeat sclerosant (STS and doxycycline) injection is done the following day under general anesthesia or sedation, and drains again are switched off for 6 h. After aspiration, the drains are removed and the patient can be discharged. LM sclerotherapy results in scarring and cyst collapse and may need to be repeated at 6-week intervals. For well-localized macrocystic LMs, sclerotherapy can be curative. For more diffuse and complex LMs, sclerotherapy can lead to much improvement, and treatments usually need to be staged. Weeping or bleeding from cutaneous vesicles can be controlled with local injection sclerotherapy, although leakage generally resumes after a short interval.

Bleomycin has been shown to be effective in many patients with LMs [21–23]. However, as results of doxycycline sclerotherapy for macrocystic LMs are excellent, bleomycin potentially offers an option for microcystic LMs. Because of reduced postsclerotherapy swelling seen with bleomycin, it has advantages for usage in locations such as the oral cavity, airway, and orbit. The amount of bleomycin injected is determined by the size of the LM. Bleomycin solution is used at a concentration of 1 mg/mL. A suggested maximum intralesional dose per treatment is 1 mg/kg or 15 mg (15 units).

Most LM sclerotherapy is done as an elective day-case procedure. Patients are monitored in hospital for up to 4 h during which time-repeated observations of the treated area are made. Admission may be needed in young infants or if the LM requires drainage and repeat injections the following day. Elective intensive care admission is needed if the LM is located in challenging areas such as the thoracic oral cavity or airway. As Bleomycin is associated with less post-sclerotherapy swelling, this can be an advantage when treating certain locations such as the tongue. Using Bleomycin may avoid the need for intensive care post-sclerotherapy.

Post-procedure Care

Following sclerotherapy, some swelling of the treated area is expected. Significant pain is unexpected and should be managed appropriately. Complications are unusual and unexpected following LM sclerotherapy. Infrequent self-limited minor bleeding can be seen into the treated cyst (during the procedure or shortly after). Rarely, skin injury with necrosis is seen with doxycycline and occurs with overfilling of superficial cysts.

At the time of discharge, the patient should be systemically well. Significant swelling at the treated site is unexpected. Provided the patient is otherwise well, tissue swelling does not preclude discharge from hospital. Patients must be able to swallow sufficient fluids and have stable and satisfactory vital functions, and minor pain must be easily controlled with oral analgesics prior to discharge. All patients should be aware of the follow-up arrangements and be provided with a contact should unexpected problems arise. Crutches or a walker for younger children may be required for a few days if treatment temporarily impairs mobility before swelling resolves. We generally caution against exercise for 2 weeks postsclerotherapy to avoid trauma to the treated area.

Follow-up

Repeat LM sclerotherapy is performed approximately every 6 weeks. Patients with small lesions are reviewed clinically and with US ahead of the next planned treatment. Once treatment is completed (shown by significant improvement on physical examination), outpatient clinical follow-up is arranged at 3 and 12 months when imaging can be repeated. If all is well, patients are then seen at infrequent intervals (every few years) throughout childhood. Patients are aware that sudden expansion of the LM may demand attendance at emergency and particularly if there is evidence of localized infection and cellulitis, as these require antibiotic treatment.

Practical Tips for LM Sclerotherapy

1. Use US and avoid routine fluoroscopic guidance for most procedures.
2. Use US to guide punctures and for real-time imaging during cyst injection.
3. Routine iodinated contrast injection (including mixing of iodinated contrast with doxycycline solution) is not required in most cases.
4. Contrast injection is done if there are concerns about associated venous malformations or phlebectasia.
5. The types/lengths of needle used for cyst access is dependent on lesion location/depth.
6. LMs can have variable intercommunications between cysts (irrespective of cyst size).
7. With cyst intercommunication, ultrasound shows movement of the injected sclerosant solution into adjacent cysts.
8. It is often difficult to aspirate fluid from all cysts that intercommunicate by one puncture. The filling volume in intercommunicating cysts is inaccurate based on aspirated volume, and it is best to judge the filling volume by continuing to inject the doxycycline until there is slight resistance or the maximum dose is reached.
9. Consider drain placement into smaller macrocysts when significant cyst intercommunications are seen. The drain (as when treating a large macrocyst) can be opened after 6 h and used for possible repeat sclerosant injection the following day.
10. Secure all drains well. No sutures are needed. Adhesive transparent dressings and external securement devices are usually successful.
11. When treating microcystic disease by injection sclerotherapy, it is useful to consider how much of the disease contains cysts suitable for injection (i.e., visible on ultrasound). With few small microcyst cavities visible on US, reduction in lesion size may be limited.
12. Lingual microcystic LMs are challenging. Bleomycin can be injected into the tongue. In babies, microcystic LM of the tongue can be injected with bleomycin (0.5 mg/kg/session every 3 weeks and review after several sessions).

Venous Malformations (VM)

VMs are the most frequent vascular malformation referred to vascular anomaly clinics and the most frequent vascular malformation treated by pediatric interventional radiologists (Fig. 14.24). They are low-flow lesions and consist of sinusoidal venous spaces with thin walls, abnormal smooth muscle cells, and variable communications with adjacent veins. In glomuvenous malformations (a VM variant), the vascular channels are lined by glomus cells [24].

VMs can arise anywhere in the body and may involve all tissue planes. Commonly, they are seen in the skin and soft tissues [3, 25]. Forty percent affect the head and neck, 40 % affect extremities, and the remainder the trunk. Visceral involvement can occur. They grow in proportion to the patient and show no regression.

VMs may be evident at birth or, more commonly, become apparent and sometimes symptomatic with pain and swelling later in childhood. Their appearance is variable including varicosities, phlebectasias, discrete spongy masses, or complex channels permeating tissues and organs (Fig. 14.24).

Most occur sporadically and are unifocal though some are multifocal or diffuse. Diffuse VMs commonly affect an entire extremity. On physical examination, they appear as soft, bluish compressible lesions, showing refilling with release of compression and increasing in size with dependency or during a Valsalva maneuver.

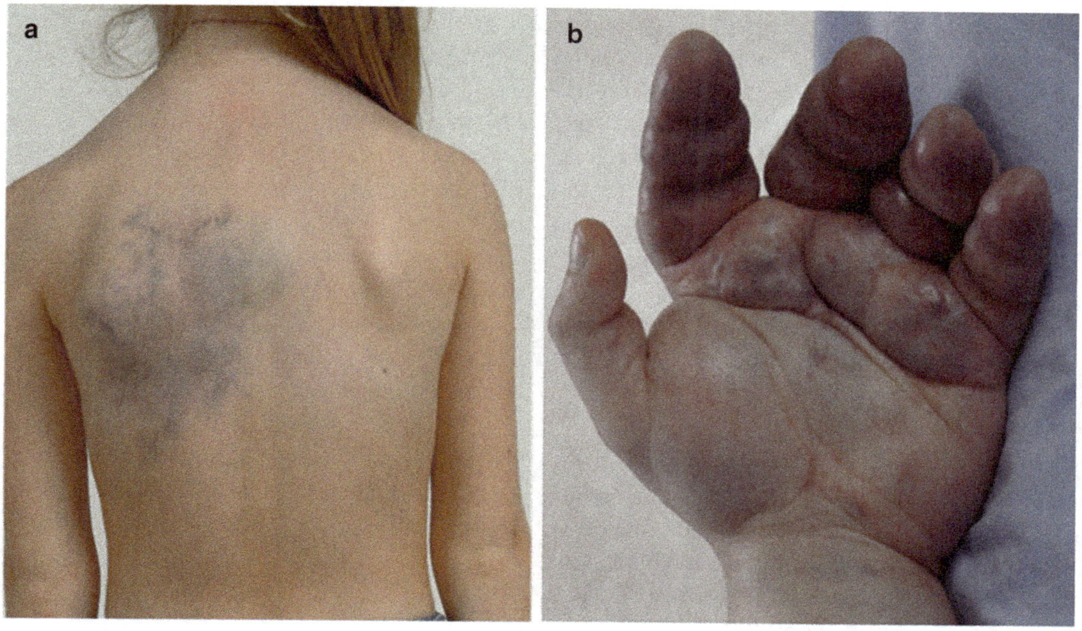

Fig. 14.24 Venous malformation (VM). Typical physical findings in 2 patients. Large periscapular VM with blue compressible swelling and network of dilated veins (**a**). VM of hand with blue compressible swelling of the palm and second to fifth fingers (**b**). The hand swellings could be emptied by compression/arm elevation and refill on release of compression/arm lowering

Up to 42 % show a localized intralesional coagulopathy, which is severe in approximately 4 % and seen particularly in those with diffuse intramuscular involvement (where significant elevated D-dimer and low fibrinogen levels can be detected in peripheral blood) [26–28]. Intralesional thrombosis occurs sometimes associated with acute pain.

Associated muscle wasting can be evident in those with diffuse disease. Involvement of bones and joints may lead to pathological fractures, recurrent hemarthroses, and arthritis with osteoarticular changes similar to hemophilia. In patients with a diffuse type of VM, pulmonary hypertension has been recently reported; however, it is unclear if this is due to recurrent silent pulmonary emboli [29].

VMs can occur throughout the gastrointestinal tract and are often multiple. When associated with VMs of the pelvis and perineum, they are more commonly located in the descending colon and rectum. Gastrointestinal bleeding, typically chronic, can cause anemia. In the "blue rubber bleb nevus" syndrome, multifocal VMs are seen in the skin (typically on the palms of the hands and soles of the feet) and soft tissues in addition to the gastrointestinal tract. The diagnosis of gastrointestinal involvement is best made by endoscopy (including wireless capsule endoscopy). Surgical and endoscopic treatment options should be considered for gastrointestinal VMs if bleeding is problematic.

VM Imaging

VMs are best imaged with US and MRI (Figs. 14.3 and 14.4) [4]. US can assess superficial and focal lesions. US typically shows a localized lesion with anechoic channels that are compressible and refill with release of transducer pressure. Variable solid elements within the lesion and sometimes hyper-reflective phleboliths can be seen. MR is highly tissue specific, with T1 hypointensity, T2 hyperintensity, and nonuniform lesional enhancement post contrast. T1 intralesional high signal is due to thrombi. Phleboliths (calcified thrombi) within VMs are seen as signal voids on T2 imaging. Phleboliths distinguish VMs from tumors and all other vascular malformations. The pattern of contrast enhancement distinguishes VMs from LMs.

Direct puncture venography (to characterize the VM) is undertaken at the time of injection sclerotherapy. Rarely, conventional venography of functional veins may be required.

VM Treatment

The indications for treatment of VMs include pain, swelling, functional impairment, bleeding (hemarthroses, gastrointestinal, and genitourinary), and cosmesis. Treatment options include injection sclerotherapy, laser techniques (usually endovenous), surgical interventions, conservative measures, and combinations of these [28]. Treatment for most VMs is not curative; however, most patients gain symptomatic relief.

Intralesional sclerotherapy is the mainstay of treatment for most VMs [3, 30, 31]. Glue injection into VMs is an alternative to sclerosant injection when postinjection surgical excision is planned. Sclerosants cause an intense inflammatory response, which can be potentially challenging in the early post-sclerotherapy period for the surgeon in the early post-sclerotherapy period [32].

For extensive VMs of the extremities, conservative management with graded compression stockings can achieve significant symptom improvement, provided they are correctly fitted, deliver adequate compression, are worn daily and replaced regularly (3–4 times/year). Compression garments will also improve the abnormal coagulation indices.

In patients with troublesome pain from intralesional thrombosis (when D-dimer levels are elevated >3 times normal), low-molecular-weight heparin (LMWH) can be considered and needs to be given by subcutaneous injection twice daily for several weeks, often resulting in excellent pain relief. D-dimer and fibrinogen levels are determined when patients have pain; large, extensive lesions; or blue rubber bleb syndrome.

VM Sclerotherapy

Pre-procedure Work-Up

With the exception of tiny, solitary VMs, D-dimer and fibrinogen levels are obtained for most patients prior to sclerotherapy or surgery. Otherwise, no special pre-procedure work-up is needed.

Most procedures are done with US guidance. If sclerotherapy is limited to small cutaneous vessels only, direct puncture without image guidance may be sufficient ("office sclerotherapy"). CT guidance is rarely needed for VM sclerotherapy unless challenging locations are treated as may occur with mediastinal, intrathoracic, or intraosseous disease.

Procedure

The lesion or part of the lesion to be treated is evaluated with US, the patient is placed in an optimum position to access the VM, and the skin is prepped.

To enlarge the VM to aid puncture, reducing outflow in an extremity VM can be done with an external tourniquet or for head/neck/shoulder areas by placing the patient in a Trendelenburg position.

The VM is then punctured with a 20–22 gauge needle (sheathed or non-sheathed). Multiple needles can be placed throughout the VM at varying depths and locations (Fig. 14.25). Backflow of venous blood must be seen before proceeding further. With extremity VMs, the tourniquet is deflated, and direct venography (using low frame rate DSA at 2 frames/s) is done at each puncture site within the VM (Fig. 14.26). The purpose of direct puncture venography is to assess the endoluminal morphology of the VM (Figs. 14.26, 14.27, and 14.28), determine its filling volume, and estimate the filling volume before possible escape is observed into functional veins. Provided the direct puncture venograms are satisfactory, sclerosant is injected at each puncture site without a tourniquet (using "road mapping" to reduce dose) (Fig. 14.26).

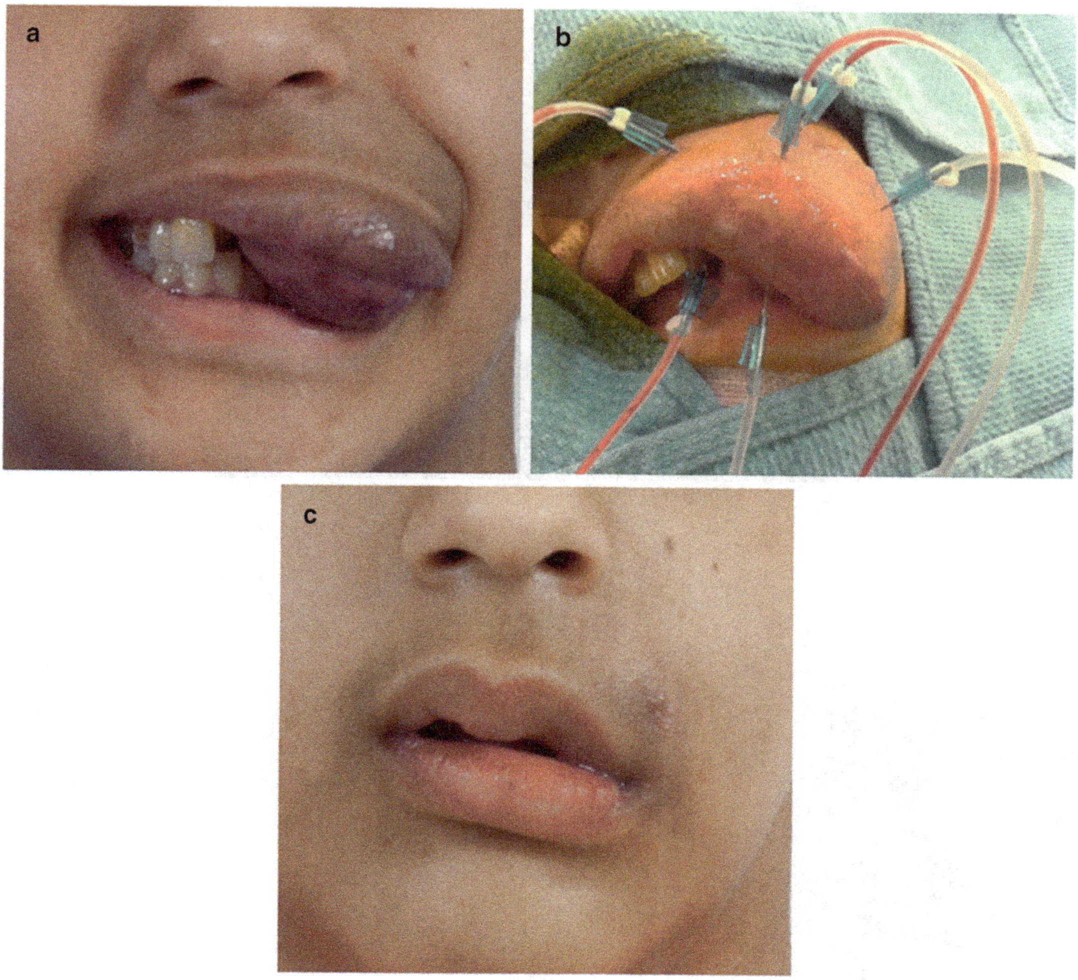

Fig. 14.25 Venous malformation (VM) sclerotherapy. Upper lip VM (**a**). Multiple punctures of the VM are made with 23 gauge butterfly needles (**b**). Good backflow of blood was obtained from all needles, direct puncture venography done, and sclerosant injected using 3 % STS foam and bleomycin. Two treatment sessions performed with an excellent postsclerotherapy result (**c**)

Sclerosant agents used for intralesional sclerotherapy into VMs include 3 % STS (sodium tetradecyl sulphate) as a foam, ethanol, and bleomycin. STS and ethanol cause endothelial damage, thrombosis, scarring, and reduction in size of the VM. Three percent STS has gained popularity in usage due to reports of fatalities and major systemic complications associated with ethanol. The maximum doses at any one treatment should not exceed 0.5 mL/kg 3 % STS liquid or 1 mL ethanol/kg body weight. STS can be easily made into a foam by agitating an equal volume of liquid and air. The injected sclerosant may be opacified with contrast; however, the foam itself acts as a "negative contrast." Occasional closure of large venous channels within the VM or draining the VM can be done using coils, glue, and endovenous laser.

Stasis in a VM is needed before bleomycin is injected to reduce washout of bleomycin. This can easily be done by injecting a small volume of 3 % STS foam immediately before the bleomycin. A suggested maximum intralesional dose of bleomycin per treatment is 1 mg/kg up to 15 mg (15 units).

Most VM sclerotherapy is done as an elective day case. Patients are monitored in the hospital

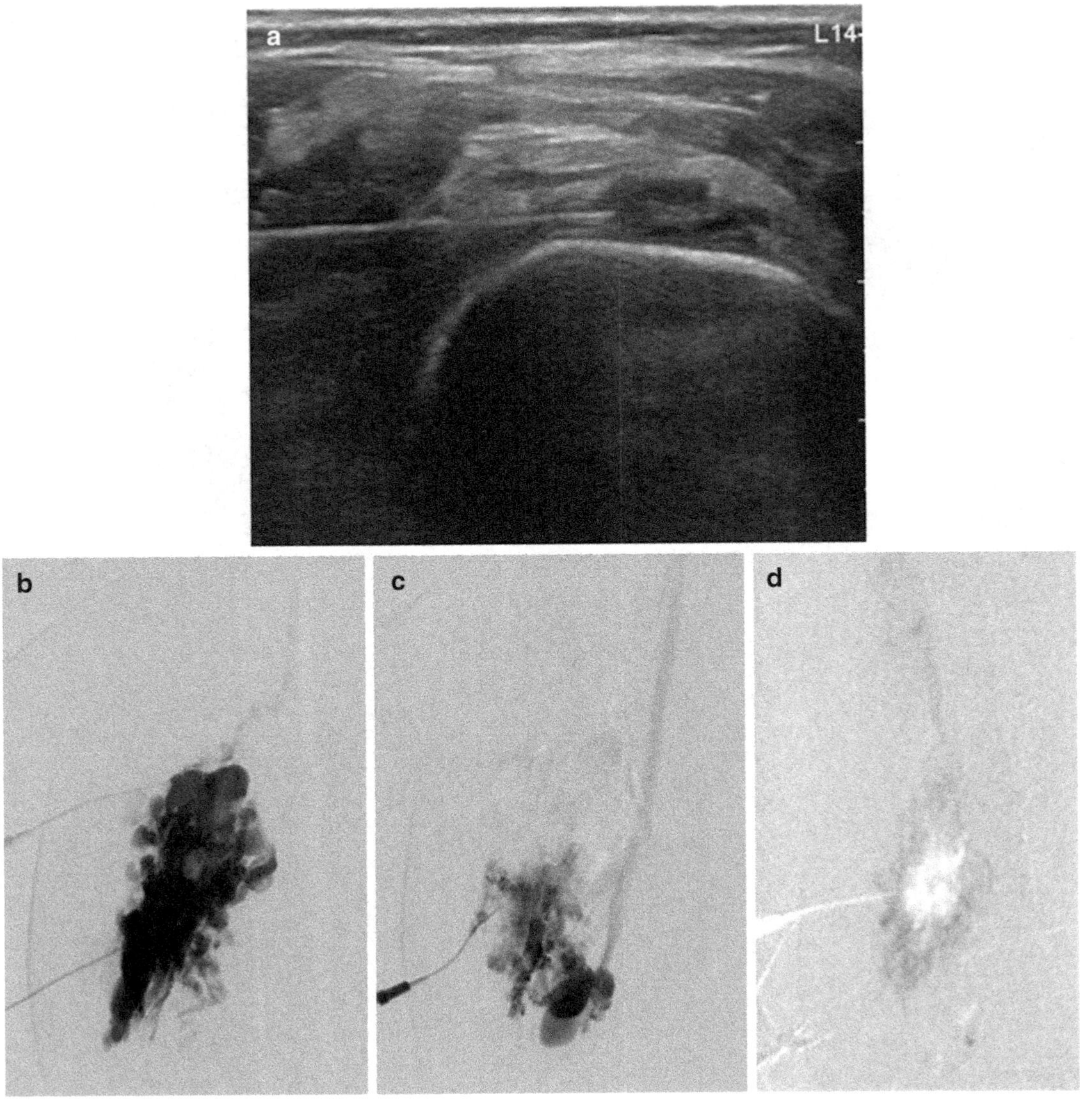

Fig. 14.26 Venous malformation (VM) sclerotherapy. Intramuscular thigh VM. Ultrasound (US) guides successful puncture of the venous channels using 20 gauge sheathed needles (**a**). After backflow of blood is obtained from the needles, direct puncture venography is done through all punctures (**b**, **c**). Sclerosant (3 % STS foam) is injected through needles showing satisfactory filling of the VM by negative contrast (**d**)

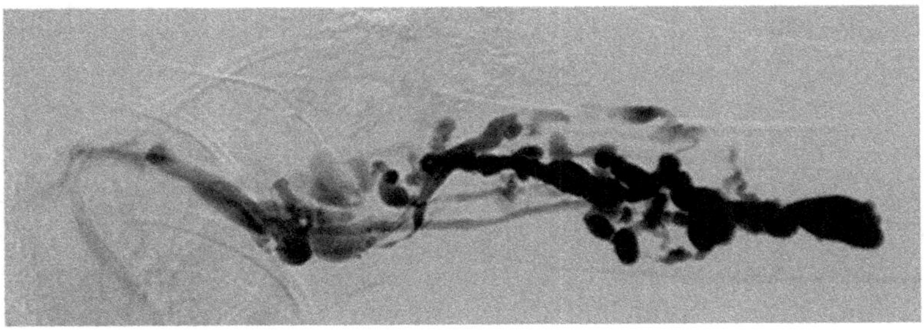

Fig. 14.27 Venous malformation (VM) venography. Patient with varicose type VM in upper extremity with long dysplastic nonfunctional channels. Venography is important in these VMs to identify the dysplastic nonfunctional channels and communications between these and the functioning veins. If there is significant flow through communications, external tourniquets may be required. If this fails, then using a multi-needle technique (Fig. 14.28) or endovascular glue and coil embolization (Fig. 14.29) may be required to control this outflow allowing successful sclerotherapy

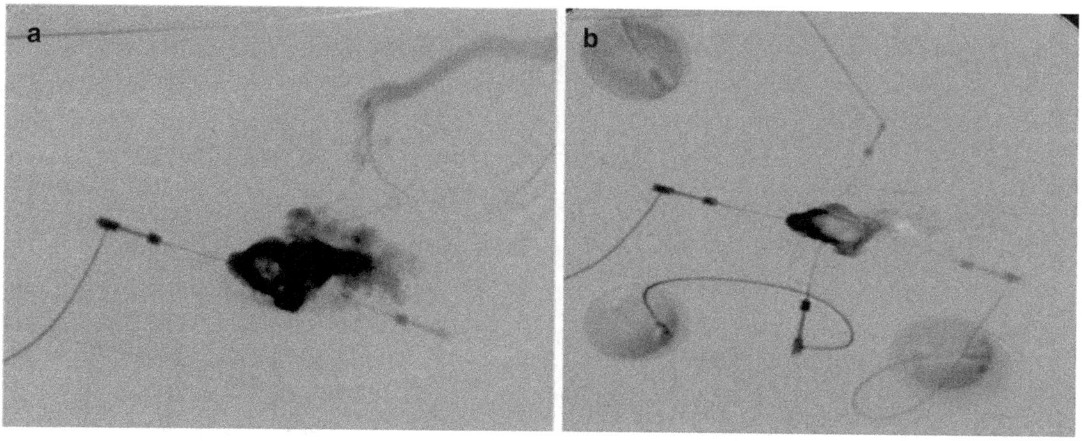

Fig. 14.28 Outflow control from venous malformation (VM). Direct puncture venography shows outflow between the VM and functioning veins (**a**). This is reduced by placing multiple needles into the VM. Contrast and sclerosant can preferentially escape through these opened needles when one is injected, reducing outflow into functioning veins (**b**)

for up to 4–6 h during which time the treated area is repeatedly assessed for skin change, discoloration, or blistering. Young infants are usually admitted overnight. Elective intensive care admission is needed if the VM to be treated is located in challenging areas such as the oral cavity including tongue or airway. In patients with disease involving entire extremities needing sclerotherapy to multiple locations, consecutive daily treatments over 2–3 days can be done provided the same location is not treated twice. For example sclerotherapy may be done to the upper arm on day 1, the forearm on day 2, and the hand on day 3, if needed.

Post-procedure Care

Following sclerotherapy, local swelling is expected and ensues immediately and progresses over several hours (eventually subsiding by 5–7 days) [32]. Pain should be managed appropriately. Significant pain after STS administration is not expected. Local tissue injury with skin and mucosal blistering is not uncommon and can be seen before the patient leaves the procedure room or within 24 h of the injection. Polysporin ointment should be used on skin blisters for 1-week post treatment. Tissue ulceration may rarely occur and should be managed in conjunction with plastic surgery.

Hydration is important post procedure to minimize the effects of hemoglobinuria which frequently occurs with STS/ethanol [33, 34]. Oral fluids are encouraged along with twice normal IV fluid maintenance given routinely for 4 h post procedure. Hemoglobinuria is managed by additional hydration with IV and oral fluids, intravenous furosemide, and occasional urine alkalinization with a sodium bicarbonate intravenous infusion. Measuring urine output as well as observing urine color during the hospital post-procedure stay is important. All complications (Table 14.3) require close observation and follow-up [33].

At the time of discharge, the patient should be systemically well. Tissue swelling is expected and does not itself preclude discharge. For example, a patient may not be able to open the eyelids when a VM of the forehead, eyebrow, or upper cheek is treated and if otherwise well can be discharged. Patients must be able to swallow sufficient fluids, have stable and satisfactory vital functions, and have normal urine output and color prior to discharge, and minor pain should be easily controlled with oral analgesics. Crutches or a walker for younger children may be required for a few days if treatment temporarily impairs mobility before swelling resolves. We generally caution against exercise for 2 weeks post sclerotherapy to avoid trauma to the treated area.

Table 14.3 Potential complications of ethanol and sodium tetradecyl sulfate

1. Sclerosant effects
Local tissue injury (blisters, tissue necrosis, neurologic injury and paralysis, compartment syndrome)
Hemoglobinuria
Venothromboembolic events
Metabolic complications (e.g., acidosis, hypoglycemia)*
Cardiorespiratory events (respiratory depression, cardiopulmonary collapse, arrhythmias)*
Seizures*
Perilesional fibrosis (muscle)
2. Coagulation derangement
3. Procedure + device risk (from catheters and implantable devices, e.g., embolic and occlusion devices)
4. Inadvertent embolization (of blood clots and embolic agents, e.g., glue)
5. Age-related risk (CNS susceptibility to alcohol in neonates)*

Regarding the sclerosant effects, (*) denotes effects observed with alcohol, whereas all other effects can be seen using both sclerosants

All patients should be aware of the follow-up arrangements and be provided with a contact if unexpected problems arise.

Follow-up

The aim of sclerotherapy is symptom relief and not necessarily significant reduction of VM distribution as shown on imaging, although the latter can sometimes be seen. VMs have a propensity for recanalization and re-enlargement. Therefore, repeat injection sclerotherapy treatments are needed in many patients. Repeat VM sclerotherapy is done approximately every 6 weeks. Those patients with small lesions are reviewed clinically and with US ahead of the next planned treatment. Once treatment is completed (shown by significant improvement in symptoms and sometimes findings on physical examination), outpatient clinical follow-up is arranged at 3 and 12 months and then at infrequent intervals (every few years) throughout childhood. Routine follow-up imaging post sclerotherapy is not always performed as it is well known that lesion residue persists despite symptom improvement. Repeat imaging however is always done when symptoms persist despite adequate treatment or when further treatment is required.

Practical Tips for VM Sclerotherapy

1. Prepare patients for expected outcomes which include tissue swelling, skin staining, and sometimes skin/mucosal blistering.
2. Check plasma D-dimer and fibrinogen levels in all patients with pain, those with diffuse VMs and blue rubber bleb nevus syndrome, and all undergoing sclerotherapy and surgery. If fibrinogen is <1 g/L, LMWH is required pretreatment to reduce intraprocedural bleeding.
3. Elevated D-dimer most likely is due to intralesional thrombosis within the VM rather than a deep venous thrombosis in functional veins.
4. Extremity tourniquets are not required for most sclerosant injections.
5. Tourniquets need to be used with caution as complications can occur. Unexpected redirection of blood flow including arterial reflux may occur with devastating tissue necrosis.
6. When using a tourniquet and its position or pressure is altered, venography should be repeated to reassess venous flow prior to sclerosant injection.
7. Tourniquets can be placed above and below the VM to occlude outflow, and if used during sclerosant injection, the tourniquet should be applied close to the VM to minimize sclerosant stasis and deep venous thrombosis in communicating deep veins.
8. Limiting the outflow from the VM into functional veins can also be achieved by placement of multiple needles into the VM (Fig. 14.28), coil embolization (Fig. 14.29), glue embolization, and endovascular laser (using, e.g., diode laser). (One of the editors (FM) has used the ClariVein catheter (Vascular Insights, New Haven, USA) for venous outflow embolization in VM therapy.)
9. Flow characteristics of sclerosant foam dispersal through a VM differ to that of liquid contrast. Meticulous road mapping and injection using DSA during sclerosant foam injection are required.

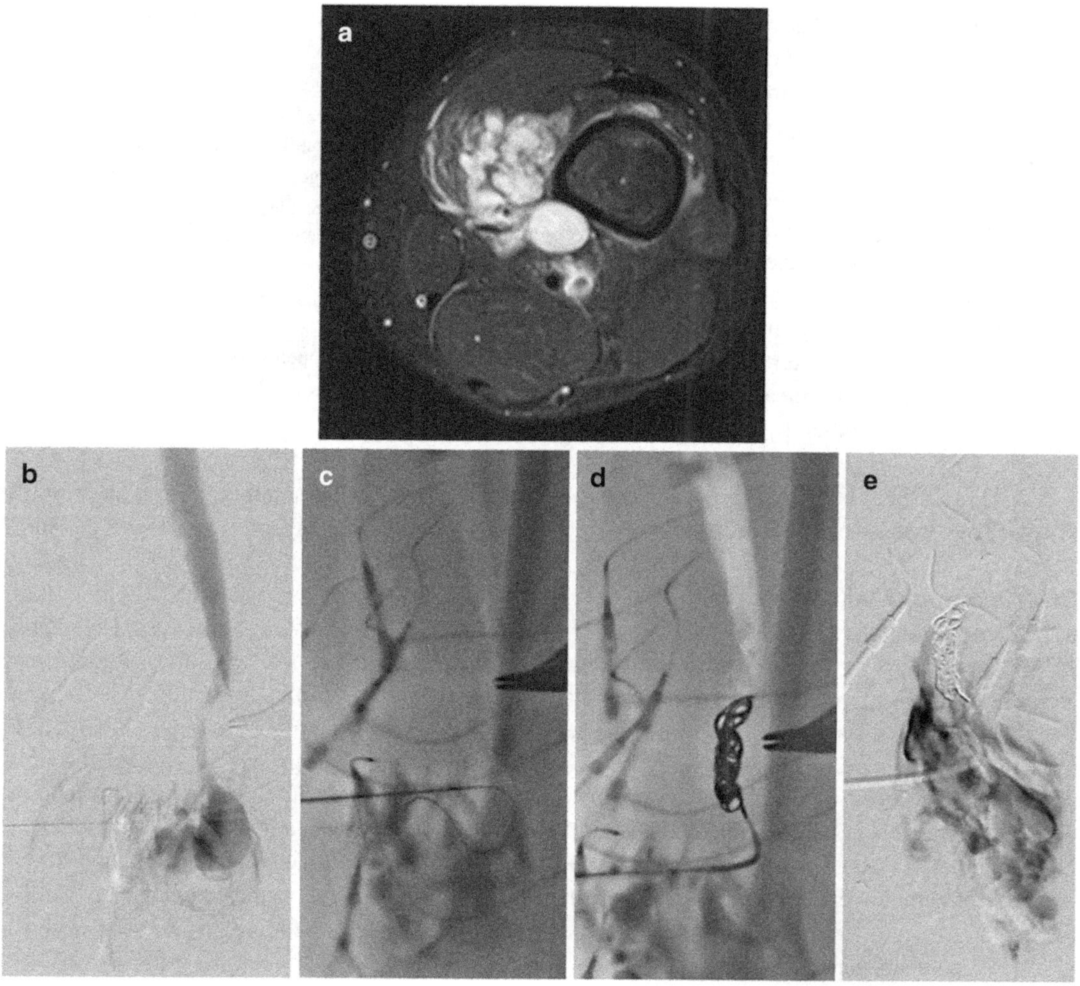

Fig. 14.29 Outflow control from venous malformation (VM). Intramuscular thigh VM (**a**). Multiple puncture venograms into the VM showed prompt drainage between the VM and the femoral vein despite an external tourniquet. One direct percutaneous puncture showed filling of a saccular channel with rapid outflow into the femoral vein (**b**). The sac was catheterized (**c**), an angiographic catheter advanced and coil embolization of the communication was done (**d**). Other communications were similarly closed, allowing for safe sclerosant injection (**e**)

10. Caution with "polypharmacy sclerotherapy." Do not add a second sclerosant (STS/ethanol) at any one site during the same treatment session if the maximum dose of the initial sclerosant (STS/ethanol) has been reached. Tissue swelling and tissue injury risk increases, including compartment syndrome.
11. Caution with unfamiliar or complex anatomic territories, e.g., paraspinal area. Meticulous venography is needed to ensure there is no communication with epidural veins prior to sclerosant injection.
12. Consider techniques to reduce the VM volume to improve the effectiveness of sclerotherapy when large "lake like" channels are present. Surgical compartmentalizing or compression of the VM by suturing the VM or endovascular coil/guidewire placement into the VM (by direct puncture or transvenous catheter) can be undertaken.
13. Consider localized sclerotherapy for patients with diffuse extremity VMs who have localized pain, despite compliance with compression garments and treated with LMWH.

14. Direct interstitial laser by percutaneous access directly into the VM (using, e.g., Nd:YAG) can provide an alternative to sclerosant injection.
15. Presurgical sclerotherapy is an option as it reduces the size of the VM and decreases bleeding during resection.
16. Patients undergoing sclerotherapy of intramuscular VMs will benefit from physiotherapy as sclerotherapy induces perilesional fibrosis. Stretching exercises, night splints, and surgical tendon release may be required to augment sclerotherapy.

Table 14.4 Schobinger clinical severity score of peripheral AVMs

Stage 1	Quiescent stage Clinical features: warm vascular stain in skin mimicking a capillary malformation
Stage 2	Expansion stage Clinical features: lesion warmer, bruits and thrills are present, and lesion is enlarging
Stage 3	Destructive stage Clinical features: ulcers, hemorrhage, bone lysis, and pain
Stage 4	Cardiac decompensation stage Clinical features: onset of cardiac failure from overload

High-Flow Vascular Malformations

Arteriovenous Malformations and Arteriovenous Fistulas

AVMs are high-flow vascular malformations that are very different to the more common low-flow vascular malformations [3]. This section focuses on the treatment of peripheral AVMs. Pulmonary AVMs are discussed in Chap. 7. Treatment of congenital arteriovenous fistulas (AVFs) is similar to that of AVMs. Differences in AVM and AVF treatment will be highlighted where applicable.

AVMs are characterized by a precapillary arteriovenous shunt, the so-called "nidus". Often multiple nidi are present in AVMs. The nidus is made up of a network of small vascular channels and differentiates AVMs from congenital AVFs, which are also high-flow vascular malformation with precapillary shunts but no nidus. AVFs single or multiple shunts. The appearance of complex AVF shunts may be confused with nidi from an AVM.

AVM shunts can be localized or extensive and commonly involve the extremities, trunk, and viscera. These lesions do not respect tissue boundaries, and AV shunting can occur in soft tissues and bone.

AVMs usually undergo slow progression in stages over many years, and during childhood, the AVM grows in proportion with the child. Schobinger staging (Table 14.4) is a clinically based severity scoring system and should be used for all peripheral AVMs. At birth, AVMs appear as a pink cutaneous skin stain and can be mistaken for a CM or the premonitory sign of an infantile hemangioma. However, high flow from AV shunting is present beneath the vascular skin stain, and this can easily be detected with Doppler ultrasound. The high flow is characterized clinically by increased growth and warmth of the affected body part, bruits, thrills, arterial aneurysms, and enlargement of draining veins (Fig. 14.30). These features become progressively evident throughout childhood. AV shunting can be confirmed by using continuous wave Doppler. Tissue ischemia, from AV shunting, results in pain and tissue necrosis with ulceration and bleeding (Fig. 14.30). High-output cardiac failure can be seen in those with significant shunts in large extensive AVMs. It is well recognized that puberty, pregnancy, and local trauma (including iatrogenic trauma) can trigger rapid expansion in these lesions with increased shunting. Proximal surgical ligation or proximal arterial embolization of feeding arteries will result in nidi recruiting a vascular supply from adjacent territories.

Functionally, AVMs and AVFs can have similar effects such as ischemia, ulceration, tissue necrosis and cardiac failure.

Imaging/Angiography

AVMs are best imaged noninvasively by MR including MRA [35]. Inflow arteries are enlarged, tortuous, and sometimes aneurysmal. Outflow veins are enlarged and tortuous. Numerous flow voids are evident on spin echo sequences. The high density of vessels is easily demonstrated including the nidi. MR provides an excellent overall map showing the distribution of the

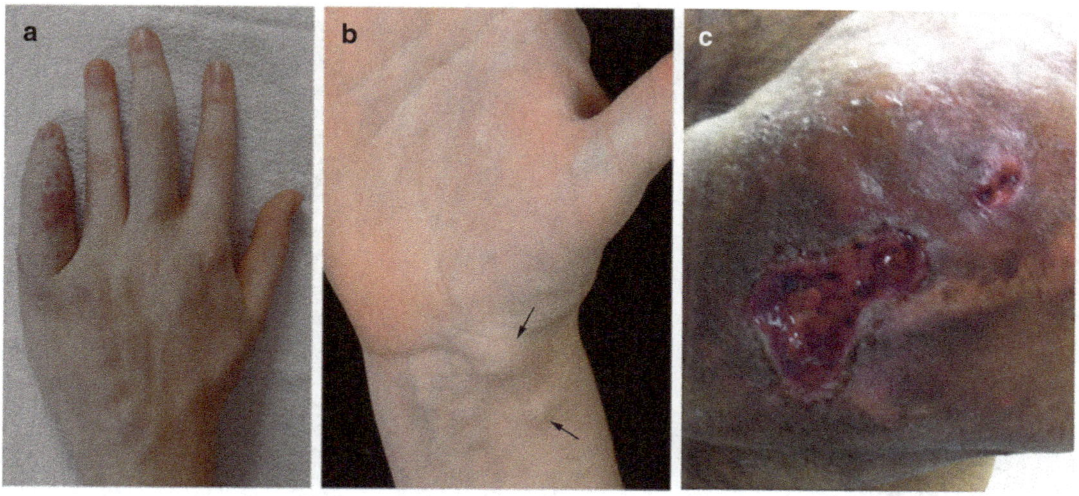

Fig. 14.30 Peripheral arteriovenous malformation (AVM). Typical physical findings in 3 patients. Tissue overgrowth with prominent draining veins (**a**), pulsatile arterial aneurysms (*arrows*) (**b**), and skin ulceration (**c**) are all clinical features of AVMs

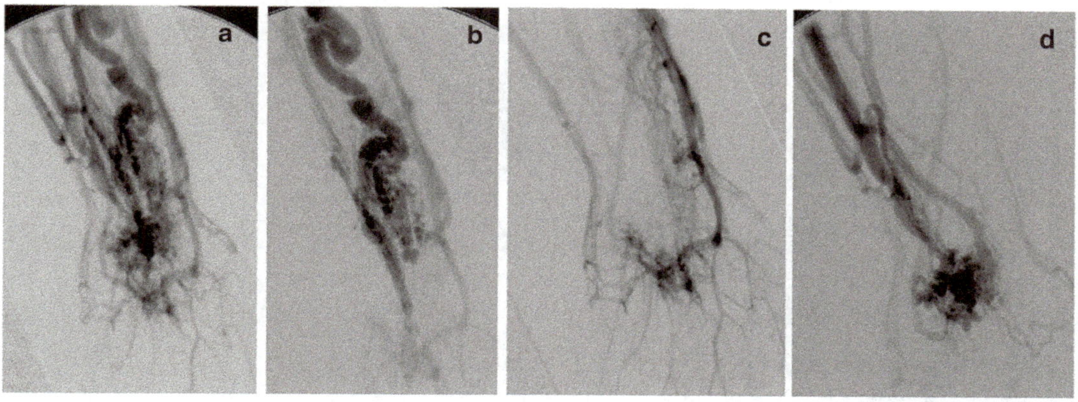

Fig. 14.31 Shunt (nidi) identification in arteriovenous malformation (AVM). Global catheter angiography can demonstrate shunts (**a**); selective catheter angiography is needed to evaluate these in detail for embolization. In this patient with an upper extremity AVM, nidi in the soft tissues of the distal forearm (**b**) and palm (**c**, **d**) were evaluated by selective catheterization of the interosseous (**b**), radial (**c**), and ulnar arteries (**d**)

disease and the tissues involved by the shunts. An important imaging feature is that in AVMs there is no evidence of a parenchymal tumor, which allows differentiation from vascular tumors which may exhibit high flow and AV shunts. Soft tissue edema in AVMs can be seen on MR surrounding the AV shunts.

Details of shunt morphology and their venous drainage are better assessed by catheter angiography and direct puncture techniques (Figs. 14.8, 14.31, 14.32, and 14.33).

Catheter angiography remains the gold standard in imaging however is not required until treatment is needed (and is usually done at the time of the first embolization). The initial catheter angiogram, for example, on a patient with a peripheral AVM should include "global" as well as "selective" angiography (Figs. 14.8 and 14.31). For extremities, "global angiography" means leaving the angiographic catheter in a high brachial or common femoral artery location for injection during image acquisition. Image acquisition should avoid bolus chasing so as to image all AV shunt. Multiple injections may be needed to cover the entire extremity. Always use a pump injection for global angiography. Selective

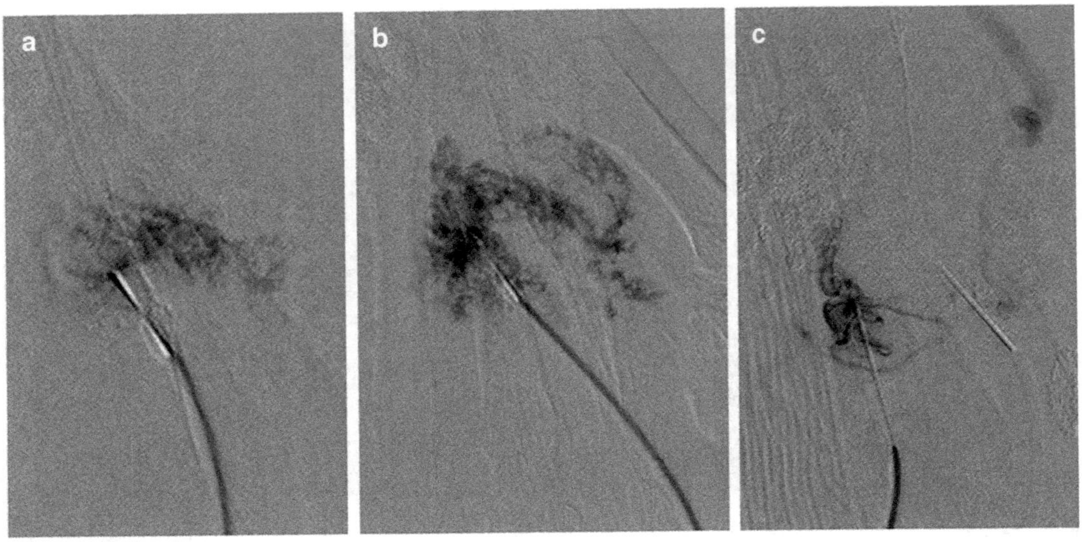

Fig. 14.32 Direct needle puncture embolization of arteriovenous malformation nidus. This nidus was present in the soft tissue of the hand and punctured using a 23-gauge butterfly needle. Contrast injection was done with good nidal filling (**a**, **b**). Non-opacified ethanol was injected. Post ethanol, contrast injection showed good closure of the shunt (**c**)

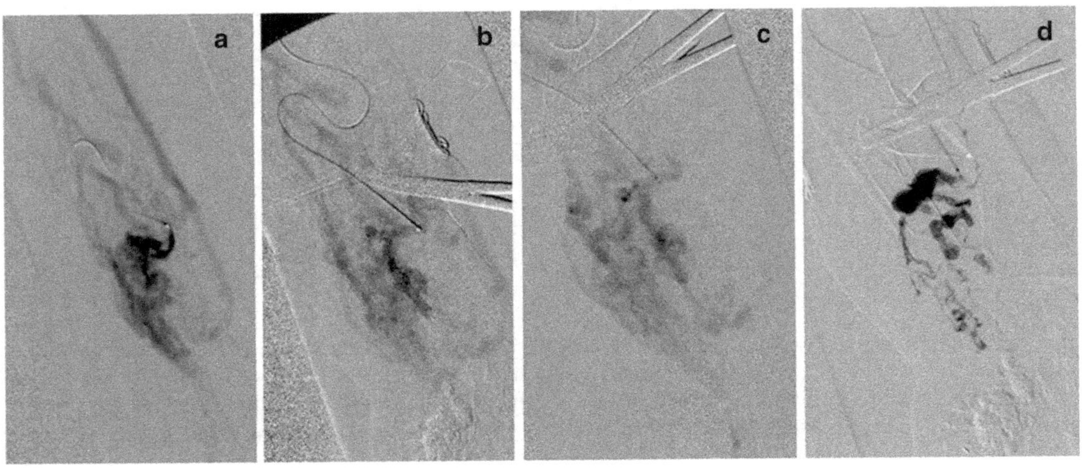

Fig. 14.33 Arterial catheter embolization of arteriovenous malformation nidus. Nidus in soft tissue of distal forearm. Contrast injection via microcatheter shows good nidal filling and prompt venous drainage (**a**). External tourniquet control near the nidus reduces venous outflow (**b**). Increasing tourniquet pressure stops venous outflow (**c**). For catheter embolization, the tourniquet pressure was maintained between that used for (**b**) and (**c**) to allow for good nidal filling with forward flow. Glue was injected (**d**). Glue polymerization occurred rapidly. Optimal nidal filling with glue would have been preferred to the proximal glue deposition as shown in (**d**); however, the angiographic result was satisfactory

angiography is done by advancing the catheter (sometimes using a microcatheter coaxially) to allow assessment of shunts in greater detail in preparation for embolization. Selective angiograms may be pump/hand injected. Hand injection may suffice if vessels are small and rate of injection can match flow to provide excellent opacification. Inject each contrast bolus over 2 s and acquire images using DSA at 3 frames/s. Diagnostic angiography should always aim to demonstrate (1) the arterial runoff throughout the extremity, (2) feeding arteries to shunts, (3) location of the shunts, (4) shunt morphology, and (4) venous drainage from the shunts (Figs. 14.8 and 14.31).

AVFs are best images by MR and MRA. However, catheter angiography remains the gold standard. Similar to AVMs, angiography for AFVs is not undertaken until intervention is necessary.

AVM Treatment Approach

The majority of AVMs will eventually require treatment because of continued lesion expansion. This can be associated with troublesome symptoms, including tissue ischemia and ulceration, pain, and sometimes cardiac overload [3].

Embolization has been the mainstay of treatment either alone or in combination with surgical excision [36, 37]. Recently, it has been suggested that well-localized "stage 1" AVMs amenable to surgical excision have better outcomes without preoperative embolization. However, as the full extent of the AVM may be underrecognized during early disease, embolization and surgery during infancy and early childhood are rarely undertaken as there is a high risk of disease progression. This propensity for progression or "recurrence" after certain treatments poses many challenges. Thrombosis, ischemia, and partial resection trigger enlargement and sometimes endothelial hyperplasia, explaining these so-called recurrences.

Many patients are observed with AVMs in their early stages and monitored carefully throughout childhood. Yearly clinical follow-up is undertaken unless urgent problems demand more frequent attention. The difficulty for many interventional radiologists is knowing when to commence embolization, how many to perform, the frequency of treatment sessions, and when to stop. All patients should be offered treatment for "stage 3" and "stage 4" AVMs. As practices vary, some patients may undergo embolization at "stage 2" (or "advanced stage 2"). For "stage 3" AVMs, once embolization is commenced, patients may require frequent treatments every 2 months. For "stage 4" AVMs, the frequency of embolization is determined by the urgency of the clinical situation. Embolization can be stopped when symptoms improve and are controlled. For "stage 2" AVM, it is less clear as to the number of treatment sessions needed and when to stop. "Stage 2" AVM has no symptoms, such as pain, that can be used to monitor effectiveness of embolization. Angiographic improvement alone is used, and follow-up angiography is therefore required. For all peripheral AVMs, there is no "quick fix," and most require repeated treatment sessions over several years. Embolization can at best provide "control" and not cure of the AVM.

The disease itself is one of the most challenging of all vascular anomalies, and all treatments including embolization are high risk [36–39]. Surgical resection if performed in selected patients with well-localized disease should be undertaken within 2–3 days of preoperative embolization of the nidus. Although angiographic embolization decreases intraoperative bleeding, it does not reduce the amount or extent of tissue resected. In those with extensive AVMs, surgical resection is not possible, and therefore embolization is the only option for symptom control. Surgical amputation may be considered for advanced extremity AVMs causing major problems threatening the affected limb or the patient's life. As cures are rarely seen, all patients should have long-term follow-up following treatment.

AVF Treatment Approach

The treatment and approach to AVFs is similar to that of AVMs as discussed above. Simple AVF can be cured with embolization. Complex AVFs with multiple shunts, like AVMs, may be incurable, and at best lesion control might be expected.

AVFs like AVMs may require sacrifice of the draining vein to allow for complete closure.

AVM Embolization

Pre-procedure Work-Up/Planning

A pre-procedure work-up is not routinely required unless the AVM is causing significant dysfunction either (1) locally (e.g., with liver AVMs, pre-procedure liver function must be assessed) or (2) generally (e.g., if there is cardiac overload, a pre-procedure cardiac assessment and echocardiogram are needed).

Although the catheter angiogram is the gold standard in mapping the AVM for embolization, it is important to review cross-sectional imaging (MR and if needed CT) and plain radiographs when AVM shunts are involving challenging locations, e.g., viscera and bone, and deep locations such as the pelvis. This can help in embolization planning. For example, identifying large draining venous channels for direct puncture embolization can be advantageous in pelvic AVMs.

The aim of endovascular treatment of AVMs is to selectively target closure of the AV shunts. These are complex procedures and nontarget closure should be avoided as (1) closure of proximal feeding arteries (either surgical or catheter embolization) results in arterial recruitment to the nidus from adjacent vascular territories leading to disease progression, (2) proximal closure of inflow arteries will compromise further embolizations, and (3) it can lead to major complications such as tissue necrosis including skin ulceration and nerve injury with paralysis.

Nidal closure and shunt reduction can be achieved by various embolization methods including:

1. Direct percutaneous puncture of the AVM nidus (for non-visceral AVMs) (Fig. 14.32)
2. Trans-arterial catheter embolization (using a coaxial catheter system with a microcatheter advanced as close to the nidus as possible) (Fig. 14.33)
3. Embolization of the venous outflow from the nidus (either by direct puncture of the vein outflow or by retrograde venous catheterization) (Fig. 14.34) [40, 41]

It is important to evaluate the catheter angiogram and decide the most appropriate method of nidal closure, sometimes employing several methods and multiple approaches (Fig. 14.35). Trans-arterial/venous and direct puncture techniques (into soft tissue/bone, depending on the shunt location) may have to be employed, and therefore familiarity with these techniques, devices, and embolic agents is essential. The angiogram will locate the position of nidi for percutaneous puncture. Sometimes ultrasound can help; however,

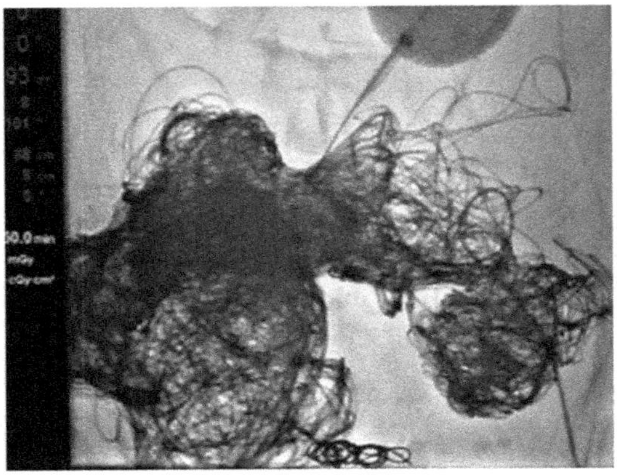

Fig. 14.34 Venous outflow embolization in arteriovenous malformation (AVM). The giant venous outflow sac from this large pelvic AVM was embolized by direct puncture and over 100 guidewires (stripped to remove the mandril cores before deployment). A large occlusion balloon was placed in the iliac vein to reduce outflow. Image courtesy of Dr. Martin Simons, Toronto Western Hospital, Toronto, Canada

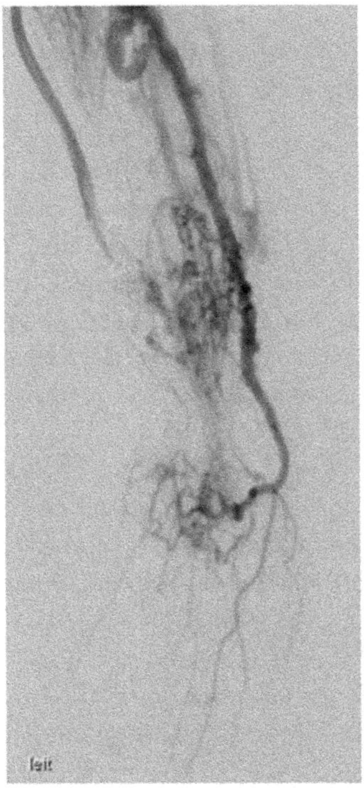

Fig. 14.35 Angiographic result of AVM embolization. Same patient as in Fig. 14.31. Embolization performed to control troublesome pain. After multiple embolizations (transcatheter and direct punctures), the pain was resolved. Post-embolization angiogram shows significant closure to shunts in the distal forearm and hand, with preservation of digital flow. Transcatheter embolization resulted in distal ulnar artery occlusion

real-time puncture of the nidus is difficult because of the numerous, small channels.

Procedure

4 or 5 Fr angiographic catheters are suitable for arterial catheterizations and can be used as outer, coaxial systems for microcatheter techniques. Larger catheters can be used if needed for venous embolizations.

Twenty-two or 23 gauge needles (such as a butterfly) can be used for direct puncture of a superficial nidus/venous end and longer needles for deeper targets. The nidus has extremely small channels and larger gauge needles will not suffice. Direct puncture of capacious venous ends of shunts can be done with larger needles such as 18 gauge sheathed needles for pelvic AVMs.

As AVMs invariably have many nidi, the question often asked is which nidus/nidi should be closed. With diffuse extremity disease, nidal closure at the location of symptoms such as pain would be appropriate. In those with cardiac overload, closure of the largest shunts initially would be appropriate.

Embolic agents used to close AV shunts include liquids and coils. The commonly used liquid embolics are ethanol and the adhesive glue *n*-butyl-2-cyanoacrylate (Histoacryl, B Braun, Melsungen AG, Germany). The nonadhesive liquid embolic ethylene vinyl alcohol copolymer (Onyx, eV3, Plymouth, MN, USA) is favored by some interventionalists. Ethanol, despite being the most destructive vascular endothelial agent, is not favored by some because of its associated life-threatening cardiopulmonary complications. However, when used appropriately, angiographic results can be excellent. Histoacryl glue and Onyx can result in satisfactory angiographic shunt closure; however, do not destroy the vascular endothelium as does ethanol. All three liquid agents can be injected by microcatheter or direct percutaneous methods. Ethanol must never be injected into visceral AVMs as the risk of parenchymal necrosis is high. Histoacryl glue is a useful alternative for visceral AVMs. In pediatrics, success has been reported for novel lifesaving neonatal liver AVM embolizations with excellent long-term outcomes. [42, 43] Traditionally coil embolization is not recommended in AVMs; however, this teaching refers to proximal arterial closure. Nidal closure, as mentioned above, can be achieved in selected cases by closing the venous end of the shunt [39, 40]. Sometimes the large capacity of the venous end demands occlusion with multiple coils or even entire guidewires to provide satisfactory closure (Fig. 14.34).

Controlled selective contrast injection (transarterial/transvenous/direct puncture) immediately before embolic injection is done using DSA to assess the volume of the nidus and the speed of flow through the nidus. For embolization, flow should be continuous and forwards through the shunt into the venous end. If flow is too rapid for safe embolization, flow control can be used to reduce arterial inflow and venous outflow. An external tourniquet for extremities or endovascular balloon occlusion techniques for other territories may be needed. With flow control, repeat contrast injections are essential prior to injection of the embolic agent. With ethanol and glue, multiple injections may be needed at different locations. Following embolic injection, contrast injection is done (via the microcatheter or direct puncture needle) to assess closure. If shunting persists, embolization is repeated until shunting is satisfactorily reduced or nidal closure is complete. A nonselective completion angiogram via the outer coaxial catheter may be required at the end of the procedure. These procedures can be lengthy, lasting several hours.

Repeated embolization procedures typically provide temporary improvement as the large number of often small-sized shunts makes it difficult to achieve complete occlusion of all. Despite this, patients can often have much symptom improvement with embolization (Fig. 14.35).

AVM embolization is usually done as an elective procedure with a 24-h post-procedure stay during which time-repeated observations should be made of the treated area and well-being of the patient maintained. Elective intensive care admission post procedure is needed if the AVM involves vital areas such as the airway or oral cavity including the tongue.

Post-procedure Care

The high complication risk associated with AVM embolization is due to the local and systemic problems related to the injected embolic agents, the catheter technique and devices used, and risks from inadvertent embolization (Table 14.2).

Following embolization, local swelling is expected and ensues immediately with progression over several hours (eventually subsiding by 5–7 days). Pain should be managed appropriately. Local tissue injury with necrosis can occur and affect skin and mucosa with early signs evident within 24 h. This needs careful follow-up and appropriate care in conjunction with plastic surgery.

Post-procedure hydration is important to minimize the effects of hemoglobinuria which frequently occurs with ethanol [34]. Oral fluids are encouraged along with twice normal IV fluid maintenance given routinely for 4 h post procedure. Hemoglobinuria is managed by additional hydration with IV and oral fluids, intravenous furosemide, and occasional urine alkalinization with a sodium bicarbonate intravenous infusion [34].

Bed rest for several hours (approximately 6 h) is recommended when arterial catheterization is performed via the femoral artery. All relevant peripheral pulses are monitored during the first 6 h post procedure. All complications (Table 14.2) require close observation and follow-up [36–39].

At the time of discharge, the patient should be systemically well. Significant swelling does not itself preclude discharge provided the patient can swallow sufficient fluids, vital functions are stable and satisfactory, minor pain is easily controlled with oral analgesics, and urine output and color are normal. Patients should be aware of follow-up arrangements and be provided with emergency contact information if unexpected problems arise. Crutches or a walker for younger children may be required for a few days if treatment temporarily impairs mobility before swelling resolves. We generally caution against exercise for 2 weeks post embolization to avoid trauma to the treated area.

Follow-up

Repeat AVM embolization is done approximately every 8 weeks (or more frequent if needed), and all patients are reassessed with history and physical exam prior to the next treatment. Once all treatments are completed (as judged particularly by symptom improvement), outpatient clinical follow-up is arranged at 3 months and then yearly throughout childhood.

Practical Tips for AVM Embolization

1. The method of embolization (transcatheter and or direct puncture) is decided at time of catheter angiography.
2. Use DSA for catheter angiography and direct puncture contrast injections.
3. For the novice, identifying the nidi is challenging (identifying draining veins and looking proximally will help identify some nidi). Superficial shunts can be seen on ultrasound.
4. Without major life-threatening bleeding, give systemic heparin (initial 100 units/kg, maximum 5,000 units, repeating 1/2 dose every 2 h to keep activated clotting time >200 s).
5. Be prepared to undertake different methods of embolization (transcatheter and direct puncture) and utilize different routes (into soft tissue and intraosseous shunts) (Figs. 14.32, 14.33, and 14.34).
6. Direct puncture into superficial soft tissue nidi can be performed when the patient has received systemic heparin.
7. Be familiar with embolics agents and their preparation including mixing and precautions needed for delivery.
8. Dextrose flushing of the catheter or puncture needle immediately before glue injection is required to prevent glue polymerization on injection.
9. Glue should be mixed with Lipiodol Ultra Fluid prior to injection.
10. The ratio of injected glue: Lipiodol is often 1:2 to 1:4 (1 part glue: 2 to 4 parts Lipiodol). This can be reversed in very high-flow lesions. Using less Lipiodol promotes faster

polymerization, needed when flow is fast and the target is close to the injection site.
11. The glue Lipiodol mixture volume for injection by microcatheter/direct puncture is dependent on the target volume of the nidus. Injection aliquots often vary between 0.2 and 2 mL. The glue mixture can be pushed using dextrose if needed. (Dextrose solutions do not cause glue polymerization.)
12. If using ethanol, aliquot volumes for injection vary between 0.2 and 2 mL/injection.
13. Tourniquets need to be used with caution as complications can occur. Unexpected redirection of blood flow may occur with devastating tissue necrosis.
14. When using a tourniquet and its position/pressure is altered, repeat contrast injection is needed prior to embolization.
15. Other practical tips are included under the section on "practical tips for catheter angiography and embolization in infants with vascular tumors."
16. Post procedure, if "skin bruising" or significant pain occurs at/near the embolization site, this may represent early tissue necrosis and careful follow-up is required.

Complex Combined Vascular Malformations

These complex disorders are often associated with regional overgrowth, commonly soft tissue and skeletal overgrowth. The eponyms applied to several of the complex malformations can cause confusion, and it is better to describe the vascular channels affected in addition to the growth abnormality. The interventional radiologist can help with symptom management in patients with these complex disorders; however, there are no cures.

Klippel–Trenaunay Syndrome

KTS is a low-flow combined vascular malformation involving abnormal capillary, lymphatic, and venous channels (CLVM) associated with soft tissue and bony hypertrophy [44, 45]. Commonly the malformation affects a single lower extremity, but it can involve more than one extremity and the trunk. This syndrome is sporadic and evident at birth and varying in severity.

The triad of physical findings needed for diagnosis are (1) a cutaneous CM, (2) VM/varicosities/phlebectasia, and (3) regional growth abnormality, commonly hypertrophy of soft tissue and bone (Fig. 14.36).

The CM component is present in the skin often as a "geographic" stain. The venous component consists of anomalous superficial embryonic veins (especially the so-called lateral marginal vein of Serville) (Fig. 14.7). Deep venous anomalies can occur such as hypoplasia and segmental atresias (Fig. 14.37). A lymphatic component (LM) is variable and includes lymph channel hypoplasia, lymphedema, and cystic LMs. Often small LMs are embedded in the surface of the cutaneous CM and can bleed intermittently.

Extremity overgrowth is obvious at birth, and although progressive, major changes after birth are unusual. Overgrowth can affect the length and girth of a limb (including the hand and foot). Yearly monitoring of leg length (done when the malformation affects the lower extremity) is needed as leg length discrepancy (LLD) can occur. X-ray monitoring of leg length is done in those children with a LLD who are older than the toddler age group to assess the need for surgical correction. Infrequently, there can be undergrowth of the affected limb.

Extremity pain is not uncommon and can be due to a variety of causes such as venous hypertension and chronic venous insufficiency, cellulitis, venous thrombosis (in superficial, deep and embryonic veins), thrombophlebitis, osseous venous malformations, arthropathy, neuropathy, and growing pain [46].

Thrombophlebitis of the anomalous veins occurs in up to 45 % of patients, and pulmonary emboli are reported in 4–25 % of patients. Pulmonary hypertension has been recently reported in KTS patients, possibly due to silent recurrent pulmonary emboli [29].

Bleeding can be problematic from the skin, genitourinary, and gastrointestinal tracts. Patients

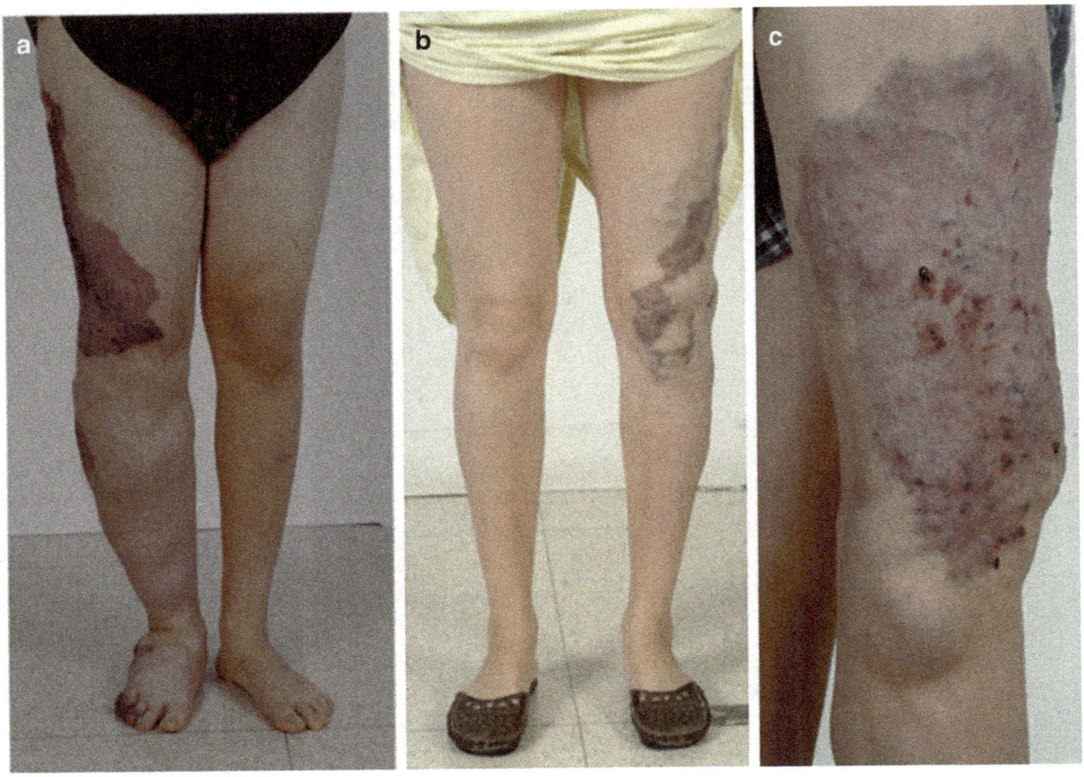

Fig. 14.36 Klippel–Trenaunay syndrome (KTS). Typical physical findings in 3 patients with lower extremity KTS; extremity overgrowth (**a**, **c**), capillary malformation/port-wine stain (**a–c**), lateral varicosities (**b**, **c**). Lymphatic malformations present on the surface of the port-wine stain (**c**) and appear as small blood-filled vesicles

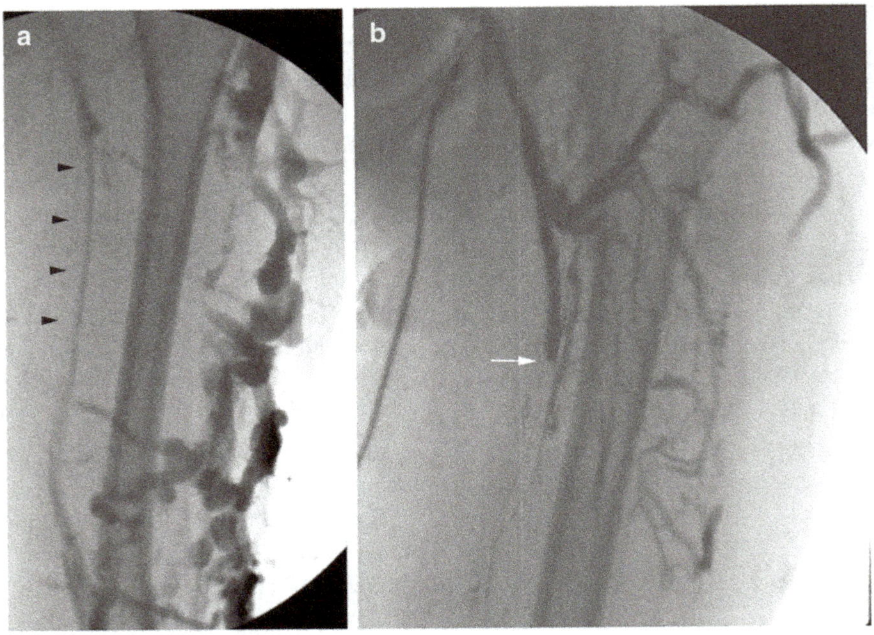

Fig. 14.37 Deep venous system in lower extremity Klippel–Trenaunay syndrome. Venograms in 2 patients showing femoral vein hypoplasia (*black arrow heads*) (**a**) and atresia (*white arrow* points to top of atretic segment) (**b**). Venography performed in (**a**) by pedal vein injection with ankle tourniquet inflation (to divert flow into deep veins) and in (**b**) by common femoral vein injection with groin compression (to promote retrograde filling). (**a**) Shows that the embryonic lateral marginal vein has multiple channels

can also be troubled with recurrent LM infections, cellulitis, and lymphedema.

KTS Imaging and Treatment

Imaging has an important role in evaluating KTS patients [3]. Radiographs including CT scanogram/digital radiography are done to measure lower extremity length discrepancies. MR can assess the type and extent of VMs and LMs and hypertrophic fatty tissue in areas of overgrowth. MRV can help define the anatomy of the deep venous system and venous anomalies, although the deep venous system may be hypoplastic with segmental atresias and therefore difficult to visualize on MRV. Occasionally, this might require further invasive assessment with conventional venography performed by a variety of techniques including conventional pedal venography, percutaneous injection of tibial veins, retrograde catheter venography, and "diversion venography." [47]

For most patients, treatment is conservative [44, 45]. When lower extremities are affected, leg lengths should be measured and a LLD managed appropriately. Specific problems have to be addressed when they arise such as infections, bleeds, thromboembolic events, and extremity pain. Graded compression stockings can be extremely helpful in those with leg enlargement, venous anomalies, venous hypertension, chronic venous insufficiency, and lymphedema. A variety of topical treatments can be effective to treat skin bleeding. Sclerotherapy can be offered to treat certain components such as focal VMs including perirectal VMs causing rectal bleeding, macrocytic LMs, and bleeding cutaneous lymphatic vesicles. Recurrence after sclerotherapy is recognized. Endovenous laser ablation or surgical removal of anomalous veins which give rise to pain or are potential sources of pulmonary emboli is an option. Symptom recurrence after surgical excision of these channels is not uncommon. In order to reduce the size of a severely enlarged extremity (particularly the leg), radical debulking of subcutaneous tissues can be undertaken. Prophylactic anticoagulation and inferior vena cava filter placement should be considered in KTS patients when they are undergoing long and complex interventions and surgery because of the known increased venothromboembolic risk.

Parkes Weber Syndrome

This is a sporadic complex combined fast-flow vascular malformation affecting the extremities and trunk and associated with a RASA-1 gene mutation [48]. In PKWS, there is a vascular skin stain, overgrowth of the affected body part, and prominent veins (Figs. 14.38 and 14.39). The extremities are commonly affected. Although it may be confused with KTS because of this triad of clinical findings, the disease may have a focal distribution as well as affecting an extremity in a more diffuse/multifocal pattern. AV shunting occurs through macro and micro AV fistulae, and varicosities result from the AV shunting. The vascular skin stain is not a true CM as in KTS and has been described as a "pseudo CM." It is most likely due to micro AV fistulae, which explains the warmth when the stain is palpated, unlike the CM in KTS. Lymphatic malformations and abnormalities of lymphatic flow may occur in PKWS. On physical examination, the condition is obvious at birth and appears as overgrowth with a "geographic" macular pink skin stain. The overgrowth may affect the entire extremity or part of an extremity. The clinical findings of high flow are characterized by localized hyperthermia, bruits, thrills, and prominent veins. Physical findings can be confirmed easily with continuous wave Doppler demonstrating AV shunting. AV shunting may lead to cardiac decompensation from volume overload.

PKWS Imaging and Treatment

MR is recommended to evaluate the overall distribution of the disease. In an affected extremity, enlarged inflow arteries and outflow veins are seen and numerous flow voids are present on spin echo sequences. Micro AV fistulae can be seen as T2 signal hyperintensity in deeper tissues such as muscle. MR will demonstrate associated lymphatic anomalies.

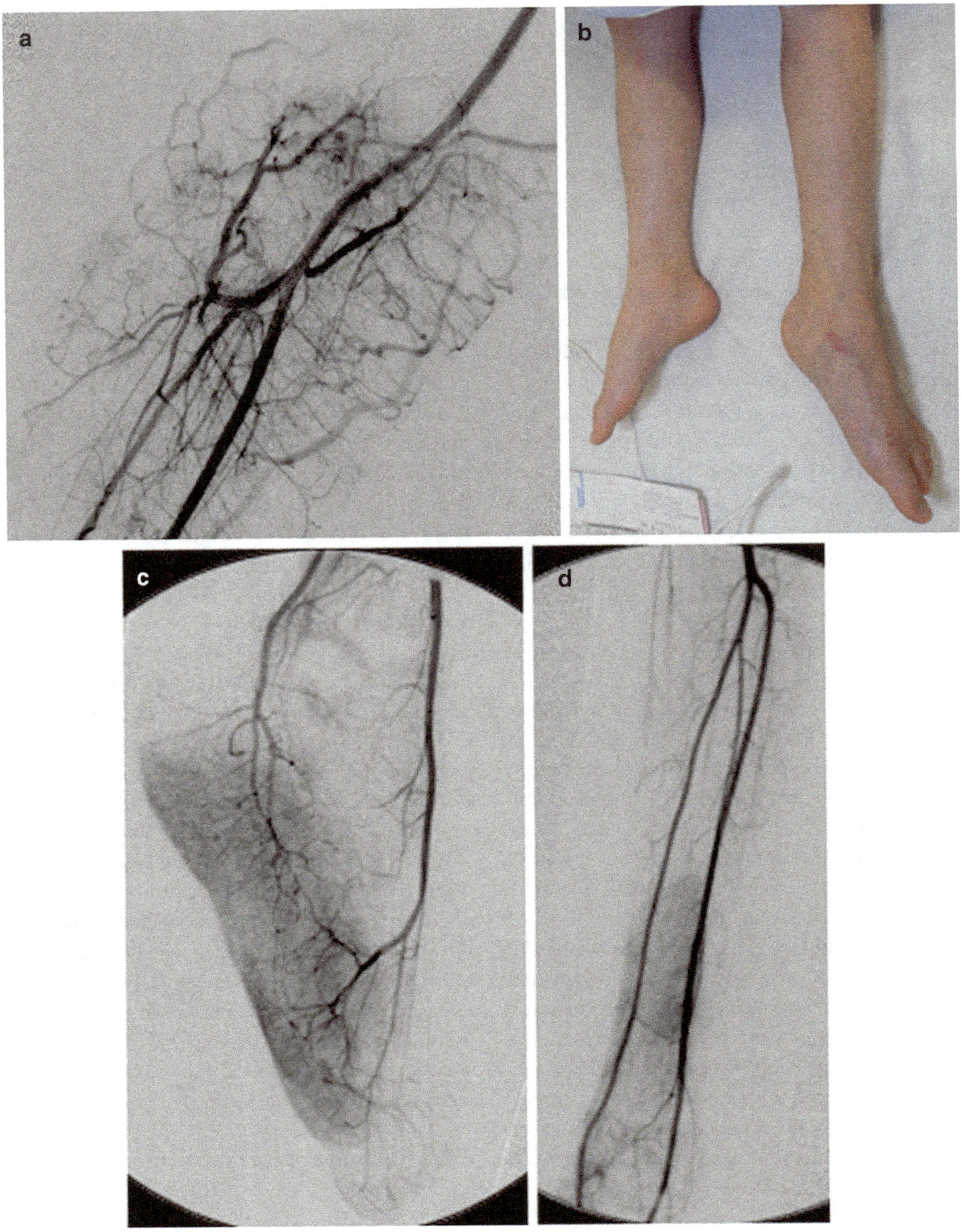

Fig. 14.38 Parkes Weber syndrome (PKWS) with micro AV fistulae (AVF). Catheter angiogram (**a**) shows numerous circumferential soft tissue micro AVFs at the elbow. Another patient (**b–d**) with enlargement of calf and foot, vascular foot stain, and dilated veins, has numerous micro AVFs in calf and foot. On angiogram, micro AVFs can appear as intense soft tissue staining (**c**, **d**)

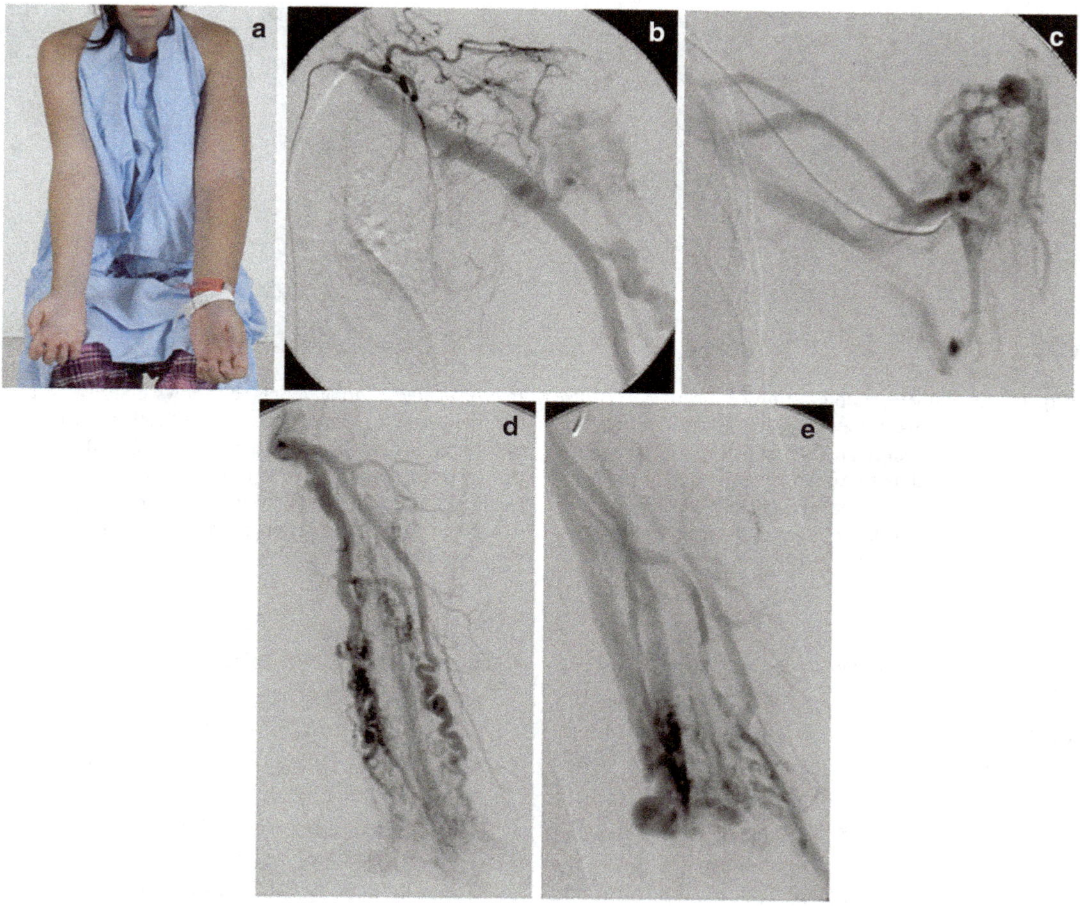

Fig. 14.39 PKWS with macro AV fistulae (AVF). Patient with enlarged left upper extremity, cardiac decompensation and "effort dyspnea" (**a**). Global subclavian angiogram shows numerous macro AVFs in supraclavicular area, around upper humerus and in the upper arm (**b–e**). Macro AVFs in the upper arm supplied by an enlarged profunda brachii artery with venous drainage into enlarged soft tissue veins and intraosseous channels in humerus

Catheter angiography is not usually undertaken unless the patient has local pain, tissue ulceration, or cardiac decompensation/cardiac failure. The catheter angiogram is important in these situations as it can identify macro AV fistulae, which may be suitable for endovascular closure, resulting in symptom improvement. Angiography should be performed as in peripheral AVMs with global and selective studies at the time of intended shunt closure. Angiography depicts enlargement of inflow arteries and draining veins and numerous AV fistulae (Figs. 14.38 and 14.39). The AV fistulae may occur throughout an entire extremity or more focally, and both macro and micro fistulae can be identified [3]. Micro AV fistulae are unsuitable for catheter embolization. Endovascular closure of macro AV fistulae reduces shunting leading to better tissue perfusion with reduced pain, aid healing of skin ulceration, and control of cardiac overload (Fig. 14.40).

Endovascular closure is performed at the time of the diagnostic catheter angiogram. Transarterial catheter embolization of the macro AV fistulae is done by embolization as close to the fistulae as possible (using coaxial techniques). However, it is important to consider other methods including direct percutaneous puncture and venous outflow closure. The angioarchitecture of an AV fistula is different to peripheral AVMs as there is no nidus, and therefore direct percutaneous

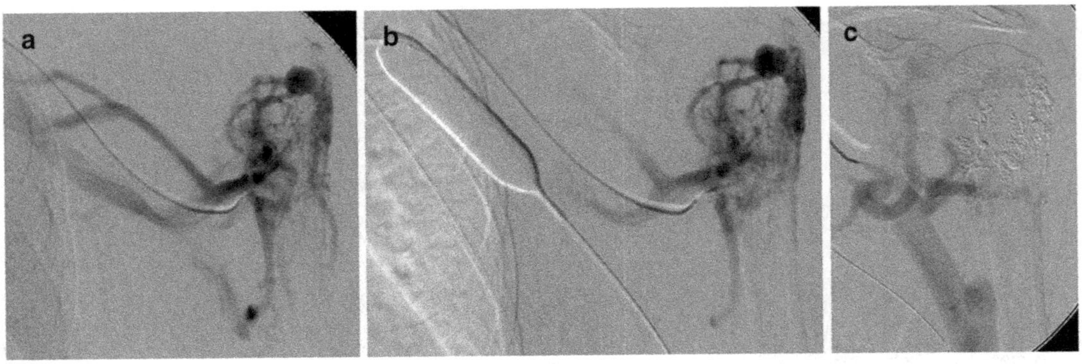

Fig. 14.40 Catheter embolization of macro AV fistulae in PKWS. Same patient as in Fig. 14.39. Selective embolization of upper humeral AVF. Selective angiography of shunt shows rapid flow (**a**). Flow was reduced with a subclavian vein occlusion balloon, placed via the femoral vein (**b**). Glue embolization was performed via a coaxial microcatheter into the shunt. (**c**) Shows good shunt closure on repeat angiography after embolization. Successful closure of AVFs (supraclavicular area, shoulder, upper arm, and forearm) using glue was done over several treatments. Embolization resulted in significant improvement of cardiac status and left upper arm reduced in size

techniques may have to be modified. Several treatment sessions may be required, the frequency of which depends on the clinical problem. Endovascular treatments are stopped when symptom control is achieved.

Both KTS and PKWS are complex vascular malformations, and although there are no cures, the interventional radiologist can provide useful therapeutic options with symptom improvement.

Chapter Summary

Overview

- ISSVA classification (Table 14.1)
  - Vascular tumors
    - Infantile hemangioma most common
    - Rarely associated with vascular malformations (e.g., PHACES)
    - Most treatments use medical therapy
  - Vascular malformations
    - Genetic etiology identified for many venous malformations
    - Sclerotherapy, embolization, and laser used

Imaging

- 80–90 % of anomalies diagnosed without imaging
- Imaging used to determine extent, flow patterns, and tissue characteristics
- US and MR most common
- X-ray and CT helpful to assess skeletal growth issues (e.g., KTS)
- Lymphangiography sometimes used to assess lymphatic channels/leaks
- Venography and angiography performed during treatment
- Vascular tumors
  - Parenchymal tumor present.
  - Variable shunts present.
  - Enlarged inflow/outflow vessels when AV shunts present.
- Vascular malformations
  - No tumor present
  - Venous malformations (VM)
    - Dysplastic veins, thrombi, and phleboliths
    - ± fluid-fluid levels
  - Lymphatic malformations (LM)
    - Cystic ± hemorrhage, and thrombi
    - Microcystic—solid and echogenic
    - ± fluid-fluid levels
  - Arteriovenous malformation (AVM)
    - Hypervascularity, shunting, and perilesional edema
    - Enlarged inflow/outflow vessels

Equipment/Drugs

Embolic Agents

- Cyanoacrylate glue—mixed with Lipiodol to control polymerization and opacify the glue
- Onyx, coils, vascular plugs, ethanol, and PVA

Sclerotherapy Agents

- Ethanol—max 1 mL/kg
- STS—max 0.5 mL/kg liquid STS, often used as foam
- Doxycycline—10 mg/mL solution; max. 300 mg babies or 1,200 mg >12 years
- Bleomycin—1 mg/kg; max 15 mg (15 units)

Prophylactic medications

- Dexamethasone—1 mg/kg, max 8 mg; decrease swelling
- Cefazolin—30 mg/kg, max 1 g; treatment of oral/orbital/anal lesions
- Ketorolac—0.5 mg/kg, max 15 mg if <16 years, for analgesia

Vascular Tumors

Infantile Hemangiomas (IH)

- Most common tumor of infants
- Cutaneous lesions often head/neck
  - Red, raised lesions
  - Ulceration and bleeding possible
- Liver, GI tract, and brain possible
  - High-output congestive heart failure possible (i.e., liver)
- Twenty percent multiple
- Three phases
  - Proliferative: rapid growth, angiogenesis; 9–12 months
  - Involuting: decease size/angiogenesis; reduced flow, fibrofatty replacement; 1 to 5–7 years
  - Involuted: fibrofatty residue, small capillaries/veins, 50 % normal appearance, no recurrence; >5–7 years

Congenital Hemangioma (CH)

- Rare, distinct from IH
- Antenatal onset, fully developed at birth
- Hypervascular tumors
- Rapidly involuting congenital hemangioma (RICH)
  - Protuberant mass
  - Resolve by 12–24 months
  - High-output cardiac failure possible
- Non-involuting congenital hemangioma (NICH)
  - Flat/slightly raised round skin lesion, telangiectasia, and pale halo
  - Persistent through life

Infantile Hepatic Hemangioma (IHH)

- Heart failure, anemia, and hepatomegaly rare
- Interventions: medical therapies (steroids, β-blockers, etc.) and embolization
- Focal
  - Often large, present antenatally
  - Regress in 12–24 months
  - Cardiac decompensation antenatally
- Multifocal
  - Three-phase life cycle as with IH (above)
  - Cardiac failure can be delayed (months)
- Diffuse
  - Massive hepatomegaly—abdominal compartment syndrome and respiratory compromise.
  - Shunting is rare.
  - Associated with hypothyroidism.

Tufted Angioma (TA), Kaposiform Hemangioendothelioma (KHE)

- Invasive tumors with variable onset
- KHE more extensive, violet color
- TA red skin plaque
- Biopsy occasionally helpful
- Kasabach–Merritt phenomenon
  - KHE and TA only
  - Thrombocytopenia (consumption)
  - Coagulopathy; decreased fibrinogen, increased D-dimer, PT/INR, and PTT
  - Steroids, vincristine used
  - Platelet transfusion given when <10,000/μL
  - 250–350 μm PVA particles used when embolization necessary

Treatment

- Cutaneous IH—if treatment required, most receive β-blockers/steroids sometime surgical resection.
  KHE with KMP—vincristine, steroids, and sometimes embolization.
- Angiography/embolization for shunting or devascularization
  - Glue, PVA, microcoils, and vascular plugs used.
  - See Practical Tips, page 191.

Low-Flow Vascular Malformations

Capillary Malformations (CM)

- Low-flow, cutaneous, pink-red stains (port-wine)
- Permanent
- No interventional role
- Can be syndromic (SWS and KTS)

Lymphatic Malformations (LM)

- Lymph containing cysts.
- Localized or infiltrating.
- Mass effect can lead to complications.
- Infection and hemorrhage can occur—treated conservatively.
- Classified based on cyst size/appearance.
  - Macrocystic—visible on imaging or > 1 cm in size.
  - Microcystic—not visible on imaging or < 1 cm in size.
- Macrocystic can be soft and partially compressible.
  - Do not refill after compression, and do not increase in size when dependent (unlike VMs).
- Sclerotherapy, surgery, laser, conservative, or medical (rapamycin) treatment options available.
- Imaging.
  - MR or US
  - Cyst fluid (êT1, éT2)
  - Enhancement (septal for macrocystic; none or ill-defined with microcystic)
  - Fluid-fluid levels (protein, blood)
- LM treatment indications.
  - Swelling, pain, infection, functional impairment, fluid leakage, and cosmesis
- LM sclerotherapy.
  - See Practical Tips.
  - US guidance and GA.
  - Day case (unless repeat sclerosis following day planned); ICU bed for high-risk areas (tongue, airway).
  - Cysts punctured and aspirated.
  - Small drains may be placed.
  - Doxycycline ± STS.
    - Replace 1/2 aspirated cyst volume with Doxycycline solution 10 mg/mL (max. dose 300 mg babies, 1,200 mg >12 years)
    - With drain: leave clamped for 4–6 h; pretreatment with STS may increase effectiveness.
    - Repeat q6weeks if necessary.
  - Bleomycin
    - As less swelling cf. doxycycline, used for oral cavity, orbits, eyelids, airway
    - Concern re: risk of pulmonary fibrosis (unlikely with low cumulative doses)
    - Max dose (per treatment): 1 mg/kg to max 15 mg
- LM post-procedure care.
  - Supportive care
  - Monitor for intracystic bleeding.
  - Assure swallowing intact, vitals stable and pain controlled before informed discharge.
- LM follow-up.
  - Sclerotherapy repeated q6wks (after US and clinical assessment)
  - Clinical follow-up at 3 and 12 months following treatment

Venous Malformations (VM)

- Frequently seen/treated by IR
- Low-flow and dysplastic venous spaces, variable venous communications
- Soft compressible mass (refills after release) and expands with Valsalva/dependent position
- Detected at birth or when symptomatic in childhood
- Occur in any location.
- Often unifocal but multifocal/diffuse forms seen.

- Grow with patient, no spontaneous regression.
- Localized intravascular Coagulopathy in 42 % (severe in 5 %).
- Injection sclerotherapy, laser, and surgical and conservative treatment options.
- Surgical/endoscopic treatment for GI VMs.
- VM imaging.
  - Phleboliths seen only in VM.
  - US—refilling with compression, variable solid elements, and phleboliths.
  - MR—êT1, éT2 with variable enhancement; éT1 with thrombus and phlebolith voids.
  - Venography (at time of treatment)
- VM treatment indications
  - Pain, swelling, functional impairment, bleeding, and cosmesis
- VM pre-procedure work-up
  - ◦ D-dimer and fibrinogen
  - ◦ If fibrinogen <1 g/L consider LMWH
- VM sclerotherapy
  - See Practical Tips, page 204.
  - GA, US guidance with fluoro (CT needed rarely).
  - Day case; ICU admission for high-risk areas (tongue, airway).
  - Consider external tourniquet or Trendelenburg to distend lesion.
  - Puncture with multiple small needles, must see venous backflow.
  - Assess morphology, volume, and escape with venogram (2 fps; without tourniquet).
  - Three percent STS foam.
    - ◦ Foam made by adding equal volume of air and agitated through 3-way stopcock.
    - ◦ Can add contrast if desired.
    - ◦ Max dose: 0.5 mL/kg liquid.
  - Ethanol.
    - ◦ Reports of intraprocedural deaths and cardiopulmonary complications have greatly decreased utilization.
    - ◦ Max dose: 1 mL/kg.
  - Bleomycin.
    - ◦ Stasis required before injection—use STS first.
    - ◦ Max dose: 1 mg/kg, maximum 15 mg.
  - Coils, glue, and endovenous laser can be used for large channels or draining veins.
- VM treatment post-procedure care
  - See complications (Table 14.2)
  - Supportive care.
  - Monitor 4–6 h; watch for skin blistering and pain.
  - Consult plastic surgery if ulceration occurs.
  - Aggressive hydration, monitor urine ± sodium bicarbonate, and furosemide for hemoglobinuria.
  - Assure swallowing intact, vitals stable, pain controlled, and urine volume/color normal before informed discharge.
- VM follow-up.
  - Recanalization and enlargement occurs.
  - Sclerotherapy repeated q6wks (after US and clinical assessment).
  - Clinical follow-up at 3 and 12 months following treatment.

High-Flow Vascular Malformations

Peripheral Arteriovenous Malformations (AVM)/ Arteriovenous Fistulas (AVF)

- AVM nidus is abnormal focus of precapillary shunt; multiple nidi often present.
- AVF: no nidus, simple, and complex forms; complex may be confused with AVM.
- Localized or extensive.
- Do not respect tissue boundaries.
- Slow progression and grows with child.
- Schobinger staging for AVM (Table 14.3).
- Signs: increased growth/warmth of area, bruits, thrills, arterial aneurysms, enlarged draining veins, tissue ischemia, ulceration, bleeding, and high-output cardiac failure.
- Exacerbated by puberty, pregnancy, and trauma.
- Embolization, surgical excision (± preoperative embolization), or amputation possible.
- Surgical ligation not helpful.
- AVM imaging/angiography.
  - MR/MRA best.

  - Enlarged inflow/outflow
  - Flow voids on spin echo
  - Surrounding edema
- Plan films/CT may be helpful with osseous involvement.
- Angiography is gold standard.
  - Detailed, global angiogram (morphology, arterial runoff, feeders, nidi, draining veins)

- AVM/AVF treatment indications.
  - Usually required for lesion progression.
  - Ischemia, ulceration, pain, and cardiac overload.
  - Threat to limb or life
- AVM treatment.
  - High rate of progression/recurrence with inappropriate treatment.
  - Repeated treatments over years.
  - Surgical excision for stage 1 suggested.
  - Stage 3, 4, and some stage 2 offered embolization.
  - Limb amputation may be required for severe disease or a non-functional limb
- AVM/AVF pre-procedure work-up.
  - LFTs for liver AVMs.
  - Echocardiogram if cardiac failure/overload.
  - Review all imaging.
- AVM/AVF embolization.
  - See Practical Tips, page 212.
  - GA.
  - Elective, 24 h admission; ICU for high-risk areas.
  - Targeted embolization of AV shunts is goal.
  - Proximal embolization results in subsequent arterial recruitment.
  - Tissue necrosis, skin ulceration, and nerve injury possible.
  - Angiography.
    - Initially to determine volume/flow through shunt.
    - If too fast consider tourniquet; repeat angio.
    - Repeat angio after each embolization and at completion.
  - Direct nidus puncture.
    - US may be helpful.
    - 22 or 23 gauge butterfly needle.
  - Coaxial, microcatheter embolization.
    - 4 or 5 Fr coaxial catheters
  - Venous outflow embolization.
    - Larger (>5 Fr) may be necessary.
    - Direct puncture with 18 gauge needles possible if large veins.
  - Ethanol, glue, and Onyx used.
  - Ethanol.
    - Narrows safety margin; destroys nidus endothelium
    - Never use in visceral AVM
    - 0.2–2 mL/injection
  - Glue/Onyx.
    - Good shunt closure but nidus endothelium not damaged.
    - Mixed with Lipiodol to control rate of polymerization (usually 1 part glue: 2–4 parts Lipiodol).
    - Dextrose flushes.
- Coils/guidewires occasionally used for high-capacity venous outflow from shunt.
- AVM/AVF post-procedure care.
  - See complications (Table 14.4).
  - Supportive care.
  - Bed rest post arteriography.
- AVM/AVF follow-up.
  - Repeat embolization q 8 weeks after clinical assessment and
  - Clinical visit at 3 months. Then yearly.

Complex-Combined Vascular Malformations

Klippel–Trenaunay Syndrome (KTS)

- Cutaneous CM, VM/varicosities/phlebectasia, and soft tissue/bone hypertrophy.
- Usually single lower extremity.
- Pain/bleeding can occur.
- No cardiac failure.
- No cure.
- KTS imaging.
  - X-ray/CT for leg length issues
  - MR—VM/LM extent; hypertrophic tissues
  - MRV—deep venous system (may require invasive imaging)
- KTS treatment.
  - Mostly conservative/symptomatic
  - Compression stockings

- Sclerotherapy—VMs and LMs.
- Closure of embryonic vein when PE potential, pain, venous hypertension.
- Anticoagulation/IVC filter with complex radiology or surgical intervention.

Parkes Weber Syndrome (PKWS)

- High-flow AV fistulae, vascular skin stain, prominent veins, and overgrowth.
- Confused with KTS.
- Focal/multifocal.
- Skin stain not CM; warm to touch.
- Lymphatic issues occur.
- Can result in cardiac failure.
- No cure.
- PKWS imaging.
  - MR—flow voids, éT2, and lymphatic abnormalities.
  - Angiography (for intervention)—large inflow/outflow vessels, fistulae, and no nidus
- PKWS treatment.
  - For pain, ulceration, or cardiac failure.
  - Microcatheter embolization of fistulae.
  - Consider direct puncture and venous outflow closure.

References

1. Enjolras O, Wassef M, Chapot R. ISSVA classifications, color atlas of vascular tumors and vascular malformations. New York: Cambridge University Press; 2007.
2. Hartemink DA, Chiu YE, Drolet BA, Kerschner JE. PHACES syndrome: a review. Int J Pediatr Otorhinolaryngol. 2009;73(2):181–7.
3. Frieden I, Enjolras O, Esterly N. Vascular birthmarks and other abnormalities of blood vessels and lymphatics. In: Schachner LA, Hansen RC, editors. Pediatric dermatology. 3rd ed, Chapter 20. St. Louis: Mosby; 2003. p. 833–62.
4. Burrows PE, Laor T, Paltiel H, Robertson RL. Diagnostic imaging in the evaluation of vascular birthmarks. Pediatr Dermatol. 1998;16(3):455–88.
5. Luu M, Frieden IJ. Hemangioma: clinical course, complications and management. Br J Dermatol. 2013;169(1):20–30.
6. Mulliken JB, Enjolras O. Congenital hemangiomas and infantile hemangiomas: missing links. J Am Acad Dermatol. 2004;50:875–82.
7. Gorincour G, Kokta V, Rypens F, et al. Imaging characteristics of two subtypes of congenital hemangiomas: rapidly involuting congenital hemangiomas and non-involuting congenital hemangiomas. Pediatr Radiol. 2005;35:1178–85.
8. Christison-Legay ER, Burrows PE, Alomari A, et al. Hepatic hemangiomas: subtype classification and development of a clinical practice algorithm and registry. J Pediatr Surg. 2007;42:62–8.
9. Kassarjian A, Zurakowski D, Dubois J, et al. Infantile hepatic hemangiomas: clinical and imaging findings and their correlation with therapy. AJR Am J Roentgenol. 2004;182:785–95.
10. McHugh K, Burrows PE. Infantile hepatic hemangioendotheliomas: significance of portal venous and systemic collateral arterial supply. J Vasc Interv Radiol. 1992;3(2):337–44.
11. Drolet BA, Trenor III CC, Brandão LR, et al. Consensus-derived practice standards plan for complicated kaposiform hemangioendothelioma. J Pediatr. 2013;163(1):285–91.
12. Enjolras O, Mulliken JB, Wassef M, et al. Residual lesions after Kasabach-Merritt phenomenon in 41 patients. J Am Acad Dermatol. 2000;42:225–35.
13. Ryan C, Price V, John P, et al. Kasabach-Merritt phenomenon: a single centre experience. Eur J Haematol. 2010;84(2):97–104.
14. Tan OT, Sherwood K, Gilchrest BA. Treatment of children with port-wine stains using the flashlamp pumped tunable dye laser. N Engl J Med. 1989;320:416–21.
15. Hassanein AH, Mulliken JB, Fishman SJ, et al. Lymphatic malformation: risk of progression during childhood and adolescence. J Craniofac Surg. 2012;23(1):149–52.
16. Cahill AM, Nijs E, Ballah D, et al. Percutaneous sclerotherapy in neonatal and infant head and neck lymphatic malformations: a single center experience. J Pediatr Surg. 2011;46(11):2083–95.
17. Shergill A, John P, Amaral JG. Doxycycline sclerotherapy in children with lymphatic malformations: outcomes, complications and clinical efficacy. Pediatr Radiol. 2012;42(9):1080–8.
18. Swetman GL, Berk DR, Vasanawala SS, et al. Sildenafil for severe lymphatic malformations. N Engl J Med. 2012;366(4):384–6.
19. Hammill AM, Wentzel M, Gupta A, et al. Sirolimus for the treatment of complicated vascular anomalies in children. Pediatr Blood Cancer. 2011;57(6):1018–24.
20. Greene AK, Perlyn CA, Alomari AI. Management of lymphatic malformations. Clin Plast Surg. 2011;38:75–82.
21. Cuervo JL, Galli E, Eisele G, et al. Lymphatic malformations: percutaneous treatment with bleomycin. Arch Argent Pediatr. 2011;109(5):417–22.
22. Bai Y, Jia J, Huang XX, et al. Sclerotherapy of microcystic lymphatic malformations in oral and facial regions. J Oral Maxillofac Surg. 2009;67(2):251–6.
23. Yang Y, Sun M, Ma Q, Cheng X, Ao J, Tian L, et al. Bleomycin A5 sclerotherapy for cervicofacial lymphatic malformations. J Vasc Surg. 2011;53(1):150–5.
24. Dompmartin A, Vikkula M, Boon LM. Venous malformation: update on aetiopathogenesis, diagnosis and management. Phlebology. 2010;25(5):224–35.

25. Hassanein AH, Mulliken JB, Fishman SJ, et al. Venous malformation: risk of progression during childhood and adolescence. Ann Plast Surg. 2012; 68(2):198–201.
26. Mazoyer E, Enjolras O, Laurian C, et al. Coagulation abnormalities associated with extensive venous malformations of the limbs: differentiation from Kasabach-Merritt syndrome. Clin Lab Haematol. 2002;24:243–51.
27. Mazoyer E, Enjolras O, Bisdorff A, et al. Coagulation disorders in patients with venous malformation of the limbs and trunk: a case series of 118 patients. Arch Dermatol. 2008;144(7):861–7.
28. Dompmartin A, Acher A, Thibon P, et al. Association of localized intravascular coagulopathy with venous malformations. Arch Dermatol. 2008;144(7):873–7.
29. Rodriguez-Manero M, Aguado L, Redondo P. Pulmonary arterial hypertension in patients with slow-flow vascular malformations. Arch Dermatol. 2010;146(12):1347–52.
30. Burrows PE. Endovascular treatment of slow-flow vascular malformations. Tech Vasc Interv Radiol. 2013;16(1):12–21.
31. Goyal M, Causer PA, Armstrong D. Venous vascular malformations in pediatric patients: comparison of results of alcohol sclerotherapy with proposed MR imaging classification. Radiology. 2002;223(3): 639–44.
32. Tieu DD, Ghodke BV, Vo NJ, Perkins JA. Single-stage excision of localized head and neck venous malformations using preoperative glue embolization. Otolaryngol Head Neck Surg. 2013;148(4):678–84.
33. Berenguer B, Burrows PE, Zurakowski D, Mulliken JB. Sclerotherapy of craniofacial venous malformations: complications and results. Plast Reconstr Surg. 1999;104(1):1–11.
34. Barranco-Pons R, Burrows PE, Landrigan-Ossar M, et al. Gross hemoglobinuria and oliguria are common transient complications of sclerotherapy for venous malformations: review of 475 procedures. AJR Am J Roentgenol. 2012;199(3):691–4.
35. Arnold R, Chaudry G. Diagnostic imaging of vascular anomalies. Clin Plast Surg. 2011;38(1):21–9.
36. Greene AK, Orbach DB. Management of arteriovenous malformations. Clin Plast Surg. 2011;38(1):95–106.
37. Lee BB, Baumgartner I, Berlien HP, et al. Consensus Document of the International Union of Angiology (IUA)-2013. Current concept on the management of arterio-venous management. Int Angiol. 2013;32(1): 9–36.
38. Yakes WF. Endovascular management of high-flow arteriovenous malformations. Semin Intervent Radiol. 2004;21(1):49–58.
39. Do YS, Yakes WF, Shin SW. Ethanol embolization of arteriovenous malformations: interim results. Radiology. 2005;235(2):674–82.
40. Jackson JE, Mansfield AO, Allison DJ. Treatment of high-flow vascular malformations by venous embolization aided by flow occlusion techniques. Cardiovasc Intervent Radiol. 1996;19(5):323–8.
41. Houbballah R, Mallios A, Poussier B, et al. A new therapeutic approach to congenital pelvic arteriovenous malformations. Ann Vasc Surg. 2010;24(8):1102–9.
42. Pollak JS, White Jr RI. The use of cyanoacrylate adhesives in peripheral embolization. J Vasc Interv Radiol. 2001;12(8):907–13.
43. Al-Saleh S, John PR, Letarte M, et al. Symptomatic liver involvement in neonatal hereditary hemorrhagic telangiectasia. Pediatrics. 2011;127(6):e1615–20.
44. Jacob AG, Driscoll DJ, Shaughnessy WJ, et al. Klippel-Trenaunay syndrome: spectrum and management. Mayo Clin Proc. 1998;73:28–36.
45. Gloviczki P, Driscoll DJ. Klippel-Trenaunay syndrome: current management. Phlebology. 2007; 22(6):291–8.
46. Lee A, Driscoll D, Gloviczki P, et al. Evaluation and management of pain in patients with Klippel-Trenaunay syndrome: a review. Pediatrics. 2005;115:744–9.
47. Ahmad I, Alomari MD. Diversion venography—a modified technique in Klippel-Trenaunay syndrome: initial experience. J Vasc Interv Radiol. 2010;21(5):685–9.
48. Revencu N, Boon LM, Mulliken JB, et al. Parkes Weber syndrome, vein of Galen aneurysmal malformation, and other fast-flow vascular anomalies are caused by RASA1 mutations. Hum Mutat. 2008; 29(7):959–65.

15 Endovascular Thrombosis Treatment

Michael Temple, Anne Marie Cahill,
and Leonardo R. Brandão

General/Background Information

While pediatric arterial and venous thrombosis was initially considered rare, recent data have shown a steady increase, particularly in the pediatric hospital setting [1–3]. Arterial thrombotic events (ATE) and venous thrombotic events (VTE) can result in significant morbidity or even death [4]. Endovascular damage related to deep venous thrombosis (DVT) can lead to post-thrombotic syndrome (PTS), a potentially debilitating condition that includes symptoms such as limb swelling, pain, discoloration, and skin ulceration described in up to 26 % of pediatric cases [5–9]. Peripheral arterial thrombosis can also cause long-term sequelae such as leg length discrepancies (in 8 %) or loss of a limb [10]. Pediatric thrombosis is most commonly iatrogenic (related to vascular access) but can be secondary to anatomic issues, thrombophilic abnormalities or an underlying disease [4].

The treatment of thrombosis is in evolution. In previous decades, anticoagulation and surgical thrombectomy were the only treatments available. Recently multiple generations of thrombolytic drugs and a number of endovascular thrombus removal techniques have been developed to improve patient outcomes. Current treatment options include anticoagulation, systemic or local or catheter-directed thrombolysis, and surgical or endovascular thrombectomy.

Limited pediatric literature and the absence of large-scale prospective trials make exact recommendations for thrombosis intervention problematic. This is further complicated by the fact that there are age-related variations in the coagulation system in pediatric patients. Thrombolysis has been shown to decrease the incidence and severity of PTS in children [11], but its safety profile has not been established to allow recommendation for widespread use. As a result, some groups are attempting to stratify DVT treatment based on potential future risk [12]. Likewise, safe and effective dosing parameters for thrombolytic administration for pediatric (or adult for that matter) patients have not been conclusively established in in vivo studies. Thrombectomy devices decrease length of treatment time and associated costs (avoid or decreased ICU time) [13, 14], but

M. Temple, M.D., F.R.C.P.(C.)
Hospital for Sick Children, University of Toronto, Toronto, ON, Canada M5G 1X8
e-mail: michael.temple@sickkids.ca

A.M. Cahill, M.B., B.ch., B.A.O. (✉)
Department of Radiology, Children's Hospital of Philadelphia, 34th and Civic Center Boulevard, Philadelphia, PA 19104, USA
e-mail: cahill@email.chop.edu

L.R. Brandão, M.D., M.Sc.
Division of Hematology/Oncology, The Hospital for Sick Children, 555 University Avenue, 10th Floor, Black Wing, Room 10412, Toronto, ON M5G 1X8, Canada
e-mail: leonardo.brando@sickkids.ca

M. Temple and F.E. Marshalleck (eds.), *Pediatric Interventional Radiology: Handbook of Vascular and Non-Vascular Interventions*, DOI 10.1007/978-1-4419-5856-3_15,

no randomized, controlled trials have been performed to recommend thrombectomy over thrombolysis [15]. These factors have led to the development of a number of treatment approaches and strategies in pediatric patients.

This chapter provides an overview of thrombosis intervention followed by more specific information relating to venous or arterial thrombosis treatment. Intervention for intracranial thrombosis and pulmonary embolism will not be specifically discussed. Further information on pulmonary embolism treatment can be found in Chap. 7.

Information regarding treatment options in this section is based on current practice models used in various institutions. In the absence of firm scientific evidence, treatment approach should be determined in conjunction with a multidisciplinary team that includes pediatric thrombosis experts, surgeons, interventional radiologists, and intensive care physicians.

Coagulation in Pediatrics

The pediatric coagulation system is extremely complex. In brief, the coagulation system provides a timely and effective response to injury called hemostasis, consisting of the formation of a thrombus (insoluble blood clot) from previously soluble substrates. The hemostatic response prevents excessive bleeding in a newly developed wound. Conversely, potentially excessive hemostatic response is controlled by several natural anticoagulant mechanisms. Both pro- and antithrombotic reactions interact and control each other under several feedback mechanisms to ensure a balanced result.

The hemostatic system in children is different to that in adults [16]. Developmental hemostasis (age-dependent variation in hemostasis) has a direct impact on the efficacy and safety of available treatment options used in children with either ATE or VTE. For example, age-related variations occur in levels of both coagulation factors (responsible for thrombus formation) and natural anticoagulant inhibitors (which downregulate thrombin formation) [17]. In addition to quantitative differences related to lower or higher circulating coagulation factor levels in comparison to adult circulating levels, qualitative changes to several coagulation-related factors have also been described. For example, plasminogen levels in newborns are 50 % of adult values and a portion of that is fetal plasminogen [18]. Thrombus from umbilical cord blood has been demonstrated to be more resistant to thrombolysis than adult thrombus [19]. Therefore, plasminogen replacement, in the form of transfusion of fresh plasma [FP], has been used to facilitate thrombolysis in neonates [19]. Given the many qualitative and quantitative discrepancies in relation to adults, developmental hemostasis becomes even more clinically relevant when we acknowledge that most therapeutic protocols used in children derive from adult practice.

Acute thrombus is composed of a "mesh" containing platelets and red blood cells trapped within a network of fibrin. Fibrin is formed from conversion of fibrinogen by thrombin. It is believed that for ATE, shear stress in combination with the injured endothelial and subendothelial layers generates a platelet-rich thrombus (white thrombus), whereas in VTE, the platelet component related to clot formation is less important (red thrombus) [20].

Fibrinolysis is a regulatory mechanism to prevent excessive clot formation where a naturally occurring protease, plasmin, breaks down fibrin. The plasmin proenzyme, plasminogen, is found in circulating plasma and bound to thrombin. Plasmin degrades fibrin, fibrinogen, factors V and VIII, and complement and can lead to hypocoaguability through excessive consumption of vital hemostatic factors. Plasmin activity is inhibited by α2-antiplasmin and α2-macroglobulin.

As thrombus ages, fibroblastic activity results in increasing organization that affects fibrinolytic treatment success rates, as less thrombin gets exposed to plasmin. In fact, both thrombectomy and thrombolysis become less successful after approximately 14 days, as the thrombus becomes increasingly organized and progressively attached to the vessel wall [14, 21, 22].

Indications/Contraindications

Conservative approaches suggest the use of endovascular thrombosis treatment as a therapeutic modality only in the instances of life-, limb-, or organ-threatening disease in adults [23]. There are currently no recommendations for invasive treatment in pediatric patients.

Intervention for arterial thrombosis is performed when muscle dysfunction and neurologic changes do not indicate imminent limb loss [24] or when surgical intervention is not technically possible (i.e., in infants and small toddlers).

Early DVT intervention improves long-term outcomes in adults. SIR guidelines currently suggest intervention for *phlegmasia cerulea dolens*, acute or subacute inferior vena cava (IVC) thrombosis with pelvic or limb symptoms and low bleeding risk, acute DVT in ambulatory patients with low bleeding risk, and symptomatic subacute and chronic iliofemoral DVT in patients with low bleeding risk [25]. Guidelines for intervention in upper limb DVT have not been created. Further discussion related to specific approaches in children is outlined in the venous and arterial sections below.

Contraindications for thrombolysis include recent surgery, recent hemorrhagic stroke, cerebral neoplasm, and active bleeding. Table 15.1 is a checklist of relative and absolute contraindications.

Preprocedure Work-Up

Imaging

Existing imaging is reviewed and further studies ordered if necessary. Thrombosis is most commonly assessed using duplex ultrasound with compression. CT or MR can be utilized for deeper structures or prior to undertaking more complex procedures such as venous recanalization. CTA is performed to assess for suspected pulmonary embolism.

Additional imaging may be required when thrombosis is related to an underlying disease. For example, a patient with DVT and a testicular tumor should undergo brain MRI (or CT) to exclude cerebral metastases prior to considering thrombolysis.

Bloodwork

Complete blood count (CBC), partial thromboplastin time (PTT), prothrombin time (PT)/international normalized ratio (INR), fibrinogen, D-dimers, blood urea nitrogen (BUN), creatinine, and blood group for potential crossmatch should be obtained.

Thrombophilia Testing

Thrombophilia testing is not routinely performed at the time of presentation. Most thrombophilic abnormalities will not have a direct impact on immediate clinical management, and acute derangements in the coagulation system can result in false-positive results. Exceptions to this approach include suspected severe deficiencies of specific coagulation inhibitors (i.e., antithrombin or protein C/S) or an inherited/acquired condition that may require longer anticoagulation due to higher risk of thrombosis recurrence (i.e., lupus anticoagulant) [26, 27].

Testing should be performed in children older than 12–18 months of age, preferably at least 4–6 weeks after anticoagulation has been discontinued. The assessment includes determination of protein S, protein C, and antithrombin deficiencies, factor V Leiden and prothrombin mutations, lupus and anticardiolipin antibodies, and elevations of factor VIII and lipoprotein (a). Thrombophilia screening likely has the greatest benefit in adolescents with spontaneous thrombosis. Thrombophilia testing in asymptomatic patients with a known family history is not indicated [28].

History and Physical

Obtain a thorough description of the acute event and timing; review risk factors for thrombosis

Table 15.1 Review of systems/labs and questions before catheter-directed thrombolysis

Neurology	Active head bleeding?	( ) Yes	( ) No
	Intracranial tumor? Spinal tumor?	( ) Yes	( ) No
	Intracranial lesion (AVM, aneurysm)?	( ) Yes	( ) No
	Seizure disorder?	( ) Yes	( ) No
	TIA? Moyamoya?	( ) Yes	( ) No
	Lumbar puncture <7 days?	( ) Yes	( ) No
	Recent neurosurgery?	( ) Yes	( ) No
	Head trauma or intracranial bleeding <2 weeks?	( ) Yes	( ) No
		( ) Yes	( ) No
Hematology	Severe thrombocytopenia (<100,000)?	( ) Yes	( ) No
	DIC? Bleeding disorder?	( ) Yes	( ) No
	Contraindication to anticoagulation?	( ) Yes	( ) No
		( ) Yes	( ) No
Acute events	Active internal bleeding?	( ) Yes	( ) No
	Recent GI or GU bleeding (<2 weeks)?	( ) Yes	( ) No
	Recent CPR?	( ) Yes	( ) No
	Massive PE with hemodynamic compromise?	( ) Yes	( ) No
	Major surgery or trauma (last 10 days)	( ) Yes	( ) No
	Recent biopsy?	( ) Yes	( ) No
		( ) Yes	( ) No
Other systems	Right to left cardiac or pulmonary shunt? HHT?	( ) Yes	( ) No
	Bacterial endocarditis or pericarditis?	( ) Yes	( ) No
	Myocardial infarction?	( ) Yes	( ) No
	Renal failure?	( ) Yes	( ) No
	Uncontrolled hypertension?	( ) Yes	( ) No
	Hepatic failure?	( ) Yes	( ) No
	Recent eye surgery? Diabetic retinopathy?	( ) Yes	( ) No
	Allergies: contrast, TPA?	( ) Yes	( ) No
	Pregnancy?	( ) Yes	( ) No
Lab values	Platelets <100,000/μL	( ) Yes	( ) No
	INR >1.6	( ) Yes	( ) No
	PTT prolonged by >4 s	( ) Yes	( ) No
	Fibrinogen <100 g/dL	( ) Yes	( ) No

Reproduced courtesy of Dr. João Amaral

and those associated with relative and absolute contraindications (see Table 15.1). Physical examination should include assessment of perfusion, neurologic status/muscle function assessment, leg circumference (for DVT), and pulses/perfusion (where applicable).

Multidisciplinary Discussion

The best treatment approach should be determined through interdisciplinary discussion between thrombosis, interventional radiology, intensive care and, when appropriate, vascular/plastic surgery services.

Commonly Used Drugs and Blood Products

Anticoagulation Drugs

Anticoagulants act by inhibiting the formation of new thrombus. The commonly encountered traditional agents, unfractionated heparin (UH) and warfarin, are now used alongside other anticoagulants such as low-molecular-weight heparin (LMWH) and various forms of antiplatelet agents (i.e., aspirin, clopidogrel, dipyridamole).

Heparin

Heparin is a polymeric glycosaminoglycan that inhibits thrombin, an enzyme necessary for thrombus formation. Due to its short half-life, ease of titration, and the ability to fully reverse its effect with protamine, UH tends to be used for acute thrombotic events, particularly in instances when the perceived risk of bleeding is elevated. To obtain therapeutic heparinization, the standard approach is to give a bolus injection of 75–100 U/kg followed by an infusion of 20 U/kg/h (28 U/kg/h if under 12 months) [29]. Several different laboratory-monitoring modalities are used in clinical practice. PTT (and sometimes activated clotting time [ACT]) and the anti-Xa assay are used to titrate the dose to the appropriate UH levels.

The use of heparinization during thrombolysis is controversial due to a possible increase in bleeding risk [5, 30]. Approaches vary from withholding heparin to administering partial (10 U/kg/h) to full heparinization.

Following intervention, the thrombosis service may commence the use of LMWH with dosing based on age-appropriate regimens and monitoring for therapeutic anti-Xa levels.

Warfarin

Warfarin is a vitamin K antagonist that suppresses synthesis of multiple vitamin K-dependent clotting factors produced by the liver (oral vitamin K antagonist [OVKA]). The complete anticoagulant effects of warfarin take several days, and vitamin K is the most commonly used reversal agent available (given either orally or intravenously, more rapid reversal with the latter). Effectiveness is monitored by assessing the international normalized ratio (INR). When an urgent reversal is necessary, factors can be supplied through administration of FFP, prothrombin complex concentrates (PCCs), or the recombinant activated factor VII (rFVIIa).

Antiplatelet Agents

The formation of a thrombus (blood clot) is divided in two phases. The initial one, in a process called primary hemostasis, is responsible for the formation of a platelet plug. Subsequently, with the participation of the coagulation factors following the coagulation cascade, a insoluble net of protein (ie. fibrin) anchoring the clot to the wound site ensues. Platelet plugs constitute a major player in the formation of thrombi, particularly in damaged vessels with high shear stress of the arterial system. Platelet plugs are formed in the following manner:

(a) Platelet adhesion—platelet-vessel wall interaction
(b) Activation—release of platelet's internal contents from their alpha and/or dense granules with amplification of the platelet-mediated prothrombotic effects
(c) Platelet aggregation—platelet-platelet interaction

Antiplatelet agents are used to target specific molecular interactions preventing thrombus formation. They are used for prophylaxis (endovascular stents, Kawasaki disease) or to prevent thrombus growth (myocardial infarction or ATE).

The most common agents used in children are aspirin, clopidogrel (i.e., Plavix®), dipyridamole, and, rarely, abciximab [31].

Aspirin

Aspirin acts by irreversibly acetylating one of the enzymes (cyclooxygenase-1 [COX-1]) responsible for the generation of one of the most potent platelet agonists, named thromboxane A_2. Its inhibition lasts for the entire platelet lifespan. In general, prevention of periprocedural bleeds in children receiving aspirin involves its discontinuation for at least 7–10 days prior to the procedures. The most common side effects are excessive bruising, gastrointestinal toxicity, and the dose-dependent Reye syndrome.

Clopidogrel

Clopidogrel (Plavix®) is part of the thienopyridine family, inhibitors of the platelet agonist,

ADP receptor $P2Y_{12}$. In general, prevention of periprocedural bleeds in patients taking Plavix involves its discontinuation for at least 7 days prior to the procedure. The most common side effects are skin rash, neutropenia, nausea and vomiting, and, rarely, thrombotic thrombocytopenic purpura.

Dipyridamole

Dipyridamole (Persantine®) is a compound commonly used in the setting of clotting prophylaxis in patients post solid organ transplant or in recipients of ventricular assistant devices. It has several mechanisms of action, including changes of adenosine uptake and potentiation of nitric oxide effect. It should also be stopped 7–10 days prior to surgery, and its most common side effects are nausea, flushing, and bleeding.

Abciximab

Abciximab (i.e., ReoPro®) is a monoclonal antibody against the most important platelet agonist relevant for platelet aggregation, glycoprotein IIb/IIIa (GPIIb/IIIa). It is one of three FDA-approved GPIIb/IIIa antagonists resulting in immediate inhibition of platelet aggregation [32]. It is usually utilized as a rescue medical therapy before adult patients are submitted to revascularization or in children, mostly with coronary artery problems (i.e., aneurysms secondary to Kawasaki disease). The major potential adverse events are bleeding and severe thrombocytopenia.

Thrombolytic Drugs

Thrombolytic agents actively break down thrombus. They act by promoting the conversion of plasminogen to plasmin that in turn breaks down fibrin. Plasminogen is found in circulating plasma and bound to fibrin within thrombus. Fibrin-specific thrombolytic agents target bound plasminogen where non-fibrin-specific agents activate both bound and free forms. The activation of free plasminogen acts to deplete plasma proteins and increases bleeding risk. Reported pediatric and adult doses are discussed in Table 15.2.

Compared to systemic administration, catheter-directed thrombolysis decreases the thrombolytics dose with a potential decrease in associated complications. Administration can be performed on a continuous or intermittent basis [33].

Tissue plasminogen activator (TPA) and urokinase are the two most widely used thrombolytics. Their efficacy and safety is similar in DVT treatment in adults [34].

TPA

TPA is a serine protease that is produced using recombinant DNA technology. TPA has high fibrin specificity with a free plasma half-life of 3–6 min and a thrombin-bound half-life of 2 h.

In vitro studies demonstrate a bell-shaped response curve to TPA concentration with the best results found using q 30 s pulse spray application of 0.01 mg/mL in rabbit thrombus [35]. TPA was originally used clinically in concentrations of 0.5–1 mg/mL. This concentration was based on solubility when TPA is dissolved in balanced salt solution. The same is not true for other types of dilutants including normal saline [36]. Lower concentrations (0.01 mg/mL) are routinely employed for treatment of DVT.

Reported pediatric doses vary widely from 0.01 to 0.5 mg/kg/h [3, 5, 37] and can be delivered systemically or by catheter-directed techniques. Local administration is effective and, as lower doses are administered, there are potential advantages regarding safety (see Table 15.2) [3, 6, 37, 38].

Urokinase

Urokinase (UK) is a direct plasminogen activator that is produced in the urothelium. The half-life is approximately 15 min. UK has a higher affinity for fibrin-bound plasminogen than free plasma plasminogen. The product is created using cell culture techniques. UK was temporarily removed from the market in the USA due to concerns over inadequate microbiologic testing. As a result, urokinase is not in common use today.

Table 15.2 Commonly used drugs in thrombosis treatment

Heparin
Unfractionated
Initial loading dose: a) anticoagulation alone: 50–100 U/kg/dose; b) Before preprocedures: 100–150 U/kg/dose
Infusion for "full" heparinization: 20 U/kg/h (28 U/kg/h if less than 12 months old[a])
Partial heparinization: 10 U/kg/h
TPA[a]
Adult (>10 years[b])
Arterial
Bolus: 4–5 mg, can repeat × 2
Infusion: 0.5–1 mg/h (at 0.5–1.0 mg/mL concentration)
DVT
Bolus: 4–10 mg[c]
Infusion: 1 mg in 100 mL NS per hour[d]
– Can increase to 2 mg/h if needed
– For bilateral lower extremity DVT, can run two catheters with 1 mg/h
Pediatric[e]
Systemic
Low dose: 0.01–0.06 mg/kg/h [3]
Regular (high) dose: 0.1–0.5 mg/kg/h [5, 6]
Catheter directed
Low dose
– Start at 0.06 mg/kg/h in neonates
– 0.03 mg/kg/h in non-neonates [3]
Arterial (non-neonates)
Bolus
– 0.1–0.2 mg/kg (5 mg maximum), can repeat × 1
Infusion
– Start at 0.03–0.1 mg/kg/h
– If not effective, can incrementally increase to systemic dose (0.5 mg/kg/h)
DVT
Bolus
– 0.1–0.2 mg/kg (5 mg maximum), can repeat × 1
Infusion
– 0.03–0.06 mg/kg/h; run at maintenance volume

[a] Optimal dose parameters for the use of tissue plasminogen activator (TPA) in children have not been established. Dose regimens indicated are for guidance only. Appropriate dose should be determined by IR and thrombosis teams on a case by case basis

[b] Given developmental hemostasis changes, "adult" dosing can be used in patients over 10 years of age

[c] Bolus dosing varies when thrombectomy devices are used. For example, 6 mg in 6 mL NS for 15 cm Trellis, 6–10 mg in 10 mL for 30 cm Trellis, and 10–20 mg in 50–100 mL NS (power-pulse spray AngioJet). Check manufacturer's current recommendations

[d] Infusion volumes (for DVT treatment) may have to be adjusted based on patient weight and clinical status

[e] Patients <10 kg fresh frozen plasma (FFP) routinely administered (10–20 mL/kg over 1–2 h) and then p.r.n. to keep fibrinogen >100 mg/dL

Reported local doses in pediatric patients range from 4,000 to 40,000 U/kg loading dose and 2,000–120,000 U/kg/h over periods of 6–9 days [5, 39–41].

Blood Products

Blood products such as packed red blood cells, FFP, or cryoprecipitate may be required to correct derangements during thrombolysis.

Plasminogen

Isolated human plasminogen is not available outside of a laboratory setting. When plasminogen levels may be low (neonates and poorly responding older children), plasminogen can be supplemented through administration of FFP to attempt to facilitate thrombolysis [16, 42, 43].

Equipment

Thrombolysis Equipment

Standard end-hole catheters can be used; however, specialized 3–5 Fr multi-side-hole infusion catheters and wires (0.035″) come in a variety of infusion lengths. Infusion catheters without a one-way end valve require a tip-occluding wire to assure preferential flow through the side holes. Pulse spray thrombolytic administration can also be performed through infusion catheters. Wires and/or catheters are used alone or in combination to allow the interventionalist to customize the infusion length based on thrombus extent.

A recent innovation, catheter-directed thrombolysis assisted by US thrombus fragmentation (EKOS EndoWave, EKOS, Bothell, WA), may potentially increase the interaction of the thrombolytic agent with the thrombus and reduce the length of thrombolytic infusion [44].

Thrombectomy Equipment

Thrombectomy devices range from simple balloons to specialized catheters and complex machines.

Balloons

Balloons were traditionally used to perform surgical thrombectomy. Fogarty balloons were inserted through a venotomy or arteriotomy and thrombus was extracted. Over-the-wire Fogarty balloons are now available. Traditional angioplasty balloons are used to fragment thrombus or treat underlying stenosis. Balloon fragmentation has been used to treat life-threatening central DVT [40]. Specialized drug delivery balloons have also been used for thrombolytic administration.

Catheters

By applying manual suction with a syringe, any large-bore catheter can be used to perform a thrombectomy. Specially designed manual suction thrombectomy catheters are available.

Specialized Thrombectomy Devices

Numerous, specialized devices have been created to aspirate, macerate, or fragment thrombus. A few of the commonly used examples include AngioJet®, Trellis®, and Arrow-Trerotola PTD®.

Aspiration devices create a vacuum directly or use high-pressure saline resulting in the creation of suction through the Bernoulli effect. The AngioJet® (MEDRAD, USA) is a rheolytic device where internal saline flow creates suction. Four to 6 Fr AngioJet catheters allow treatment of vessels ranging in size from coronary arteries to large veins involved in DVT.

Another device that is in widespread use today is a pharmacomechanical isolation thrombectomy catheter Trellis® (Covidien, USA) available in 6 and 8 Fr sizes. The device uses two balloons to isolate a segment of thrombosed vessel. Thrombolytic agent is then injected between the balloons and is agitated with a sine wave generator by the intervening wire segment. The thrombus fragments are then aspirated prior to deflating the balloons to avoid the risk of distal embolization (Fig. 15.1).

The Arrow-Trerotola PTD® (Teleflex, USA) is an example of a mechanical thrombectomy device that is FDA approved for arterial and venous thrombectomy. It has primarily been used to treat hemodialysis grafts. This device a motor-driven fragmentation device rotating when

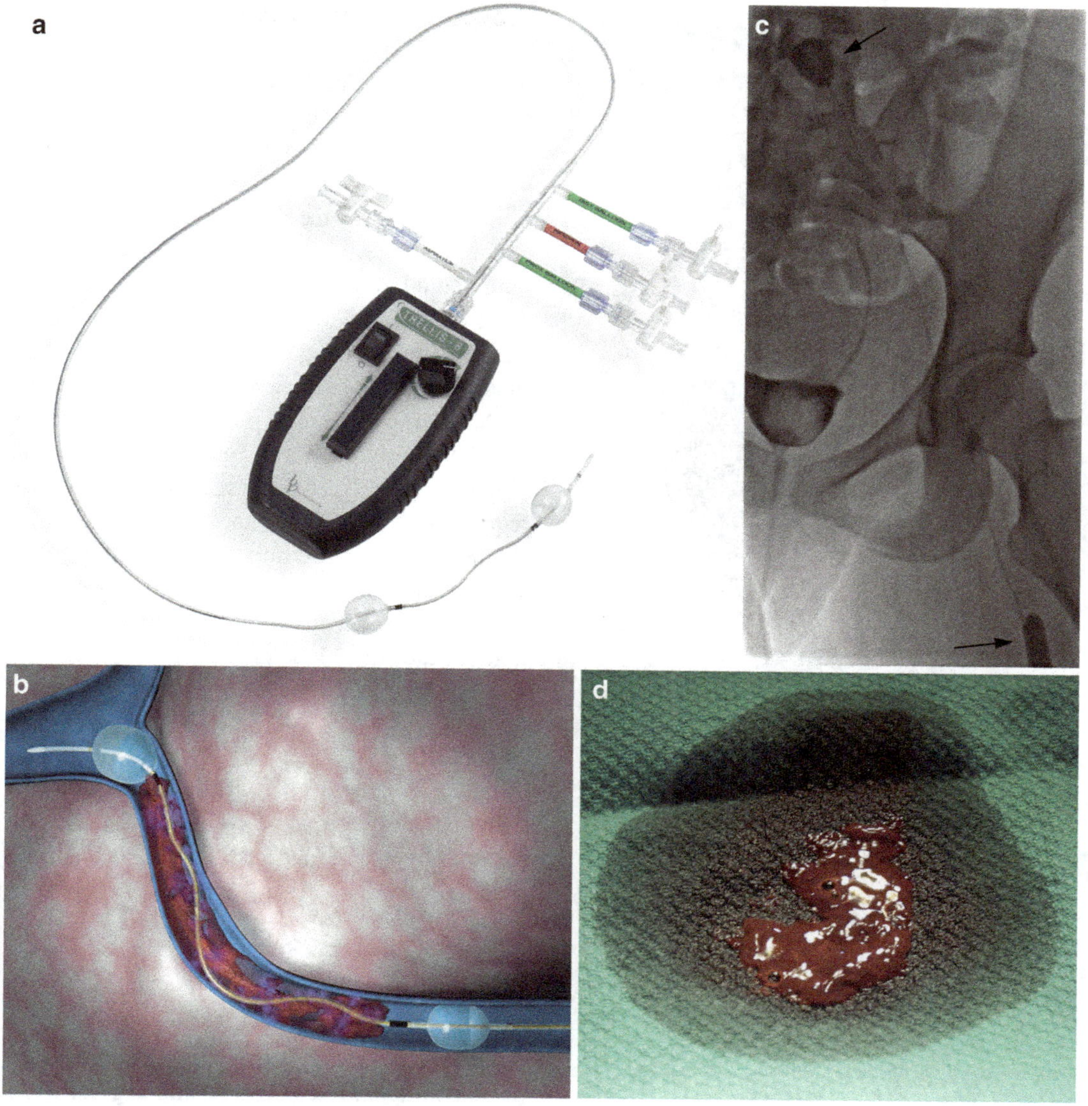

Fig. 15.1 Trellis™ peripheral infusion system. (**a**) Overview of device demonstrates balloons used to isolate a segment of thrombus. Thrombolytic is sequestered between the balloons, agitated with the motor-driven wire, and aspirated. (**b**) Computer-generated representation of device in use. (**c**) Fifteen-year-old female with iliofemoral DVT undergoing treatment with Trellis™. The balloons (*arrows*) isolate the thrombus during treatment. (**d**) Image of thrombus fragment obtained after aspiration. With permission © Covidien AG, 2013

deployed at 3,000 rpm. The fragmented thrombus can then be evacuated through the compatible 7 Fr introducer sheath or larger sheath [45].

Other approaches such as ultrasound wires [46] and high-intensity focused ultrasound/histotripsy [47, 48] have been described but are not in widespread use at this time.

Some thrombectomy devices can cause fragmentation of thrombus resulting in pulmonary embolism or hemolysis leading to hemoglobinuria and the possibility of renal impairment.

Chronic Thrombosis

Treatment of chronic thrombosis can be accomplished and have benefit even years after the index thrombotic event [49, 50]. Recanalization can be accomplished using a sharp needle (see Fig. 9.16, Chap. 9) or

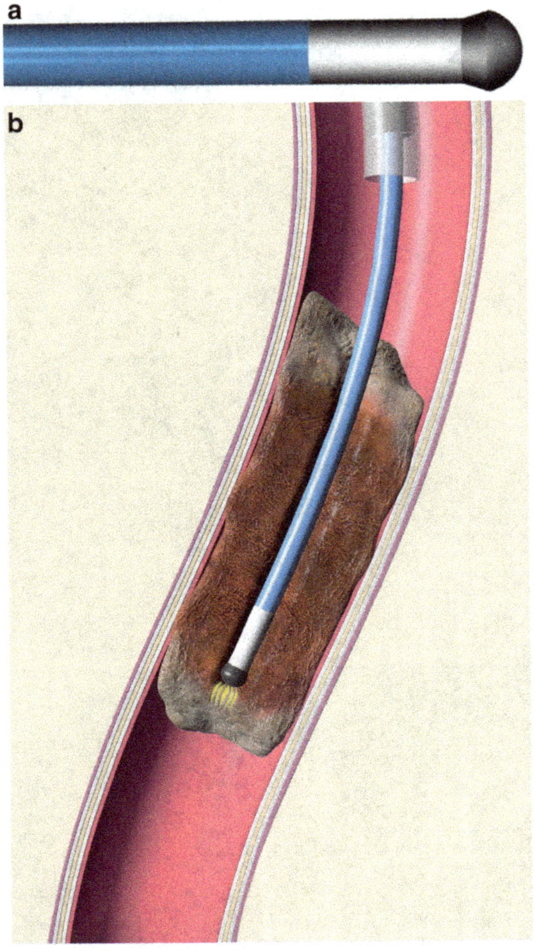

Fig. 15.2 (**a**) Graphic representation of RF tip of wire. (**b**) Radiofrequency energy is used to create a channel through fibrotic regions of chronic thrombus. With permission. © Baylis Medical Company Inc. 2013

specialized equipment such as a radiofrequency wire (Fig. 15.2) [51, 52].

Procedure Technique

Below is a basic outline of endovascular thrombosis management. The exact steps are dictated by the specific approach being utilized. More detailed information for venous and arterial thrombosis intervention is included in the sections below.

Procedure Preparation

Informed consent is obtained. For younger patients, assent should be obtained where appropriate. An ICU bed is booked if thrombolysis might continue after procedure. When using a thrombectomy device that can cause hemolysis, administration of (isotonic) double-maintenance fluid should be considered to reduce the risk of renal tubular toxicity. Pharmacy should be contacted to allow adequate preparation time and timely delivery of lytic agent.

An arterial line can be placed to allow invasive blood pressure monitoring and easy collection of blood samples. Thrombolysis patients who will require ICU admission and ongoing bloodwork should undergo insertion prior to infusion of TPA to minimize potential bleeding complications. A large-bore IV is placed for administration of fluids and blood products.

Sedation

Sedation/anesthesia is based on the needs of the patient, procedure, and institutional availability/practice. See Chap. 3.

Positioning

Arterial interventions are performed with the patient in supine position. Positioning for DVT intervention is determined by the access route. The patient is placed in prone position when accessing the popliteal vein and supine position for the femoral vein, posterior tibial vein (or other patent calf vein), or upper extremity access. If an IVC filter is being placed, the patient may need to be repositioned during the procedure. Some operators avoid this issue by inserting the filter through a popliteal approach with the patient in prone position [53].

Filter Insertion

Placement of IVC filters during thrombosis treatment is controversial. Insertion of IVC filters has

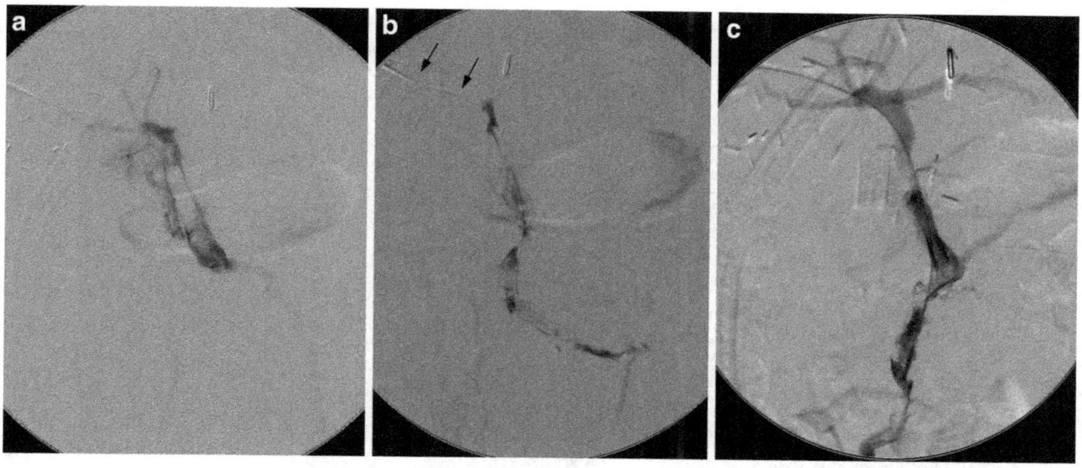

Fig. 15.3 Portal vein thrombosis following liver transplantation. (**a**, **b**) A transhepatic catheter (*arrows*) demonstrates portal and superior mesenteric vein thrombosis. (**c**) Following pulse spray thrombolysis, thrombectomy, and 48 h of TPA infusion, portal vein flow has been restored. Thrombus in the splenic vein (not shown) completely resolved, thus providing adequate flow to maintain portal vein patency

been demonstrated to decrease the incidence of pulmonary embolism in patients undergoing endovascular VTE treatment [53]. When used, venous filters are placed at the beginning of the procedure. In very small patients filters may not open fully resulting in concerns related to the overall length and efficacy. Chaudry et al. described successful, uncomplicated IVC filter insertion performed in three patients with an IVC diameter less than 1 cm [54]. Filter insertion techniques are described in Chap. 11.

Vascular Access

The location of thrombus, the type of vessel involved (artery vs. vein), the vessel size, and the potential for causing further (iatrogenic) thrombosis affect the choice of access site and route.

Whenever possible, antegrade access below the level of thrombosis is utilized for DVT treatment. This minimizes the potential for creating further valvular damage and improving efficacy by allowing establishment of venous inflow and outflow.

Transhepatic access is used for portal vein interventions (Fig. 15.3). Alternatively, antegrade access through the superior mesenteric vein can be obtained during laparoscopy if a combined surgical-radiological approach is desired.

As there are no valves within the arterial system, an antegrade or retrograde approach can be used.

Insertion of a vascular sheath will minimize the potential for vessel damage related to catheter changes and provides an infusion port for administration of drugs and contrast. The size of vascular sheath is based on the device and/or balloon used (3–9 Fr).

Define Thrombus Extent

DSA venography/angiography is used to define the extent of thrombosis and the presence of collateral pathways (Figs. 15.4a–c and 15.5a, b). This information helps determine the best procedural method. For example, escape of lytic agent through large collaterals around an area of DVT may make use of the Trellis less desirable than other devices.

The use of a wire and catheter used to perform angiography or venography can improve treatment outcomes and can be predictive of success. Rotation of the wire and/or catheter can be used to fragment the thrombus to increase surface area available to react with the lytic agent. The ability

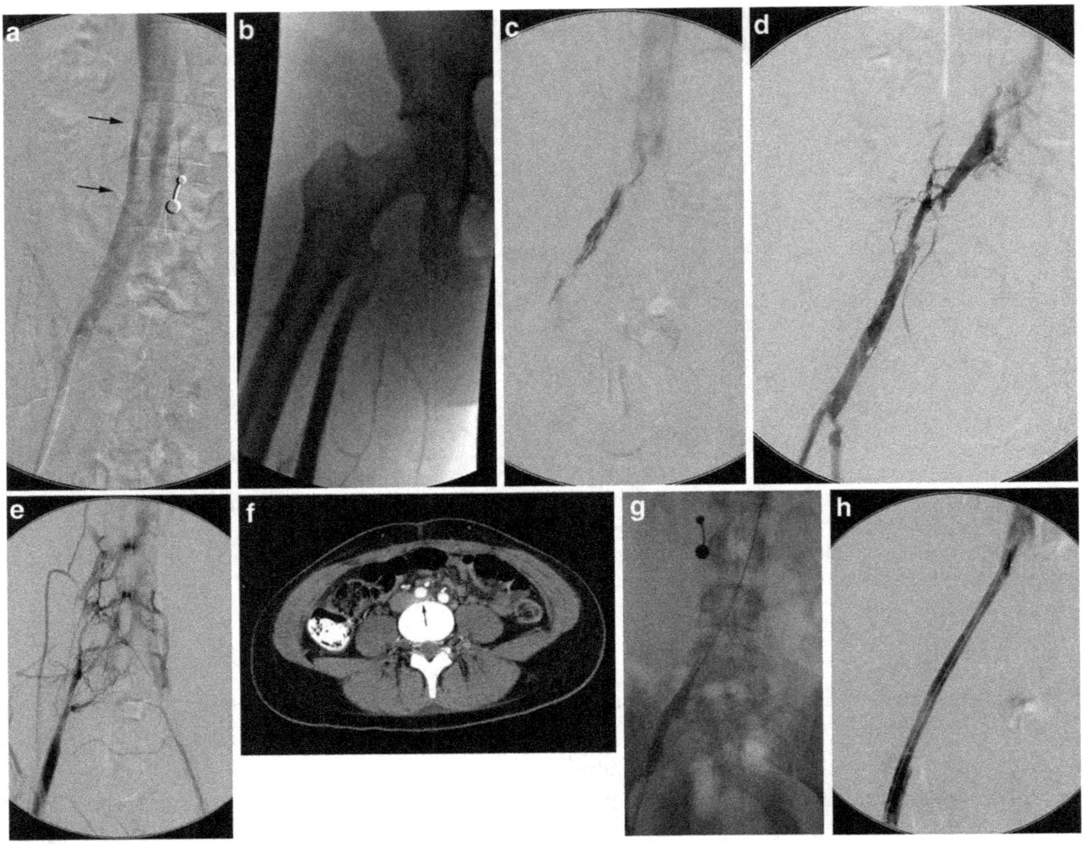

Fig. 15.4 May-Thurner: Fifteen-year-old female with acute left leg swelling, recent change in oral contraceptives, and multiple family members with DVT and PE. (**a**) Femoral venogram obtained prior to IVC filter insertion demonstrates free floating IVC thrombus (*arrows*) arising from left common iliac vein. An IVC filter was placed using a jugular approach. (**b**, **c**) DSA venography shows left iliofemoral thrombosis (patient is prone). (**d**) Near-complete thrombus resolution following AngioJet power-pulse spray thrombolysis and thrombectomy. (**e**) After TPA infusion, thrombosis has cleared but normal antegrade flow through the common iliac has not been reestablished. (**f**) CT demonstrates external compression of right CFA on left CFV (*arrow*) consistent with May-Thurner syndrome. (**g**) Several episodes of unsuccessful venoplasty were undertaken prior to placing a 14 mm wall stent (**h**)

to pass a wire through an area of arterial thrombosis is a predictor of success in arterial interventions [55]. This underlines a basic tenet of thrombosis treatment: success is dependent upon the ability to establish both inflow and outflow.

Initial Lytic Administration

When not proceeding directly to thrombectomy, thrombolytic agents can be administered using lacing or pulse spray techniques or with some thrombectomy devices. During the initial administration, single or multiple doses of lytic agent are given. Multiple doses are administered at 15–30 min intervals (to allow time for the lytic agent to act).

Lacing is the injection of lytic agent throughout the length of a thrombus (usually through an end-hole catheter). To perform pulse spray thrombolysis, small aliquots are injected under high pressure to force the lytic agent deeper into the thrombus to improve efficacy. Traditional pulse spray is performed with a multi-side-hole catheter (Fig. 15.6). Certain AngioJet catheters perform an automated version called power-pulse spray.

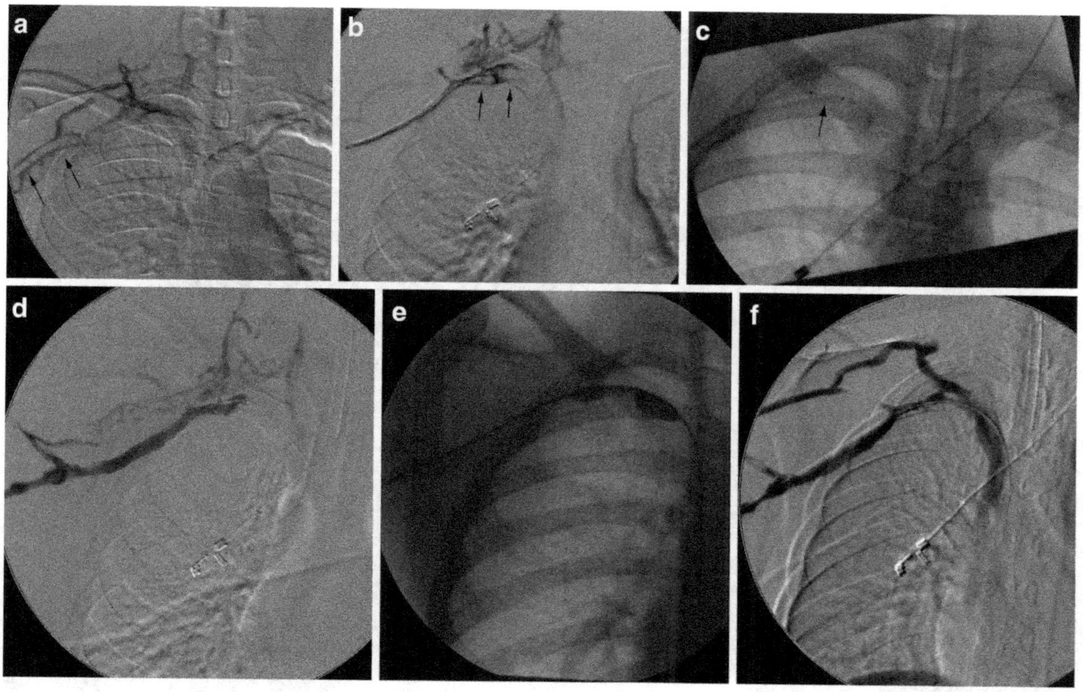

Fig. 15.5 Paget-Schroetter: Fourteen-year-old baseball player with 3-day history of right arm pain and swelling. (**a**, **b**) Axillary and subclavian vein thrombosis (*arrows*) demonstrated on venogram. (**c**) Power-pulse spray thrombolysis and AngioJet© thrombectomy performed resulting in (**d**) near-complete clearance. (**e**, **f**) Venoplasty was performed resulting in reestablishment of flow. The patient was referred for urgent surgical assessment but required two further episodes of thrombectomy and venoplasty

Other approaches include intermittent administration directly into thrombus [33] or through a specialized isolation thrombectomy device (Fig. 15.1c).

Thrombectomy

When used, a thrombectomy device is inserted to disrupt, macerate, or remove thrombus (Fig. 15.5c). The choice of thrombectomy device is dependent upon institutional availability and thrombus location and extent. Venography is used to assess progress and determine if further intervention is necessary (Figs. 15.4d and 15.5d).

Thrombectomy devices should be used according the manufacturers recommendations while being mindful of the differences in treatment of pediatric patients. For example, appropriate thrombectomy times for adults could result in significant hemolysis or relatively high volumes of blood loss related to the lower total blood volume.

Reversible bradycardia has been reported with use of the AngioJet device [56]. Possible mechanisms include adenosine or potassium release from hemolysis. Most bradycardic episodes resolve within seconds of stopping active thrombectomy. As such, short pulses of thrombectomy are used after breaking through the most proximal portion of the thrombus during DVT treatment. Use in the pulmonary arteries has lead to profound bradycardia and death [57] theorized to be secondary to an effect on regional stretch receptors. As such, recommendations for use of AngioJet in pulmonary embolism range from "not indicated" [57] to "can be considered but suggest concomitant pacemaker insertion" [58].

Lytic Infusion

Infusion catheters and wires can be used alone or in combination. As such, the length of the infusing segment(s) can be customized to administer lytic

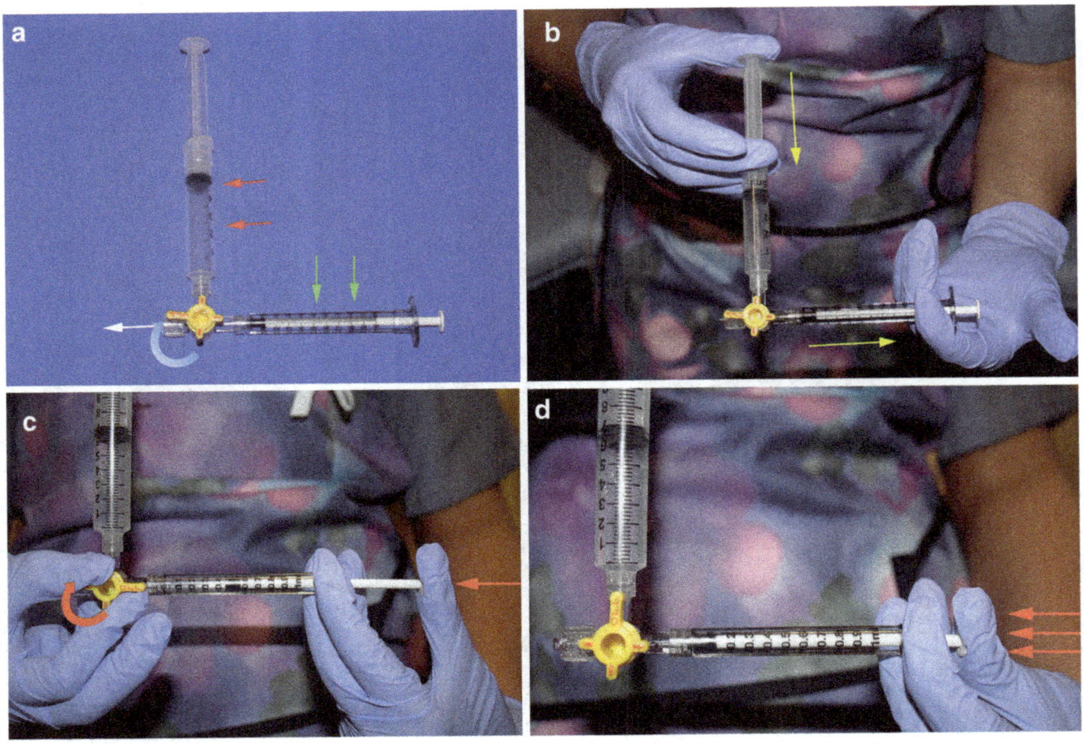

Fig. 15.6 Pulse spray thrombolysis technique. (**a**) A 3-way stopcock is used to connect a reservoir syringe containing the full dose of TPA (*red arrows*) and a sturdy, small (1 mL) syringe (*green arrows*) for injections. The infusion catheter (not shown) attaches at the *white arrow*. (**b**) The injection syringe is filled with a small volume (0.1–0.3 mL) of TPA (*yellow arrows*). (**c**) Push the plunger of the injection syringe against the closed 3-way stopcock to generate pressure (*red arrow*). (**d**) While maintaining pressure, the stopcock is opened causing the plunger of the injection syringe to quickly depress (*red arrows*), causing TPA to be forcefully ejected through the infusion catheter

throughout the length of the thrombus while avoiding infusion into unaffected portions of the vessel.

The choice of dose, concentration, and the rate and volume of infusion is optimized based on the location (arterial vs. venous, large vs. small vessel) and patient age. See Table 15.2 for a description of dose levels.

The choice to provide full, partial, or no heparinization is made at the discretion of the radiologist and hematologist. Heparin administration during thrombolysis has been associated with an increased risk of bleeding [5, 25, 59]. However, vessel reocclusion is common following endovascular treatment in pediatric patients [59]. This finding supports more aggressive anticoagulation, but research is needed before recommendations can be made.

Ongoing Evaluation

Thrombosis intervention is a dynamic process and ongoing evaluation is required to allow changes in thrombolytic dose or repositioning of a catheter to take place as the thrombus load and extent change. While bedside ultrasound can be performed, a DSA contrast study provides the most accurate information regarding the residual thrombus burden. During thrombolysis, the patient is transferred from intensive care to the imaging suites for intermittent assessment (every 4–24 h) (Fig. 15.4e). The catheters are removed when the thrombus has resolved or when it is felt that thrombolysis would be of no further benefit. The vascular sheath can be left in place for heparin infusion and for bloodwork.

While there is some controversy [25], q 4–6 h bloodwork is obtained to monitor coagulation parameters (CBC, INR, PTT, fibrinogen, D-dimers). Symptomatic bleeding or blood value derangements may require supplementation with cryoprecipitate, FFP, or blood transfusion. In case of severe acquired hypofibrinogenemia due to marked consumption, the use of plasma-derived fibrinogen concentrates may be warranted.

Dilatation/Stent Placement

Underlying anatomic causes of thrombosis are sometimes defined following resolution of thrombosis. When a significant lesion is identified, dilatation ± stent placement is considered. Given the long life expectancy in pediatric patients, stents are not placed as readily as in adults. Pediatric interventional radiologists will often assess the outcome of dilatation alone prior to consideration of stent placement (Figs. 15.4f–h and 15.5d–f).

Postprocedure Care/Follow-Up

Due to the high rate of rethrombosis in pediatric patients [59], therapeutic heparin levels should be attained as soon as possible after the intervention is complete. Patients are switched from UH to a longer-acting anticoagulant (LMWH, OVKA) shortly afterward. Antiplatelet agents may also be added at the discretion of the thrombosis team.

Thrombectomy-associated hemolysis can lead to hemoglobinuria and potential renal damage. In these patients, hyperhydration should be performed and the urine monitored for the presence of blood. BUN and creatinine should be assessed in the presence of hematuria.

The patient is followed by the thrombosis service to monitor anticoagulation. Thrombophilia testing is undertaken as described in the section above.

Patients who underwent IVC filter insertion should be followed to assure the filter is removed as soon as possible.

Appropriate long-term follow-up by interventional radiology has not yet been defined. Collaborative studies to determine outcomes and appropriate multidisciplinary follow-up would be beneficial.

Table 15.3 Indications/contraindications for venous thrombosis intervention

1. Strong indications for thrombolytic therapy in neonates and children:
(a) Life-, limb-, or organ-threatening thrombosis
– Arterial or venous thrombosis causing tissue ischemia
– SVC syndrome due to thrombosis
– Massive PE with cardiovascular collapse
– Bilateral renal vein thrombosis
– Cerebral sinovenous thrombosis with progressive neurologic deficits
– Large atrial thrombi
– Congenital heart disease with shunt obstruction
2. Intermediate indications in neonates and children:
(a) Acute obstructive iliofemoral or IVC thrombosis
(b) Anatomic compressive syndromes
– May-Thurner syndrome
– Paget-Schroetter syndrome
Contraindications to thrombolytic therapy in neonates and children:
1. Major surgery 7–10 days
2. Active bleeding
3. CNS surgery/ischemia/bleeding/trauma within 30 days
4. Seizures within 48 h
5. Inability to maintain platelet count >50,000/μL
6. Inability to maintain fibrinogen >100 mg/dL
7. Uncontrolled hypertension

Source: Elsevier

Venous Thrombosis

Indications/Contraindications [2, 60]

Indications and contraindications are included in Table 15.3.

Preprocedure Work-Up

Imaging

As stated in the section above, the patient's existing imaging studies should be reviewed and further studies ordered if warranted. When venous thrombosis is secondary to an underlying disease such as malignancy, additional imaging may be warranted to exclude an intracranial metastasis. The extent of the thrombosis should be detailed by a preprocedure imaging study. In children, due to their small-size duplex, US may be the most easily accessible modality to determine the extent of thrombosis. The SIR guidelines for lower extremity thrombus recommend venographic imaging whenever possible for complete thrombus extent but alternatively US assessment for calf vein thrombus and MR/CT imaging for iliofemoral thrombus [25].

Bloodwork

Prior to venous thrombolysis basic hematological parameters such as a CBC, PTT, INR, fibrinogen, D-dimers, factors, BUN, and creatinine should be performed.

Thrombophilia testing is undertaken as described in the section above.

History and Physical

A venous thrombosis history should include thorough description of the acute thrombosis event and timing and prior history of DVT and review of risk factors for thrombosis and those associated with relative and absolute thrombolysis contraindications (see Tables 15.1 and 15.3) and any coexisting morbidities. A physical examination should be performed including assessment of extent of the extremity edema, perfusion, neurologic status, extremity circumference, and pulses. The presence of *phlegmasia cerulea dolens* increases the risk of arterial insufficiency and compartment syndrome and the ultimate risk of venous gangrene and amputation [25].

Multidisciplinary Discussion

Interdisciplinary discussion between thrombosis team, interventional radiology, and, when appropriate, vascular surgery services should be undertaken to determine the best treatment approach for the patient depending on extent of thrombosis, duration of symptomatology, and patient risk factors.

Equipment

- General thrombolysis equipment is outlined in the section above.
- Thrombolysis catheters, as previously stated, are small-bore catheters (3–5 Fr) which can be placed across the thrombosed segment in younger children facilitating the infusion of low-dose thrombolytic directly into the clot, thereby reducing the risk of major bleeding [5]. A bolus of thrombolytic therapy such as 4–10 mg (TPA) may be initially infused over 10 min through the infusion catheter.
- More recently catheter-directed thrombolysis assisted by US thrombus fragmentation (EKOS EndoWave, EKOS, Bothell, WA) may potentially further reduce the length of thrombolytic infusion [44].
- All pharmacomechanical devices are effective in the acute clot setting (<14 days) as clot extraction is maximal [14].
- The AngioJet system offers the advantage of a small sheath (4 Fr) for access to smaller-sized vessels in the pediatric population.
- The Trellis Peripheral Infusion System is particularly useful in acute short-segment venous thrombosis and utilizes a technique called "isolated thrombolysis" [61]. The advantage of this device in children includes the presence of occlusion balloons that are inflated proximal and distal to the thrombus to confine the thrombolytic agent to the treatment area and thereby limit systemic delivery and complications. In addition the diameter of the proximal and distal balloons varies from 5 to 16 mm and the treatment segments from 15 to 30 cm allowing for flexibility in treatment segments. TPA dosing of 3–5 mg for the 15 cm length and 5–10 mg for the 30 cm length administered over 5–10 min is recommended within the treatment segment [22]. The device is currently available in 6 and 8 Fr diameters.
- In the setting of subacute/chronic clot (15 to >28 days), one should consider the combination of catheter-directed infusion therapy and pharmacomechanical therapy to increase clot retrieval [14].

Procedure Technique

Basic procedural technique is discussed in the section above. Potential issues with mechanical rheolytic thrombectomy devices include volume overload, hemolytic anemia, hyperkalemia, and bradycardia from adenosine release especially in younger children. In general these issues are more likely in venous thrombolysis due the larger size of vessels and greater clot burden than in arterial thrombosis. A potential technique to reduce the risk of bradycardia from mechanical thrombectomy may be to mechanically remove the more central portion of the clot toward the end of thrombolysis to reduce systemic adenosine release (i.e., leave a 1–2 cm "cap" of thrombus until the end).

Excessive blood loss is also a consideration especially in smaller children. Close monitoring of the effluent is advised to ensure that clot fragments and not fresh blood is being extracted. The estimated blood loss calculation is recommended to be half the total effluent at the end of the thrombolysis session.

Rheolytic catheters are available in a variety of French sizes and types, and the ability to perform pharmacomechanical thrombolysis, i.e., "power-pulse" mode, is limited to specific catheters not including the smaller French sizes.

The vascular access created for endovascular techniques can be used for adjunctive therapies such as angioplasty and venous stenting when required especially for venous compression syndromes [59, 62, 63].

In the setting of venous thrombolysis angioplasty will play a large role in restitution of flow, more so than arterial thrombolysis. The access sheath placed should be sized with a view to delivery and removal of the maximal-sized balloon angioplasty catheter required particularly in the setting of a compression syndrome.

Venographic confirmation of a compression syndrome can be performed once restoration of flow is achieved.

Stenting has greater long-term implications in children. In lower extremity compression syndromes (i.e., May-Thurner), stenting should be considered in the setting of failed venous angioplasty (Fig. 15.4h) [63].

In upper extremity compression syndrome (i.e., Paget-Schroetter), stenting does not play a role due to the high risk of stent fracture and occlusion. Prompt surgical decompression of the thoracic outlet ± vein grafting is advised post thrombolysis. Repeat interval venography and venoplasty may be required (Fig. 15.5f) [59, 64].

Postprocedure Care

Basic postprocedure care is discussed in the section above. Patients undergoing thrombolysis need close monitoring of coagulation parameters such as PTT, INR, platelets, and fibrinogen, initially every 4 h. If fibrinogen decreases to <100 mg/dL, the thrombolytic dose is adjusted accordingly to reduce the risk of systemic hemorrhage.

Biochemical parameters such as potassium, urine macroscopic hemoglobin, hemoglobin, and hematocrit should be performed to assess the presence of systemic hemolysis and blood loss.

When partial heparinization is utilized during thrombolysis, varying strategies are utilized. Unfractionated heparin can be administered based on weight (i.e., 10 U/kg/h) or titrated to achieve specific anti-Xa levels or PTT in the low therapeutic range (60–80 s[1]). At cessation of thrombolysis, heparin infusion is increased (to 20 U/kg/h) and titrated to achieve a PTT range of 80–100 s (Footnote 1) as quickly as possible to reduce the risk of rethrombosis. At the discretion of the hematology service, patients may initially be transitioned from unfractionated heparin to LMWH and finally to warfarin for 3–6 months.

Patients with lower extremity venous thrombosis are advised to wear a below the knee, low to medium compression garment for life [65].

[1] Note that there is variation in PTT values between institutions. Correlate recommendations with target values for your institution.

Follow-Up

Patients undergo hematological follow-up at 1 month post procedure and annually thereafter for PTS assessments. Thrombophilia testing is performed as discussed in the Preprocedure Work-up section above.

At the discretion of the hematology team interval imaging, either MRV or US may be performed to confirm patency and thereafter as clinically indicated. Ultrasound is limited in the iliac/IVC region due to reduced visualization.

In addition, clinic visits is recommended after anticoagulation cessation may also occur for screening of PTS development. Such visits usually occur at 12–18-month intervals.

Arterial Thrombosis

General/Background Information

Arterial thrombosis is encountered less commonly in the pediatric population than venous thrombosis and is often related to catheterization [66]. Other causes include sepsis, cardiac disease, underlying coagulation abnormality, and transplant-related issues [29, 67–70]. Table 15.4 outlines arterial thrombosis in children. Common causes in neonates include dehydration, maternal diabetes, sepsis, cardiac disease, or placental embolism.

Prompt diagnosis and administration of treatment is essential to minimize risk of limb or organ loss.

Table 15.4 Etiology of arterial thrombosis

Commonly described causes of arterial thrombosis in children:
1. Catheterization
(a) Angiography
(b) Umbilical artery catheters
(c) Peripheral arterial catheters
2. Congenital heart disease
(a) Postsurgical—heart valves, Blalock-Taussig shunt, post Fontan or other shunt procedure, PDA ligation
(b) Underlying disease—PDA, VSD, cardiomyopathy
3. Infection
(a) Haemophilus influenza meningitis
(b) Pneumonia
(c) Infective endocarditis
(d) Sepsis
4. Transplant
(a) Liver
(b) Renal
5. Trauma
6. Vascular
(a) Takayasu's arteritis
(b) Kawasaki disease
(c) Behçet's disease
(d) Polyarteritis nodosa
7. Congenital disorders
(a) Thrombophilia
(b) Hyperlipidemia
(c) Hyperhomocysteinemia
8. Heparin-induced thrombocytopenia

Indications/Contraindications

Surgery is the treatment of choice for a limb at imminent risk. Interventional techniques are used when the limb is marginally threatened, patient vessels are too small for surgical intervention, or there is a need to treat thrombosis at a capillary/tissue level (Figs. 15.7 and 15.8). SIR guidelines for treatment of lower limb ischemia in adults recommend interventional treatment for category IIa and surgery for IIb ischemia as defined in Table 15.5 [24].

Noninvasive treatment methods should also be considered. Anticoagulation remains a good first-line treatment when limbs are not at imminent risk. Heparin has been found to effectively treat arterial thrombosis in approximately 71 % of patients following cardiac catheterization [71]. Hyperbaric oxygen therapy has been reported to successfully treat posttransplant hepatic arterial thrombosis in pediatric patients [72]. In neonates, in whom a spastic vascular component post catheter insertion may also play a role in acute arterial obstruction, the topical application of a vasodilator may be beneficial (i.e., topical nitroglycerin 2 % ointment) [73].

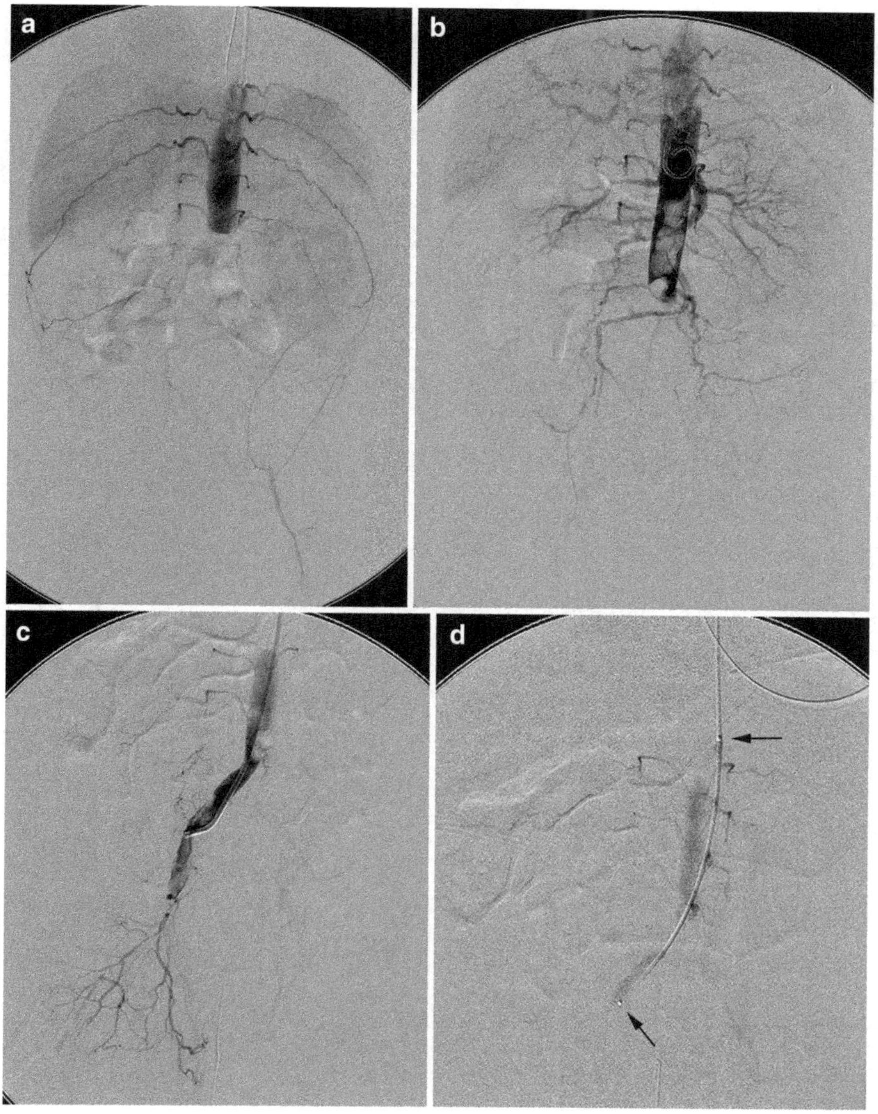

Fig. 15.7 Three-day-old infant of diabetic mother with life-threatening aortic thrombosis. The patient was too ill to undergo surgical thrombectomy so thrombolysis was undertaken. (**a**) Aortogram (via brachial artery) shows complete obstruction of aorta. Note poor celiac flow, absent superior mesenteric flow, and reconstitution of left common femoral artery. (**b**) TPA boluses and manual aspiration resulted in fragmentation of aortic thrombus and improved renal and mesenteric flow. (**c**) With further aspiration and dissolution, the right common iliac artery was accessed. (**d**) Radiopaque markers (*arrows*) delineate the area of TPA infusion on a thrombolysis catheter. The neonate died secondary to complications of intestinal ischemia

Preprocedure Work-Up

The preprocedure work-up takes place as outlined in the section above. Careful attention should be paid to the neurologic and perfusion status of affected limbs—a change in status may necessitate a change in treatment approach. Compartment syndrome can result from muscular reperfusion. Orthopedic surgery should be consulted when arterial thrombolysis is performed.

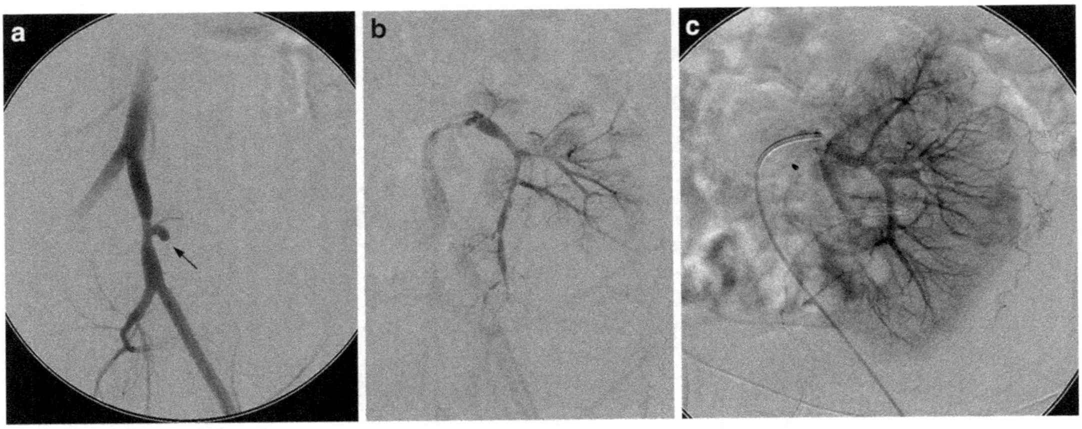

Fig. 15.8 (**a**) RAO view shows complete occlusion of (transplant) renal artery (*arrow*). (**b**) After three TPA boluses, flow to major arteries has been reestablished. Note the lack of perfusion secondary to small vessel thrombosis. (**c**) Parenchymal perfusion improved dramatically after TPA infusion

Table 15.5 Clinical categories of clinical limb ischemia

			Findings		Doppler	
Category	Description	Prognosis	Sensory loss	Motor deficit	Arterial	Venous
I	Viable	No immediate threat	None	None	Audible	Audible
II	Threatened					
IIa	Marginal	Salvageable if promptly treated	Minimal (toe) or none	None	Inaudible	Audible
IIb	Immediate	Salvageable if immediately revascularized	More that toes, rest pain	Mild/moderate	Inaudible	Audible
III	Irreversible	Major tissue loss or permanent nerve damage inevitable	Profound, anesthetic	Profound, paralysis (rigor)	Inaudible	Inaudible

Reprinted with permission from Rutherford RB, Baker JD, Ernst C, Johnston KW, Recommended standards for reports dealing with lower extremity ischemia: revised version. Porter JM, Ahn S, Jones DN., J Vasc Surg. 1997 Sep; 26(3):517–38 [78]

Equipment

Equipment for arterial thrombectomy and thrombolysis is described in the section above.

Compared with DVT, arterial therapy is generally performed in smaller vessels and will require the use of smaller, repurposed equipment. For example, thrombectomy catheters designed for use in coronary arteries (through a 4 Fr sheath) can be used to perform thrombectomy in small peripheral vessels, or 0.035″ infusion wires can be used in the place of larger (3–5 Fr) infusion catheters. Microcatheters have been used to perform catheter-directed thrombolysis of hand vessels in a neonate [74].

Procedure Technique

The basic approach to treatment is outlined in the section above. While thrombectomy is commonly performed, patients will often require thrombolysis for complete resolution. Again, the level of anticoagulation during intervention is controversial. Frequent (q 4–24 h) imaging follow-up is performed until resolution of thrombosis or no further benefit is felt to be possible.

As there are no valves, arterial access can be obtained using an antegrade or retrograde approach based on patient size and anatomy or area to be treated and available equipment. For example, a teenager with thrombosis of the dorsalis pedis artery may require antegrade puncture of his ipsilateral femoral artery in order for an infusion catheter to reach the treatment area. The same lesion in a toddler could also be approached through a retrograde puncture of the contralateral femoral artery.

The rate of thrombolytic infusion for arterial thrombosis is much lower, and the concentration is much higher than that used in DVT treatment (see Table 15.2 for dose and rate information). Arterial flow, especially in the presence of capillary/tissue level thrombosis can be quite slow (Fig. 15.8).

Postprocedure Care

Careful sensory and motor function assessment and monitoring of pulses is performed frequently while undergoing active treatment in the intensive care unit.

Full anticoagulation should be instituted as quickly as possible after completion of the intervention. Change to a long-acting anticoagulant and platelet inhibitor is instituted in conjunction with the thrombosis service.

As pediatric arteries are prone to spasm, concurrent administration of a vasodilator (such as a calcium channel blocker) can be considered [75–77]. The patient should also be monitored for signs of compartment syndrome that can occur with arterial reperfusion.

Follow-Up

Patients undergo hematological follow-up at 2 weeks post procedure and annually thereafter for screening for peripheral arterial insufficiency assessment. Thrombophilia testing is performed as discussed in the Preprocedure Work-up section above.

Chapter Summary

Thrombosis Overview

Background

- Increasing incidence
- Significant morbidity/mortality
- Anticoagulation, systemic or local thrombolysis, and surgical or percutaneous thrombectomy possible
- Very limited pediatric literature

Pediatric Coagulation

- Developmental hemostasis can impact treatment approach
- Efficacy of thrombosis intervention decreases after 2 weeks

Indications/Contraindications

- See Tables 15.1 and 15.3

Preprocedure Work-Up

- Imaging
  - Review pertinent imaging
  - Obtain head MRI if there is possible CNS abnormality before thrombolysis
- Bloodwork
  - CBC, INR, PTT, fibrinogen, D-dimers, blood group and hold
  - BUN, creatinine
  - Thrombophilia testing
    - 4–6 weeks after anticoagulation (for most)
    - >12–18 months of age
- History/physical
  - Risk factors (Table 15.2)
  - Leg circumference (DVT), neurologic assessment, perfusion, pulses
- Multidisciplinary discussion
  - Thrombosis, intensive care, vascular/plastic/orthopedic surgery

Equipment/Drugs

- Drugs
  - See Table 15.2 for commonly used drugs
- Blood products
  - RBC, FFP, or cryoprecipitate for specific derangements

   - Consider plasminogen administration (FFP) to facilitate thrombolysis
- Thrombolysis equipment
   - Catheters—3–5 Fr end-hole, multiple side-hole infusion catheters
   - Wires—infusion wires available
   - Specialized—ultrasound-enhanced catheter
- Thrombectomy equipment
   - Balloons (Fogarty, venoplasty balloons)
   - Catheters—large bore
   - Specialized devices—(e.g., AngioJet, Trellis, etc.)

Procedure Technique

1. Patient preparation
   (a) Consent
   (b) Consider double-maintenance fluid and bladder catheterization if there is chance of hemoglobinuria
   (c) Arterial/IV access
   (d) Sedate vs. GA
2. Filter insertion
   (a) Controversial in DVT treatment
   (b) See Chap. 11
3. Vascular access
   (a) Antegrade preferred for DVT
   (b) Vascular sheath (3–9 Fr)
4. Define thrombus
   (a) DSA—thrombus extent, collaterals
5. Initial lytic administration
   (a) Lacing, pulse spray, power-pulse spray
   (b) Allow 15–30 min between multiple doses
6. Thrombectomy
   (a) Keep small pediatric blood volume in mind
   (b) Monitor for bradycardia
7. Thrombolysis
   (a) Infusion catheter/wire based on anatomy and extent of clot
   (b) ICU admission
   (c) Concomitant heparinization controversial
8. Ongoing evaluation
   (a) DSA q 4–24 h to monitor progress
   (b) Blood: CBC, coagulation parameters q 4–6 h
9. Dilatation/stent placement
   (a) Treat underlying hemodynamically significant lesions
   (b) Dilatation preferred over stenting in pediatric patients

Postprocedure Care

- High rate of early rethrombosis
   - Reestablish therapeutic anticoagulation
   - Imaging to monitor outcome
- Monitor for renal issues if hemolysis possible
- Appropriate long-term IR follow-up not established

Venous Thrombosis

Procedure

- Thrombolysis
   - 3–5 Fr catheters placed through thrombus
   - 4–10 mg TPA bolus over 10 min
- Thrombectomy
   - Clear distal thrombus initially leaving central "cap" with rheolytic devices (decrease bradycardia)
- Venoplasty
   - Often required in May-Thurner and Paget-Schroetter
   - Stenting may be required in May-Thurner but contraindicated in Paget-Schroetter

Postprocedure Care

- Below knee, low to medium compression garment
- Thrombosis follow-up at 1 month
- MRV/US to assess ongoing patency

Arterial Thrombosis

Background

- Usually iatrogenic
- Consider noninvasive methods of treatment
- Intervention undertaken when limb at risk (not imminently) or surgery not possible

Procedure

- Antegrade or retrograde access
- Thrombectomy used but thrombolysis often required
- Slower infusion rates (0.5–2 mL/h) compared to DVT treatment (50–100 mL/h in adults)
- Consider vasodilator if spasm is present
- Follow pulses, neurologic assessment
- Monitor for compartment syndrome

References

1. Andrew M, David M, Adams M, Ali K, Anderson R, Barnard D, et al. Venous thromboembolic complications (VTE) in children: first analyses of the Canadian Registry of VTE. Blood. 1994;83(5):1251–7. PubMed PMID: 8118029. Epub 1994/03/01.eng.
2. Raffini L, Huang YS, Witmer C, Feudtner C. Dramatic increase in venous thromboembolism in children's hospitals in the United States from 2001 to 2007. Pediatrics. 2009;124(4):1001–8. PubMed PMID: 19736261. Epub 2009/09/09.eng.
3. Wang M, Hays T, Balasa V, Bagatell R, Gruppo R, Grabowski EF, et al. Low-dose tissue plasminogen activator thrombolysis in children. J Pediatr Hematol Oncol. 2003;25(5):379–86. PubMed PMID: 12759624. Epub 2003/05/22.eng.
4. Monagle P, Adams M, Mahoney M, Ali K, Barnard D, Bernstein M, et al. Outcome of pediatric thromboembolic disease: a report from the Canadian Childhood Thrombophilia Registry. Pediatr Res. 2000;47(6):763–6. PubMed PMID: 10832734. Epub 2000/06/01.eng.
5. Albisetti M. Thrombolytic therapy in children. Thromb Res. 2006;118(1):95–105. PubMed PMID: 16709478. Epub 2006/05/20.eng.
6. Gupta AA, Leaker M, Andrew M, Massicotte P, Liu L, Benson LN, et al. Safety and outcomes of thrombolysis with tissue plasminogen activator for treatment of intravascular thrombosis in children. J Pediatr. 2001;139(5):682–8. PubMed PMID: 11713447. Epub 2001/11/20.eng.
7. Goldenberg NA. Long-term outcomes of venous thrombosis in children. Curr Opin Hematol. 2005; 12(5):370–6. PubMed PMID: 16093782. Epub 2005/08/12.eng.
8. Hausler M, Hubner D, Delhaas T, Muhler EG. Long term complications of inferior vena cava thrombosis. Arch Dis Child. 2001;85(3):228–33. PubMed PMID: 11517106. Pubmed Central PMCID: 1718896. Epub 2001/08/23.eng.
9. Goldenberg NA, Donadini MP, Kahn SR, Crowther M, Kenet G, Nowak-Gottl U, et al. Post-thrombotic syndrome in children: a systematic review of frequency of occurrence, validity of outcome measures, and prognostic factors. Haematologica. 2010; 95(11):1952–9. PubMed PMID: 20595095. Pubmed Central PMCID: 2966919. Epub 2010/07/03.eng.
10. Taylor LM Jr, Troutman R, Feliciano P, Menashe V, Sunderland C, Porter JM. Late complications after femoral artery catheterization in children less than five years of age. J Vasc Surg. 1990;11(2):297–304; discussion 304–6. PubMed PMID: 2405199. Epub 1990/02/01.eng.
11. Goldenberg NA, Durham JD, Knapp-Clevenger R, Manco-Johnson MJ. A thrombolytic regimen for high-risk deep venous thrombosis may substantially reduce the risk of postthrombotic syndrome in children. Blood. 2007;110(1):45–53. PubMed PMID: 17360940. Pubmed Central PMCID: 1896126. Epub 2007/03/16.eng.
12. Goldenberg NA, Knapp-Clevenger R, Manco-Johnson MJ. Elevated plasma factor VIII and D-dimer levels as predictors of poor outcomes of thrombosis in children. N Engl J Med. 2004;351(11):1081–8.
13. Kim HS, Patra A, Paxton BE, Khan J, Streiff MB. Adjunctive percutaneous mechanical thrombectomy for lower-extremity deep vein thrombosis: clinical and economic outcomes. J Vasc Interv Radiol. 2006; 17(7):1099–104.
14. Lin PH, Zhou W, Dardik A, Mussa F, Kougias P, Hedayati N, et al. Catheter-direct thrombolysis versus pharmacomechanical thrombectomy for treatment of symptomatic lower extremity deep venous thrombosis. Am J Surg. 2006;192:782–8.
15. Karthikesalingam A, Young EL, Hinchliffe RJ, Loftus IM, Thompson MM, Holt PJ. A systematic review of percutaneous mechanical thrombectomy in the treatment of deep venous thrombosis. Eur J Vasc Endovasc Surg. 2011;41:554–65.
16. Parmar N, Albisetti M, Berry LR, Chan AK. The fibrinolytic system in newborns and children. Clin Lab. 2006;52(3–4):115–24. PubMed PMID: 16584057. Epub 2006/04/06.eng.
17. Andrew M, Paes B, Milner R, Johnston M, Mitchell L, Tollefsen DM, et al. Development of the human coagulation system in the full-term infant. Blood. 1987;70(1):165–72. PubMed PMID: 3593964. Epub 1987/07/01.eng.
18. Ries M. Molecular and functional properties of fetal plasminogen and its possible influence on clot lysis in the neonatal period. Semin Thromb Hemost. 1997;23(3):247–52. PubMed PMID: 9255905. Epub 1997/01/01.eng.
19. Andrew M, Brooker L, Leaker M, Paes B, Weitz J. Fibrin clot lysis by thrombolytic agents is impaired in newborns due to a low plasminogen concentration. Thromb Hemost. 1992;68(3):325–30. PubMed PMID: 1440499. Epub 1992/09/07.eng.
20. Grabowski EF. Thrombolysis, flow, and vessel wall interactions. J Vasc Interv Radiol. 1995;6(6 Pt 2 Suppl):25S–9. PubMed PMID: 8770839. Epub 1995/11/01.eng.
21. Mewissen MW, Seabrook GR, Meissner MH, Cynamon J, Labropoulos N, Haughton SH. Catheter-directed thrombolysis for lower extremity deep venous thrombosis: report of a national multicenter registry. Radiology. 1999;211(1):39–49. PubMed PMID: 10189452. Epub 1999/04/06.eng.
22. O'Sullivan GJ. The role of interventional radiology in the management of deep venous thrombosis: advanced therapy. Cardiovasc Intervent Radiol. 2011; 34(3):445–61. PubMed PMID: 20927522. Epub 2010/10/12.eng.
23. Monagle P, Chan AK, Goldenberg NA, Ichord RN, Journeycake JM, Nowak-Gottl U, et al. Antithrombotic therapy in neonates and children: Antithrombotic Therapy and Prevention of Thrombosis, 9th ed: American College of Chest Physicians Evidence-Based Clinical Practice Guidelines. Chest. 2012;141

(2 Suppl):e737S–801. PubMed PMID: 22315277. Pubmed Central PMCID: 3278066. Epub 2012/02/15.eng.
24. Patel NH, Krishnamurthy VN, Kim S, Saad WE, Ganguli S, Walker TG, et al. Quality improvement guidelines for percutaneous management of acute lower-extremity ischemia. J Vasc Interv Radiol. 2013;24(1):3–15. PubMed PMID: 23273693. Epub 2013/01/01.eng.
25. Vedantham S, Thorpe PE, Cardella JF, Grassi CJ, Patel NH, Ferral H, et al. Quality improvement guidelines for the treatment of lower extremity deep vein thrombosis with use of endovascular thrombus removal. J Vasc Interv Radiol. 2009;20:S227–39.
26. Kenet G, Nowak-Gottl U. Hemostasis and thrombosis in pediatric patients: special issues and unique concerns. Semin Thromb Hemost. 2011;37(7):721–2. PubMed PMID: 22187393. Epub 2011/12/22.eng.
27. Young G, Albisetti M, Bonduel M, Brandao L, Chan A, Friedrichs F, et al. Impact of inherited thrombophilia on venous thromboembolism in children: a systematic review and meta-analysis of observational studies. Circulation. 2008;118(13):1373–82. PubMed PMID: 18779442. Epub 2008/09/10.eng.
28. Raffini L. Thrombophilia in children: who to test, how, when, and why? Hematology Am Soc Hematol Educ Program. 2008:228–35. doi: 10.1182/asheducation-2008.1.228. PubMed PMID: 19074088. Epub 2008/12/17.Eng.
29. Price VE, Chan AK. Arterial thrombosis in children. Expert Rev Cardiovasc Ther. 2008;6(3):419–28. PubMed PMID: 18328000. Epub 2008/03/11.eng.
30. Semba CP, Murphy TP, Bakal CW, Calis KA, Matalon TA. Thrombolytic therapy with use of alteplase (rt-PA) in peripheral arterial occlusive disease: review of the clinical literature. The Advisory Panel. J Vasc Interv Radiol. 2000;11(2 Pt 1):149–61. PubMed PMID: 10716384. Epub 2000/03/15.eng.
31. Israels SJ, Michelson AD. Antiplatelet therapy in children. Thromb Res. 2006;118(1):75–83. PubMed PMID: 16709476. Epub 2006/05/20.eng.
32. Hofmann LV, Razavi M, Arepally A, Reginelli JP, Resar J, Geschwind JF, et al. GPIIb-IIIa receptor inhibitors: what the interventional radiologist needs to know. Cardiovasc Intervent Radiol. 2001;24(6):361–7. PubMed PMID: 11907740. Epub 2002/03/22.eng.
33. Chang R, Horne III MK, Shawker TH, Kam AW, Chen EA, Joe GO, et al. Low-dose, once-daily, intraclot injections of alteplase for treatment of acute deep venous thrombosis. J Vasc Interv Radiol. 2011; 22:1107–16.
34. Grunwald MR, Hofmann LV. Comparison of urokinase, alteplase, and reteplase for catheter-directed thrombolysis of deep venous thrombosis. J Vasc Interv Radiol. 2004;15(4):347–52. PubMed PMID: 15064337. Epub 2004/04/06.eng.
35. Bookstein JJ, Bookstein FL. Augmented experimental pulse-spray thrombolysis with tissue plasminogen activator, enabling dose reduction by one or more orders of magnitude. J Vasc Interv Radiol. 2000; 11(3):299–303. PubMed PMID: 10735423. Epub 2000/03/29.eng.
36. Semba CP, Weck S, Patapoff T. Alteplase: stability and bioactivity after dilution in normal saline solution. J Vasc Interv Radiol. 2003;14(1):99–102. PubMed PMID: 12525593. Epub 2003/01/15.eng.
37. Yee DL, Chan AK, Williams S, Goldenberg NA, Massicotte MP, Raffini LJ. Varied opinions on thrombolysis for venous thromboembolism in infants and children: findings from a survey of pediatric hematology-oncology specialists. Pediatr Blood Cancer. 2009;53(6):960–6. PubMed PMID: 19544387. Epub 2009/06/23.eng.
38. Leary SE, Harrod VL, de Alarcon PA, Reiss UM. Low-dose systemic thrombolytic therapy for deep vein thrombosis in pediatric patients. J Pediatr Hematol Oncol. 2010;32(2):97–102. PubMed PMID: 20118811. Epub 2010/02/02.eng.
39. Giacoia GP. High-dose urokinase therapy in newborn infants with major vessel thrombosis. Clin Pediatr (Phila). 1993;32(4):231–7. PubMed PMID: 8462236. Epub 1993/04/01.eng.
40. Robinson A, Fellows KE, Bridges ND, Rome JJ. Effectiveness of pharmacomechanical thrombolysis in infants and children. Am J Cardiol. 2001;87:496–9, A8.
41. Strife JL, Ball Jr WS, Towbin R, Keller MS, Dillon T. Arterial occlusions in neonates: use of fibrinolytic therapy. Radiology. 1988;166(2):395–400. PubMed PMID: 3336714. Epub 1988/02/01.eng.
42. Manco-Johnson MJ. How I, treat venous thrombosis in children. Blood. 2006;107(1):21–9. PubMed PMID: 16099882. Pubmed Central PMCID: 1895344. Epub 2005/08/16.eng.
43. Bassareo PP, Fanos V, Iacovidou N, Mercuro G. Antiplatelet therapy in children: why so different from adults? Curr Pharm Des. 2012;18(21):3019–33. PubMed PMID: 22385057. Epub 2012/03/06.Eng.
44. Parikh S, Motarjeme A, McNamara T, Raabe R, Hagspiel K, Benenati JF, et al. Ultrasound-accelerated thrombolysis for the treatment of deep vein thrombosis: initial clinical experience. J Vasc Interv Radiol. 2008;19(4):521–8. PubMed PMID: 18375296. Epub 2008/04/01.eng.
45. Lee KH, Han H, Lee KJ, Yoon CS, Kim SH, Won JY, et al. Mechanical thrombectomy of acute iliofemoral deep vein thrombosis with use of an Arrow-Trerotola percutaneous thrombectomy device. J Vasc Interv Radiol. 2006;17(3):487–95. PubMed PMID: 16567673. Epub 2006/03/29.eng.
46. Atherton ME, Culp WC, Brown AT, Erdem E. Successful intravascular ultrasound thrombolysis of dural sinus thrombosis with pre-existing subarachnoid and intraparenchymal hemorrhages. Interv Neuroradiol. 2010;16:455–8.
47. Maxwell AD, Owens G, Gurm HS, Ives K, Myers Jr DD, Xu Z. Noninvasive treatment of deep venous thrombosis using pulsed ultrasound cavitation therapy (histotripsy) in a porcine model. J Vasc Interv Radiol. 2011;22(3):369–77.

48. Siegel RJ, Luo H. Ultrasound thrombolysis. Ultrasonics. 2008;48:312–20.
49. O'Sullivan GJ, Semba CP, Bittner CA, Kee ST, Razavi MK, Sze DY, et al. Endovascular management of iliac vein compression (May-Thurner) syndrome. J Vasc Interv Radiol. 2000;11(7):823–36. PubMed PMID: 10928517. Epub 2000/08/06.eng.
50. Razavi MK, Hansch EC, Kee ST, Sze DY, Semba CP, Dake MD. Chronically occluded inferior venae cavae: endovascular treatment. Radiology. 2000;214(1):133–8. PubMed PMID: 10644112. Epub 2000/01/22.eng.
51. Guimaraes M, Schonholz C, Hannegan C, Anderson MB, Shi J, Selby Jr B. Radiofrequency wire for the recanalization of central vein occlusions that have failed conventional endovascular techniques. J Vasc Interv Radiol. 2012;23(8):1016–21. PubMed PMID: 22739648. Epub 2012/06/29.eng.
52. Iafrati M, Maloney S, Halin N. Radiofrequency thermal wire is a useful adjunct to treat chronic central venous occlusions. J Vasc Surg. 2012;55(2):603–6. PubMed PMID: 22104339.Epub 2011/11/23.eng.
53. Sharifi M, Bay C, Skrocki L, Lawson D, Mazdeh S. Role of IVC filters in endovenous therapy for deep venous thrombosis: the FILTER-PEVI (Filter Implantation to Lower Thromboembolic Risk in Percutaneous Endovenous Intervention) Trial. Cardiovasc Intervent Radiol. 2012;35(6):1408–13. PubMed PMID: 22271078. Epub 2012/01/25.eng.
54. Chaudry G, Padua HM, Alomari AI. The use of inferior vena cava filters in young children. J Vasc Interv Radiol. 2008;19:1103–6.
55. Kandarpa K. Technical determinants of success in catheter-directed thrombolysis for peripheral arterial occlusions. J Vasc Interv Radiol. 1995;6(6 Pt 2 Suppl):55S–61. PubMed PMID: 8770843. Epub 1995/11/01.eng.
56. Dwarka D, Schwartz SA, Smyth SH, O'Brien MJ. Bradyarrhythmias during use of the AngioJet system. J Vasc Interv Radiol. 2006;17(10):1693–5. PubMed PMID: 17057013.Epub 2006/10/24.eng.
57. Kuo WT, Gould MK, Louie JD, Rosenberg JK, Sze DY, Hofmann LV. Catheter-directed therapy for the treatment of massive pulmonary embolism: systematic review and meta-analysis of modern techniques. J Vasc Interv Radiol. 2009;20(11):1431–40. PubMed PMID: 19875060. Epub 2009/10/31.eng.
58. Jaff MR, McMurtry MS, Archer SL, Cushman M, Goldenberg N, Goldhaber SZ, et al. Management of massive and submassive pulmonary embolism, iliofemoral deep vein thrombosis, and chronic thromboembolic pulmonary hypertension: a scientific statement from the American Heart Association. Circulation. 2011;123(16):1788–830. PubMed PMID: 21422387. Epub 2011/03/23.eng.
59. Goldenberg NA, Branchford B, Wang M, Ray Jr C, Durham JD, Manco-Johnson MJ. Percutaneous mechanical and pharmacomechanical thrombolysis for occlusive deep vein thrombosis of the proximal limb in adolescent subjects: findings from an institution-based prospective inception cohort study of pediatric venous thromboembolism. J Vasc Interv Radiol. 2011;22(2):121–32. PubMed PMID: 21216157. Pubmed Central PMCID: 3058325. Epub 2011/01/11.eng.
60. Monagle P, Chalmers E, Chan A, DeVeber G, Kirkham F, Massicotte P, et al. Antithrombotic therapy in neonates and children: American College of Chest Physicians Evidence-Based Clinical Practice Guidelines (8th Edition). Chest. 2008;133(6 Suppl): 887S–968. PubMed PMID: 18574281.Epub 2008/07/24.eng.
61. O'Sullivan GJ, Lohan DG, Gough N, Cronin CG, Kee ST. Pharmacomechanical thrombectomy of acute deep vein thrombosis with the Trellis-8 isolated thrombolysis catheter. J Vasc Interv Radiol. 2007;18(6):715–24. PubMed PMID: 17538133. Epub 2007/06/01.eng.
62. Thompson JF, Winterborn RJ, Bays S, White H, Kinsella DC, Watkinson AF. Venous thoracic outlet compression and the Paget-Schroetter syndrome: a review and recommendations for management. Cardiovasc Intervent Radiol. 2011;34(5):903–10. PubMed PMID: 21448772. Epub 2011/03/31.eng.
63. Raffini L, Raybagkar D, Cahill AM, Kaye R, Blumenstein M, Manno C. May-Thurner syndrome (iliac vein compression) and thrombosis in adolescents. Pediatr Blood Cancer. 2006;47(6):834–8. PubMed PMID: 16365865. Epub 2005/12/21.eng.
64. Molina JE, Hunter DW, Dietz CA. Protocols for Paget-Schroetter syndrome and late treatment of chronic subclavian vein obstruction. Ann Thorac Surg. 2009;87(2):416–22. PubMed PMID: 19161749. Epub 2009/01/24.eng.
65. Biss TT, Kahr WH, Brandao LR, Chan AK, Thomas KE, Williams S. The use of elastic compression stockings for post-thrombotic syndrome in a child. Pediatr Blood Cancer. 2009;53(3):462–3. PubMed PMID: 19459199. Epub 2009/05/22.eng.
66. Monagle P, Newall F, Barnes C, Savoia H, Campbell J, Wallace T, et al. Arterial thromboembolic disease: a single-centre case series study. J Paediatr Child Health. 2008;44(1–2):28–32. PubMed PMID: 17803664. Epub 2007/09/07.eng.
67. Balci YI, Unal S, Gumruk F, Cetin M, Ozkutlu S, Gurgey A. Nonstroke arterial thrombosis in children: Hacettepe experience. Blood Coagul Fibrinolysis. 2008;19:519–24.
68. Coombs CJ, Richardson PW, Dowling GJ, Johnstone BR, Monagle P. Brachial artery thrombosis in infants: an algorithm for limb salvage. Plast Reconstr Surg. 2006;117:1481–8.
69. Price V, Massicotte MP. Arterial thromboembolism in the pediatric population. Semin Thromb Hemost. 2003;29(6):557–65. PubMed PMID: 14719172. Epub 2004/01/14.eng.
70. Streif W, Monagle P, South M, Leaker M, Andrew M. Spontaneous arterial thrombosis in children. J Pediatr. 1999;134:110–2.
71. Ino T, Benson LN, Freedom RM, Barker GA, Aipursky A, Rowe RD. Thrombolytic therapy for

femoral artery thrombosis after pediatric cardiac catheterization. Am Heart J. 1988;115:633–9.
72. Grover I, Conley L, Alzate G, Lavine J, Van Hoesen K, Khanna A. Hyperbaric oxygen therapy for hepatic artery thrombosis following liver transplantation: current concepts. Pediatr Transplant. 2006;10(2):234–9. PubMed PMID: 16573613. Epub 2006/04/01.eng.
73. Baserga MC, Puri A, Sola A. The use of topical nitroglycerin ointment to treat peripheral tissue ischemia secondary to arterial line complications in neonates. J Perinatol. 2002;22(5):416–9. PubMed PMID: 12082481. Epub 2002/06/26.eng.
74. Theile RJ, Coombs CJ. Microvascular and thrombolytic revascularization of an arm in a 32-week-gestation neonate: case report and review of the literature. J Reconstr Microsurg. 1996;12(8): 539–42. PubMed PMID: 8951122. Epub 1996/11/01.eng.
75. Neff KW, Dinter D, Schaible T, Lehmann KJ, Duber C. Intraarterial subclavian artery thrombolysis in a neonate. AJR Am J Roentgenol. 2001;177(2):446–8. PubMed PMID: 11461880. Epub 2001/07/20.eng.
76. Temple M, Williams S, John P, Chait P, Connolly B. Percutaneous treatment of pediatric thrombosis. Eur J Radiol. 2005;53:14–21.
77. Watkins S, Yunge M, Jones D, Kiely E, Petros AJ. Prolonged use of tissue plasminogen activator for bilateral lower limb arterial occlusion in a neonate. J Pediatr Surg. 2001;36:654–6.
78. Rutherford RB, Baker JD, Ernst C, Johnston KW, Porter JM, Ahn S, Jones DN. Recommended standards for reports dealing with lower extremity ischemia: revised version. J Vasc Surg. 1997;26(3):517–38.

16 Vascular Interventions: Lymphangiography and Thoracic Duct Embolization

Michael Temple and Ganesh Krishnamurthy

Introduction

The lymphatic system plays an essential role in fluid transport within the body. To support cellular respiration, the circulatory system transports oxygen, carbon dioxide, nutrients, and waste products to and from cells throughout the body. This delivery is facilitated by exchange of fluid (plasma) and solutes across capillary membranes (secondary to the Starling forces of hydrostatic and osmotic pressure). The process is not 100 % efficient and results in a small net outflow of fluid from the capillaries into the tissues. In adults, the extracellular lymphatic fluid volume is approximately 12 L [1], and the thoracic duct carries around 2.5 L of this excess fluid from the tissues back into the venous system daily [2]. Secondary lymphatic system functions include fat transport from the small intestines and presentation of antigens to immune cells within lymph nodes.

In the 1950s, radiologists developed diagnostic lymphangiography to investigate primary and secondary cancers and suspected lymphatic abnormalities. The procedure was technically challenging and time-consuming, requiring isolation and puncture of a lymphatic duct on the dorsum of the foot. Following development of cross-sectional imaging (CT and MRI), lymphangiography fell out of favor.

Recently, however, there has been a resurgence in the use of lymphangiography related to development of percutaneous embolization methods to treat lymphatic leaks and technical simplification of the procedure. Constantin Cope pioneered thoracic duct and lymphatic vessel interventions [3–6] that have now been reported in pediatric patients [7]. The development of intranodal contrast administration has greatly simplified the procedure [8, 9].

Lymphatic leaks can be either congenital or acquired. The congenital or the idiopathic leak can be divided further into two major categories: (1) occlusion of the upper part of the thoracic duct with development of compensatory collaterals and (2) chylous leak in the presence of a lymphatic malformation. The hypothesis for thoracic duct occlusion is subclinical trauma, which leads to the development of multiple lymphatic collaterals. If one of these collaterals abuts a serous surface (pleural, pericardial, or peritoneal), it can rupture and then result in chylous leak.

Acquired causes are related to either direct or surgical trauma, tumor, and radiation therapy. Lymphatic leaks in the pediatric age group are most often related to surgical intervention.

M. Temple, M.D., F.R.C.P.(C.)
Hospital for Sick Children, University of Toronto, Toronto, ON, Canada M5G 1X8
e-mail: michael.temple@sickkids.ca

G. Krishnamurthy, M.D., D.N.B. (✉)
The Children's Hospital of Philadelphia, 34th Street and Civic Center Boulevard, Philadelphia, PA 19104, USA
e-mail: krishnamurthy@email.chop.edu

M. Temple and F.E. Marshalleck (eds.), *Pediatric Interventional Radiology: Handbook of Vascular and Non-Vascular Interventions*, DOI 10.1007/978-1-4419-5856-3_16,

The loss of large volumes of lymphatic fluid leads to loss of proteins and lymphatic cells that can eventually lead to death [6, 10]. Conventional treatments including dietary fat restriction and octreotide administration are not always successful [11]. Identification of the exact location of the duct during surgical thoracic duct ligation can be quite difficult and limits the success of the technique [10]. Another limitation of surgical intervention is the inability to accurately identify the site of lymphatic leak. Ligating the duct above the leak or causing redistribution or increasing lymphatic collaterals can worsen symptoms. Thoracic duct embolization represents a minimally invasive, accurate, and effective treatment method.

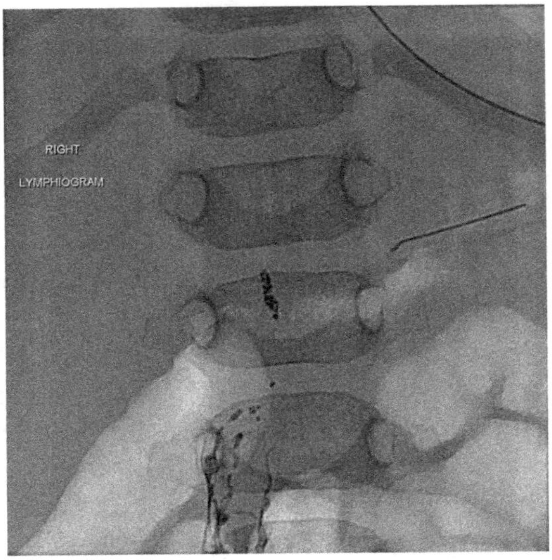

Fig. 16.1 Cisterna chyli. A linear collection of oily contrast drops opacifies the cisterna chyli overlying the L2 vertebral body

Anatomy

The lymphatic vessels form a unidirectional fluid transport system. Valves located in the ducts function to provide antegrade lymphatic flow. Endothelial microvalves are also theorized to exist [12].

Lymphatic capillaries are diffusely distributed in tissues throughout the body. They coalesce to form larger lymphatic channels that include lymph nodes distributed along the pathways. Fluid from the lower extremities is carried through the iliac and lumbar lymphatics. These networks meet with lymphatic channels from the liver and intestines and form a lakelike cavity, the cisterna chyli that drains through the thoracic duct. The thoracic duct enters the venous system usually at the junction between the left jugular and subclavian veins. Lymph from the left arm, chest, and face joins the thoracic duct. The right arm, face, and chest drain through the smaller right lymphatic duct.

The cisterna chyli is variable in shape with ovoid or triangular configurations being the most commonly encountered. It often lies anterior to the L1–L2 vertebral bodies, to the right of the aorta and posterior to the right crus of the diaphragm (Fig. 16.1).

Small lymphatic-venous connections are normally present but are not visualized unless an obstruction is present (Fig. 16.2) [13–15].

Indications/Contraindications

Lymphangiography is performed for both diagnostic and interventional purposes. The most common indication for intervention is chylothorax following cardiac surgery that is not

Fig. 16.2 Lymphatic disruption to treat congenital chyloperitoneum. (**a**) Ultrasound (US) shows large-volume fluid collection. Fetal urinary drain placed to decompress chyloperitoneum in utero became displaced into the abdomen (*white arrow*). (**b**) US used to insert a 22-G Angiocath into the groin lymph node. (**c**) FLASH and (**d**) MIP MR images showing dilated lumbar collaterals (*yellow arrowheads*) perirenal lymphatic leak (*yellow arrow*) and opacification of the azygous vein through lymphovenous channels (*white arrowheads*). (**e**) Delayed FLASH image shows accumulation of peritoneal contrast and "staining" of the perilymphatic tissues. (**f**) Fluoroscopic freeze frame image showing location of leaking lymphatic vessel. Note "chaser" technique used to access pelvic node. (**g**) AP and (**h**) lateral images show 22-G needles used to disrupt the leaking duct. (**i**) Chest radiography performed 48 h after lymphangiogram shows passage of Lipiodol to jugular lymph nodes (*black arrow*). (**j**) US image 4 months after procedure shows near complete resolution of ascites

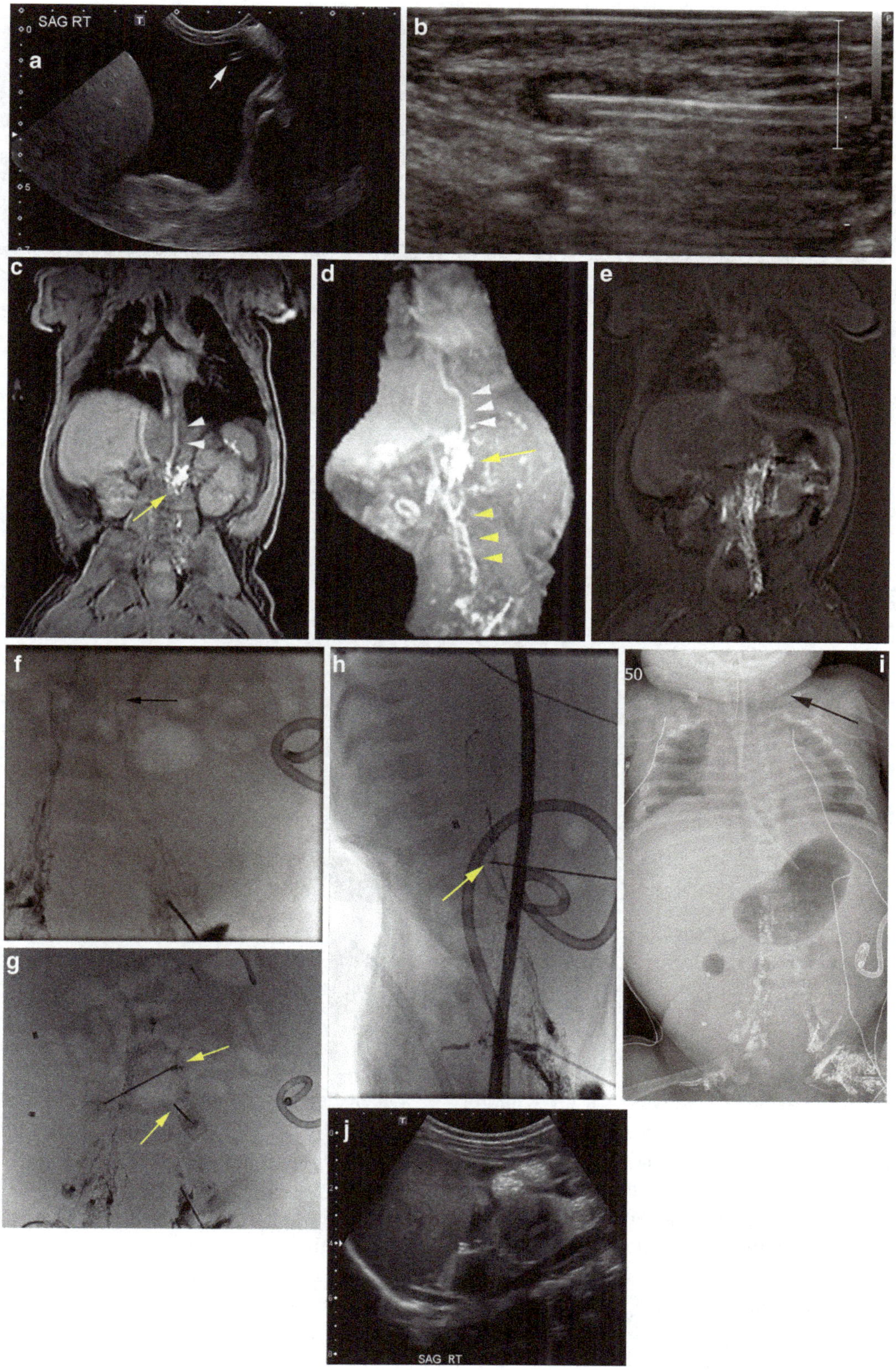

Fig. 16.2 (continued)

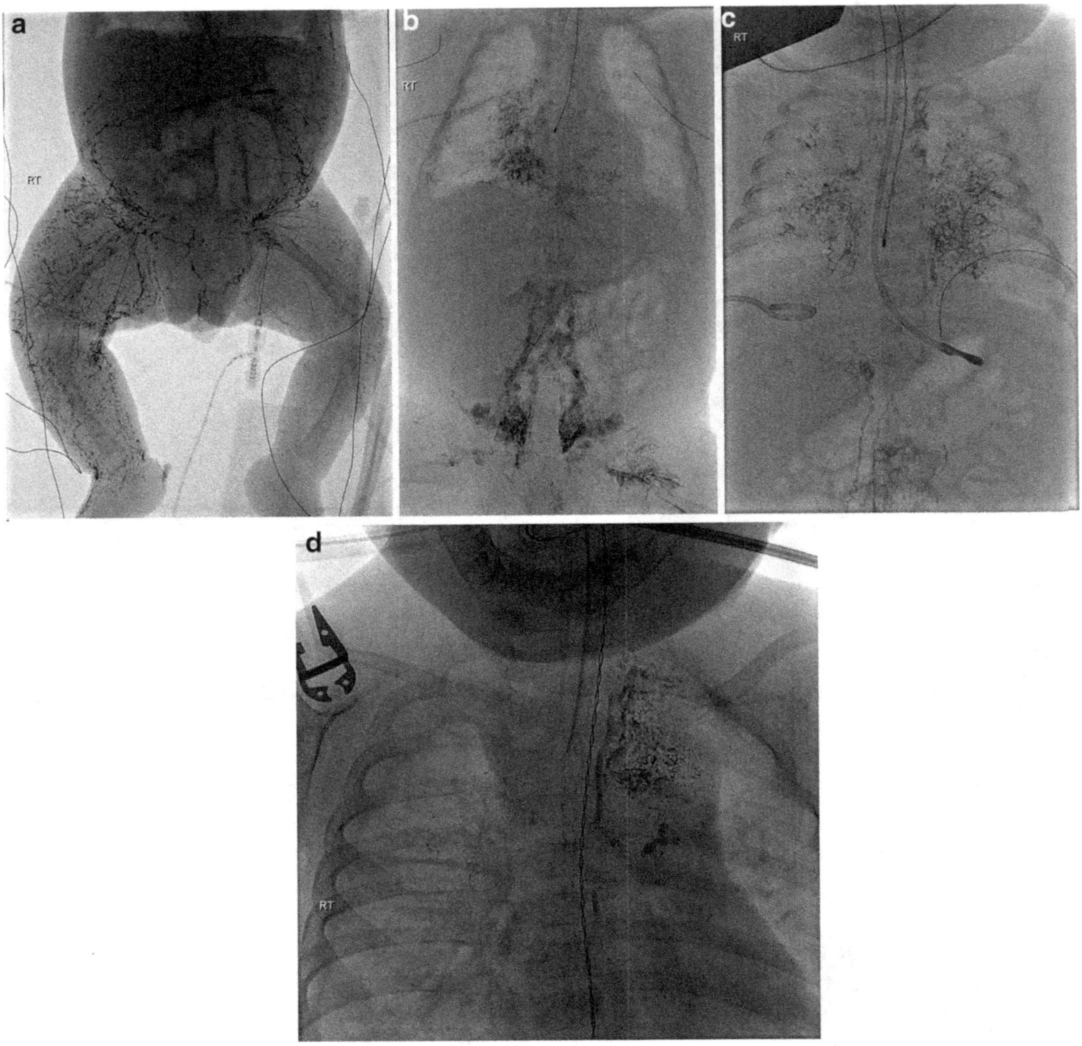

Fig. 16.3 Lymphatic ectasia. (**a**, **b**) Lipiodol injection demonstrates abnormal lymphatic flow down the legs and around the abdominal wall in patient with severe lymphatic ectasia and absence of central lymphatic ducts. (**c**) Congenital lymphatic ectasia with abnormal retroperitoneal and bronchial lymph channels. (**d**) Congenital ectasia with peribronchial channels that were the cause of chylothorax

controlled by conservative measures and/or after failed surgical thoracic duct ligation. There are many diagnostic indications including characterization of lymphatic abnormalities or determination of the location of thoracic, abdominal, or pelvic lymphatic leaks (Figs. 16.2c–f, 16.3, and 16.4a). There are numerous reports of cessation of lymphatic drainage following diagnostic lymphangiography with oil-based contrast [16–18].

Other than uncorrectable coagulopathy, there are no specific contraindications to performing lymphangiography. However, use of oily contrast is absolutely contraindicated in patients with an active right-to-left cardiac shunt due to the risk of arterial embolization. Water-soluble contrast should be used in any patient with an intracardiac shunt. However, in unusual cases, oil-based contrast could be considered in patients who have only a potential shunt (e.g., patent foramen ovale

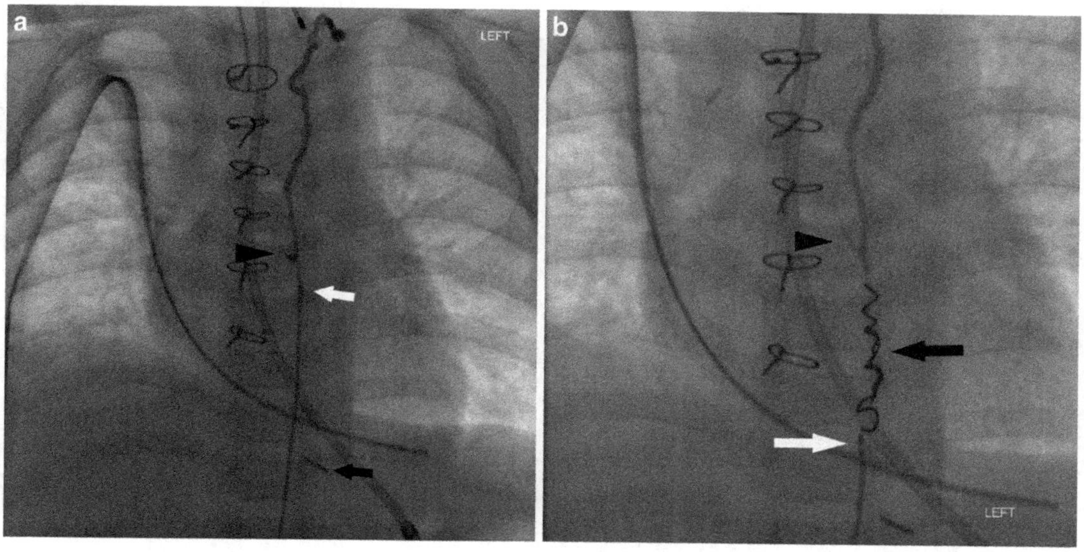

Fig. 16.4 Thoracic duct embolization with coil. (**a**) The thoracic duct was opacified using a microcatheter (*white arrow*) delineating a pericardial lymphatic leak (*black arrowhead*). Note the site of previously attempted surgical ligation (*black arrow*). (**b**) A coil was deployed in the thoracic duct (*black arrow*)

with no active shunting detected), but the possibility of arterial embolization must be discussed with the patient. Oil-based contrast can cause pneumonitis [19, 20] so caution must be exercised in patients with limited respiratory reserve. Patients with impaired renal function are not candidates for MR lymphangiogram study with gadolinium injection.

Equipment

- For intranodal injection in the groin:
  - 25-G-long needle, short connecting tube, 5 mL syringe
- For pedal access:
  - Surgical microscope/magnifying surgical loupes, methylene blue, local anesthetic, scalpel, and surgical dissection equipment
  - 30-G Cook Lymphangiography needle (Cook Medical, Bloomington, USA)
  - Local anesthetic
- Contrast media:
  - Gadolinium (diluted 1:1–1:2 with normal saline [21][1])
  - Oil-based contrast (Lipiodol, EZ EM, Montréal, Canada)
  - Water-soluble contrast with high iodine content (Omnipaque 350, GE Healthcare, Fairfield, USA)—used if right-to-left shunts are present
- For embolization:
  - 22-G-long Chiba needle (tip is bent slightly for easy maneuverability)
  - Sturdy wire with floppy tip (0.018″ V-18 ControlWire guidewire, Boston Scientific, Natick, USA)
  - High-flow 2.3F short-length microcatheter—(65 cm 2.3F Rapid Transit, Boston Scientific, Natick, USA)
  - Various embolization coils, cyanoacrylate glue, tantalum powder

[1] At author's institution, 0.1 mL/kg of Gadovist® is diluted with 0.2 mL/kg NS.

Pre-procedure Workup

No specific blood work is necessary although complete blood count (CBC) with group and hold can be considered.

Procedure Technique

General anesthesia is required for both diagnostic and interventional components of the procedure. When intervention is undertaken, wide-spectrum antibiotic prophylaxis to cover for potential bowel transgression is recommended [22]. Dynamic MR lymphangiography is becoming increasingly utilized for lymphatic leak localization and characterization [21, 23].

The diagnostic procedure can be performed either by direct intranodal injection or pedal lymphatic duct cannulation. Intranodal injection of contrast is the preferred technique as it has many advantages over the pedal cannulation technique. Intranodal injection is easier to perform, less time-consuming, and hence less radiation exposure to the child. Better contrast opacification of the thoracic duct can be obtained by accessing multiple nodes in the groin region and by accessing nodes bilaterally. Pedal duct cannulation requires a high level of skill and training to access the tiny lymph vessel, and success rates are not high. Accessing the lymphatic vessels in both pedal regions can be very time-consuming and takes a long time for the contrast to flow from the pedal region to the thoracic duct region. The technique of pedal duct cannulation is still important, as it is the only method to demonstrate lymphatic leaks in the groin region following multiple groin punctures related to vascular access for cardiac catheterizations and interventions (Fig. 16.5).

The diagnostic lymphangiogram by intranodal injection can be performed using either MRI or fluoroscopy. At the current time, MR lymphangiogram with intranodal injection of dilute gadolinium is becoming the method of choice for diagnostic assessment [21]. In many cases, MR lymphangiography provides additional information regarding the cause of lymphatic leaks without exposure to ionizing radiation (Figs. 16.2c–e and 16.6).

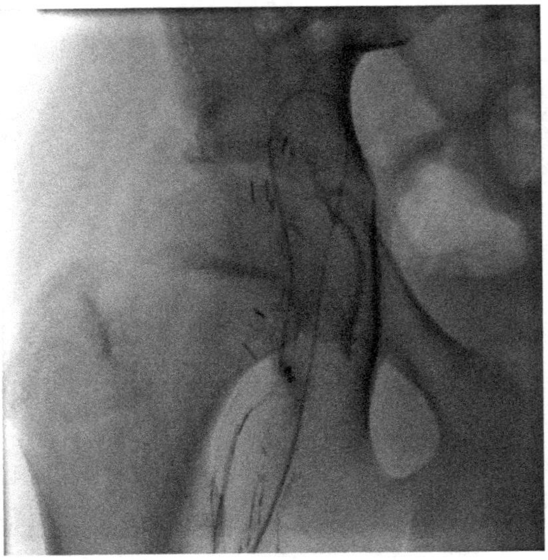

Fig. 16.5 Lymphatic leak following cardiac catheterization. Pedal access is required to perform lymphangiography when a lymphatic leak is suspected in the groin area

Diagnostic Lymphangiogram with Intranodal Access

A high-frequency linear probe is used to introduce the tip of a small (21–25 G) needle or angiocatheter into the medulla of a lymph node in the inguinal area (Fig. 16.2b). A small test injection with saline can help to demonstrate that the needle tip is in an appropriate position and there is no extravasation. Contrast must be injected slowly to assure that you do not "blow" the node allowing contrast to leak into the surrounding tissues. Injection rates of oil-based contrast around 0.1–0.2 mL/min are described in adult patients [17, 18, 24]. Reported injection volumes of oil-based contrast range from 0.3 to 0.5 mL in infants [7], 1–6 in children [25], and 1–8 mL (with a maximum of 14 mL) in adults [25].

For MR lymphangiography, the *angiocatheter* is stabilized using a clear dressing and the patient is moved to the MRI machine. Coronal thin

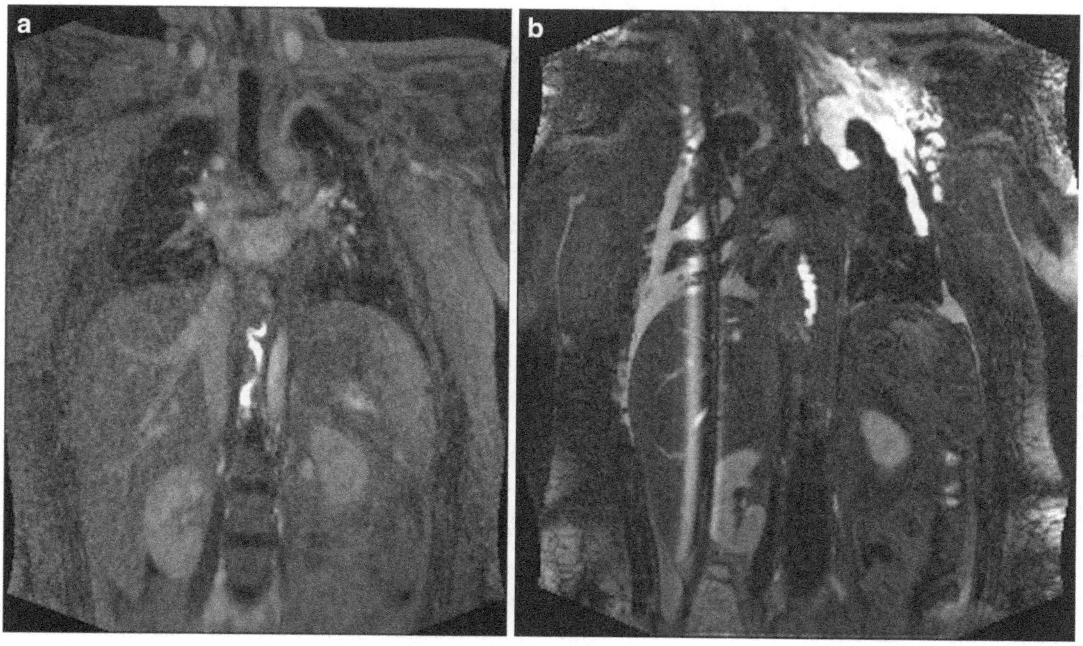

Fig. 16.6 MR lymphangiogram. (**a**) Early and (**b**) delayed FLASH MR images were obtained. The delayed image shows the contrast leak and accumulation within the left pleural space

section volumetric T1-weighted FLASH sequence images are obtained at regular intervals during the contrast injection (Figs. 16.2c and 16.6a). Delayed images are also obtained which better demonstrate the leak and accumulation of contrast in the serous cavities if present (Figs. 16.2e and 16.6b).

If extravasation occurs during nodal injection under fluoroscopy or if the contrast is not sufficient to opacify the thoracic dust/cisterna chyli, a node "chaser technique" is used wherein a higher node in the chain along the iliac vessels can be accessed either by ultrasound or fluoroscopy (Figs. 16.2g, h and 16.7). Since a thin-bore 25-G needle is used, the risk of vascular injury is minimal when a pelvic node is accessed.

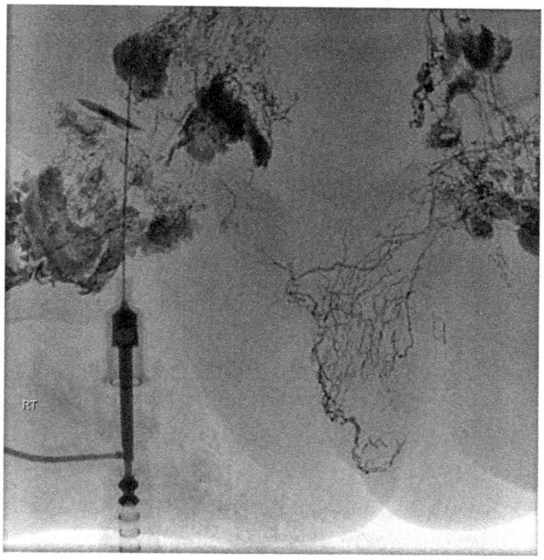

Fig. 16.7 "Chaser" technique. A 25-G needle has been inserted into a left iliac chain node to promote opacification of the lymphatic chain

Pedal Duct Cannulation

To facilitate visualization of a lymphatic duct prior to cannulation, methylene blue is injected in the web spaces between the toes. When a duct has been identified on the dorsum of the foot, local anesthetic is injected, and a transverse incision is made in the overlying skin. Blunt dissection is used to gently free the duct. A surgical microscope or loupes can be helpful to help cannulate the duct with a 30-G lymphangiography catheter (Cook

Medical, Bloomington, USA). When successfully accessed, a suture is drawn around the needle to help it fix in place during contrast injection.

Thoracic Duct Embolization

Contrast is slowly administered during the embolization procedure (Figs. 16.2, 16.4, and 16.8). If the diagnostic study was performed using MRI, additional Lipiodol is injected through the same needles after transfer to the fluoroscopy table. Often the cisterna chyli is transiently opacified with a few drops of contrast (Fig. 16.1). To improve visualization, high-dose radiation fluoroscopy with the grid is used. The cisterna chyli is punctured with a 22-G Chiba needle. Bending the tip of the needle slightly can provide more maneuverability making the puncture easier. When possible, a right-sided approach is used to minimize the risk of injuring the aorta.

A relatively rigid wire with a flexible tip is then used to gently probe through the end of the needle in an attempt to pass cranially into the thoracic duct. When accessed, a high-flow microcatheter is advanced over the wire (Figs. 16.4a and 16.8b). Water-soluble contrast is injected to visualize the duct and attempt to delineate the area of leakage (Figs. 16.4a and 16.8c). When a focal leak is identified, the catheter is advanced beyond the area and a coil is deployed across the site, whenever possible. Following the coil embolization, a second embolization with glue is carried out proximal to the deployed coils. If the catheter cannot be advanced, the anatomy does not allow exact targeting or a focal leak is not identified, cyanoacrylate glue mixed with Lipiodol (1:1) glue, and/or tantalum powder can be injected to fill the ducts as the catheter is withdrawn (Fig. 16.8d).

In many cases, after delineating the leak, accessing the cisterna chyli might not be possible. In these cases, disruption of the duct by the needle will be sufficient to redistribute the flow of lymph and thus stop the life-threatening chylothorax or pericardial leak [5, 26, 27].

If the patient has chyloperitoneum and a leak is identified below the level of the cisterna chyli, one can attempt to access a dilated duct below the level of the leak and embolize through a catheter as previously described. Otherwise, attempted disruption of the visualized ducts below the level can be attempted with fluoroscopy or CT (Fig. 16.2) [5, 26, 27].

Retrograde thoracic duct access (utilizing a reverse curve or coaxial catheter) and embolization have been described [28].

Post-procedure Monitoring

Following the procedure, supportive care is provided. The patient is monitored for signs of infection or bleeding. When a patient with a potential right-to-left cardiac shunt has had oil-based contrast administered (see description in "Indications/Contraindications" section), they should remain intubated for several hours after the procedure to minimize potential intracardiac pressure changes that may occur with extubation/recovery.

Complications and Outcomes

Extravasation of oil-based contrast has been reported to cause local irritation [29, 30].

Lymphatic duct puncture can result in damage to any intervening structure (depending on path and location) including the liver, bowel, blood vessels, ureter, and pancreas.

Lymphatic duct intervention works by redirecting lymph from embolized or damaged vessels into other (hopefully intact) collateral channels. It can take several weeks to determine if a procedure has been successful. Lymph redistribution may be unsuccessful or can result in worsening of output from the site of leakage or a change in location (i.e. chyloperitoneum can develop following chylothorax treatment) [31]. Changes in lymphatic flow dynamics can lead to complications such as diarrhea or leg swelling [32].

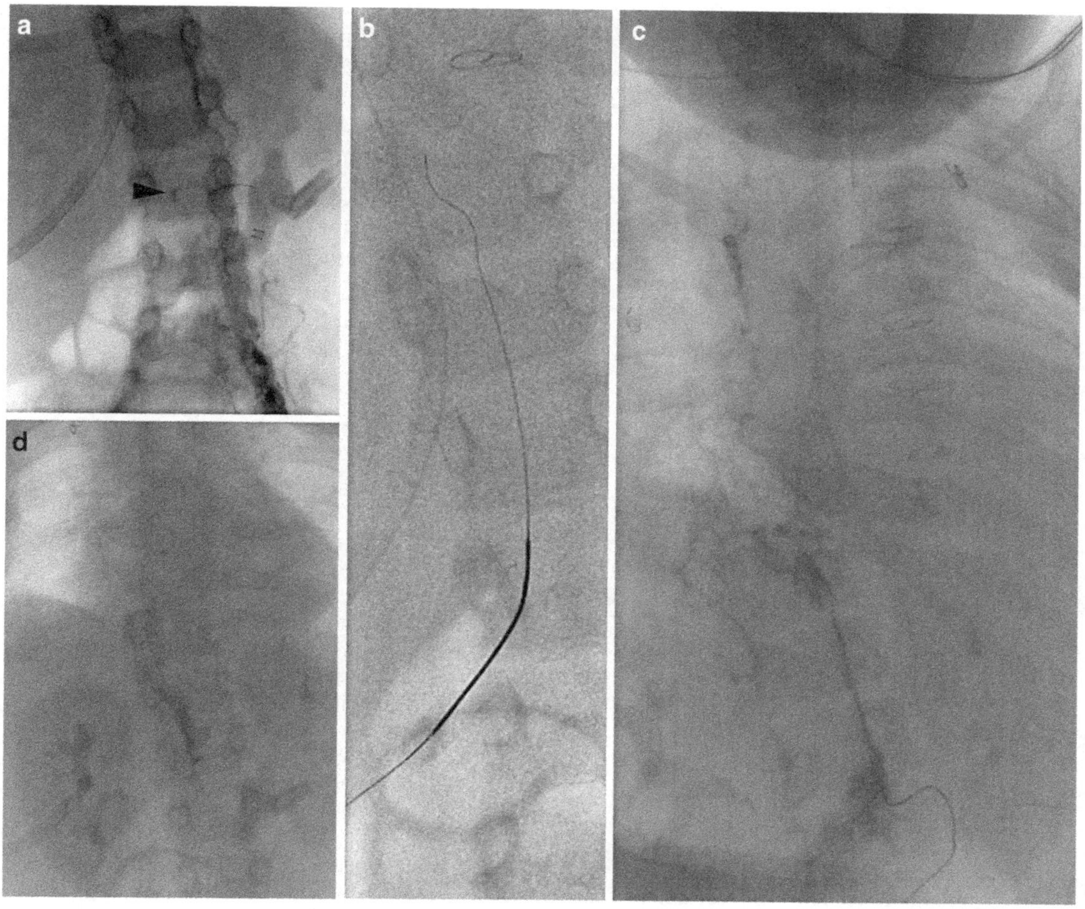

Fig. 16.8 Thoracic duct embolization (TDE) with glue. (**a**) Fluoroscopic image shows cisterna chyli (CC) transiently opacified with water-soluble contrast in patient with a fenestrated Fontan. (**b**) CC accessed with 0.018″ V-18 wire and Rapid Transit microcatheter. (**c**) Contrast injection shows diffuse lymphatic collaterals but site of right chylothorax was not identified. (**d**) Appearance following administration of cyanoacrylate glue (diluted 1:2 with Lipiodol and tantalum powder added). The patient developed chylous ascites 3 weeks after TDE that resolved after 4 months

Follow-Up

Pediatric lymphatic intervention is a rapidly evolving but relatively new procedure. As such, no specific follow-up regimen has been determined. In summary, pediatric lymphatic intervention is a rapidly evolving but relatively new procedure that is very effective in treating life-threatening lymphatic leaks and often represents the only option when surgical intervention has failed.

Chapter Summary

Background

- Lymphatic system essential in fluid homeostasis
- Lymphatic leaks
  - Congenital—occlusion, lymphatic malformation
  - Acquired—postsurgical, trauma, radiation, tumor

Anatomy

- Unidirectional fluid transport
- Cisterna chyli (CC) formed by iliac/lumbar, hepatic, and intestinal lymphatics
- Thoracic duct carries lymph from CC to left jugular/subclavian vein
- Right lymphatic duct drains right arm, chest, and face

Indications

- Diagnostic—characterization of lymphatic abnormalities, localization of leaks
- Interventional—embolization of leaks

Contraindications

- Uncorrectable coagulopathy
- Oil-based contrast contraindicated with right-to-left cardiac shunt

Equipment

Pre-procedure Workup

- CBC, group and hold

Procedure Technique

- General anesthesia
- Obtain access
  - Intranodal access—US guidance, easy, 21–25-G needle
  - Pedal—technically challenging, 30-G lymphangiography catheter
- Diagnostic lymphangiogram
  - Dynamic MR lymphangiography (1:1–1:2 gadolinium to normal saline)
  - Fluoroscopy with oil-based or water-soluble contrast
    - Lipiodol—0.1–0.2 mL/min in adults; volume, 0.3–0.5 mL in infants, 1–6 mL in children, 1–8 mL (max 14 mL) in adults
- Embolization/duct disruption
  - CC often difficult to visualize
  - Chiba needle, 0.018″ stiff wire, high-flow microcatheter
    - Water-soluble contrast to visualize leak
    - Coil above leak if possible, follow with glue; can glue without coiling if area not accessible or leak site not identified
- If unable to access duct, needle used to attempt to disrupt duct

Post-procedure Monitoring

- Supportive

Complications/Outcomes

- Contrast extravasation associated with local irritation
- Damage to intervening structures (bowel, liver, blood vessels, pancreas, etc.)
- Change in chyle output or location
- Diarrhea, leg swelling

Follow-Up

- Not currently established

References

1. Olszewski WL. The lymphatic system in body homeostasis: physiological conditions. Lymphat Res Biol. 2003;1(1):11–21; discussion 21–4.
2. Mallick A, Bodenham AR. Disorders of the lymph circulation: their relevance to anaesthesia and intensive care. Br J Anaesth. 2003;91(2):265–72.
3. Cope C. Percutaneous thoracic duct cannulation: feasibility study in swine. J Vasc Interv Radiol. 1995; 6(4):559–64.
4. Cope C. Percutaneous transabdominal embolization of thoracic duct lacerations in animals. J Vasc Interv Radiol. 1996;7(5):725–31.
5. Cope C, Salem R, Kaiser LR. Management of chylothorax by percutaneous catheterization and embolization of the thoracic duct: prospective trial. J Vasc Interv Radiol. 1999;10(9):1248–54.
6. Cope C, Kaiser LR. Management of unremitting chylothorax by percutaneous embolization and blockage of retroperitoneal lymphatic vessels in 42 patients. J Vasc Interv Radiol. 2002;13(11):1139–48.
7. Itkin M, Krishnamurthy G, Naim MY, Bird GL, Keller MS. Percutaneous thoracic duct embolization as a treatment for intrathoracic chyle leaks in infants. Pediatrics. 2011;128(1):e237–41.
8. Nadolski GJ, Itkin M. Feasibility of ultrasound-guided intranodal lymphangiogram for thoracic duct embolization. J Vasc Interv Radiol. 2012;23(5):613–6.
9. Rajebi MR, Chaudry G, Padua HM, Dillon B, Yilmaz S, Arnold RW, et al. Intranodal lymphangiography: feasibility and preliminary experience in children. J Vasc Interv Radiol. 2011;22(9):1300–5.
10. Ferguson MK, Little AG, Skinner DB. Current concepts in the management of postoperative chylothorax. Ann Thorac Surg. 1985;40(6):542–5.
11. Bonner W. A review of the nutritional management of chyle leakage in adults. J Hum Nutr Diet. 1998; 11(2):105–14.

12. Trzewik J, Mallipattu SK, Artmann GM, Delano FA, Schmid-Schonbein GW. Evidence for a second valve system in lymphatics: endothelial microvalves. FASEB J. 2001;15(10):1711–7.
13. Farrell WJ. Lymphangiographic demonstration of lymphovenous communication after radiotherapy in Hodgkin's disease. Radiology. 1966;87(4):630–4.
14. Bruna J. Collateral lymphatic circulation. Eur J Plast Surg. 2000;20(6):321–5.
15. Stamp GF, Peters AM. Peripheral lymphovenous communication in lymphoedema. Nucl Med Commun. 2012;33(7):701–7.
16. Kawasaki R, Sugimoto K, Fujii M, Miyamoto N, Okada T, Yamaguchi M, et al. Therapeutic effectiveness of diagnostic lymphangiography for refractory postoperative chylothorax and chylous ascites: correlation with radiologic findings and preceding medical treatment. AJR Am J Roentgenol. 2013;201(3):659–66.
17. Matsumoto T, Yamagami T, Kato T, Hirota T, Yoshimatsu R, Masunami T, et al. The effectiveness of lymphangiography as a treatment method for various chyle leakages. Br J Radiol. 2009;82(976):286–90.
18. Yamagami T, Masunami T, Kato T, Tanaka O, Hirota T, Nomoto T, et al. Spontaneous healing of chyle leakage after lymphangiography. Br J Radiol. 2005;78(933):854–7.
19. Goff AM, Gaensler EA. Respiratory distress syndrome following lymphangiography. Respiration. 1971;28(1):89–97.
20. Silvestri RC, Huseby JS, Rughani I, Thorning D, Culver BH. Respiratory distress syndrome from lymphangiography contrast medium. Am Rev Respir Dis. 1980;122(4):543–9.
21. Krishnamurthy R, Hernandez A, Kavuk S, Annam A, Pimpalwar S. Dynamic magnetic resonance lymphangiography (MRL): a new technique to image the central conducting lymphatics (CCL). J Vasc Interv Radiol. 2013;24(4):S28.
22. Chen E, Itkin M. Thoracic duct embolization for chylous leaks. Semin Intervent Radiol. 2011;28(1):63–74.
23. Praveen A, Sreekumar K, Nazar P, Moorthy S. Technical note: thoracic duct embolization for treatment of chylothorax: a novel guidance technique for puncture using combined MRI and fluoroscopy. Indian J Radiol Imaging. 2012;22(2):89–92.
24. Gomez FM, Martinez-Rodrigo J, Marti-Bonmati L, Santos E, Forner I, Lloret M, et al. Transnodal lymphangiography in the diagnosis and treatment of genital lymphedema. Cardiovasc Intervent Radiol. 2012;35(6):1488–91.
25. LLC G. Lipiodol product insert. Available from: http://www.fda.gov/downloads/Drugs/DrugSafety/DrugShortages/UCM213187.pdf.
26. Binkert CA, Yucel EK, Davison BD, Sugarbaker DJ, Baum RA. Percutaneous treatment of high-output chylothorax with embolization or needle disruption technique. J Vasc Interv Radiol. 2005;16(9):1257–62.
27. Litherland B, Given M, Lyon S. Percutaneous radiological management of high-output chylothorax with CT-guided needle disruption. J Med Imaging Radiat Oncol. 2008;52(2):164–7.
28. Mittleider D, Dykes TA, Cicuto KP, Amberson SM, Leusner CR. Retrograde cannulation of the thoracic duct and embolization of the cisterna chyli in the treatment of chylous ascites. J Vasc Interv Radiol. 2008;19(2 Pt 1):285–90.
29. Redman HC. Dermatitis as a complication of lymphangiography. Radiology. 1966;86(2):323–6.
30. Mansfield DC, Zeki SM, Mackenzie JR. Case report: extravasation of lipiodol—a complication of dacryocystography. Clin Radiol. 1994;49(3):217–8.
31. Gaba RC, Owens CA, Bui JT, Carrillo TC, Knuttinen MG. Chylous ascites: a rare complication of thoracic duct embolization for chylothorax. Cardiovasc Intervent Radiol. 2011;34 Suppl 2:S245–9.
32. Laslett D, Trerotola SO, Itkin M. Delayed complications following technically successful thoracic duct embolization. J Vasc Interv Radiol. 2012;23(1):76–9.

Section V

Nonvascular Interventions: Biopsy

Percutaneous Biopsies in Children 17

Krijn P. van Lienden and Rick R. van Rijn

General/Background Information

According to the Society of Interventional Radiology Standards of Practice Committee, image-guided percutaneous biopsy is defined as placement of a needle or needles into a suspected abnormal target site for the purpose of obtaining tissue or cells for diagnosis [1]. In contrast to the adult clinical setting, image-guided biopsies in the pediatric population have not yet reached a full level of acceptance [2]. One of the main differences is the need for general sedation in most of the patients, this as childhood oncology has a peak in the young pediatric population. Of all cases of childhood cancer under the age of 15 years, approximately 50 % are diagnosed below the age of 5 years [3]. In children, in contrast to adults, hematological malignancies and tumors of the central nervous system account for the majority of all cancers (Fig. 17.1).

In pediatric oncology there seems to be hesitance among clinicians and pathologists to use percutaneous image-guided biopsies, and therefore, surgical excision biopsies are frequently obtained. In many international oncology protocols, such as the SIOP E*p*SSG trial, surgical biopsies are actually mandatory. The rationale for this has always been that a surgical biopsy will always yield enough material for the diagnosis and biological studies. As in most cases general anesthesia is mandatory, clinicians are reluctant to risk an insufficient and therefore nondiagnostic percutaneous biopsy. It is interesting to note that in most of these clinical discussions, the literature evidence related to the value of image-guided percutaneous biopsies on the one hand and risk related to surgical biopsies on the other hand is underexposed (Fig. 17.2) [4].

There is ample evidence that in the hands of capable (pediatric) interventional radiologists, percutaneous core needle biopsies (CNB) can be as diagnostic as surgical biopsies. A retrospective study was performed in the Department of Interventional Radiology, Great Ormond Street Hospital for Children (London, UK) [5]. In this study 37 consecutive CNB procedures, of a primary ($N=20$) or recurrent ($N=10$) tumor or lymph nodes ($N=7$), were performed in 24 children. The CNB procedures from the 30 tumors and the seven lymph nodes were 100 % diagnostic.

In this chapter the indications, contraindications, materials, and techniques of needle biopsy will be discussed.

K.P. van Lienden, M.D., Ph.D.
R.R. van Rijn, M.D., Ph.D. (✉)
Department of Radiology, Emma Children's Hospital, Academic Medical Center Amsterdam, 1 Meirbergdreef 9, Amsterdam 1105AZ, The Netherlands
e-mail: k.p.vanlienden@amc.uva.nl; r.r.vanrijn@amc.uva.nl

M. Temple and F.E. Marshalleck (eds.), *Pediatric Interventional Radiology: Handbook of Vascular and Non-Vascular Interventions*, DOI 10.1007/978-1-4419-5856-3_17,

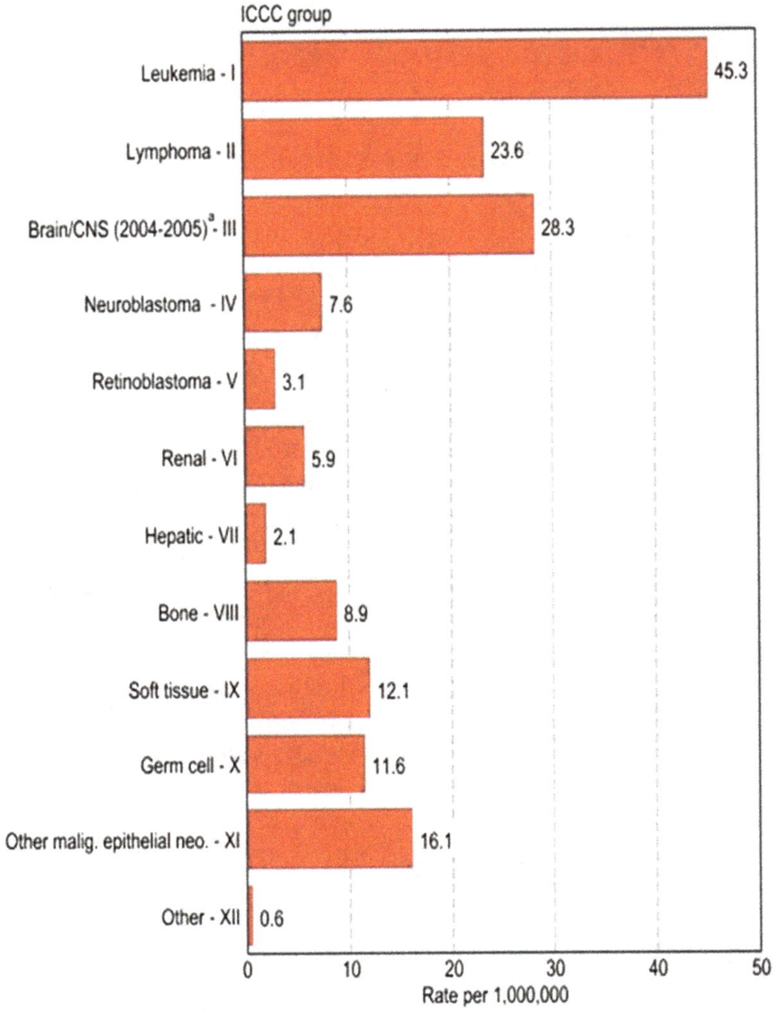

Fig. 17.1 Childhood cancer: SEER incidence rates 2002–2006 by ICCC Group (includes Group III benign brain (2004–2006) and myelodysplastic syndromes) under 20 years of age, both sexes, all races (Data: The Surveillance, Epidemiology, and End Results [SEER] Program of the National Cancer Institute [NCI]). All material in this report is in the public domain and may be reproduced or copied without permission. From Horner MJ, Ries LAG, Krapcho M, Neyman N, Aminou R, Howlader N, Altekruse SF, Feuer EJ, Huang L, Mariotto A, Miller BA, Lewis DR, Eisner MP, Stinchcomb DG, Edwards BK (eds). SEER Cancer Statistics Review, 1975–2006, National Cancer Institute. Bethesda, MD, http://seer.cancer.gov/csr/1975_2006/, based on November 2008 SEER data submission, posted to the SEER web site, 2009 [62]

Indications/Contraindications

Indications

The indication for image-guided biopsy is to obtain tissue for cytologic or histological examinations from an organ [1, 6]. There are four main categories, which serve as an indication for image-guided biopsy:

- In case of a mass or focal lesion, to establish the benign or malignant nature of a lesion
- To stage patients with known or suspected malignancy when local spread or distant metastasis is suspected
- To obtain material for microbiological analysis in patients with known or suspected infections
- To determine the nature and extent of diffuse parenchymal diseases

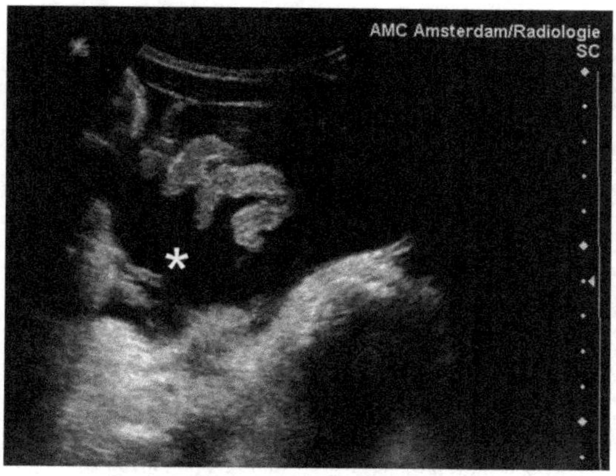

Fig. 17.2 Abdominal ultrasound study of a 10-year-old girl who underwent a surgical biopsy of a right adrenal gland neuroblastoma and postsurgically became anemic. The study shows a massive hematoperitoneum

Contraindications

Abnormal Coagulation Time

Normally biopsies of superficial structures, for instance, in the groin and the neck, can be taken without any coagulation studies. When bleeding occurs, manual compression will achieve hemostasis.

For all chest and abdominal biopsies as well as for all deep-seated lesions, standard partial thromboplastin time (PTT) and prothrombin time (PT) and a platelet count should be obtained.

An uncorrected bleeding diathesis is a contraindication for biopsies, especially those taken from parenchymatous organs (liver, spleen, and kidney). Patients using nonsteroidal anti-inflammatory drugs, e.g., aspirin, are advised to stop medication and defer the biopsy for 10 days. However, a study by Atwell showed no significant association between aspirin use within 10 days before biopsy and significant bleeding after biopsy of any specific organ [7].

Ascites

Ascites is thought to be a risk factor for bleeding after liver biopsies; however, literature, obtained from adult studies shows no statistically significant higher risk of minor or major bleeding complications after image-guided percutaneous liver biopsies in the presence of perihepatic ascites, given a normal coagulation status [8, 9].

Single Native Kidney

The presence of a single native kidney is by many nephrologists considered to be an absolute contraindication to percutaneous image-guided biopsy [10, 11]. The rationale is that if a serious adverse event would occur, the patient might become anephric. With regard to these adverse events, one can think of persistent AV fistulas or persistent hemorrhage, leading to a partial or even complete nephrectomy. Interestingly percutaneous biopsies of renal transplant, even non-image guided, are a standard procedure in everyday pediatric transplant nephrology.

Absence of Safe Percutaneous Approach

Overlying bone or bowel structures can be the cause of a contraindication for safe percutaneous approach. Bear in mind, during planning of the biopsy approach, that ultrasonography (US)-guided biopsies have the advantage that overlying bowel loops, can sometimes be pushed aside using compression with the transducer, so a safe approach can be created. In case of an overlying colonic loop, deflation using a needle has been shown to be a safe method to obtain a free pathway [12]. Fine needle biopsies using fine needles (20–22G) can safely transgress bowel loops.

Preprocedural Work-Up

Preprocedural Imaging

Proper preprocedural imaging is a key factor in the success of an image-guided biopsy. The interventional radiologists should be fully aware of all prior imaging before any interventional procedure is planned and performed. A European study among CIRSE members showed that 27 % spent more than 80 % of their time on interventional radiology alone [13]. There is an international movement towards a separate specialty in which minimal invasive surgery and interventional radiology are merged into one specialty [14]. This increasing sub-specialization in radiology has the inherent hazard that diagnostic and interventional radiology become two different entities within one single radiological department and that patients might enter the department of interventional radiology for procedures without the interventional radiologist fully aware of the preprocedural imaging and the clinical setting of the patient.

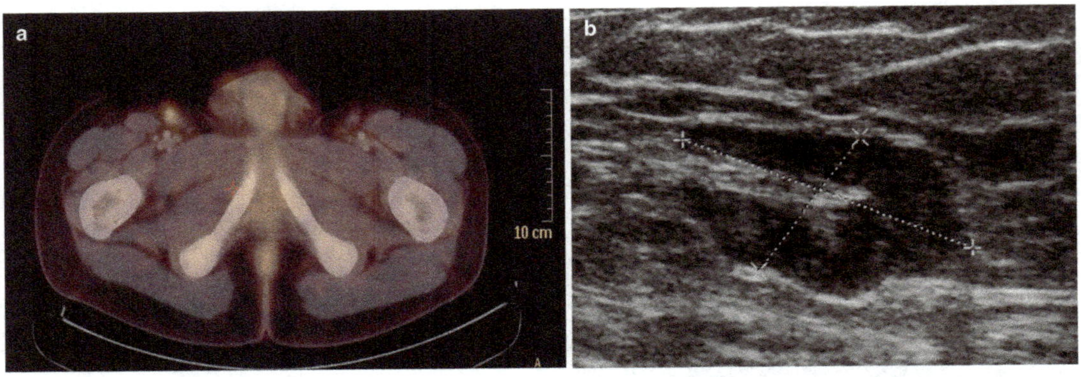

Fig. 17.3 (**a**) A 17-year-old male with an osteosarcoma of the right distal femur; PET-CT shows FDG uptake in a lymph node in the right groin. In a multidisciplinary meeting it was decided that for adequate staging purposes a percutaneous biopsy of this lymph node would be performed. (**b**) Ultrasonography of the same lymph node shows an enlarged lymph node with a normal fat center. Based on this ultrasound study, the interventional radiologist, who was not present at the multidisciplinary meeting, decided that the lymph node was most likely reactive and enlarged and to be refrained from biopsy. As a consequence the patient *later* had to be upstaged and treated with a high risk protocol

In case of ultrasound-guided biopsies, it is imperative that the interventional radiologist performs the preprocedural ultrasound study. This study will allow for the assessment of safe approach and feasibility of the ultrasound-guided biopsy. He/she should also be aware of relevant clinical discussions in order not to interfere with a treatment plan previously decided upon in, e.g., a specialist panel (Fig. 17.3a, b).

Informed Consent, Sedation, and Patient Preparation

Informed Consent

Before starting any interventional procedure, the indication for the biopsy, the technique used, and the possible postprocedural complications and discomforts must be explained to the parents and whenever necessary to the child. In the Netherlands informed consent obtained from the patient is mandatory in children over 12 years of age. It is also the interventional radiologist's duty to assess if it is possible to perform the biopsy under sedation or that general anesthesia should be used.

Sedation

One of the hallmarks of pediatric radiological interventions is the need for sedation in combination with analgesia. Where in the adult population local anesthesia will mostly suffice, this will almost never be the case in children. This aspect of the interventional procedure may be one of the reasons for the lower level of acceptance of interventional radiology in children.

In case of biopsies under general anesthesia, close collaboration between the anesthesiologist and the interventional radiologist is mandatory. The anesthesiologists will be able to obtain a period of apnea which can offer a window of opportunity to biopsy smaller lung, liver, or renal lesions.

Following an interventional procedure, the children should be observed and, depending on the intervention, feeding can be started but only if the child has regained full consciousness.

Patient Preparation

All patients must have an intravenous access prior to the start of the intervention. The appropriate personnel must have undertaken all preparations for sedation. The patient must be positioned in a comfortable position without compromising the puncture site, e.g., lateral decubitus for a native renal biopsy. The skin must be scrubbed and sterilized with alcohol. Sterile drapes are used around the puncture site.

The use of sterile gowns, facial shields, and goggles should comply with local regulations. The use of sterile gloves is absolutely mandatory in all cases.

Equipment

Imaging Systems

Ultrasonography

US is the most widely used technique to guide percutaneous biopsies. For US-guided CNB, the patient needs to be covered with surgical draping and the ultrasound probe placed in a sterile polyethylene, latex-free transducer cover. The choice of the probe depends on the location of the mass to be biopsied, but a probe with a high frequency and thus high resolution has a distinct preference over a probe with a lower frequency.

The biopsy itself can be performed with free hand, i.e., the radiologist guides the biopsy needle under US guidance; this allows for maximum flexibility but it requires both a steady hand and experience. A second technique is the use of a biopsy adaptor attached to the head of the ultrasound probe, which guides the needle (Fig. 17.4). When the biopsy adaptor is used, the needle follows the path that is overlain over the ultrasound image by special biopsy software, thus possibly allowing for a highly accurate biopsy (Fig. 17.5). There are some studies in adults, mainly in breast imaging, with conflicting results [15, 16]. A phantom-based study by Phal et al. showed that although probe-guided biopsies were faster to perform, 20 s faster (95 % confidence interval, −35 to −5 s; $P=0.01$), sample quality showed no difference between techniques [17]. Therefore the choice between these techniques is solely based on personal preference.

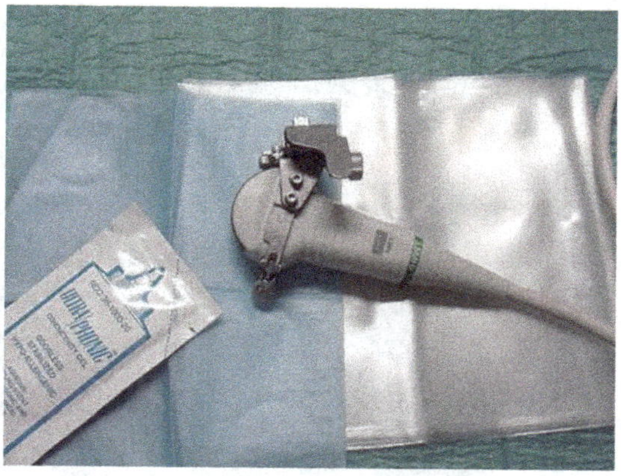

Fig. 17.4 Non-disposable biopsy guide attached to 7.5 MHz curvilinear probe

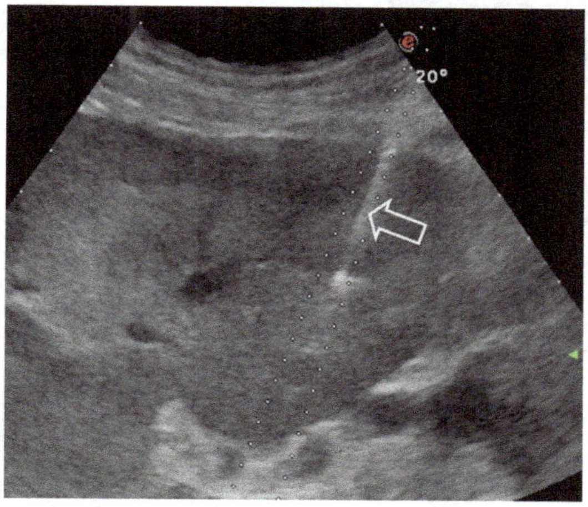

Fig. 17.5 Liver biopsy using US guidance; the tru-cut needle (*arrow*) is positioned between the projected trajectories (*dotted lines*)

Computed Tomography

Computed tomography (CT)-guided biopsy is a well-established technique, but given the associated radiation dose, it should be reserved for those cases where US-guided biopsy is not feasible [18].

The lesion is first localized with a focused CT scan with, in relation to the lesion, relatively thick slices; prior to the scan, radiopaque markers are placed on the patient. After the lesion has been localized, the location for needle entry is marked on the skin using the light beam from the CT scanner. The needle is introduced and subsequent, as few as possible, focal scans are performed to confirm the needle position (Fig. 17.6a, b).

There are systems available that allow for CT fluoroscopy; however, the use of this technique is ill advised in children as it generates a relatively high radiation dose compared to the technique described above. In all cases of CT-guided biopsy, the need of CT guidance should be weighed against the radiation risk [18].

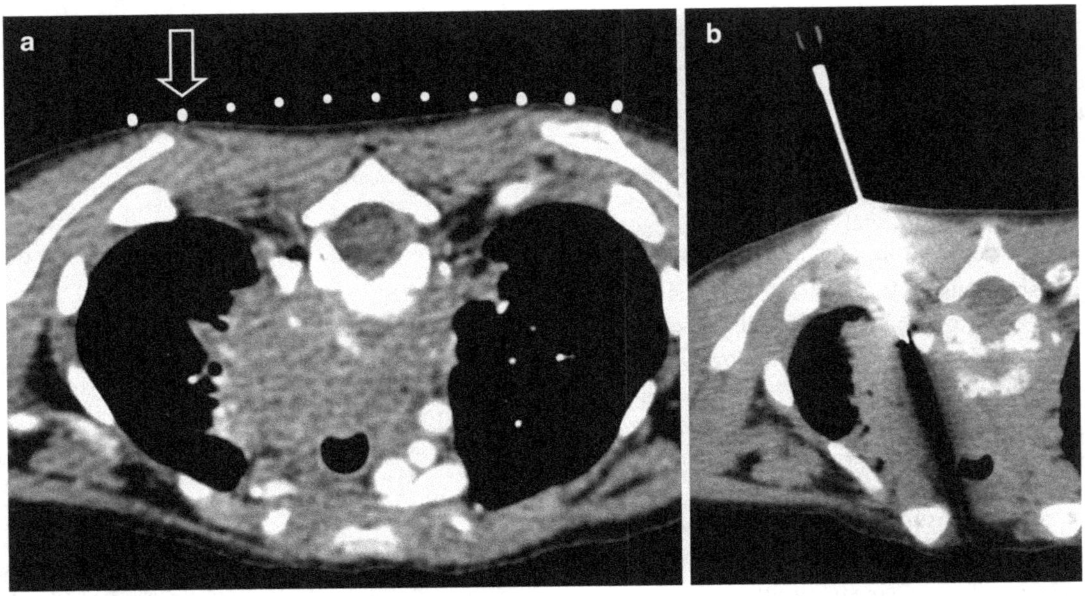

Fig. 17.6 (**a**) The use of grid (*arrow*) in a CT-guided thoracic biopsy. The grid is used to plan the biopsy and is removed prior to biopsy in order to obtain a sterile environment. (**b**) Thoracic CT-guided biopsy in a 5-year-old boy with chronic granulomatous disease. MRI showed spondylodiscitis with an adjacent soft tissue mass

Magnetic Resonance Imaging

The use of magnetic resonance imaging (MRI)-guided biopsies in children has been described in literature, but its use is extremely rare [19–21]. MRI-guided biopsies can be done either according to protocols used in CT-guided biopsies whereby the patient is shifted in and out of the magnetic bore or in a real-time environment. For the latter an "open" MRI is needed; for this purpose a midfield open system or more widely known as "double doughnut" MRI, e.g., SIGNA SP/I (GEMS, Milwaukee, WI, USA), has been developed. This enables access to the patient in an almost natural position for the interventional radiologist. Another option is the use of a biplanar magnet design, e.g., Philips Panorama (Philips Medical Systems, Best, Netherlands); in these systems two magnets are separated by fixed supports. These systems limit patient access, and the interventional radiologist cannot work in a natural position; however, due to its design the MRI system can be used for diagnostic work as well. The latter will make it possible for more centers to buy and run an open MRI. The future of MRI-guided interventional radiology could be a suite in which it is possible to move the MRI in and out of the angiography suite.

Besides specific, and sometimes dedicated, MR systems, MRI-guided biopsies require MR-compatible anesthesia equipment and biopsy sets (e.g., normal surgical blades are not acceptable and need to be replaced by non-ferromagnetic, plastic, or ceramic blades) [22, 23].

In light of the highly specific demands of MRI-guided interventions, only specialized centers will be able to perform this procedure, and therefore, further discussion of this technique is outside the scope of this chapter.

Biopsy Systems

Fine Needle Aspiration

Introduction

Fine needle aspiration (FNA) is a relatively easy procedure that, in most instances, can be performed in a regular ultrasound suite. FNA in pediatrics is mainly used in case of suspected

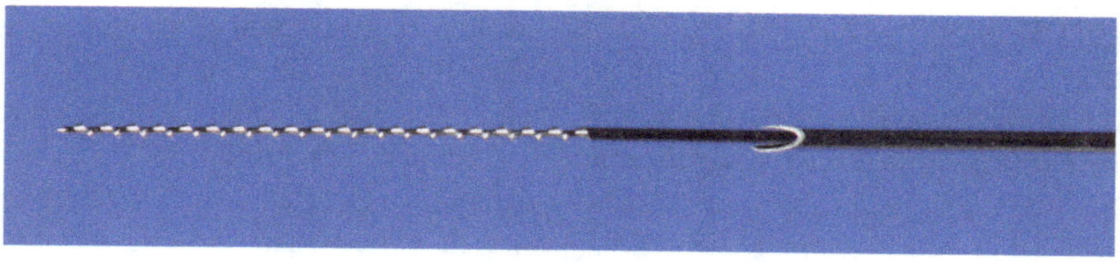

Fig. 17.7 Rotex needle, thin screw needle in an outer needle with a diameter of either 0.8 or 1 mm

infection, where it actually is the first technique of choice, where a culture is requested but drainage is not necessary. In case of oncology it is widely used to assess tumor spread to adjoining or distant lymph node stations. In case of nodal disease of the thyroid gland, FNA is also the main method of choice. In almost all other instances, core needle biopsy will be the preferred method. Finally deeper-located lesions, such as pancreatic lesions (extremely rare in children), will be more approachable for FNA than CNB, for example, using a transgastric approach.

Technique and Materials

For FNA a standard IV needle and syringe are used. Some radiologists prefer to place a line between the needle and the syringe in which case the radiologist handles the needle and the radiological technician handles the syringe. If an FNA procedure has to be done single-handed, special syringe grips are available.

As FNA is relatively nontraumatic, general sedation is mostly not needed. We do however make liberal use of EMLA cream (lidocaine 2.5 % and prilocaine 2.5 %), which is topically applied at the puncture site and gives local analgesia. EMLA cream has been shown to be a safe and effective pain relief in children undergoing procedures such as venipunctures and lumbar punctures [24, 25]. We should however not forget that part of this effect can also be ascribed to the placebo effect and that the application should be done with attention to this effect [26].

In case of FNA we feel that it is imperative that there is a direct feedback from a pathologist. In our clinic we routinely have a pathology assistant in the room for immediate assessment of the quality of the aspirated material.

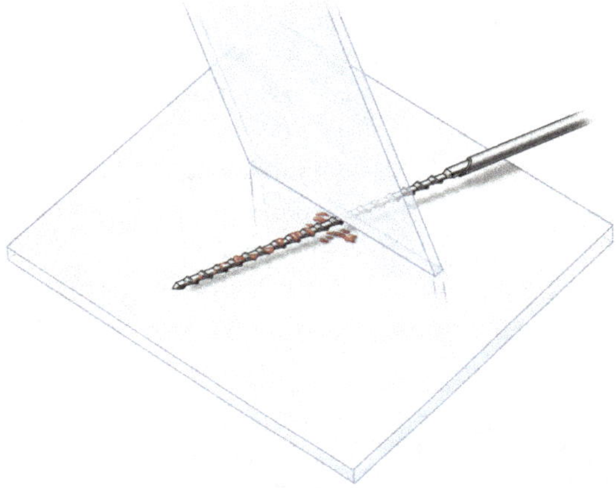

Fig. 17.8 The collected material can be retrieved by rotating the screw needle against the edge of a glass slide

Fine Screw Needle Biopsy

Introduction

Although originally developed for pulmonary biopsies, we have a strong preference for the use of Rotex® needle screw biopsies (Ursus Medical AB, Stockholm, Sweden) in case of well-vascularized organs/tissues such as the thyroid or lymph node. Compared to FNA less admixture of blood cells is seen in the sample, yielding a biopsy with a higher sensitivity.

Technique and Materials

The Rotex® needle consists of an outer guide needle and an inner threaded needle (Fig. 17.7). The outer needle is advanced into the lesion after which the inner threaded needle is "screwed" into the lesion; after advancing the outer needle to the tip of the inner needle, the needles are removed. Along the tread of the needle, the tissue is captivated, leading to a higher yield in comparison to FNA. The collected material can be retrieved by rotating the screw needle against the edge of a glass slide (Fig. 17.8).

Core Needle Biopsy

Introduction

Core needle biopsy (CNB) is the technique of choice in case of an oncological work-up; in contrast to FNA CNB will yield more material, and with the increasing use of staining techniques, marker studies, and genetic analysis, clinicians need more and more tissue samples.

Technique

For CNB one can choose for either a cutting-edge or the so-called "tru-cut" needle with or without an automated biopsy device (Fig. 17.9a–c). Numerous variants of both devices are on the market, with personal experience usually guiding the choice for a specific device. A much-used technique is working coaxially. A needle is advanced into or near to the lesion, the biopsy needle is inserted, and biopsies are taken. Using this technique multiple passes are easily possible with a low risk of spill and thus avoiding potential complications of the procedure. A second advantage is that due to the coaxial needle configuration, hemostatic material can be deposited into the needle tract. This has been reported to be a very effective technique for reducing the risk of CNB-induced hemorrhage, especially in liver lesions.

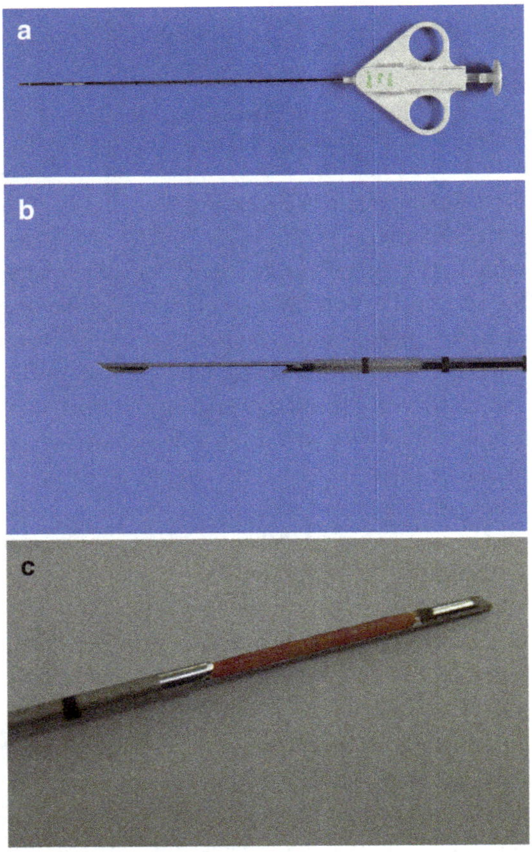

Fig. 17.9 (**a**) Disposable biopsy gun. (**b**) Detail of biopsy needle. (**c**) 18G needle containing a biopsy specimen

Although one would expect a significant difference in complication rates of blind versus image-guided biopsies, relatively few studies have been performed to demonstrate this. Nobili et al. reported a retrospective analysis on 140 biopsies (64 blind versus 76 ultrasound guided) in which 95 % of the blind biopsies and 100 % of the ultrasound-guided biopsies were of diagnostic quality [27]. Moreover, in the blind biopsy population, three patients developed significant hemorrhage versus none in the ultrasound-guided population.

FNA Versus CNB Versus Surgical Biopsies

As medicine is more and more becoming an evidence-based science, it is important that percutaneous biopsy techniques are adequately validated. Several studies into the effectiveness of FNA and CNB in children have been published [4, 28, 29]. In a meta-analysis by Sebire et al., overall biopsy quality was sufficient to make a diagnosis of 94 % (95 % CI 92–96 %) [4]. The diagnostic accuracy rate in cases with adequate material was 94 % (95 % CI 92–96 %). Complications requiring treatment occurred in 1 %.

One issue which should also be addressed relates to the economics of medicine. Lachar et al. studied the cost-effectiveness of core needle biopsy versus surgical biopsy in adult lymphoma patients [30]. In their study CNB established a pathological diagnosis deemed sufficient to begin treatment for primary and recurrent lymphomas in most cases. CNB, compared with a surgical biopsy, yield a cost savings of more than 75 %.

Procedural Technique

Liver

Percutaneous Liver Biopsy

Dependent on the preference of the radiologist, the location of the liver lesion, and whether it is a focal or a diffuse liver biopsy, the biopsy can be guided by computed tomography or ultrasound [28].

In case of diffuse liver disease, in most cases, a midaxillary route is chosen. With deep inspiration, the caudal border of the pleural sinus can be identified to avoid a transpleural puncture. After local anesthetic infiltration of the skin and the liver capsule, two biopsies are taken in expiration. Dependent of the age and size of the child, 18 or 16G biopsy needles should be used.

In case of focal liver lesions, the shortest path is chosen; in our experience the best biopsies are taken from the edge of the lesion to avoid nonrepresentative material caused by central necrosis. If possible, it is advised to approach the target lesion through a "cuff" of normal liver tissue to decrease the risk of bleeding (Fig. 17.10). The normal liver tissue will tamponade a possible bleeding. If an intercostal route is used, one should puncture over the rib to avoid a bleeding from an intercostal artery or vein, as they are located directly below the rib.

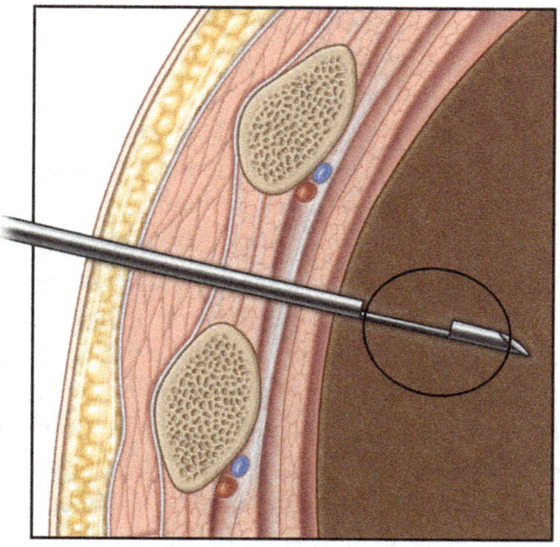

Fig. 17.10 Hepatic biopsy procedure using intercostal approach. Note that the intercostal artery runs just below the rib

When multiple biopsies must be taken, a coaxial technique is advised, in which case the guiding outer needle passes the liver capsule only once, after which more biopsies can be taken through the coaxial guiding needle. A second advantage is that due to the coaxial needle configuration, hemostatic material can be deposited into the needle tract. This has been reported to be a very effective technique for reducing the risk of CNB-induced hemorrhage, especially in liver lesions [28, 31]. One should be aware that even this effective and safe technique has a risk for the patient, as a case of dislodged embolization material has been described in literature [32].

Patients should be warned that after a liver biopsy, they temporarily can experience some referred right shoulder pain. After the biopsy, patients should have bed rest for 1–2 h. Vital signs must be monitored. If a pneumothorax is suspected, a chest X-ray must be obtained.

Transjugular Hepatic Biopsy

Particularly in patients with diffuse liver abnormalities, ascites, and coagulopathy with a platelet count of less than 50,000/μL or an INR of more than 1.5, transjugular liver biopsies are a safe alternative when a percutaneous route is contraindicated [28].

The right jugular vein is punctured and a sheath is placed. The right hepatic vein is accessed with a cobra-shaped catheter and a Terumo wire (Terumo, Eschborn, Germany) under fluoroscopy guidance. The biopsy set is very similar to the TIPS set. After introducing the introducer sheath in the right hepatic vein, a rigid guiding cannula is positioned approximately 2–3 cm from the IVC. The biopsy needle is introduced. After the cannula is turned in anterior direction, the biopsy needle is advanced into the liver parenchyma, the mechanism is fired, and 18G biopsies are taken. The biopsies can be monitored by ultrasound.

The success rate of this transjugular procedure is 98 %. Major complications are rare; minor complications are described in 2–5 % [33].

Pancreas

In childhood pancreatic tumors, the main reason for biopsies, are extremely rare. If present in the majority of cases, the biopsy can relatively safely and easily be performed by gastroenterologists using endoscopic ultrasound-guided techniques [34]. Given the high overall accuracy of this technique, percutaneous image-guided biopsies should, if possible, be avoided [35]. This as the latter due to interposition of bowel loops carries a higher risk of complications.

Spleen

Historically biopsies of splenic lesions have been considered to be relatively complex. Due to the anatomical position of the spleen and its high vascularity, the risk of hemorrhagic complications was considered to be high. However, with modern imaging techniques biopsy of the spleen can safely be performed. The aim of splenic biopsies will in most cases be the determination of parenchymal lesions or staging of malignant lymphoma [29, 36]. In general an 18G tru-cut needle will be used for splenic biopsies.

Muraca et al. reviewed their experience in a series of 30 children aged 6 months to 15.3 years (mean, 7.0 years); there were focal lesions in 27 and homogeneous splenomegaly in three patients [29]. In this study a diagnosis was obtained in 25 children (83 %), a false-negative result in two children (7 %), and in three children (10 %) the biopsy was nondiagnostic.

Liang et al. evaluated 43 splenic biopsies for focal lesions ($N=27$ [16 single, 11 multiple]) or diffuse splenomegaly ($N=15$) in 42 patients. There was a random allocation to either an 18G cutting or a 21G needle biopsy. The accuracy of US-guided spleen biopsy in their study was 85.7 %, and the 18G biopsies had a higher diagnostic accuracy ($P<0.05$) and required fewer needle passes ($P<0.05$), without a significant difference in the overall complication rate [37].

Kidney

Although in daily clinical practice non-imaging-guided renal biopsies are still performed by clinicians, we feel that this practice should be discontinued. Although one would expect a significant difference in complication rates of blind versus image-guided biopsies, relatively few studies have been performed to demonstrate this. Maya et al. retrospectively analyzed 129 renal biopsies (65 were US guided and 64 were performed by blind technique and all biopsies were performed in an adult population) [38]. They found that in US-guided biopsies significantly more glomeruli were found and less large hematomas occurred and these biopsies were in 100 % diagnostically adequate.

In children the indications for renal biopsies range from generalized parenchymal disease (e.g., glomerulonephritis or nephrotic syndrome) to focal lesions (e.g., renal tumors) [4, 39, 40]. In case of generalized parenchymal disease, in general, two tissue samples of adequate size will suffice. In case of a renal tumor, the number of samples will be higher, especially if additional examinations, such as genetic marker studies, are planned. In these cases close collaboration between the treating pediatric oncologist and the radiologist is mandatory. In case of an oncological biopsy, care should be taken to biopsy through the retroperitoneal space, in order to avoid spread to the peritoneal cavity in case of post-biopsy hemorrhage, and the procedure should be performed using a coaxial technique, in order to decrease the risk of tumor seeding.

In renal biopsies care must be taken to avoid perforating the capsule, i.e., the core should be taken from the cortex only (in case of generalized disease) or from the tumor. This as trauma to the capsule will increase the risk of postprocedural hemorrhage. The approach should be from laterodorsal, in order to stay clear of the colon, and the biopsy needle angle should be either very steep or very shallow (Fig. 17.11).

In case of patients in whom percutaneous renal biopsy is contraindicated because of abnor-

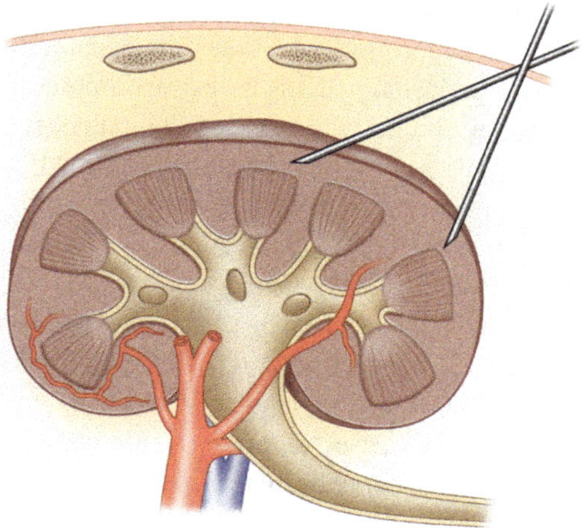

Fig. 17.11 In renal biopsy approach the biopsy needle angle should be either very steep or very shallow [39]

mal clotting, thrombocytopenia, and a single functioning kidney, a transjugular biopsy can be performed [41]. This procedure can safely be performed in experienced hands and in older children, as the available systems are not suited for small children, in those cases where a pathological diagnosis is critical to clinical management.

The major complications from a percutaneous renal biopsy consist of hemorrhage and/or the development of an arteriovenous fistula [39, 42–44]. Minor hematuria after renal biopsies is a common finding in up to 7 % of patients and this requires no intervention [43, 44]. It is sometimes advocated to perform a post-biopsy ultrasound 1 h after the biopsy; however, literature shows that the absence of a perinephric hematoma after a biopsy is indicative of an uncomplicated procedure; in contrast the presence of a perinephric hematoma is not predictive for a clinical relevant hematoma [45, 46]. In case of a major perinephric hematoma or the development of a significant arteriovenous fistula, radiological intervention may be warranted [42, 47, 48].

As renal biopsies are relatively safe procedures, it can, in patients without comorbidity, be performed in an outpatient clinic [49].

Chest and Lung Biopsies

Indications for biopsies from the chest, mediastinum, and lung consist of evaluation of a solitary pulmonary lung lesion, evaluation of multiple lesions in suspected metastatic disease, and evaluation of focal infection and pleural and mediastinal masses.

Poor cooperation caused by uncontrollable cough, severe underlying lung disease, severe pulmonary hypertension (particularly for central lesions), and bleeding diathesis (platelet count <50,000/μL/INR > 1.5) are contraindications for biopsies of the chest and lung.

Ultrasound guidance can be used for masses in the chest wall, in the pleura, and in the anterior mediastinum and for pleural-based nodules. This is the authors' preference.

However, most intrapulmonary and hilar lesions as well as mediastinal masses cannot be seen with US, and in those cases CT guidance is necessary. CT imaging can help to plan the needle course avoiding vital vascular structures, fissures, and bullae. Additional information can be obtained on the aspect of the mass (necrotic parts), therefore improving the biopsy yield.

For most biopsies of pleural masses and tumors of the chest wall, a single needle puncture technique can be used. For all other biopsies, a coaxial needle system is advised to obtain multiple tissue samples, using a single pleural puncture. This reduces the risk for a pneumothorax.

After cleansing the skin and covering the puncture site with sterile drapes, the skin and subcutaneous tissue are injected with lidocaine. The guiding needle is used to check the direction of the puncture course. When the procedure is CT guided, the use of a marker grid can be very helpful (Fig. 17.6a). When the needle is positioned in the right direction, the parietal pleura is passed and the needle is advanced in the direction of the target lesion (Fig. 17.6b). When possible the outer needle is positioned 2–3 mm in the edge of the tumor. Now multiple biopsies can be obtained. Normally a 22G needle aspiration biopsy obtains adequate tissue samples for diagnosing a malignancy (e.g., Cook, Bloomington, IN). In a coaxial system, a 19G outer needle is used. It is useful to have a cytopathologist present on site for immediate processing of the biopsy. It improves the biopsy yield, and when infection is suspected, extra material can be taken for further microbiological evaluation. For further differentiation of the tumor, e.g., suspected lymphoma, histological CNB are needed. For this an 18G cutting needle with spring-activated handle is used with a 16G guiding needle.

A CT-guided procedure is advised for biopsies of mediastinal masses. A full contrast-enhanced scan of the chest should be made to identify the target lesion in relation to all the surrounding vascular structures in the mediastinum (aorta, pulmonary artery, and particularly the internal mammary artery and vein).

If the procedure is CT guided, a single slice should be made at the end of the procedure at the level of the puncture site. If no pneumothorax is seen, the patient can be brought to the ward for observation and can be discharged after 2 h. A small, asymptomatic pneumothorax does not require any treatment, and the patient can be discharged after 4 h if free of symptoms. Symptomatic pneumothoraces (dyspnea, chest pain, size more than 30 % or increasing over time) must be treated. A pleural drainage with a 6–10 Fr pleural drain is performed, and the air is aspirated using a three-way stopcock. The patient must be admitted for further evaluation. If there is no air leakage several hours after the initial drainage, the drain can be removed and the patient can be discharged [50].

A pneumothorax is a quite common complication (5–60 %); risk factors are large needle size, traversing multiple pleural surfaces/fissures, multiple biopsies, and underlying lung disease [51].

Hemorrhage and hemoptysis are rare and mostly self-limiting. If the hemoptysis is moderate, the patient is turned on his lateral side in decubitus position, with the punctured lung downwards to prevent blood getting in to the contralateral lung.

Musculoskeletal

Where bone and soft tissue biopsies in adults usually can be performed under local anesthesia, pediatric bone biopsies should always be performed under general anesthesia.

In preparation of the biopsy, it is very important that all available previous imaging is carefully studied to help and plan the biopsy and to prevent unnecessary biopsies because of obvious benign lesions. The risk of complications should be weighed against the added value of the biopsy.

The most important indications for biopsies include establishing whether musculoskeletal lesions are benign or malignant (e.g., primary bone tumor, metastatic disease), determining the nature and extent of systemic disease (e.g., connective tissue disease), determining the nature of soft tissue masses, and microbiological analysis in patients with suspected infection.

Percutaneous bone biopsy should be discouraged when the location of the lesion is inaccessible (e.g., odontoid bone, anterior arch of C1), when there's the risk of soft tissue infection and bone contamination, or when there's a known coagulopathy.

Most bone biopsies are performed under CT guidance, sometimes in combination with fluoroscopy. The needle tract must be very carefully chosen, in collaboration with the orthopedic surgeon, to avoid damage to soft tissue structures like tendons, nerves, and vascular and visceral structures and to ensure that the needle tract will be excised in future surgery. This is especially important when limb-sparing surgery is considered [52]. Biopsies of the long bones could be best taken orthogonal to the cortex to avoid deflection of the needle and damaging soft tissue structures.

Biopsies of the vertebrae can be best taken by a transpedicular route or an intercostovertebral route, depending on the level, avoiding damage to segmental nerve branches. In pelvic biopsies, one should be careful in the sacral area, avoiding damage to the lumbosacral or femoral nerve plexus.

Soft tissue biopsies can be taken with 14–18G tru-cut biopsy needles. For bone biopsies, the authors usually use a 14G trephine needle or a14G Bonopty coaxial screw needle. Reported accuracy of musculoskeletal biopsy under image guiding is in the range of 94 % [53]. Reported complications varied from 0.2 to 1 % and include pain, hematoma, bone fracture, and infection [54]. Site-specific complications like pneumothorax and vascular and spinal cord injury are rare.

Miscellaneous

Lymph Nodes

Lymphadenopathy is quite common in children and in most cases the nodes are reactive. However, there are cases in which a diagnosis is deemed necessary, e.g., in case of staging oncology. In these cases FNA can be used as a first diagnostic modality. In the case of palpable lymph nodes, US guidance for FNA is not necessary.

Head and Neck

In pediatrics, (non-)palpable lesions in the region of the head and neck include a wide differential diagnosis including inflammatory lesions and both benign and malignant neoplasm (in contrast to adults, both malignant and benign epithelial neoplasms are rare in children). In these cases image-guided FNA plays an important role. It has been shown that FNA has a high sensitivity and specificity, with an almost negligible risk for the patient [55]. In adults the successful use of CNB in these patients has also been described [56]. And although this technique can safely be used in children, we feel that if a cytopathologist is available, FNA is the preferred technique in children.

Postprocedural Care

Complications

Complications from image-guided percutaneous biopsies can broadly be divided into two categories: generic and organ specific [1]. Generic complications are defined as complications common to all biopsies and include bleeding, infection, and unintended organ injury.

Organ-specific complications are defined as complications that are only associated or most commonly associated with biopsy of a specific organ. An example of an organ-specific complication is a pneumothorax after a lung biopsy; this is clearly related to the biopsied organ, but it can inadvertently also occur after other biopsies, e.g., a biopsy of the breast [57].

Complications, if they occur, should be coded according to the Society of Interventional Radiology Standards of Practice Committee (Table 17.1). A radiologist involved in pediatric biopsies should, in our opinion, also be able to treat the complications following this procedure. This implies that he/she should be able to perform transcatheter arterial embolization, a technique which has been proven to be highly successful [48, 58].

Table 17.1 Classification of complications by outcome [61]

Minor complications
A. No therapy, no consequence
B. Nominal therapy, no consequence; includes overnight admission for observation only
Major complications
C. Require therapy, minor hospitalization (<48 h)
D. Require major therapy, unplanned increase in level of care, prolonged hospitalization (>48 h)
E. Permanent adverse sequelae
F. Death

Biopsy Material

Histological core biopsies, whatever size, can be placed on a Petri disk with a blotter, wetted with saline or cell culture medium. Whenever the biopsies are not directly processed the same day by the pathologist, it could be kept in a small container with formaldehyde.

FNAB must be spread on a glass slide and dried. Ideally there is a cytologic technician available directly in the puncture suite, in order to process the material directly and can give feedback on the quality of the material and if more biopsies are needed for diagnosis.

Although slightly superfluous, it is of utmost important that labeling of the biopsy specimen is done with care.

Follow-Up

In case of FNA there is no need for follow-up. For CNB it strongly depends on the anatomical location and the related risk where the biopsy was performed; in case of a possible post-biopsy hemorrhage, clinical observation is advised. In all other cases the patient would be allowed to return home after sedation has fully worn off and the anesthesiologist deems it safe to leave the hospital.

Further Comments

Now that image-guided percutaneous biopsy has established itself as an effective and safe technique, the next step should be the definition of quality guidelines. In the USA the Society of Interventional Radiology published quality improvement guidelines for adult image-guided biopsies [1]. In these guidelines the authors present complication thresholds (Table 17.2). The authors state that as the published complication rates are mainly assessed in large series (of several hundred patients), they choose to recommend complication-specific thresholds set at twice the published complication-specific rates. Although there is something to be said in favor of this viewpoint, the suggested complication rate thresholds will not be acceptable for pediatricians and parents. In our viewpoint the Society for Pediatric Interventional Radiology should play a pivotal role in defining complication rate thresholds for pediatric percutaneous biopsies.

Perhaps a controversial topic, one which might not be expected in a pediatric interventional radiology book, is the question: who should perform the image-guided biopsies? Based on the relative scarcity of radiological equipment and the high cost of both purchase and maintenance, this has historically been a field of expertise dedicated to radiologists. For CT and MRI one might expect that this, in general, will remain so for the coming decades. However, in case of ultrasonography, the decreasing total cost of ownership will lead to more and more physicians, other than radiologists, that are buying their own ultrasonography systems. There are hardly any studies that deal with this specific topic. Lieu, a pathologist, published a study on 500 consecutive adult cases, 415 patients with average age of 50.5 years (range 10–89), of image-guided FNA and CNB in adults performed by a pathologist [59]. In total 395 (79 %) non-palpable masses were biopsied; the locations of these lesions were as follows: thyroid 189 (48 %), breast 144 (36 %), head and neck 47 (12 %), and 15 other (not specified) lesions. In this study the biopsy was diagnostic in, respectively, 97.4 % (thyroid), 100 % (breast), 98 % (head and neck), and 100 % in other sites. Overall the biopsy was diagnostic in 98.6 % of cases. One can only wonder, when we will see the emergence of the "interventional pathologist?"

Finally, although less than an issue in adult radiology, we need to be aware of overdiagnosis. In 2010, Hall published a paper in *Radiology* entitled "Identification, Biopsy, and Treatment of Poorly Understood Premalignant, In Situ, and Indolent Low-Grade Cancers: Are We Becoming Victims of Our Own Success?" [60]. In this paper the effects of increasing screening on the one hand (a topic which is less of a focus in pediatrics) and increasing imaging sensitivity on the other hand (definitely an issue in pediatrics) with regard to increasing numbers of percutaneous biopsies, often yielding no diagnosis or a benign diagnosis, are discussed. As we are better equipped to find small lesions, percutaneous biopsies in adults on borderline, preinvasive, or low-grade cancers are now increasingly being performed. In pediatric interventional radiology we should learn from our adult colleagues and avoid this pitfall.

Table 17.2 Major complications for image-guided percutaneous biopsy [1]

Major complications	Reported rate (%)	Suggested threshold (%)
Bleeding (requiring transfusion or intervention)		
Large needle (18G or larger)	5–10	10
Small needle (19G or smaller)	3	6
Fine needle (21G or smaller)	0.1–2.0	2
Infection (requiring hospitalization or specific therapy)		
All biopsies (sterile)	1	2
Peritonitis (requiring hospitalization or specific therapy)		
Abdominal biopsies	1.5	2
Hemoptysis (requiring hospitalization or specific therapy)		
Lung biopsies	0.5	1
Pneumothorax (requiring chest tube)		
All biopsies (other than lung)	0.5	1
Lung biopsies	5	10

Chapter Summary

Indications

- Diagnosis
  - Benign versus malignant
  - Staging
  - Microbiology sampling
  - Parenchymal disease

Contraindications

- Uncorrectable bleeding diathesis
- Lack of safe access route
- Ascites
- Single native kidney
- Uncontrollable cough, severe lung disease, severe pulmonary hypertension

Equipment

- US, fluoroscopy, CT, MRI
- Needle
  - Fine
  - Screw needle
  - Core
  - Specialized—bone, transjugular
- Transport medium—depends on tissue being sampled and institutional practices
  - Formaldehyde
  - Cell transport medium
  - Special handling requirements for metabolic samples, metal determination

Preprocedural Work-Up

- Preprocedural imaging
- Informed consent
- Blood work
- Consider ordering blood ± having in room for high-risk procedures

Patient Preparation

- GA versus sedation
  - GA with apnea may be necessary for small lesions
- IV started
- Positioned appropriately
- Prep area

Technique

- Liver
  - CT or US
  - Avoid transpleural puncture
  - 16–18G needle
  - Consider coaxial technique and tract embolization
- Transjugular liver
  - When percutaneous biopsy is unsafe
  - TIPS or LAB set
  - Monitor with fluoroscopy ± ultrasound
- Pancreas
  - Endoscopic biopsy preferred
- Spleen
  - 18G needles
- Kidney
  - Ultrasound better than blind biopsy
  - Two samples for renal disease, more samples for neoplastic lesion
  - Retroperitoneal, posterolateral approach (especially with neoplastic lesion)
  - Consider coaxial
  - Transjugular renal biopsy can be performed
  - Hemorrhage or AV fistula occasionally need intervention
- Chest and lung
  - US for anterior mediastinum and pleural-based nodules, CT for all others
  - Coaxial technique to decrease pneumothorax risk
  - 18–20G core needle, 22G aspiration needle
  - Monitor for postprocedural pneumothorax
  - When bleeding occurs, place puncture site down to protect contralateral lung
  - Consider double endotracheal intubation for high-risk lung biopsy
- Musculoskeletal
  - GA
  - Careful evaluation of imaging
  - CT ± fluoroscopy for bone
  - Must assure appropriate access site if limb reconstruction or surgical resection possible

Postprocedural Care

- Monitor for complications—bleeding, infection, nontarget tissue damage

References

1. Gupta S, Wallace MJ, Cardella JF, Kundu S, Miller DL, Rose SC. Quality improvement guidelines for percutaneous needle biopsy. J Vasc Interv Radiol. 2010;21(7):969–75.
2. Kwan SW, Bhargavan M, Kerlan Jr RK, Sunshine JH. Effect of advanced imaging technology on how biopsies are done and who does them. Radiology. 2010; 256(3):751–8.
3. Stiller CA, Draper GJ. The epidemiology of cancer in children. In: Voute PA, Barrett A, Stevens MCG, Caron HN, editors. Cancer in children: clinical management. 5th ed. New York: Oxford University Press; 2005. p. 1–16.
4. Sebire NJ, Roebuck DJ. Pathological diagnosis of pediatric tumours from image-guided needle core biopsies: a systematic review. Pediatr Radiol. 2006; 36(5):426–31.
5. Chowdhury T, Barnacle A, Haque S, et al. Ultrasound-guided core needle biopsy for the diagnosis of rhabdomyosarcoma in childhood. Pediatr Blood Cancer. 2009;53(3):356–60.
6. ACR–SIR–SPR practice guideline for the performance of image-guided percutaneous needle biopsy (PNB) (2013) http://www.acr.org/~/media/1D9E3F3 270CF44F8A2E994C94F2F0FAC.pdf date accessed 10-2-14.
7. Atwell TD, Smith RL, Hesley GK, et al. Incidence of bleeding after 15,181 percutaneous biopsies and the role of aspirin. AJR Am J Roentgenol. 2010;194(3): 784–9.
8. Murphy FB, Barefield KP, Steinberg HV, Bernardino ME. CT- or sonography-guided biopsy of the liver in the presence of ascites: frequency of complications. AJR Am J Roentgenol. 1988;151(3):485–6.
9. Little AF, Ferris JV, Dodd III GD, Baron RL. Image-guided percutaneous hepatic biopsy: effect of ascites on the complication rate. Radiology. 1996;199(1): 79–83.
10. Health and Public Policy Committee. Clinical competence in percutaneous renal biopsy. American College of Physicians. Ann Intern Med. 1988;108(2):301–3.
11. Wickre CG, Golper TA. Complications of percutaneous needle biopsy of the kidney. Am J Nephrol. 1982;2(4):173–8.
12. Wiebe S, Cohen J, Connolly B, Chait P. Percutaneous decompression of the bowel with a small-caliber needle: a method to facilitate percutaneous abdominal access. AJR Am J Roentgenol. 2005;184(1):227–9.
13. Keeling AN, Reekers JA, Lee MJ. The clinical practice of interventional radiology: a European perspective. Cardiovasc Intervent Radiol. 2009;32(3):406–11.
14. Shlomovitz E, Amaral JG, Chait PG. Image-guided therapy and minimally invasive surgery in children: a merging future. Pediatr Radiol. 2006;36(5):398–404.
15. Ward ST, Shepherd JA, Khalil H. Freehand versus ultrasound-guided core biopsies of the breast: reducing the burden of repeat biopsies in patients presenting to the breast clinic. Breast. 2010;19(2):105–8.
16. Hatada T, Ishii H, Ichii S, Okada K, Yamamura T. Ultrasound-guided fine-needle aspiration biopsy for breast tumors: needle guide versus freehand technique. Tumori. 1999;85(1):12–4.
17. Phal PM, Brooks DM, Wolfe R. Sonographically guided biopsy of focal lesions: a comparison of freehand and probe-guided techniques using a phantom. AJR Am J Roentgenol. 2005;184(5):1652–6.
18. Brenner DJ, Elliston CD, Hall EJ, Berdon WE. Estimated risks of radiation induced fatal cancer from pediatric CT. AJR Am J Roentgenol. 2001;176: 289–96.
19. Schulz T, Trobs RB, Schneider JP, Hirsch W, Schmidt F, Kahn T. MR imaging-guided percutaneous procedures in children. Acad Radiol. 2005;12(9): 1128–34.
20. Schulz T, Trobs RB, Schneider JP, et al. Pediatric MR-guided interventions. Eur J Radiol. 2005;53(1): 57–66.
21. Kuhn JP, Langner S, Hegenscheid K, et al. Magnetic resonance-guided upper abdominal biopsies in a high-field wide-bore 3-T MRI system: feasibility, handling, and needle artefacts. Eur Radiol. 2010;20(10): 2414–21.
22. Zangos S, Muller C, Mayer F, et al. [Retrospective 5-year analysis of MR-guided biopsies in a low-field MR system]. Rofo. 2009;181(7):658–63.
23. Schenck JF. The role of magnetic susceptibility in magnetic resonance imaging: MRI magnetic compatibility of the first and second kinds. Med Phys. 1996;23(6):815–50.
24. Lindh V, Wiklund U, Hakansson S. Assessment of the effect of EMLA during venipuncture in the newborn by analysis of heart rate variability. Pain. 2000;86(3): 247–54.
25. Kapelushnik J, Koren G, Solh H, Greenberg M, DeVeber L. Evaluating the efficacy of EMLA in alleviating pain associated with lumbar puncture; comparison of open and double-blinded protocols in children. Pain. 1990;42(1):31–4.
26. Lurngnateetape A, Tritrakarn T. Placebo effect of eutectic mixture of lidocaine and prilocaine (EMLA) cream in reducing venepuncture pain in children. Ann Acad Med Singapore. 1994;23(4):465–9.
27. Nobili V, Comparcola D, Sartorelli MR, et al. Blind and ultrasound-guided percutaneous liver biopsy in children. Pediatr Radiol. 2003;33(11):772–5.
28. Hoffer FA. Liver biopsy methods for pediatric oncology patients. Pediatr Radiol. 2000;30(7):481–8.
29. Muraca S, Chait PG, Connolly BL, Baskin KM, Temple MJ. US-guided core biopsy of the spleen in children. Radiology. 2001;218:200–6.
30. Lachar WA, Shahab I, Saad J. Accuracy and cost-effectiveness of core needle biopsy in the evaluation of suspected lymphoma: a study of 101 cases. Arch Pathol Lab Med. 2007;131:1033–9.
31. Kaye RD, Towbin RB. Imaging and intervention in the gastrointestinal tract in children. Gastroenterol Clin North Am. 2002;31(3):897–923.

32. Riddle C, Ahmed B, Doyle J, Connolly BL. Migration of Gelfoam to the gallbladder after liver biopsy. Pediatr Radiol. 2008;38(7):806–9.
33. Mammen T, Keshava SN, Eapen CE, et al. Transjugular liver biopsy: a retrospective analysis of 601 cases. J Vasc Interv Radiol. 2008;19(3):351–8.
34. Salla C, Chatzipantelis P, Konstantinou P, Karoumpalis I, Pantazopoulou A, Dappola V. Endoscopic ultrasound-guided fine-needle aspiration cytology diagnosis of solid pseudopapillary tumor of the pancreas: a case report and literature review. World J Gastroenterol. 2007;13(38):5158–68.
35. Muller MF, Meyerberger C, Bertschinger P, Schaer R, Marincek B. Pancreatic tumors: evaluation with endoscopic US, CT, and MR imaging. Radiology. 1994;190:745–51.
36. Tam A, Krishnamurthy S, Pilsbury EP, et al. Percutaneous image-guided splenic biopsy in the oncology patient: an audit of 156 consecutive cases. J Vasc Interv Radiol. 2008;19:80–8.
37. Liang P, Gao Y, Wang Y, Yu X, Yu D, Dong B. US-guided percutaneous needle biopsy of the spleen using 18-gauge versus 21-gauge needles. J Clin Ultrasound. 2007;35(9):477–82.
38. Maya ID, Maddela P, Barker J, Allon M. Percutaneous renal biopsy: comparison of blind and real-time ultrasound-guided technique. Semin Dial. 2007;20(4): 355–8.
39. Roebuck DJ. Genitourinary intervention in children. Pediatr Radiol. 2011;41(1):17–26.
40. Vujanic GM, Kelsey A, Mitchell C, Shannon RS, Gornall P. The role of biopsy in the diagnosis of renal tumors of childhood: results of the UKCCSG Wilms tumor study 3. Med Pediatr Oncol. 2003;40(1): 18–22.
41. See TC, Thompson BC, Howie AJ, et al. Transjugular renal biopsy: our experience and technical considerations. Cardiovasc Intervent Radiol. 2008;31(5): 906–18.
42. Riccabona M, Schwinger W, Ring E. Arteriovenous fistula after renal biopsy in children. J Ultrasound Med. 1998;17(8):505–8.
43. Hergesell O, Felten H, Andrassy K, Kuhn K, Ritz E. Safety of ultrasound-guided percutaneous renal biopsy-retrospective analysis of 1090 consecutive cases. Nephrol Dial Transplant. 1998;13(4):975–7.
44. Sinha MD, Lewis MA, Bradbury MG, Webb NJ. Percutaneous real-time ultrasound-guided renal biopsy by automated biopsy gun in children: safety and complications. J Nephrol. 2006;19(1):41–4.
45. Ishikawa E, Nomura S, Hamaguchi T, et al. Ultrasonography as a predictor of overt bleeding after renal biopsy. Clin Exp Nephrol. 2009;13(4):325–31.
46. Waldo B, Korbet SM, Freimanis MG, Lewis EJ. The value of post-biopsy ultrasound in predicting complications after percutaneous renal biopsy of native kidneys. Nephrol Dial Transplant. 2009;24(8): 2433–9.
47. Novellas S, Chevallier P, Motamedi JP, Kurzenne JY, Berard E, Bruneton JN. Superselective embolization of a post-biopsy renal pseudoaneurysm in a 13-month-old infant. Pediatr Radiol. 2006;36(8):874–6.
48. Pappas P, Constantinides C, Leonardou P, et al. Biopsy-related hemorrhage of renal allografts treated by percutaneous superselective segmental renal artery embolization. Transplant Proc. 2006;38(5):1375–8.
49. Al MA, Al-Akash S. Safety of percutaneous renal biopsy as an outpatient procedure in pediatric patients. Ann Saudi Med. 2006;26(4):303–5.
50. Brown KT, Brody LA, Getrajdman GI, Napp TE. Outpatient treatment of iatrogenic pneumothorax after needle biopsy. Radiology. 1997;205(1): 249–52.
51. Perlmutt LM, Johnston WW, Dunnick NR. Percutaneous transthoracic needle aspiration: a review. AJR Am J Roentgenol. 1989;152(3):451–5.
52. Liu PT, Valadez SD, Chivers FS, Roberts CC, Beauchamp CP. Anatomically based guidelines for core needle biopsy of bone tumors: implications for limb-sparing surgery. Radiographics. 2007;27(1): 189–205.
53. Murphy WA, Destouet JM, Gilula LA. Percutaneous skeletal biopsy 1981: a procedure for radiologists—results, review, and recommendations. Radiology. 1981;139(3):545–9.
54. Carrasco CH, Wallace S, Richli WR. Percutaneous skeletal biopsy. Cardiovasc Intervent Radiol. 1991; 14(1):69–72.
55. Rapkiewicz A, Le BT, Simsir A, Cangiarella J, Levine P. Spectrum of head and neck lesions diagnosed by fine-needle aspiration cytology in the pediatric population. Cancer. 2007;111(4):242–51.
56. Pfeiffer J, Kayser G, Technau-Ihling K, Boedeker CC, Ridder GJ. Ultrasound-guided core-needle biopsy in the diagnosis of head and neck masses: indications, technique and results. Head Neck. 2007;29:1033–40.
57. Meyer JE, Smith DN, Lester SC, et al. Large-core needle biopsy of nonpalpable breast lesions. JAMA. 1999;281(17):1638–41.
58. Perini S, Gordon RL, LaBerge JM, et al. Transcatheter embolization of biopsy-related vascular injury in the transplant kidney: immediate and long-term outcome. J Vasc Interv Radiol. 1998;9(6):1011–9.
59. Lieu D. Cytopathologist-performed ultrasound-guided fine-needle aspiration and core-needle biopsy: a prospective study of 500 consecutive cases. Diagn Cytopathol. 2008;36:317–24.
60. Hall FM. Identification, biopsy, and treatment of poorly understood premalignant, in situ, and indolent low-grade cancers: are we becoming victims of our own success? Radiology. 2010;254:655–9.
61. Cardella JF, Bakal CW, Bertino RE, et al. Quality improvement guidelines for image-guided percutaneous biopsy in adults. J Vasc Interv Radiol. 2003;14(9 Pt 2):S227–30.
62. Horner MJ, Ries LAG, Krapcho M, Neyman N, Aminou R, Howlader N, Altekruse SF, Feuer EJ, Huang L, Mariotto A, Miller BA, Lewis DR, Eisner MP, Stinchcomb DG, Edwards BK, editors. SEER cancer statistics review, 1975–2006. Bethesda, MD: National Cancer Institute. http://seer.cancer.gov/csr/1975_2006/, based on November 2008 SEER data submission, posted to the SEER web site, 2009.

Section VI

Nonvascular Interventions: Fluid Drainage

Drainage Procedures in Children 18

Mark J. Hogan

Background

Image-guided drainage is a common procedure in a pediatric interventional radiology practice and the treatment of choice for many conditions [1]. As in adult practice, both primary and postoperative fluid collections have been successfully treated by image-guided techniques resulting in improved patient care [1–17]. Drainage can be performed in almost any organ system. While the techniques in children are similar to those in adults, there are several important differences. The etiologies of abscesses and fluid collections may be different [1, 3–5, 7–11]. Radiation protection is paramount in the pediatric population requiring alteration of both imaging and technique [18–20]. Children have different sedation and anesthetic requirements [21, 22]. In addition, children may be much smaller than adults. This has both advantages and disadvantages and may require/allow for alteration of the procedural techniques.

In children, the most common cause of abdominal abscesses is appendicitis [1–3, 23–27]. Abscesses may be identified at presentation or after surgery. Abscesses from appendicitis are more common in children as the diagnosis may be harder to make leading to delayed surgery and an increased risk of perforation (Figs. 18.1 and 18.2) [25, 26, 28–30]. Other common fluid collection etiologies in the abdomen include cerebrospinal fluid pseudocyst, posttraumatic collections, pancreatic fluid collections, acalculous cholecystitis, ovarian cysts in neonates, and abscesses due to Crohn's disease or necrotizing enterocolitis (Figs. 18.3, 18.4, 18.5, and 18.6) [4–6, 31].

Etiologies outside of the abdomen include pleural and pulmonary collections, joint effusions (septic or sterile), soft tissue infections from cellulitis, osteomyelitis, suppurative adenitis, para-tonsillar and other neck abscesses, and congenital lesions such as lymphatic malformations, thyroglossal duct cysts, and branchial cleft cysts (Figs. 18.7 and 18.8) [7–10].

Indications/Contraindications

Drainage of any of these collections should only be performed when [32]:

1. There is a suspicion of infection.
2. There is a need for fluid characterization.
3. The collection is causing symptoms sufficient to warrant drainage.

Contraindications are all relative. Any coagulopathies should be evaluated and corrected if possible. If safe access is not possible due to vital organs such as bowel surrounding the abscess, surgical treatment may be preferable if the approach cannot be altered to avoid these

M.J. Hogan, M.D. (✉)
Department of Radiology, Nationwide Children's Hospital, The Ohio State University, 700 Children's Drive, Columbus, OH 45205, USA
e-mail: mark.hogan@nationwidechildrens.org

M. Temple and F.E. Marshalleck (eds.), *Pediatric Interventional Radiology: Handbook of Vascular and Non-Vascular Interventions*, DOI 10.1007/978-1-4419-5856-3_18,

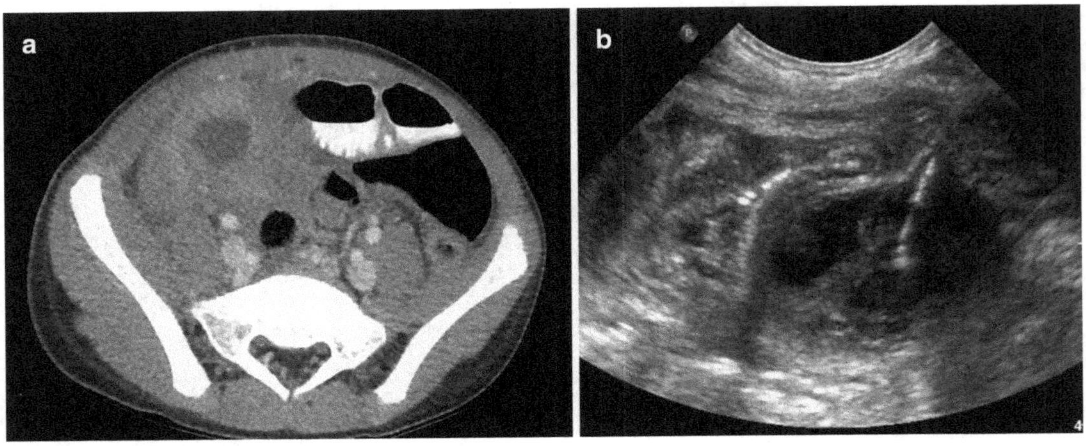

Fig. 18.1 A CT scan shows a right lower quadrant abscess in this patient with perforated appendicitis (**a**). Using ultrasound guidance, this abscess was accessed and drained (**b**)

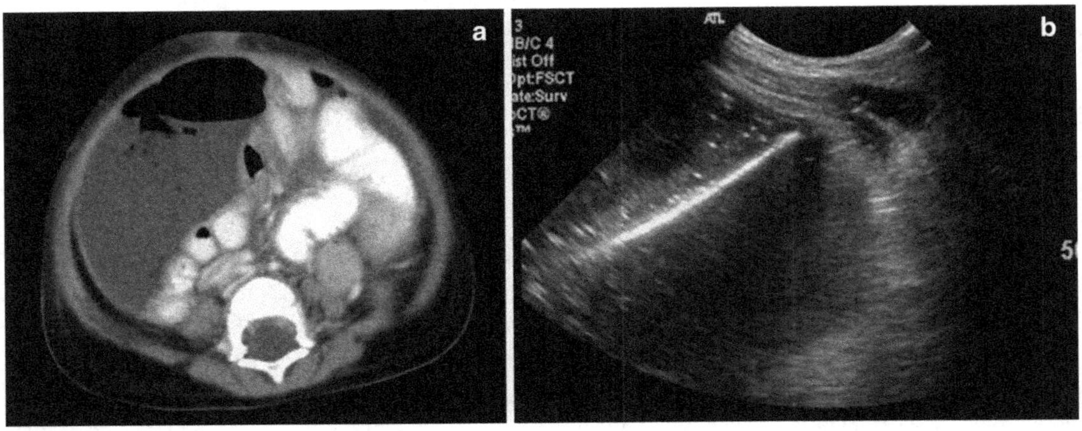

Fig. 18.2 Persistent fever after appendectomy. A large right lower quadrant abscess is identified with CT (**a**), with subsequent ultrasound-guided drainage (**b**)

structures. As with all procedures, the benefits of drainage should be weighed with regard to the patient's overall clinical status.

Preprocedure Evaluation

It is important that the interventional radiologist be involved in defining the protocols used in imaging patients that might benefit from image-guided treatment. It is important that these imaging studies be tailored to the patients' symptoms, possible diagnoses, and potential treatment options including the best access approach. If a CT scan is the study of choice, it should be done with the lowest radiation dose possible and be performed to answer all of the necessary questions listed above. CT may be the fastest, the least operator dependent, and the easiest choice; however, there is a significant radiation dose and risk [18–20]. For abdominal pain greater than 48 h, a CT with intravenous and enteric (oral and/or rectal) contrast best identifies all abscesses and possible interposed bowel. Ultrasound eliminates radiation-associated risk, but is a time-intensive procedure, may be limited to the available window that is hampered by bone or gas, and can be difficult to learn. Ultrasound may be adequate for superficial lesions or in neonates, and MRI is useful in bone or some soft tissue abscesses [11, 33].

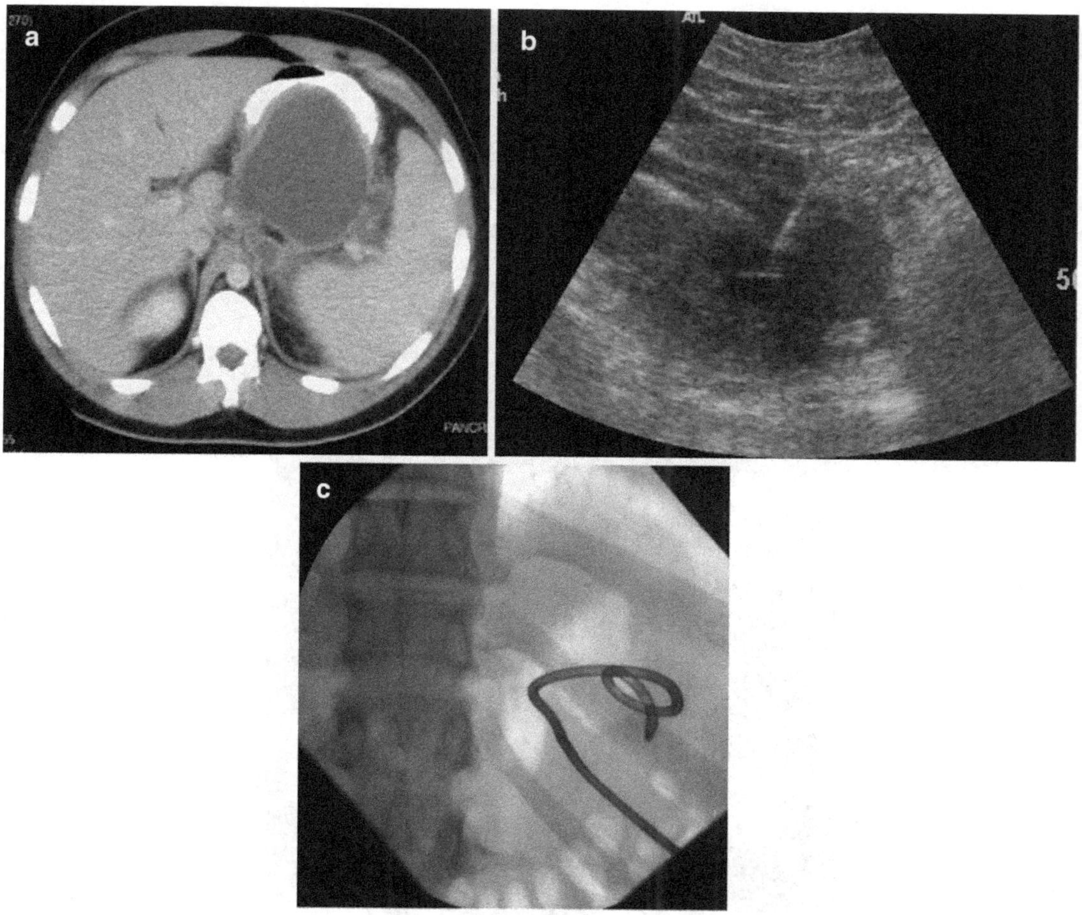

Fig. 18.3 This child had medication-induced pancreatitis and persistent fevers. The CT scan shows a pseudocyst arising from the pancreas (**a**). Utilizing ultrasound guidance (**b**), the pseudocyst was accessed and a drain placed with fluoroscopic guidance (**c**)

Routine coagulation parameters are not typically checked unless there is a suspicion of coagulopathy. General guidelines are that elective procedures can be performed safely with a platelet count of >50,000 platelets/μL, PT<18, PTT<32, and an INR<1.5.

Many patients are on antibiotics prior to the drainage procedure due to concerns of infection. If not, prophylactic antibiotics may be indicated as manipulation of an infected collection may precipitate sepsis.

Equipment

The vast majority of collections can be drained with ultrasound guidance, which has several advantages. This avoids radiation exposure to the patient, and real-time imaging allows for multiple approaches and increases safety. However, proper ultrasound equipment is needed. Patients can vary in size from less than 1 kg to greater than 200 kg. Therefore, multiple different transducers (including endocavitary probes) must be available ranging from 3 to 10 MHz or greater MHz, and the interventionalist should be familiar with and able to use all of them.

CT guidance may be indicated if the collection is inadequately visualized with ultrasound; however, it is rarely needed (Fig. 18.9a, b). If CT is used, the exposure should be limited, and CT fluoroscopy techniques minimized [18].

Fluoroscopy may be useful during wire placement, tract dilation, and catheter deployment; however, many pediatric interventional radiologists substitute ultrasound guidance during these steps to eliminate unnecessary radiation.

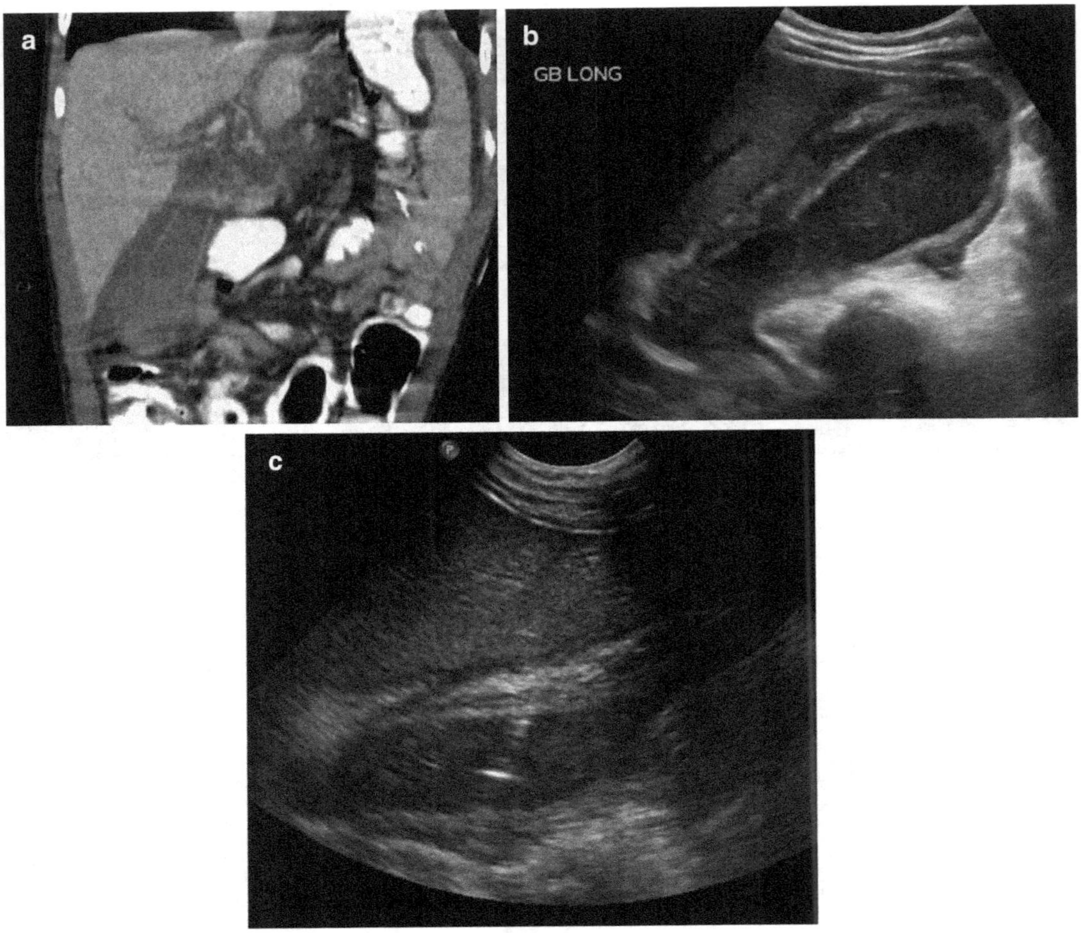

Fig. 18.4 This patient had sepsis after trauma. The CT scan shows an enlarged gallbladder with a thickened wall (**a**). This appearance of acalculous cholecystitis is confirmed with ultrasound (**b**). Ultrasound guidance was used to place a drain (**c**)

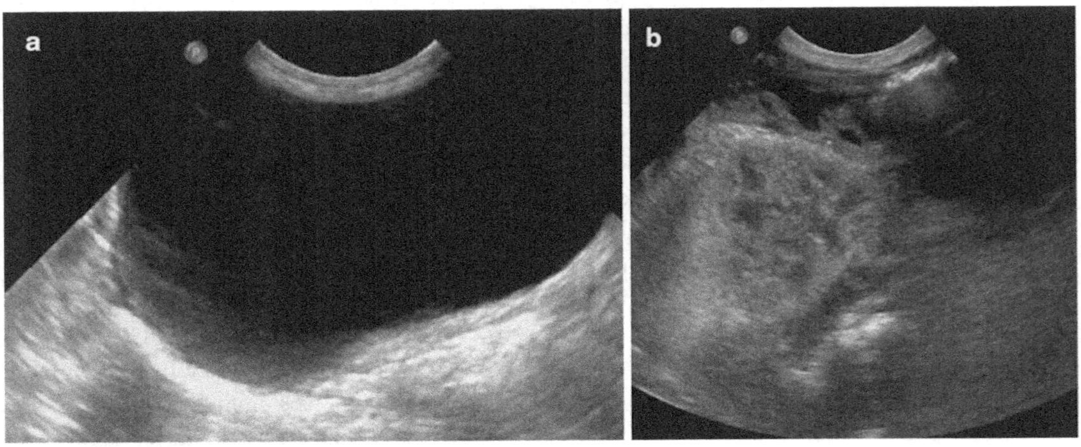

Fig. 18.5 This neonate has a large ovarian cyst due to prior transplacental maternal hormones (**a**). While these typically resolve over time, when they are over 4–6 cm in size, there is a risk of torsion. Ultrasound is used to drain the cyst completely (**b**)

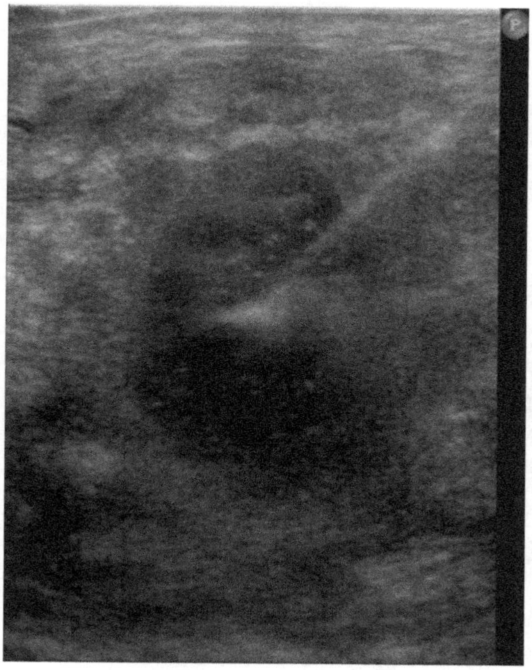

Fig. 18.6 Ultrasound is used to aspirate this abscess from necrotizing enterocolitis. The procedure was performed portably in the neonatal intensive care unit

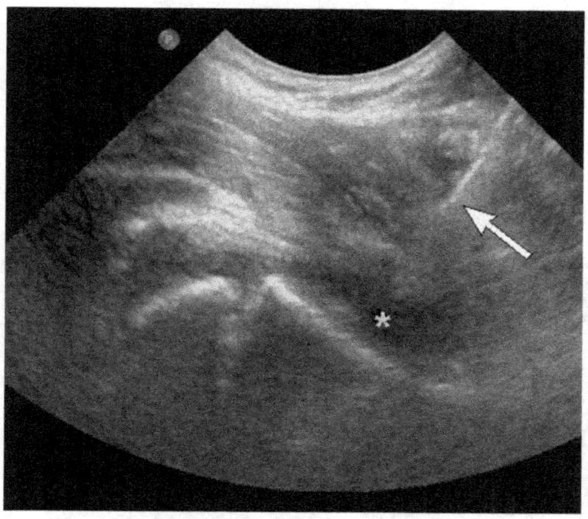

Fig. 18.7 Joint effusion is identified in the hip. Ultrasound is used to guide aspiration to evaluate for a septic joint

Most collections are accessible with standard needle and wire techniques. Both standard and micropuncture needles should be available. Standard drainage catheters (8–14 Fr) are typically placed, but smaller catheters (5 or 6 Fr) can be used for small collections. The size of the catheter is estimated by the expected fluid characterization and by any fluid aspirated during the initial puncture. Catheters also come with different loop diameters, and the appropriate choice must be made based on the size of the collection.

Procedure Technique

Most children will not be able to cooperate with the procedure without sort form of sedation or anesthesia to ensure a successful and safe outcome. Sedation or anesthesia is often the most difficult and dangerous portion of the procedure [21, 22]. Although select situations and patients may require only local anesthetic administration, most will likely require a higher level of sedation than in adults, and possibly general anesthesia with intubation. The interventionalist must help plan for this and decide what level of support the patient needs, given patient age and pain tolerance, difficulty of the procedure, and expected level of pain from the procedure. The interventional radiologist must be trained and experienced with multiple medications including dosages and antagonists, as well as life support and resuscitation methods. Topical anesthetic creams are useful adjuncts for patients undergoing conscious sedation to lessen the painful sensation caused by local anesthetic infiltration (see Chaps. 2 and 3 for more information).

The choice of which type of imaging is used for guidance is based on which modality provides for the safest procedure with the highest likelihood of success. Ultrasound guidance is by far the most common in children. The smaller body habitus in most children allows for better visualization during imaging guidance. The multiplanar capability of freehand imaging allows for many choices of access site and trajectory. As discussed previously, ultrasound eliminates the radiation risk. However, ultrasound may not be the optimal imaging modality in certain circumstances. Interposed air or bone may preclude visualization of the fluid collection, requiring alternative guidance. In obese patients, ultrasound may not provide adequate visualization.

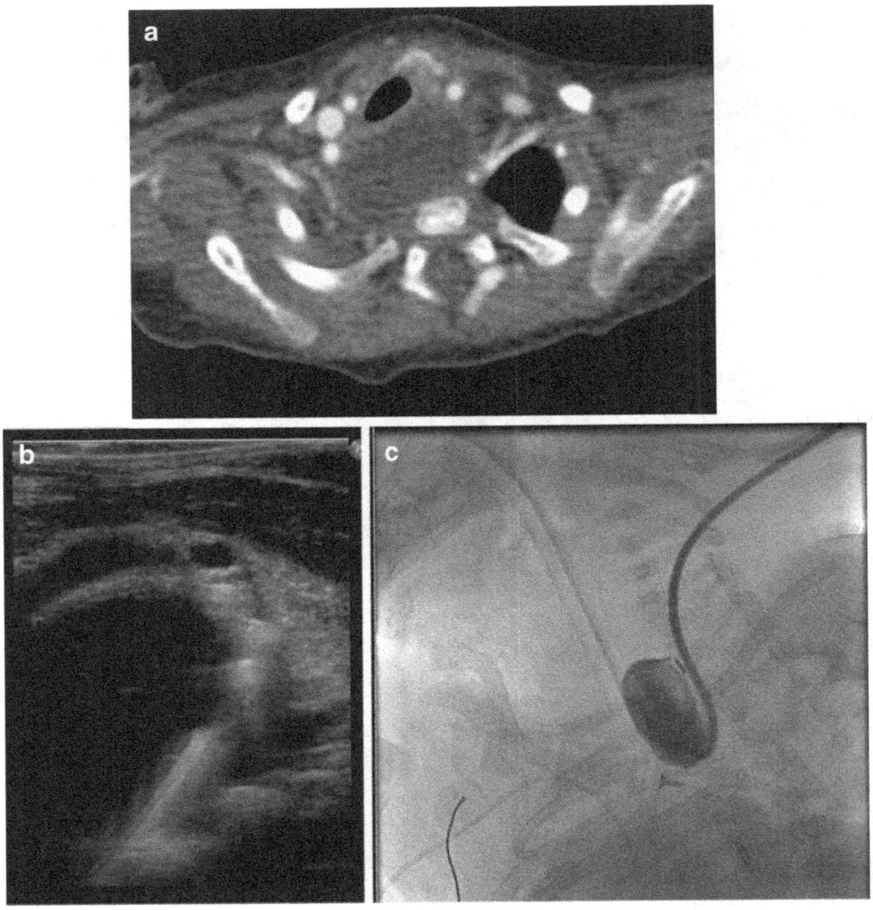

Fig. 18.8 This patient has an infected esophageal duplication cyst seen on CT (**a**). A micropuncture type set is used to access the cyst with ultrasound guidance (**b**). After drain placement (**c**), the patient had sclerotherapy on this cyst

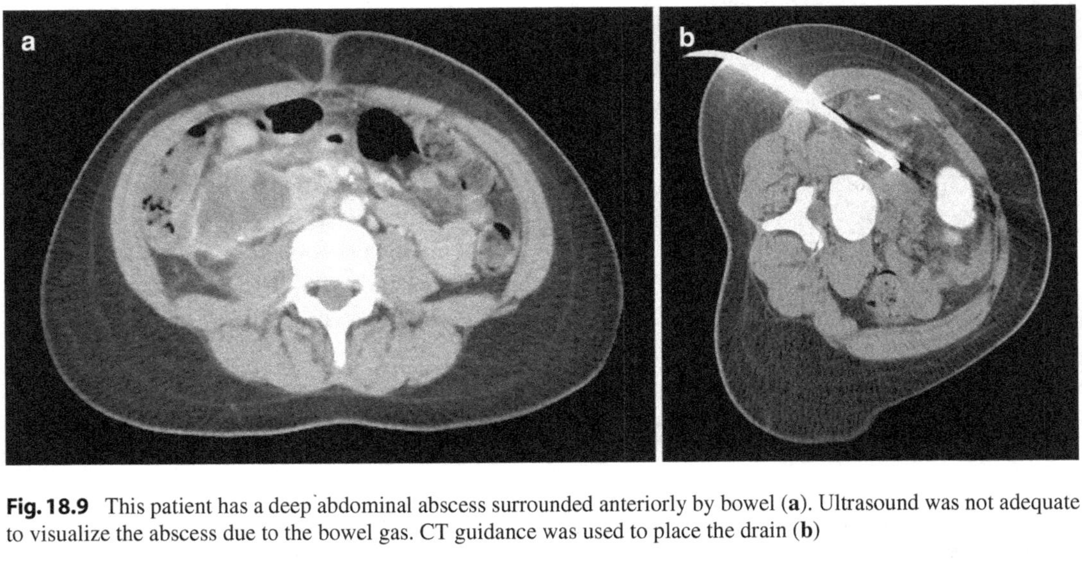

Fig. 18.9 This patient has a deep abdominal abscess surrounded anteriorly by bowel (**a**). Ultrasound was not adequate to visualize the abscess due to the bowel gas. CT guidance was used to place the drain (**b**)

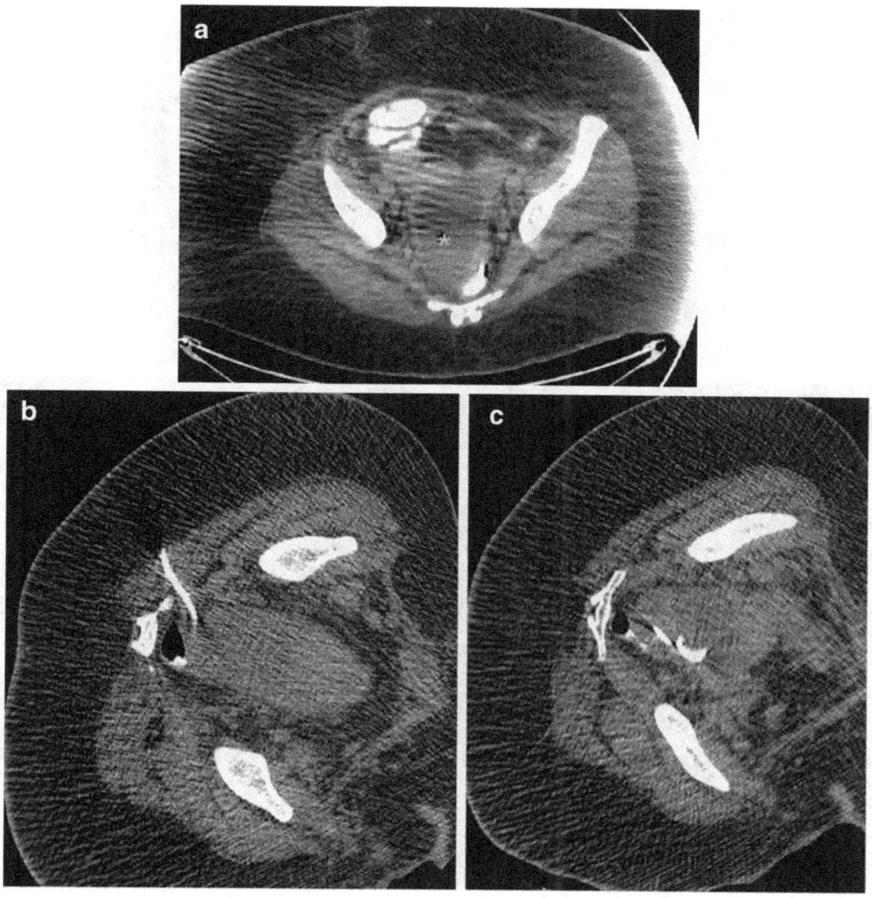

Fig. 18.10 Pelvic abscess in a pediatric patient after bariatric surgery. The initial CT shows the pelvic abscess (**a**). CT guidance was used to place the transgluteal drain (**b** and **c**)

In addition, certain techniques and situations may be better performed with alternative guidance. Transgluteal drainage can be performed with ultrasound, but may be easier with CT (Fig. 18.10a–c) [17]. CT-guided drainage of pneumothoraces or pneumatoceles in the lung may be better with CT or fluoroscopic guidance.

Prior to the procedure, ultrasound scanning should be performed by the interventional radiologist. This will help determine the appropriate transducer to use, the best window, and allow for optimization of gain, depth, field of view, and focal zone.

For most drainage procedures, a standard percutaneous approach with the Seldinger technique is used. Micropuncture sets allow puncture with a 21- or 22-gauge needle. Typically a 0.018-in. wire is advanced over which an introducer is placed. The introducer allows advancement of a 0.035-in. wire. This wire can be used for tract dilation and catheter guidance. This may be important in areas with a small window of access. Alternatively, a larger needle that accepts a 0.035-in. wire can be used primarily. Specialized or altered techniques in children are utilized when imaging demonstrates a potential complication such as interposed organs, bowel, or blood vessels or when another approach is easier to perform such as in deep pelvic abscesses or small collections such as some congenital malformations [10, 12–14, 34].

For deep pelvic abscesses, transgluteal and transrectal approaches are both possible in children, but the transgluteal approach may have a higher

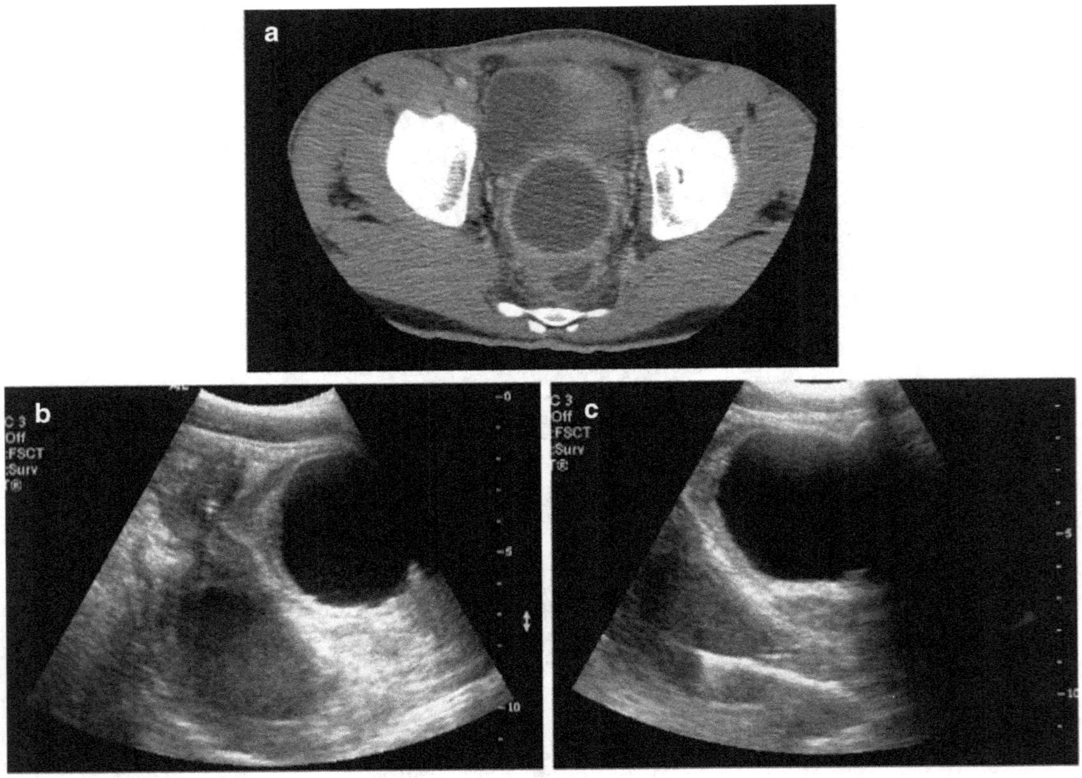

Fig. 18.11 There is a deep pelvic abscess in this patient after perforated appendicitis (**a**). Transabdominal scanning demonstrates the abscess deep to the bladder (**b**). Utilizing this ultrasound position for guidance, a needle is advanced transrectally into the abscess for drainage (**c**)

risk of hemorrhage or pain [12–14, 16, 17, 34]. The ability to advance a transrectal transducer depends on the size of the patient and the transducer. Teenagers can usually be treated with transrectal guidance, while younger children might need transabdominal guidance. General anesthesia is recommended for transrectal drainage [35].

With transabdominal guidance, the transducer is typically placed in a sagittal orientation over the lower midline abdomen (Fig. 18.11a–c). Filling the bladder with saline via a catheter may provide a better window for visualization. Several techniques have been described to safely advancing a needle and subsequently a drain into the abscess without injuring the rectal mucosa [12–14]. The stylet from the drain may be removed, and the blunt catheter tip advanced into the rectum with a trocar technique employed. Alternatively, a type of tube may be first placed with ultrasound guidance into the rectum. Enema tips, the stiffener from the abscess drain, and the plastic tubes that come from the manufacturer to protect the needles in the package can be used. When the introducer abuts the abscess, the needle is placed through the channel and then advanced into the abscess. Once the needle is in the abscess, the catheter is placed in standard fashion. The entire procedure is performed with ultrasound guidance.

Alternatively, depending on the patient's size and the size of the endocavitary probe, transrectal ultrasound imaging can be performed. Utilizing a needle guide, access can be gain to the pelvic abscess via a transrectal approach and real-time

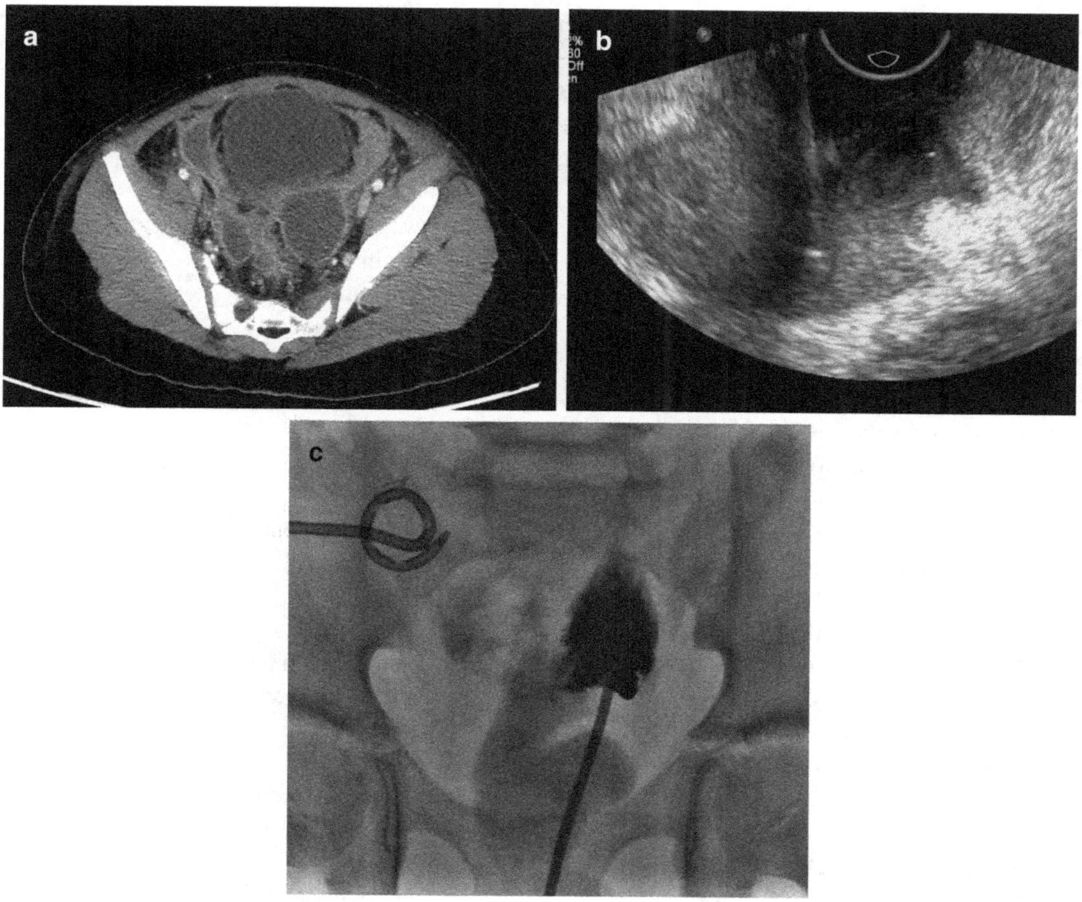

Fig. 18.12 This patient's CT shows a pelvic abscess from appendicitis (**a**). Transrectal ultrasound shows the abscess well and allows for image-guided access (**b**). The final catheter placement (**c**). An additional drain had been placed transabdominally, and there is residual contrast in the colon from the patient's CT scan

imaging (Fig. 18.12a–c). The Seldinger technique is then used to advance a drain.

Small collections such as congenital neck lesion may be difficult to access via standard techniques. As an alternative, ultrasound is used to advance a 14-gauge intravenous style catheter into the lesion. After removing the stylet, a 5-Fr drain can be advanced directly through the catheter and into the collection. When the tip of the drain advances past the end of the catheter, the stiffener is slowly pulled back while simultaneously advancing the drain. The pigtail forms in the collection, typically guided with ultrasound. The 14-gauge catheter is then pulled back out of the collection, the drain secured with sutures or an adhesive device, and a sterile dressing placed.

Catheter securement can be achieved with sutures or adhesive devices depending on patient age and the site of drainage. Adhesive devices work well for abdominal drains, but small areas such as the neck may not allow adequate skin area to apply the device and sutures may be useful. Sutures may also be useful in a patient that is likely to try and remove the drain. Adhesive devices may be applied to the leg and used to secure transrectal drains.

Postprocedure Care

Daily rounds are made on all drainage patients. There is no consensus regarding routine catheter flushing or the value of suction versus gravity drainage. The culture results should be noted, with changes in the antibiotics if appropriate. When drainage reduces to less than 10 mL/day (5 mL/day in infants), the drain may be removed if sepsis has resolved [1]. Follow-up imaging is not typically needed unless the patient remains febrile or significant tube output continues. Prolonged tube drainage may indicate a fistula and tube injection with fluoroscopy should be performed.

Expected Outcomes and Complications

Percutaneous drainage is successful in 81–100 % of patients [1–3, 6–8, 12–17, 27, 31, 34–36] and usually completes within 3 days. Complications from drainage procedures are reported in up to 11 % of patient with catheter migration being the most common [1–3, 6–8, 12–17, 27, 31, 34–36]. Other risks include hemorrhage, bacteremia or sepsis, and injury to the bowel, pleura, or other organs, all of which occur in less than 5 % of patients [1–3, 6–8, 12–17, 27, 31, 34–36].

Vascular injury can occur with any needle puncture. With appendiceal abscesses, the inferior epigastric artery may be interposed. The interventionalist should routinely try to identify its position prior to puncture. In addition, bleeding has been described as more common in adult patients with a transgluteal approach [16, 31, 36]. While not described in children, the interventionalist also needs to be aware of this potential risk.

Chapter Summary

Background

- Common procedure.
- Technique similar to adults.
- Etiology.
  - Abdominal.
    - Appendicitis.
    - CSF pseudocyst.
    - Trauma.
    - Pancreatic fluid.
    - Acalculous cholecystitis.
    - Ovarian cyst.
    - Crohn's.
    - Necrotizing enterocolitis.
  - Pleural.
    - Pneumonia.
  - MSK.
    - Joint effusion (sterile, septic).
    - Soft tissue—cellulitis.
    - Osteomyelitis.
  - Neck.
    - Suppurative adenitis.
    - Para-tonsillar abscess.
  - Congenital.
    - Thyroglossal duct.
    - Branchial cleft.
    - Lymphatic malformations.

Indications

- Suspicion of infection
- Fluid characterization
- Symptomatic collection

Contraindications

- Coagulopathy
- Lack of safe access route

Preprocedure Evaluation

- Review imaging
- CBC, PTT, and INR if there is a suspicion of coagulopathy
- Consider prophylactic antibiotics

Equipment

- Ultrasound, fluoroscopy, CT
- Drainage catheters

- 5–14 Fr
- Varying loop diameters

Technique

- Sedation or GA in most
- Appropriate positioning
- Standard Seldinger or micropuncture technique
- Ultrasound adequate for most procedures
  - Monitor placement with fluoroscopy or ultrasound
- CT or fluoroscopy often helpful for pneumothorax, pneumatocele, and lung abscess
- Transrectal or transgluteal approach for deep pelvic abscesses
- Catheter securement important especially in small children
- Tips
  - 5-French catheters can be inserted directly through a 14-gauge intravenous cannula when access is difficult
  - Transrectal or transabdominal ultrasound used for transrectal drainage

Postprocedure Care

- Daily rounds (until tube out)
- Remove when drainage <10 mL/day (5 mL/day in infants) and sepsis resolved
- Consider repeat imaging for ongoing fever or drainage issues
- Prolonged drainage (especially feculent in appearance) may indicate fistula
  - Perform tube injection with fluoroscopy

Outcomes

- Successful in 80–100 %
- Complications
  - Catheter migration
  - Hemorrhage
  - Bacteremia, sepsis
  - Injury to nearby organs
  - Vascular injury

References

1. Hogan MJ. Appendiceal abscess drainage. Tech Vasc Interv Radiol. 2003;6(4):205–14.
2. Price MR, Haase GM, Sartorelli KH, Meagher Jr DP. Recurrent appendicitis after initial conservative management of appendiceal abscess. J Pediatr Surg. 1996;31(2):291–4.
3. Curran TJ, Muenchow SK. The treatment of complicated appendicitis in children using peritoneal drainage: results from a public hospital. J Pediatr Surg. 1993;28(2):204–8.
4. Coley BD, Shiels 2nd WE, Elton S, Murakami JW, Hogan MJ. Sonographically guided aspiration of cerebrospinal fluid pseudocysts in children and adolescents. AJR Am J Roentgenol. 2004;183(5):1507–10.
5. Sidhu MK, Hogan MJ, Shaw DW, Burdick T. Interventional radiology for paediatric trauma. Pediatr Radiol. 2009;39(5):506–15. Epub 2008 Dec 17.
6. Hultman CS, Herbst CA, McCall JM, Mauro MA. The efficacy of percutaneous cholecystostomy in critically ill patients. Am Surg. 1996;62(4):263–9.
7. Feola GP, Shaw CA, Coburn L. Management of complicated parapneumonic effusions in children. Tech Vasc Interv Radiol. 2003;6(4):197–204.
8. Hogan MJ, Coley BC. Interventional radiology treatment of empyema and lung abscesses. Paediatr Respir Rev. 2008;9(2):77–84.
9. Aliabadi P, Baker ND, Jaramillo D. Hip arthrography, aspiration, block, and bursography. Radiol Clin North Am. 1998;36(4):673–90.
10. Shiels 2nd WE, Kang DR, Murakami JW, Hogan MJ, Wiet GJ. Percutaneous treatment of lymphatic malformations. Otolaryngol Head Neck Surg. 2009;141(2):219–24.
11. Zamzam MM. The role of ultrasound in differentiating septic arthritis from transient synovitis of the hip in children. J Pediatr Orthop B. 2006;15(6): 418–22.
12. Rao S, Hogan MJ. Trocar transrectal abscess drainage in children: a modified technique. Pediatr Radiol. 2009;39:982–4.
13. Pereira JK, Chait PG, Miller SF. Deep pelvic abscesses in children: transrectal drainage under radiologic guidance. Radiology. 1996;198:393–6.
14. Alexander AA, Eschelman DJ, Nazarian LN, Bonn J. Transrectal sonographically guided drainage of deep pelvic abscesses. AJR Am J Roentgenol. 1994;162(5):1227–30.
15. Gervais DA, Brown SD, Connolly SA, et al. Percutaneous imaging guided abdominal and pelvic abscess drainage in children. Radiographics. 2004;24:737–54.
16. Gervais DA, Hahn PF, O'Neill MJ, Mueller P. CT-guided transgluteal drainage of deep pelvic abscesses in children: selective uses as an alternative to transrectal drainage. AJR Am J Roentgenol. 2000;175(5):1393–6.
17. Cahill AM, Kaye RD, Towbin RB, et al. Pelvic abscess drainage in children: the trans-gluteal approach. Pediatr Radiol. 2003;33(Suppl):S81 (abstr).
18. Sidhu M, Goske M, Coley B, et al. Image gently, step lightly: increasing radiation dose awareness in pediatric interventions through an international social marketing campaign. J Vasc Interv Radiol. 2009;20:1115–9.
19. Slovis T. Radiation safety. In: Reid J, editor. Pediatric radiology. Cleveland, OH: Cleveland Clinic Center for Online Medical Education and Training; 2006.

20. Linton OW, Mettler Jr FA. National conference on dose reduction in CT, with an emphasis on pediatric patients. AJR Am J Roentgenol. 2003;181(2): 321–9.
21. Cravero JP, Blike GT, Beach M, et al. Incidence and nature of adverse events during pediatric sedation/anesthesia for procedures outside the operating room: report from the Pediatric Sedation Research Consortium. Pediatrics. 2006;118:1087–96.
22. Lasson A, Lundagårds J, Lorén I, Nilsson PE. Appendiceal abscesses: primary percutaneous drainage and selective interval appendectomy. Eur J Surg. 2002;168(5):264–9.
23. Sivit CJ, Applegate KE. Imaging of acute appendicitis in children. Semin Ultrasound CT MR. 2003;24(2): 74–82.
24. Newman K, Ponsky T, Kittle K, et al. Appendicitis 2000: variability in practice, outcomes, and resource utilization at thirty pediatric hospitals. J Pediatr Surg. 2003;38(3):372–9.
25. Weyant MJ, Eachempati SR, Maluccio MA, et al. The use of computed tomography for the diagnosis of acute appendicitis in children does not influence the overall rate of negative appendectomy or perforation. Surg Infect. 2001;2(1):19–23.
26. Mullins ME, Rhea JT, Novelline RA. Review of suspected acute appendicitis in adults and children using CT and colonic contrast material. Semin Ultrasound CT MR. 2003;24(2):107–13.
27. Jamieson DH, Chait PG, Filler R. Interventional drainage of appendiceal abscesses in children. AJR Am J Roentgenol. 1997;169(6):1619–22.
28. Patrick DA, Janik JE, Janik JS, et al. Increased CT scan utilization does not improve the diagnostic accuracy of appendicitis in children. J Pediatr Surg. 2003;38(5):659–62.
29. Stephen AE, Segev DL, Ryan DP, et al. The diagnosis of acute appendicitis in a pediatric population: to CT or not to CT. J Pediatr Surg. 2003;38(3):367–71.
30. Even-Bendahan G, Lazar I, Erez I, et al. Role of imaging in the diagnosis of acute appendicitis in children. Clin Pediatr. 2003;42(1):23–7.
31. Shuler FW, Newman CN, Angood PB, et al. Nonoperative management for intra-abdominal abscesses. Am Surg. 1996;62(3):218–22.
32. Bakal CW, Sacks D, Burke DR, Cardella JF, Chopra PS, Dawson SL, Drooz AT, Freeman N, Meranze SG, Van Moore Jr A, Palestrant AM, Roberts AC, Spies JB, Stein EJ, Towbin R. Quality improvement guidelines for adult percutaneous abscess and fluid drainage. J Vasc Interv Radiol. 2003;14:S223–5.
33. Rozovsky K, Hiller N, Koplewitz BZ, Simanovsky N. Does CT have an additional diagnostic value over ultrasound in the evaluation of acute inflammatory neck masses in children? Eur Radiol. 2010;20(2):484–90.
34. Walser E, Rzaz S, Hernandex A, Ozkan O, Kathuria M, Akinci D. Sonographically guided transgluteal drainage of pelvic abscesses. AJR Am J Roentgenol. 2003;181:498–500.
35. Koral K, Derinkuyu B, Gargan L, Lagomarsino EM, Murphy JT. Transrectal and fluoroscopy-guided drainage of deep pelvic collections in children. J Pediatr Surg. 2010;45(3):513–8.
36. Harisinghani MG, Gervais DA, Hahn PF, et al. CT-guided transgluteal drainage of deep pelvic abscesses: indications, technique, procedure-related complications, and clinical outcome. Radiographics. 2002;22(6):1353–67.

19 Empyema Drainage

David Rea

Introduction

Childhood empyema is an uncommon but serious complication of pneumonia occurring in one in 150 children hospitalized with pneumonia, affecting 3.3 per 100,000 children [1]. Recent epidemiological data demonstrates an increased incidence of pneumonia in Europe and North America [2, 3]. The principal aims of empyema treatment are control of sepsis and restoration of normal pulmonary function to prevent lung trapping by fibrous pleural peel [4–6]. The optimal treatment for childhood empyema remains a challenge as there are few well-powered randomized controlled trials comparing the variety of treatment options. Current therapeutic options include systemic intravenous antibiotics alone or in combination with thoracocentesis, chest drain insertion with or without instillation of fibrinolytics, and surgical treatments such as video-assisted thoracoscopic surgery (VATS) and thoracotomy. On the basis of the best available level one evidence, management of childhood empyema by interventional radiology (IR) techniques uses less invasive therapies, results in similar lengths of stay, and has similar success and complication rates when compared to surgical treatments such as VATS and thoracotomy [7, 8]. Treatment approaches adopted in individual hospital centers may vary depending on the level of interventional radiology and surgical coverage. Appropriate treatment algorithms should be developed in each pediatric unit to expedite patient care utilizing less invasive interventional radiology techniques first and referring to surgery where the child does not improve with initial nonoperative measures. This approach will result in most children being managed by image-guided therapies and treatment failures being referred early for surgical management.

Indications/Contraindications

Indications

As a general rule, collections resulting in severe respiratory compromise which are large and/or increasing in size should be drained. The 2005 British Thoracic Society (BTS) guidelines advise drainage of effusions that are enlarging or compromising respiratory function [4]. The guidelines detail a clinical severity assessment based on bedside parameters such as temperature, respiratory rate, intercostal recession, and ability to feed (Table 19.1).

D. Rea, M.D., M.Ch., M.R.S.C.I., F.F.R.R.C.S.I. (✉)
Department of Radiology, Our Lady's Children Hospital, Crumlin, Dublin 12, Ireland
e-mail: david.rea@olchc.ie

M. Temple and F.E. Marshalleck (eds.), *Pediatric Interventional Radiology: Handbook of Vascular and Non-Vascular Interventions*, DOI 10.1007/978-1-4419-5856-3_19,

Table 19.1 Clinical severity assessment from 2005 British Thoracic Society (BTS) guidelines

Clinical severity assessment	Mild	Severe
Infants	Temperature <38.5 °C, respiratory rate <50 per min, mild recession, taking full feeds	Temperature >38.5 °C, respiratory rate >70 per min, moderate/severe recession, unable to feed
Older children	Temperature <38.5 °C, respiratory rate <50 per min, mild breathlessness, no vomiting	Temperature >38.5 °C, respiratory rate >50 per min, severe difficulty breathing, nasal flaring, cyanosis, grunting respiration, dehydration

Contraindications

There are no absolute contraindications for percutaneous small-bore pigtail drain insertion. While coagulopathy and thrombocytopenia are important clinical concerns, they are uncommon and most children can be adequately improved by transfusion of appropriate blood products so that a relatively low-risk procedure such as image-guided small-bore catheter placement is safe and feasible.

The presence of a hydropneumothorax on the preprocedural imaging should raise the possibility of underlying parenchymal necrosis or abscess formation and a greater risk for protracted chest drainage due to the presence of a bronchopleural fistula. While these findings are not a contraindication to drain insertion, the requirement for protracted chest drainage in these clinical circumstances needs to be clearly discussed with the referring service and the child's parents prior to embarking on the procedure.

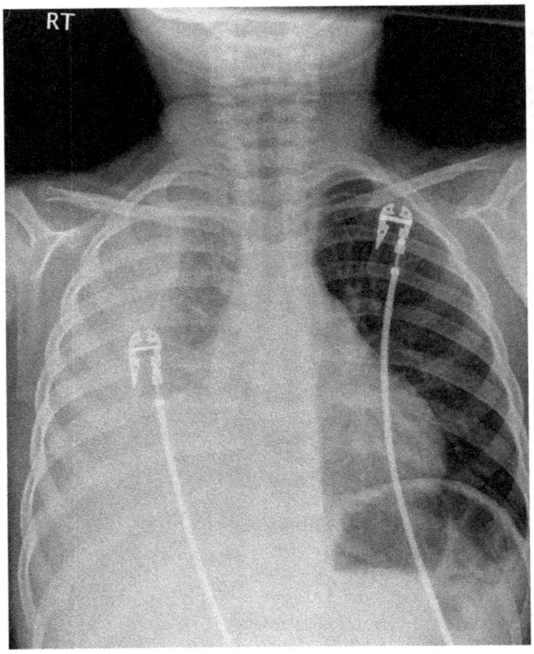

Fig. 19.1 Frontal chest radiograph of a 22-month-old child with a fever and tachypnea revealing a right middle and lower lobe pneumonia and a lentiform extrapulmonary parapneumonic effusion

Preprocedural Workup

Laboratory Workup

Children presenting with symptoms severe enough to warrant referral to a pediatric interventional radiology service will usually already have undergone prior laboratory investigations. In most cases, a complete blood count, differential, and routine blood biochemistry should be available. Almost all cases show a leukocytosis as the principal abnormal finding. Thrombocytopenia and coagulopathy are uncommon in this patient population. Most practitioners would not advocate that a coagulation profile be performed routinely on all children, as the diagnostic yield in otherwise healthy children who are not on anticoagulation therapy is extremely limited and poorly cost efficient.

Imaging Workup

There is limited published evidence regarding the appropriate imaging pathway to choose in investigation of pediatric empyema [9]. A frontal chest radiograph is the optimal initial imaging test (Fig. 19.1). There is no role for a routine lateral chest radiograph. While the radiology literature

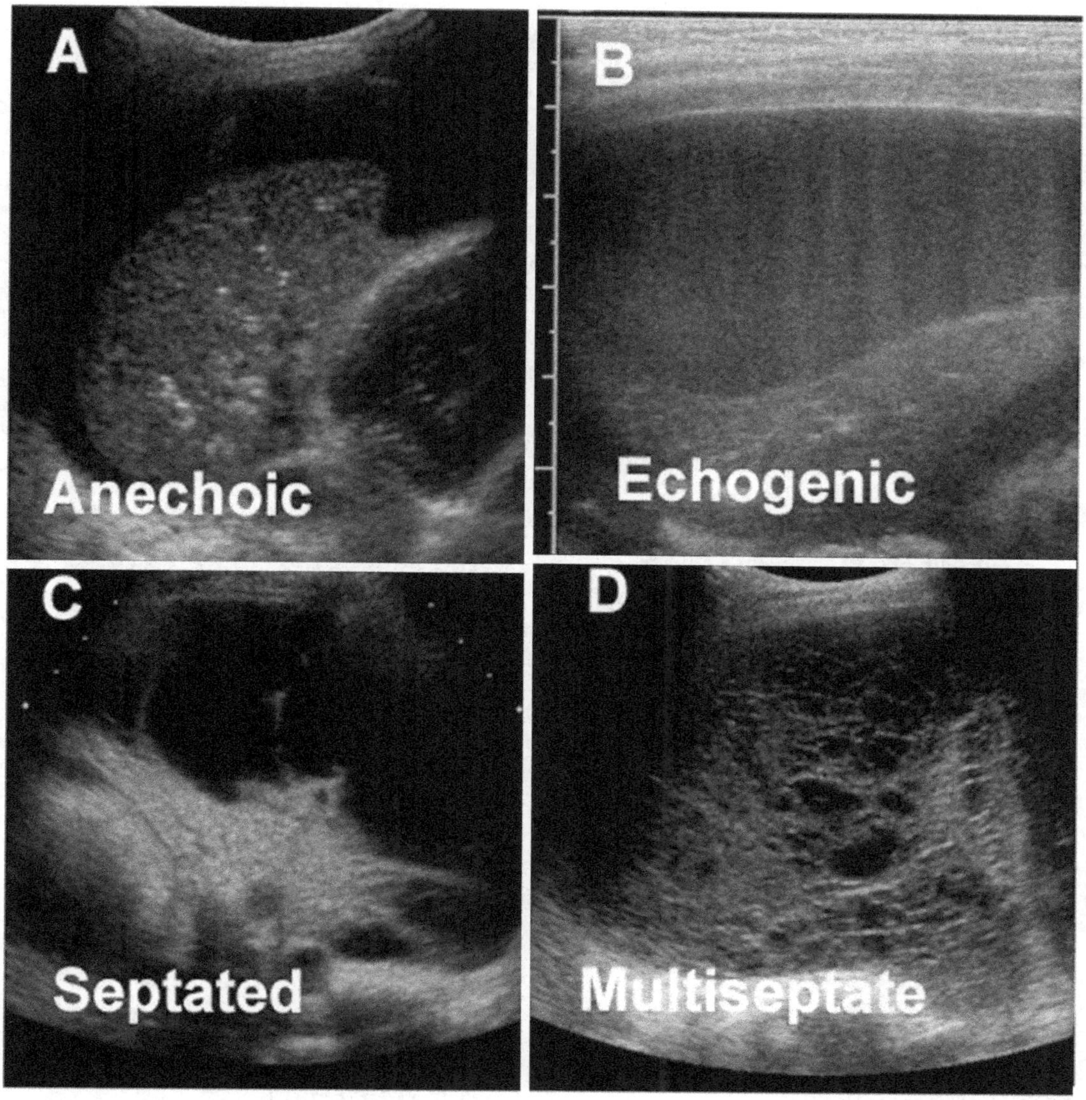

Fig. 19.2 A spectrum of the findings seen during chest ultrasonography in pediatric empyema. (**a**) Sonographic image of an anechoic pleural collection. (**b**) Sonographic image of an echogenic pleural collection. (**c**) Sonographic image of a septate pleural collection. (**d**) Sonographic image of a multiseptate "honeycomb" pleural collection

historically describes decubitus films as a useful test to define whether a pleural collection is free or loculated, it involves ionizing radiation and requires additional radiographs in an ill and often uncooperative child. The most useful imaging investigation is chest ultrasound as it can confirm the presence of pleural fluid and assess the nature of the fluid. Ultrasound also has additional benefits in that it is easily portable, does not involve use of ionizing radiation, and allows a dynamic view of the lung and pleural space. Ultrasound allows visualization of the nature of the collection to see if the fluid is anechoic, echogenic, septated, or a complex organizing pleural collection and to assess for the presence of a pleural peel (Fig. 19.2). The evidence regarding the ability of ultrasound to predict the success of pleural drainage is mixed, with some papers suggesting that the grade of the pleural collection allows prediction of success of the intervention and length of stay [10, 11], while others have found no such link [12]. The anecdotal experience of many interventional radiologists suggests that as pleural collections become more septated over time, the probability that small-bore catheter insertion alone will have a low probability of treatment success without the addition of fibrinolytics.

CT has a limited role in imaging children with empyema. While CT defines more parenchymal abnormalities than chest radiographs, this rarely alters management. CT is unable to predict clinical outcome, may require an anesthetic, and requires exposure to ionizing radiation [12]. CT should be reserved as a problem-solving tool for a child who has complicated parenchymal disease and who remains febrile and unwell despite an adequately placed drainage catheter. CT is often requested by thoracic surgeons prior to embarking on VATS or decortication. The BTS guidelines acknowledge this fact although this approach is not supported by any systematic studies [4].

Equipment

A list of equipment required for the procedure is listed in Table 19.2.

Table 19.2 Equipment

• Sterile skin preparation and drapes
• Local anesthesia, syringes, and needles
• Sterile probe cover
• 8-MHz curvilinear probe (footprint fits in rib space for interventions)
• Access to fluoroscopy during the procedure is helpful but not vital
• 21-gauge "micropuncture" access for children under 10 kg (6 months)
• Access needle (16-gauge IV cannula, 19-G needle) for all other children
• 0.035-in. standard floppy guidewire for children under 6 months
• 0.035-in. stiff guidewire for older or obese children
• Number 11 scalpel blade
• Over the wire dilators sized appropriately for the drain to be inserted
• <20 kg 8.5-French pigtail-type locking catheter
• >20 kg 10–14-French pigtail-type locking catheter
• Sterile sample containers for microbiological analysis
• Underwater seal system and access to low-pressure suction
• Clear dressing for pigtail site (allows chest U/S follow-up)
• Tape/dressings for securing heavy underwater seal drainage tube

Procedure Technique

Anesthesia

Children with compromised respiratory function due to their empyema may not be fit for general anesthesia, although at most institutions, controlled sedation under the supervision of anesthesiologist or staff appropriately trained in administering sedation to ill children is often adequate to allow drain placement.

Patient Positioning

Most pleural drainage procedures can be performed with the child in a supine position. Occasionally, it may be necessary to position a child on its side or partially rolled forward to access a specific location within the pleural space that has been identified on the preprocedural imaging.

Aseptic Preparation

Full aseptic procedures should be employed when inserting a drainage catheter into the pleural space. This includes a formal surgical scrub prior to gowning, gloving up for the procedure, and placing a sterile probe cover over the chosen ultrasound probe. The most common skin preparation agents used today include products containing iodophors or chlorhexidine gluconate. There is increasing evidence that skin preparation with alcohol-based chlorhexidine preparations is associated with reduced risk of surgical or drain site infection [13, 14]. If alcohol-based skin preparations are used, then appropriate time needs to elapse to allow the alcohol to evaporate prior to draping. Care needs to be taken not to allow excess pooling of skin preparation agents behind the child as this can make the child cold and may result in skin injury or breakdown [15].

Image Guidance

Image-guided needle placement is advocated even in cases where a very large pleural collection is present. A curvilinear probe is adequate to allow visualization for almost all chest drain insertions from neonates to larger teenagers as this probe has a small footprint to facilitate easy access to the puncture site. Most experienced interventional radiologists would advise taking a few moments at the beginning of the procedure before a child is sedated for the operator to evaluate the pleural space for themselves as this may save the need to resite or replace a badly positioned drainage catheter later.

Drainage Catheter Insertion

The vast majority of children who require a drainage catheter range between 3 and 5 years of age. For this group, once the appropriate site has been chosen, an IV cannula or access needle that will allow insertion of a 0.035-in. wire can be used to access the pleural space. Infants younger than 10 kg or 6 months constitute a significantly smaller group of children who require drainage, but their reduced size poses concerns as a large-bore IV cannula fills the rib space and may pose a greater risk of injury to the intercostal vessels. In this subgroup, some practitioners advocate use of a 21-gauge micropuncture type set to initially place a 0.018-in. wire and, through use of a coaxial system, upsize to a 0.035-in. guidewire. There is no published evidence to support either approach. Irrespective of the size of needle used, an ultrasound-guided needle puncture directed posteriorly and over the rib is required to avoid injury to the intercostal vessels. Once the sheathed needle has been placed within the collection, the sharp inner stylet may be removed, and through the outer cannula, a sample may be

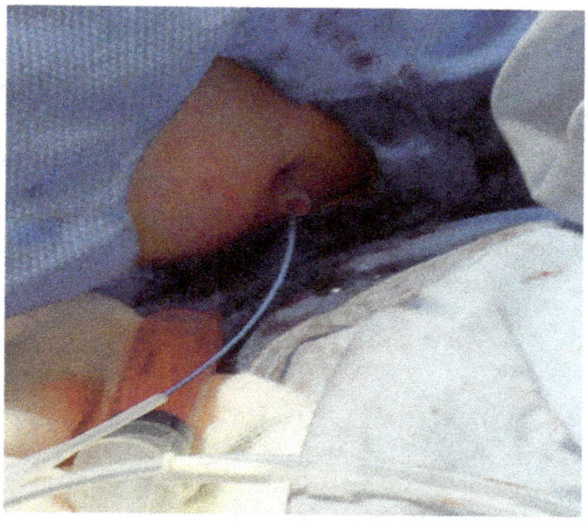

Fig. 19.3 Following image-guided placement of the sheathed needle, the sharp is removed and a sample of fluid taken for microbiological analysis. A guidewire has been placed to allow tract dilatation

obtained for microbiological analysis (Fig. 19.3). Local anesthesia should be given to the puncture site after a successful puncture has been performed. An incision is created at the puncture site to facilitate dilator and drain passage through the skin and subcutaneous soft tissues. A 0.035-in. guidewire is then placed through the outer cannula into the pleural space. In older children a stiff 0.035-in. wire is often required due to the risk of kinking or bending the guidewire during tract dilatation. Children less than 10 kg or 6 months generally require only a standard 0.035-in. floppy guidewire. Passage of the guidewire may be easy or more resistant depending on the degree of loculation. The operator should never advance the wire against resistance unless they can see where it is going using fluoroscopy and are confident that this is safe. Manipulation of the wire has been advocated as a means of breaking up pleural loculations; however, this can lead to wire kinking and does not generally lead to increased drainage compared to the use of fibrinolytics. Once there is adequate purchase of wire within the pleural space serial size, appropriate dilatation of the tract is performed with over the wire dilators. Finally, a pigtail-type locking small-bore drainage catheter may be inserted over the guidewire and the wire removed once the device is appropriately positioned, secured,

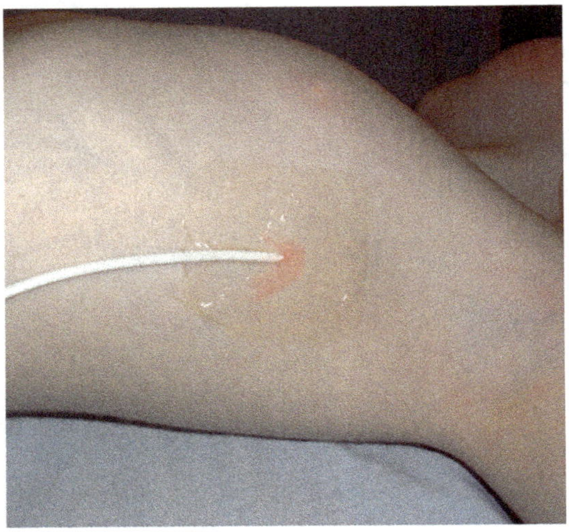

Fig. 19.4 Once the pigtail catheter has been formed, the catheter should immediately be secured and placed on underwater seal drainage

and attached to underwater seal drainage with low-pressure 10–20 cm H_2O suction. Use of a large clear self-adhesive dressing over the portion of the catheter immediately adjacent to the entry site allows chest ultrasound be performed at the drain site which is useful for patient follow-up (Fig. 19.4).

Choice of Drain Size

The prior surgical tradition was for the use of large-bore chest tubes. The published literature suggests that small-bore drainage catheters are successful in draining empyema in 80–94 % of patients [16–18]. The size of drain used is probably not critical for two reasons. Firstly, the volume of pleural fluid removed is released in a relatively controlled fashion to prevent re-expansion pulmonary edema. The BTS guidelines suggest clamping the drain for 1 h after 10 mL/kg of fluid has drained [4]. Secondly, most institutions attach a two- or three-way tap to the drain to facilitate access to the drain for injection of fibrinolytics or to flush the catheter. This action statistically reduces the flow rates of the catheter [19]. In the clinical setting, where the rate of flow from the catheter is controlled by intermittently occluding it and also by attaching a device which reduces the rate of flow, then the size of the catheter is not a critical decision point. Many interventional radiologists use empiric protocols based on weight to determine the size of catheter. Most of these protocols use smaller (8.5–10Fr) catheters for children under 20 kg and larger catheters for children over 20 kg.

Fibrinolytic Therapy

Based on the available pediatric evidence, there is no evidence that VATS is more effective than fibrinolytic treatment and because fibrinolytic treatment is less invasive and less expensive, it should be the preferred local therapy for children with empyema. Fibrinolytic therapies are not required where the pleural collections are purely anechoic. A fibrinolytic agent should be considered where the collection is echogenic, minimally septated, or a complex organizing collection [20]. In view of concerns regarding anaphylaxis, streptokinase is not in routine use. Recombinant tissue plasminogen activator (r-TPA) is the preferred agent in North America and most of Europe, while urokinase appears to be the preferred drug in the United Kingdom. Optimal dosing, regimens, and duration of therapy with either agent remain controversial. r-TPA dose varies between institutions and can be either weight based (0.1 mg/kg) or empiric (2 or 4 mg). The TPA is administered and normal saline (10–25 mL) is injected into the chest drain which is clamped for 1 h, then opened, and placed back on 10–20 cm H_2O suction. Most centers have a once a day TPA regimen, but some centers may give the drug up to three times daily for up to 3 days or until tube output is less than 50 mL per day prior to reassessing with ultrasound [20]. Urokinase is used at a dose of 40,000 units in 40 mL of saline reduced to 10,000 units in 10 mL saline for children less than 1 year. The most common regimen is twice daily instillations into the pleural space for 3 days and then to reassess with ultrasound [16].

Postprocedure Care

The child should be reviewed by the radiology service that provided the intervention at least once daily for the duration that the drain remains in situ. Parameters such as drain output, fever, and oxygen requirement should be followed on daily radiology rounds. Simple drain care to ensure that the drain is not blocked and oscillates via the underwater seal system is mandatory on each clinical radiology review. If the child has not improved clinically or has had a poorer than expected drain output at 48–72 h, then repeat imaging should be considered. Repeat imaging should include plain chest radiography and chest ultrasound to assess both the pulmonary parenchyma and more importantly the pleural space. CT should be reserved as a problem-solving tool for a child who has complicated parenchymal disease and who remains febrile and unwell despite an adequately placed drainage catheter. Where the repeat imaging reveals an adequately placed drain and a persistent collection and the child remains unwell, then a surgical consult should be considered to see if VATS or a formal thoracotomy and decortication is required.

Follow-Up

The long-term prognosis for childhood empyema is good [21], and children usually demonstrate a complete clinical recovery, and their chest radiographs return to normal usually within 3–6 months [4]. Unless there is an underlying background lung disorder such as cystic fibrosis, no specific long-term follow-up is necessary.

Conclusion

Most children who contract a complicated parapneumonic effusion or empyema have an excellent outcome irrespective of the intervention provided. Interventional radiology techniques are less invasive, result in similar lengths of stay, and have comparable success rates and complications when compared to surgical approaches such as VATS or thoracotomy. The treatment approaches adopted in individual hospital centers may vary depending on the level of interventional radiology and surgical cover. Appropriate treatment algorithms should be developed in each pediatric unit to expedite patient care utilizing less invasive interventional radiology techniques first and referring to surgery if the child does not improve with initial nonoperative measures. Using this approach, the majority of children can be treated using less invasive image-guided therapies, and treatment failures can be referred promptly to the surgical services for second-line therapy.

Chapter Summary

Indications

- Respiratory compromise
- Increasing size of collection

Contraindications

- Uncorrectable coagulopathy

Preprocedure Workup

- CBC
- Coagulation workup not usually warranted
- CXR ± ultrasound

Equipment

- See Table 19.1—page X

Postprocedure Care

- Daily evaluation
  - Output
  - Patency

Follow-Up

- None specific

References

1. Hardie W, Bokulic R, Garcia VF, Reising SF, Christie CD. Pneumococcal pleural empyemas in children. Clin Infect Dis. 1996;22(6):1057–63. PubMed PMID: 8783710.
2. Eastham KM, Freeman R, Kearns AM, Eltringham G, Clark J, Leeming J, Spencer DA. Clinical features, aetiology and outcome of empyema in children in the north east of England. Thorax. 2004;59(6):522–5. PubMed PMID: 15170039; PubMed Central PMCID: PMC1747032.
3. Schultz KD, Fan LL, Pinsky J, Ochoa L, Smith EO, Kaplan SL, Brandt ML. The changing face of pleural empyemas in children: epidemiology and management. Pediatrics. 2004;113(6):1735–40. PubMed PMID: 15173499.
4. Balfour-Lynn IM, Abrahamson E, Cohen G, Hartley J, King S, Parikh D, Spencer D, Thomson AH, Urquhart D. Pediatric pleural diseases subcommittee of the BTS standards of care committee. BTS guidelines for the management of pleural infection in children. Thorax. 2005;60 Suppl 1:i1–21. PubMed PMID: 15681514; PubMed Central PMCID: PMC1766040.
5. Jaffé A, Balfour-Lynn IM. Management of empyema in children. Pediatr Pulmonol. 2005;40(2):148–56. Review. PubMed PMID: 15965900.
6. Russell-Taylor M. Bacterial pneumonias: management and complication. Paediatr Respir Rev. 2000;1(1):14–20. Review. PubMed PMID: 16263437.
7. Sonnappa S, Cohen G, Owens CM, van Doorn C, Cairns J, Stanojevic S, Elliott MJ, Jaffé A. Comparison of urokinase and video-assisted thoracoscopic surgery for treatment of childhood empyema. Am J Respir Crit Care Med. 2006;174(2):221–7. Epub 2006 May 4. PubMed PMID: 16675783.
8. St Peter SD, Tsao K, Spilde TL, Keckler SJ, Harrison C, Jackson MA, Sharp SW, Andrews WS, Rivard DC, Morello FP, Holcomb 3rd GW, Ostlie DJ. Thoracoscopic decortication vs tube thoracostomy with fibrinolysis for empyema in children: a prospective, randomized trial. J Pediatr Surg. 2009;44(1):106–11; discussion 111. Erratum in: J Pediatr Surg. 2009;44(9):1865. Rivard, Doug C [added]; Morello, Frank P [added]. PubMed PMID: 19159726.
9. Calder A, Owens CM. Imaging of parapneumonic pleural effusions and empyema in children. Pediatr Radiol. 2009;39(6):527–37. Epub 2009 Feb 6. Review. PubMed PMID: 19198826.
10. Ramnath RR, Heller RM, Ben-Ami T, Miller MA, Campbell P, Neblett 3rd WW, Holcomb GW, Hernanz-Schulman M. Implications of early sonographic evaluation of parapneumonic effusions in children with pneumonia. Pediatrics. 1998;101(1 Pt 1):68–71. PubMed PMID: 9417153.
11. Shankar S, Gulati M, Kang M, Gupta S, Suri S. Image-guided percutaneous drainage of thoracic empyema: can sonography predict the outcome? Eur Radiol. 2000;10(3):495–9. PubMed PMID: 10757003.
12. Jaffe A, Calder AD, Owens CM, Stanojevic S, Sonnappa S. Role of routine computed tomography in pediatric pleural empyema. Thorax. 2008;63(10):897–902. Epub 2008 May 20. PubMed PMID: 18492739.
13. Lepor NE, Madyoon H. Antiseptic skin agents for percutaneous procedures. Rev Cardiovasc Med. 2009 Fall;10(4):187–93. Review. PubMed PMID: 20065928.
14. Darouiche RO, Wall Jr MJ, Itani KM, Otterson MF, Webb AL, Carrick MM, Miller HJ, Awad SS, Crosby CT, Mosier MC, Alsharif A, Berger DH. Chlorhexidine-alcohol versus povidone-iodine for surgical-site antisepsis. N Engl J Med. 2010;362(1):18–26. PubMed PMID: 20054046.
15. Upadhyayula S, Kambalapalli M, Harrison CJ. Safety of anti-infective agents for skin preparation in premature infants. Arch Dis Child. 2007;92(7):646–7. Review. PubMed PMID: 17588981; PubMed Central PMCID: PMC2083764.
16. Thomson AH, Hull J, Kumar MR, Wallis C, Balfour Lynn IM. Randomised trial of intrapleural urokinase in the treatment of childhood empyema. Thorax. 2002;57(4):343–7. PubMed PMID: 11923554; PubMed Central PMCID: PMC1746300.
17. Maskell NA, Davies CW, Nunn AJ, Hedley EL, Gleeson FV, Miller R, Gabe R, Rees GL, Peto TE, Woodhead MA, Lane DJ, Darbyshire JH, Davies RJ, First Multicenter Intrapleural Sepsis Trial (MIST1) Group. U.K. controlled trial of intrapleural streptokinase for pleural infection. N Engl J Med. 2005;352(9):865–74. Erratum in: N Engl J Med. 2005;352(20):2146. PubMed PMID: 15745977.
18. Keeling AN, Leong S, Logan PM, Lee MJ. Empyema effusion: outcome of image-guided small-bore catheter drainage. Cardiovasc Intervent Radiol. 2008;31(1):135–41. Epub 2007 Oct 18. PubMed PMID: 17943347.
19. Macha DB, Thomas J, Nelson RC. Pigtail catheters used for percutaneous fluid drainage: comparison of performance characteristics. Radiology. 2006;238(3):1057–63. PubMed PMID: 16505398.
20. Hogan MJ, Coley BD. Interventional radiology treatment of empyema and lung abscesses. Paediatr Respir Rev. 2008;9(2):77–84; quiz 84. Epub 2008 May 12. Review. PubMed PMID: 18513667.
21. McLaughlin FJ, Goldmann DA, Rosenbaum DM, Harris GB, Schuster SR, Strieder DJ. Empyema in children: clinical course and long-term follow-up. Pediatrics. 1984;73(5):587–93. PubMed PMID: 6718113.

Section VII

Nonvascular Interventions: Gastrointestinal

20 Gastrointestinal Interventions in Children

Dimitri A. Parra and Michael Temple

Introduction

Gastrointestinal (GI) interventions comprise a large component of nonvascular interventions in children. This chapter includes the most common pediatric GI interventions: balloon dilatation and enterostomy access.

Esophageal Dilatation

In the pediatric population, esophageal stenosis is almost always benign in etiology. The origin can be congenital, due to an esophageal web, for example, or secondary to external causes as seen following caustic ingestion.

Indications/Contraindications

The most frequent indication for radiologic intervention in the pediatric esophagus is postsurgical stenosis following repair of tracheoesophageal fistulae [1–3]. The patient usually develops difficulty swallowing that is detected by the surgeon or pediatrician. Dilation of a stricture in the early postoperative phase can damage or rupture an anastomosis, so it is important for the interventional radiologist and surgeon to discuss each patient on a case-by-case basis. Intervention four to six weeks after surgery is usually considered safe.

Preprocedure Workup

At the time of initial referral, an upper GI study will help plan the procedure by identifying the level of stenosis and the degree of obstruction (Fig. 20.1). Determination of coagulation factors and prophylactic antibiotic administration is usually not necessary.

Technique

Esophageal dilatation can be performed on an outpatient basis. Patients are admitted the same day and kept NPO according to the anesthetic guidelines of the institution. The patient is anesthetized and placed in the supine position. The placement of an endotracheal tube helps avoid aspiration of contrast during the procedure. Intubation is particularly important when treating a stenosis in the cervical or upper thoracic esophagus. A 0.035″ floppy-tip guidewire is inserted

D.A. Parra, M.D. (✉)
Department of Medical Imaging,
Image Guided Therapy, The Hospital for Sick Children, University of Toronto, 555 University Avenue, Toronto, ON, Canada M5G 1X8
e-mail: dimitri.parra@sickkids.ca

M. Temple, M.D., F.R.C.P.(C.)
Hospital for Sick Children, University of Toronto, Toronto, ON, Canada
e-mail: michael.temple@sickkids.ca

M. Temple and F.E. Marshalleck (eds.), *Pediatric Interventional Radiology: Handbook of Vascular and Non-Vascular Interventions*, DOI 10.1007/978-1-4419-5856-3_20,

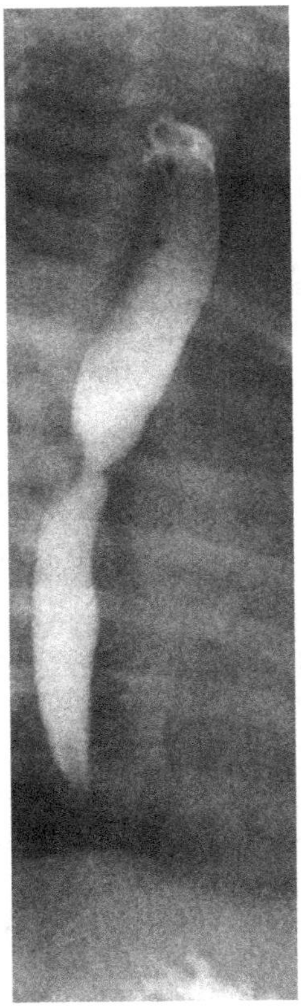

Fig. 20.1 Upper GI study. Stenosis of the upper thoracic esophagus is demonstrated with water-soluble contrast

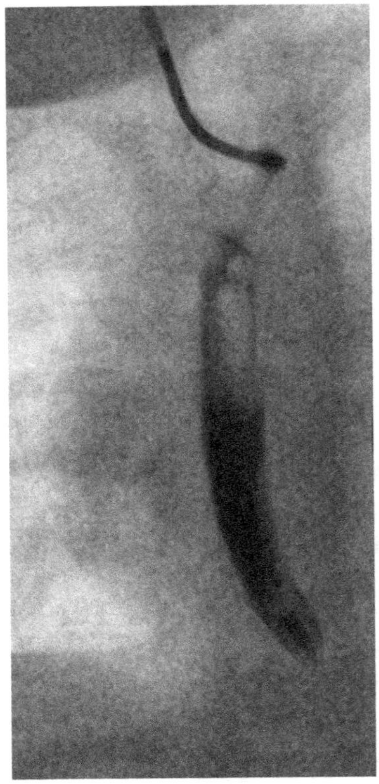

Fig. 20.2 Localization of stenosis. Contrast is injected through a catheter to demonstrate the level of the stenosis

through the mouth or nostril into the upper esophagus. The guidewire is manipulated into the distal esophagus with a guiding catheter (4 or 5 Fr JB1, Bernstein, etc.). A pullback esophagogram is performed through the guiding catheter to define the level of stenosis (Fig. 20.2) and estimate the diameter of the stenosis and esophagus. If there has been great difficulty advancing the wire through the area of stenosis, this step can be avoided as a pullback esophagogram may result in loss of access. After readvancing the guidewire into the stomach and removing the guiding catheter, an angioplasty balloon is advanced to the area of concern. The balloon is dilated using hand pressure or an inflating device (Fig. 20.3). The degree of dilatation and balloon size is determined at the discretion of the radiologist. A 3 or 4 mm balloon may be used for initial dilation of an extremely tight stenosis to decrease the likelihood of esophageal rupture. Often a 5 or 6 mm is used for the first intervention in the average anas-

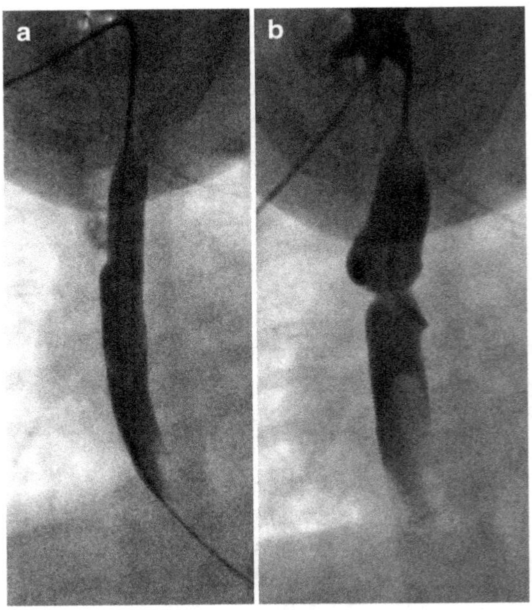

Fig. 20.3 Esophageal dilatation. (**a**) The stenosis is dilated with a balloon. (**b**) Contrast check following dilatation demonstrates a residual stenosis but no extravasation. Note the reflux of contrast into the hypopharynx

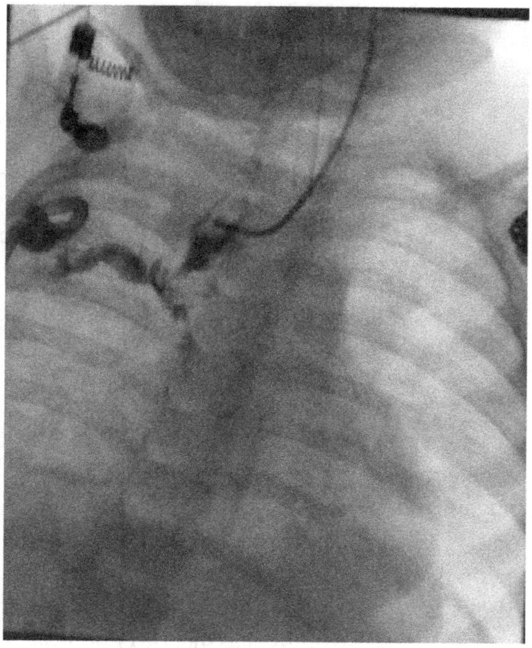

Fig. 20.4 Esophageal leak. Infant several weeks post-TEF repair with tight esophageal anastomotic stenosis. Following balloon dilatation, contrast is noted leaking into the pleural space

tomotic stenosis; sequential dilatation with larger balloons, up to the diameter of the esophagus, can be performed during subsequent procedures. The balloon is inflated until the waist is effaced, and the balloon can be increased in size as many times as needed. An esophagogram should be performed after the dilatation. Mucosal tears and esophageal perforation are known complications of this procedure (Fig. 20.4).

Patients with esophageal stenosis secondary to epidermolysis bullosa (EB) require extremely careful dilatation. Extensive use of lubricant on the balloon and catheter/guidewire should be ensured to decrease the risk of esophageal blisters in this group of patients [1, 4]. In addition, care must be taken so that the balloon does not move or slide during dilatation in order to decrease shear stress on the tissues.

Retrograde access can be considered in patients with both a significant esophageal stenosis and a gastrostomy tube. Catheterization through the stomach can be used to negotiate through the stenosis in a retrograde manner as the distal esophagus tends to be normal in caliber [5].

Mitomycin C has been utilized as an agent to prevent restenosis in patients with resistant stenoses. This chemotherapy medication is applied in the area of stenosis during the dilatation. While preliminary experience shows promise, more studies are needed to evaluate this approach [5, 6]. Likewise, the use of bioabsorbable [5] and removable [7, 8] stents has been described for treatment of difficult recurrent stenosis.

Postprocedure Care

After an uncomplicated procedure, the patient is kept NPO for 2 h followed by slow introduction of drinking with sips of water. If tolerated, a clear fluid diet can be initiated and the patient is then advanced to a soft food diet the next day. If no complications are identified, the patient is discharged home six hours after the procedure. Patients with epidermolysis bullosa or those who underwent difficult dilatation may require a longer NPO period, slower introduction of food, and possibly overnight admission.

In cases of mucosal tears, the patient is admitted overnight, and a chest X-ray is obtained to exclude pneumomediastinum or pleural effusion. Usually, no further intervention is required. Small mucosal tears can be followed clinically while maintaining the patient on a clear fluid diet for a few days. If the esophageal injury is more significant, an upper GI study using water-soluble contrast is obtained in the early phase. The decision to advance the diet is based on the results of this study. If an esophageal wall perforation is noted, the patient should be kept NPO until documentation of closure of the defect. An NG tube may be used to provide feeds if conservative management is undertaken. Antibiotic coverage should be considered in the presence of postoperative fever. Drainage of pleural effusion or mediastinal fluid collections may be required. Surgery is rarely needed.

Dilatation of the Duodenum and Colon

Duodenal and colonic image-guided balloon dilatations (and stenting) have been described in the literature [9, 10]. In the pediatric population, they have been used to treat benign duodenal strictures secondary to peptic ulcer disease or congenital webs and to manage colonic strictures due to necrotizing enterocolitis [11] or postsurgical changes. The decision to perform an image-guided dilatation should be undertaken on a case-by-case basis and with involvement of all teams taking care of the patient. The technique is essentially the same as the one described for an esophageal dilatation; however depending in the location of the stenosis, it can be difficult to advance a guidewire for anatomic and technical reasons. Endoscopy can be of great help in some difficult anatomic situations. Limited information is available about outcomes in these patients; however, the technique seems promising (Fig. 20.5).

Gap Studies

A gap study or gapogram is performed to estimate the length of the atretic portion of the esophagus prior to surgery in patients with esophageal atresia. The gap can be estimated using CT [12–14] or fluoroscopy. A gapogram can be performed without tension, relying on reflux to outline the lower esophageal pouch or with tension using instrumentation to assess the gap when under tension [15].

To perform a gapogram using instrumentation, the presence of a gastrostomy is necessary to obtain access into the lower portion of the esophagus. A guiding catheter along with a guidewire is inserted per mouth or nose and it is manipulated into the deepest portion of the upper esophagus. The same process is performed through the gastrostomy into the lower portion of the esophagus. The gap between both catheters is measured using a radiopaque ruler under fluoroscopy (Fig. 20.6).

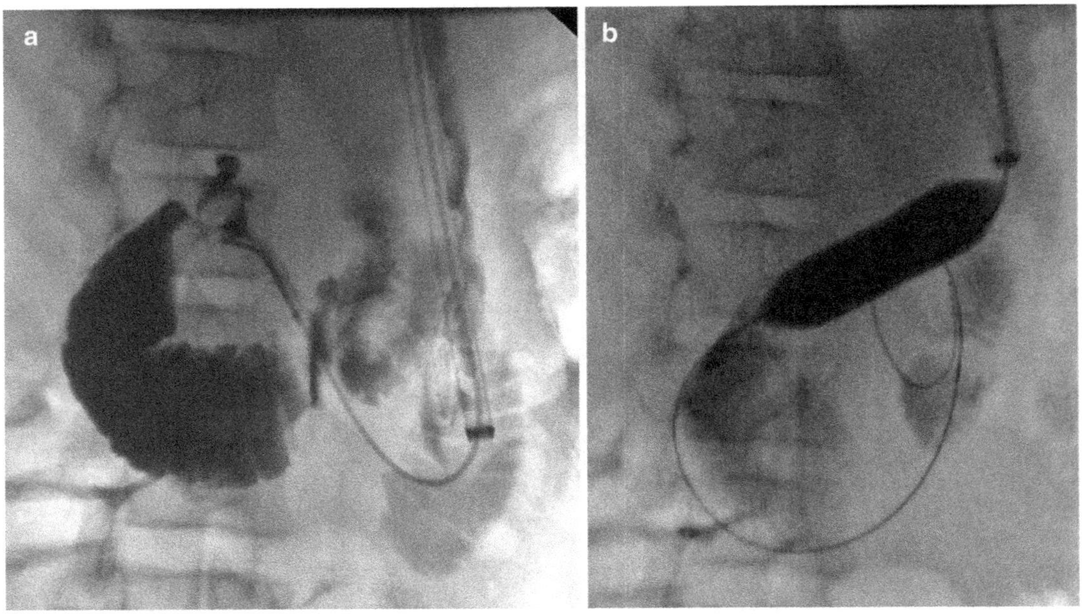

Fig. 20.5 Duodenal dilatation. (**a**) Catheter injection delineates a stenosis involving the first part of the duodenum. (**b**) The involved area is dilated with a balloon

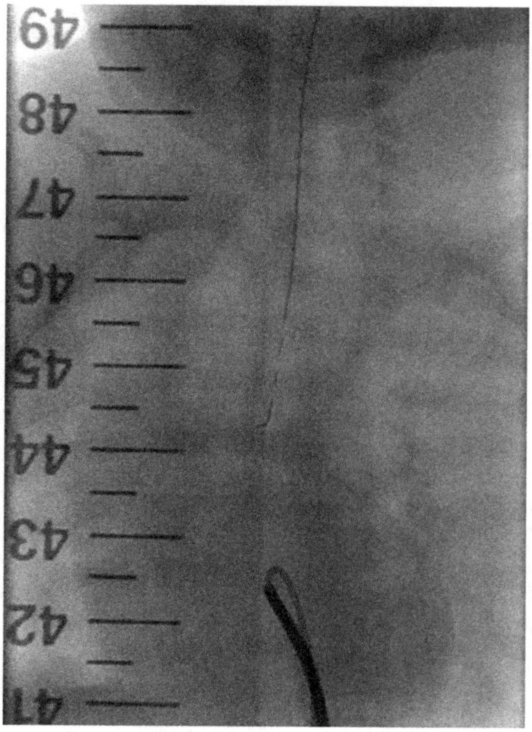

Fig. 20.6 GAP study. The distance between the upper and lower portions of the esophagus is measured using a catheter placed via a gastrostomy and the "NG" tube seen in the upper esophageal pouch

Gastrostomy and Gastrojejunostomy

Primary insertion of gastrostomy (G) and gastrojejunostomy (GJ) tubes and their ongoing care make up a large proportion of the procedures performed by the pediatric interventional radiologist. G tubes allow administration of enteral nutrition and drug administration directly into the stomach. GJ tubes allow administration of nutrition into the proximal jejunum in patients at risk of aspiration.

Two major image-guided techniques exist for initial gastric access: retrograde and antegrade tube insertion. Using the retrograde technique, small-bore catheters (G or GJ) are inserted via the abdominal wall using the Seldinger technique. When the antegrade technique is used, a large-bore PEG (endoscopy) G tube is pulled from the mouth through the abdominal wall. The choice of technique varies by institution and/or patient need. There are advantages and disadvantages to both techniques (Table 20.1).

Indications/Contraindications

The main indication for placement is the inability to tolerate feeding by mouth or to maintain adequate nutritional intake for various reasons including acute and chronic diseases [3, 12]. Gastrostomy tubes are occasionally inserted to allow glucose administration in metabolic patients or drug administration. Emergency gastrostomy is rarely performed to decompress a markedly distended stomach in a ventilated neonate with a distal tracheoesophageal fistula (Fig. 20.7).

Gastrojejunostomy tubes are an alternative for safe delivery of nutrition in patients with gastroesophageal reflux disease who are at risk of aspiration and/or have gastrointestinal dysmotility [13]. Percutaneous or surgical placement of jejunostomy tubes is rarely required.

There are a few absolute contraindications that include uncorrectable coagulopathy and ascites [12]. Patients who have undergone recent VP shunt revision should be booked after 4 weeks to decrease the risk of infection [14].

Preprocedure Workup

The preprocedure evaluation is very important to assess the need for insertion and to involve the family in the use of this long-term device. In our institution, a pediatrician and a specialized nurse practitioner assess every patient. The past medical history is reviewed as well as the indications for the G or GJ tube insertion. The parents are encouraged to attend to a G tube class where the nurse practitioners explain the procedure of insertion and care of the device in a simple and didactic way. Consent is obtained in the interventional radiology clinic.

If there is a significant anatomic abnormality in the abdomen or the patient has undergone upper abdominal surgery, a preprocedure "mapping" with ultrasound and fluoroscopy may be helpful to decide if the procedure is technically feasible.

Table 20.1 Comparison of antergrade and retrograde gastrostomy technique

	Antegrade gastrostomy	Retrograde gastrostomy
Sedation/anesthesia	– Required	– Can be performed with local anesthesia only
	– Larger caliber tube—more pain post insertion?	– Smaller caliber tube—less pain post insertion?
Esophageal instrumentation	– Placement of NG tube required for gastric insufflation	– Placement of NG tube required for gastric insufflation
	– Large bumper on tube can cause transient tracheal compression	
Gastric fixation	– None required	– 1–3 retention sutures placed
		– Usually ferromagnetic—can interfere with MRI
Sterility	Tube passes through oropharynx and esophagus. Higher potential for peritonitis/cellulitis?	Tube passes through prepped abdominal wall. Less potential for peritonitis/cellulitis?
Displacement	Large internal fixator makes accidental removal difficult	Cope loop helps prevent accidental removal but has higher potential than antegrade
Maintenance	Less maintenance post insertion	More maintenance post insertion
	– Larger diameter tubes are less likely to block	– Smaller diameter tubes have higher blocking potential
	– Bumper decreases dislodgement issues but can erode through tract	– Mobility can result in higher dislodgement rates

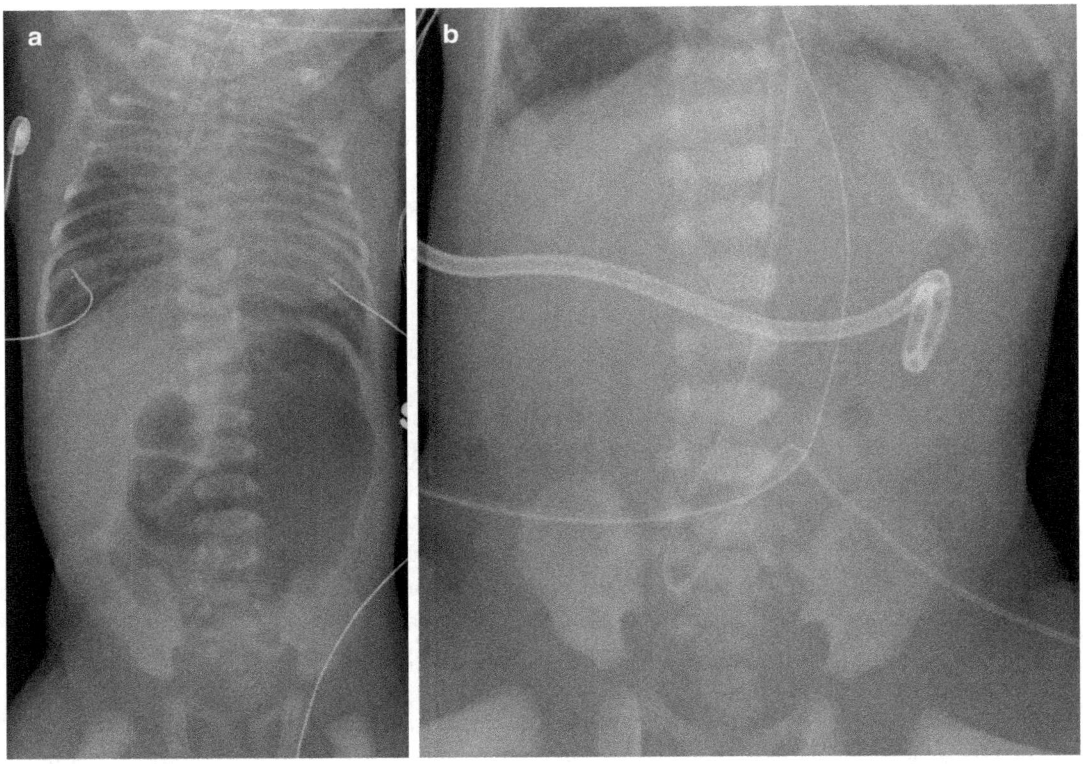

Fig. 20.7 Decompressing gastrostomy. (**a**) Massive gastric distention related to ventilation in this infant with a distal tracheoesophageal fistula further compromised respiratory status. (**b**) Complete gastric decompression following emergent gastrostomy tube insertion

The patient is admitted the same day and kept NPO according to the anesthetic guidelines of the institution. Any anticoagulation medication is stopped as necessary. In patients undergoing active chemotherapy or who have liver dysfunction, determination of platelet levels and coagulation factors should be considered. The procedure should be performed when optimal coagulation status is achieved.

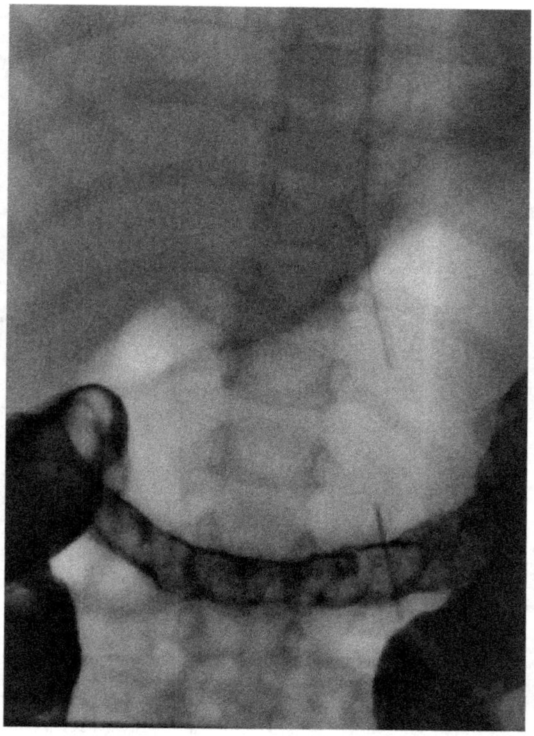

Fig. 20.8 Colon opacification. A barium enema helps avoid inadvertent colon puncture

Equipment

- Fluoroscopy ± ultrasound
- 18G needle
- Glucagon
- NG tube
- 0.035″ Guidewire
- Retention suture
- Dilator
- Directional catheter
- G or GJ tube

There are a large variety of G, GJ, and combined G/GJ tubes available. Choice depends on institutional and patient-based factors.

Gastrostomy (G) Tube Insertion

The techniques of primary gastrostomy access are described below.

Retrograde Technique

The retrograde technique originally described by Preshaw [16] is widely used. The procedure is performed under general anesthesia, sedation, or local anesthesia as required. The patient is placed in the supine position. A dose of prophylactic antibiotics is given (cefazolin 30 mg/kg). A nasogastric tube is inserted. The liver, splenic and costal margins are marked on the skin using sonographic guidance. A barium enema is performed delineating the transverse colon (water-soluble contrast can also be used) (Fig. 20.8). The anterior abdomen is prepped and draped in a sterile fashion. Glucagon is given IV at the discretion of the interventional radiologist to improve the gastric distention (usually 0.2–0.5 mg according to the weight) [12]. In patients on a ketogenic diet, glucagon cannot be administered. The stomach is inflated through the nasogastric tube. In cases of distal esophageal atresia, the stomach can be insufflated through a small-gauge needle introduced under ultrasound guidance. A site for the puncture is chosen in the abdominal wall using fluoroscopic guidance. The ideal position is lateral to the rectus abdominal muscle and a finger's width below the costal margin. If it is not possible in this location, the G tube can be placed in the midline. If not possible in either location, the third option is through the rectus or oblique abdominal muscles according to the specific anatomic conditions. If this is the case, special attention should be taken to avoid puncturing the superior epigastric vessels. If a ventriculoperitoneal shunt is present, the puncture should be performed as far as possible from it (ideally more than 5 cm). Once the site is

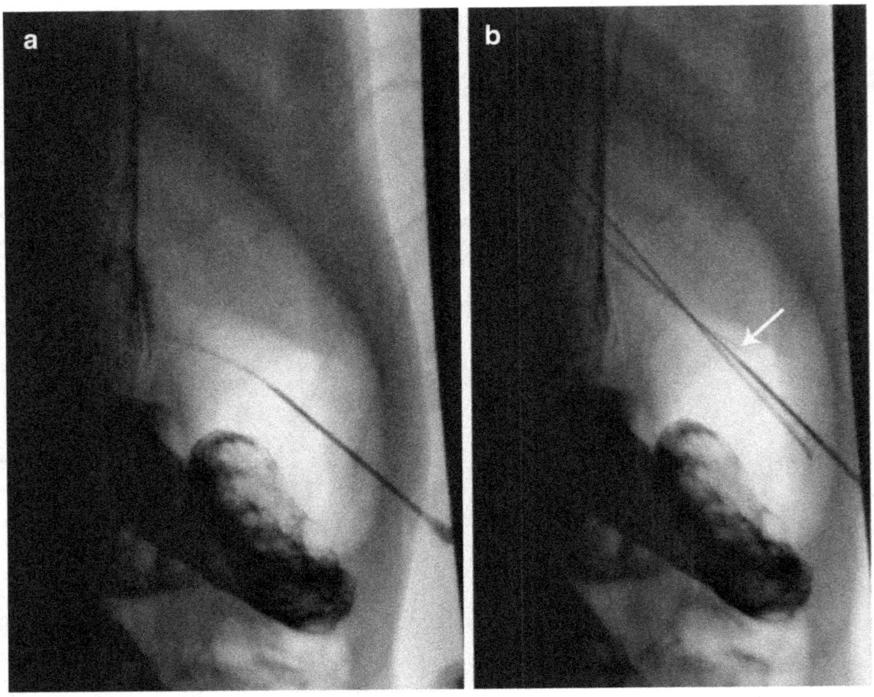

Fig. 20.9 Gastric access. (**a**) Contrast injection demonstrates appropriate intraluminal location following gastric puncture. (**b**) A 0.035″ wire is used to displace a retention suture into the stomach (*arrow*) for retrograde tube placements

chosen, local anesthetic is infiltrated with a 25–27-G needle and a small incision is performed in the skin with a sterile blade. The stomach is punctured with an 18-G needle, preloaded with a pediatric retention suture. Access to the gastric lumen is achieved with fluoroscopic guidance; however, in cases with difficult anatomy, ultrasound can be added to help guide the puncture. A 0.035″ guidewire is inserted through the needle and advanced into the gastric cavity deploying the retention suture (Cope Pediatric Gastrointestinal Suture Anchor Set, Cook) (Fig. 20.9). The tract is dilated up to the desired size, and the G tube is advanced into the gastric cavity and the guidewire is removed. Gentle and constant traction should be applied to the retention suture during the dilatation and insertion process, to keep control of the gastric wall and prevent pneumoperitoneum or migration of the catheter into the peritoneal space. If the thread breaks, a second puncture to insert a new retention suture may be required; however, the 8–14 Fr G tube can be inserted through either site. If a moderate to large pneumoperitoneum is detected, it can be aspirated with a 27-G needle under fluoroscopic guidance in the lateral view (Fig. 20.9). A small amount of free air in the peritoneal cavity is usually reabsorbed without any intervention. If the transverse colon or an air-filled bowel loop is covering the stomach, the intraluminal air can be aspirated using a 27-G needle to open a window for percutaneous access into the stomach (Fig. 20.10).

The G tube position is checked by injecting contrast and obtaining fluoroscopic views at different angles (Fig. 20.11). The retention suture is secured using a roll of gauze, and the site is covered with gauze and tape.

Antegrade Technique

The stomach is insufflated through an NG tube and punctured with an 18-G needle. Precautions for needle puncture are the same as described in the

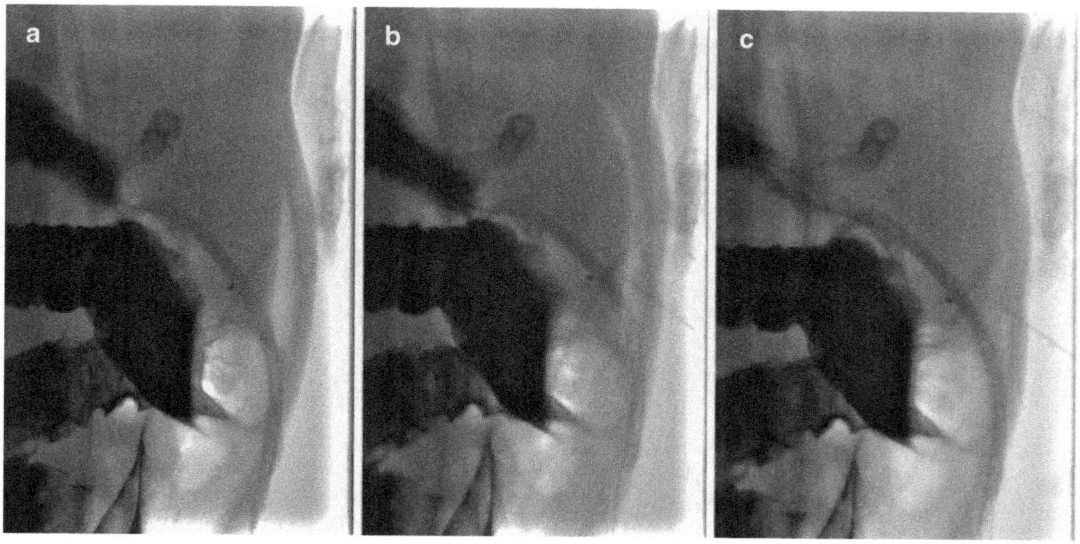

Fig. 20.10 Aspiration of pneumoperitoneum. (**a**) Lateral view following gastrostomy insertion demonstrates penumoperitoneum in a child with limited respiratory reserve. (**b**) A 27G needle is introduced into that area and (**c**) the air is aspirated

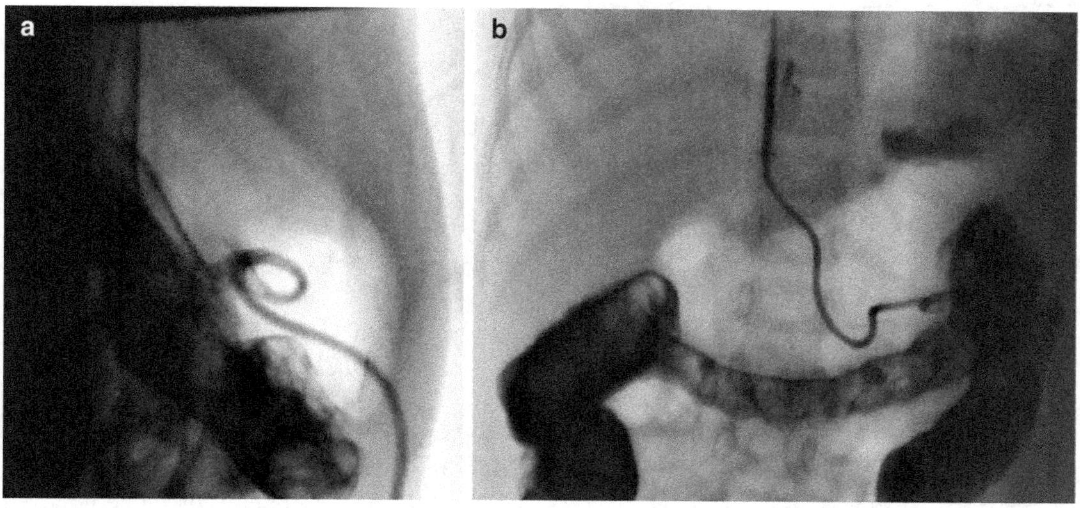

Fig. 20.11 Verification of tube location. Lateral (**a**) and AP (**b**) projections demonstrate the gastrostomy tube to be appropriately located

previous section. The supplied "folded" wire (Fig. 20.13a) is inserted through the needle into the gastric lumen. A gooseneck snare is used to capture the wire and pull it out through the mouth (Fig. 20.12). The PEG-type G tube is attached to the wire (Fig. 20.13a, b) and pulled via the mouth and esophagus through the abdominal wall. Care must be taken during passage of the G tube as the large "bumper" or internal fixator can damage the teeth during passage through the mouth or compress the trachea resulting in temporary respiratory compromise. The tube is pulled until the bumper is in continuity with the abdominal wall and it sits snugly (Fig. 20.14). After placing an external fixator, the tube is cut to an appropriate length and a feeding adapter is inserted (Fig. 20.15).

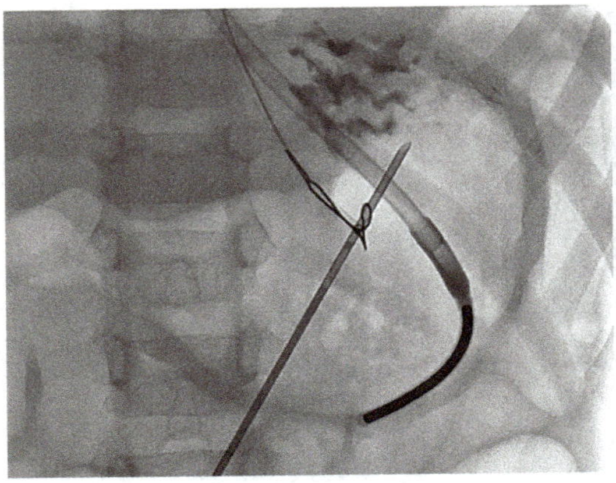

Fig. 20.12 Intragastric snaring. Following gastric puncture, the gooseneck wire was closed around the needle prior to inserting the supplied folded wire. The wire will then be pulled out through the mouth

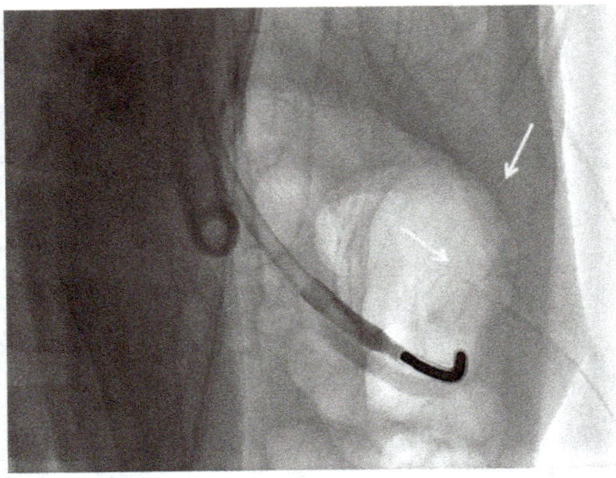

Fig. 20.14 PEG tube in place. The PEG tube has been pulled through the abdominal wall until the bumper was in apposition with the gastric wall (*arrow*). An NG tube is also present on this lateral image

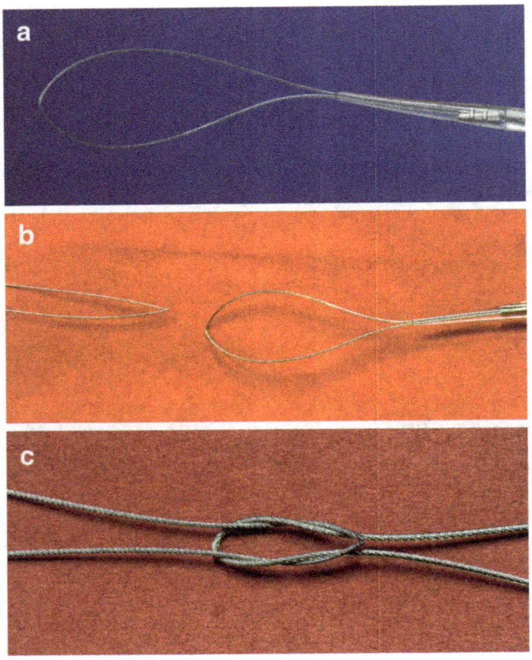

Fig. 20.13 Preparing the PEG tube. (**a**) The end of the PEG tube has a wire loop arising from the tapered, dilator tip. (**b**) The folded wire from the abdomen (left) and the PEG tube's wire loop (*right*) are shown. (**c**) The wire and loop are secured together. The loop of the PEG was inserted through the center of the folded wire; the distal end of the PEG was passed through the loop and the resulting knot was tightened. *Courtesy of Dr. Ganesh Krishnamurthy*

Gastrojejunostomy Tube Insertion

For primary gastrojejunostomy, the technique for accessing the stomach is the same as described above. When using retrograde gastric access technique, a 4- or 5-Fr guiding catheter is advanced into the stomach over the guidewire (instead of the G tube). When antegrade technique is used, a catheter and guidewire are inserted through the PEG tube (Fig. 20.16). The catheter and guidewire are then used to cannulate the proximal jejunum, and the GJ tube is advanced over the wire (Fig. 20.17). Extra care should be taken with small patients to avoid undue stress on the tissues that can lead to duodenal perforation (Fig. 20.18). In instances where a NJ tube is in place, it can be removed over an exchange length 0.035″ guidewire, keeping this wire as a guide into the small bowel, after gastric access is obtained.

Some infants who require NJ tube feeding will tolerate feeding via a G tube as the gastroesophageal junction may become competent after the NJ is removed. If necessary, a G tube can be converted to a GJ tube at any time with no need of sedation [5].

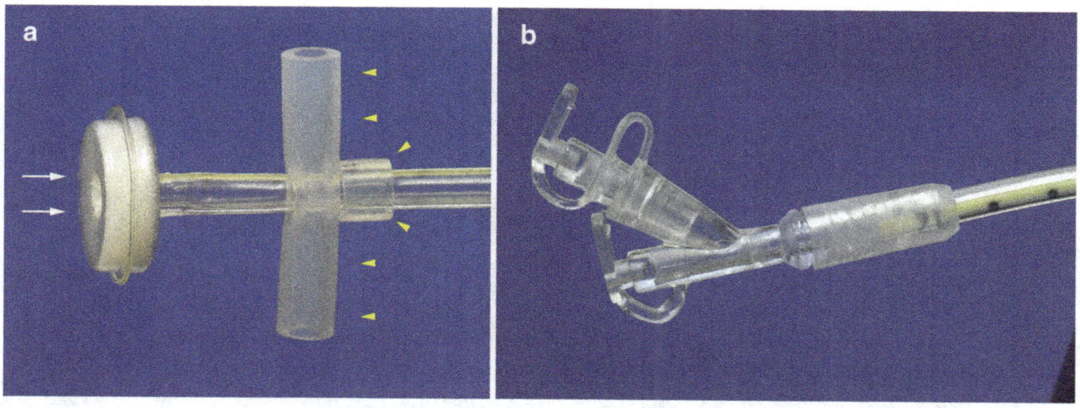

Fig. 20.15 PEG tube configuration. (**a**) The internal fixator of the PEG tube (*white arrows*) fits snugly against the abdominal wall to avoid inadvertent removal. An external fixator (*yellow arrowheads*) is attached after placement to avoid inward migration of the catheter. (**b**) A feeding adapter is fixed to the end of the shortened PEG tube. The adapter forms a tight seal to seal a small air channel that keeps the internal fixator turgid. *Courtesy of Dr. Ganesh Krishnamurthy*

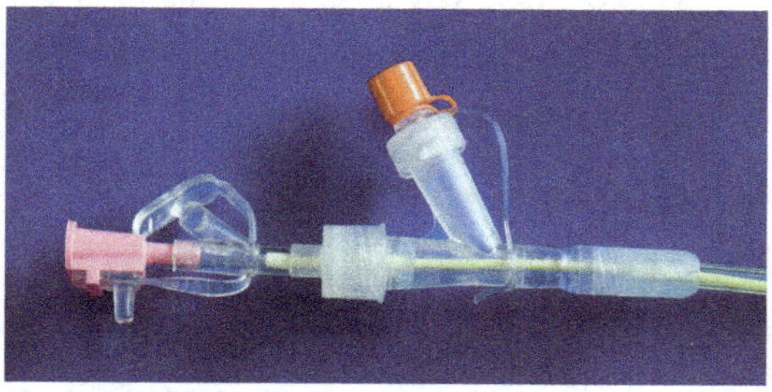

Fig. 20.16 GJ tube through PEG tube. A specialized adapter provides a gastric port and insertion of a gastrojejunal tube (*yellow* with *pink cap*) through the PEG tube. Images provided courtesy of Dr. Ganesh Krishnamurthy

Postprocedure Care

The patient is transferred to the postanesthesia care unit. If glucagon was given, blood glucose levels are measured 1 and 4 hours after administration. After the patient is fully awake and pain is controlled, he/she is transferred to the ward. The NG tube is left to drainage. Feeds are started in patients with antegrade tubes when bowel sounds return. Patients with retrograde tubes are kept NPO for at least 12 hours. After this period of time, 5 mL of an electrolyte solution is administered via the G tube Q 2 h if bowel sounds are present. If this amount of fluid is tolerated, the feeds are slowly started following a plan designed by the dietician. The interventional radiology team follows the patient daily until full feeds are reached. The retention suture is cut 14 days after the insertion.

When possible, the catheter should not be electively changed during the first 4–6 weeks due to immaturity of the tract. After this period of time, maintenance of the G tube is performed as needed. Button G tubes are the preferred device for some families. They are placed as soon as the tract is mature and has been upsized to 12 Fr (smallest device currently available). Parents are provided with a Foley catheter one size smaller than the G tube. They are instructed to insert the Foley into the mature tract if the G tube accidentally comes out to ensure that the tract is kept patent.

Complications

Complications had been described in 5–9 % of patients [12]. Peritonitis has been described in 3 % of the patients and can be a life-threatening complication. In the presence of symptoms such as fever and abdominal discomfort, there should be a low threshold to start wide spectrum antibiotics, stop feeds, and check the position of the catheter.

Glucagon use causes an initial elevation of serum glucose. Potentially profound, rebound hypoglycemia can result in fasted patients with

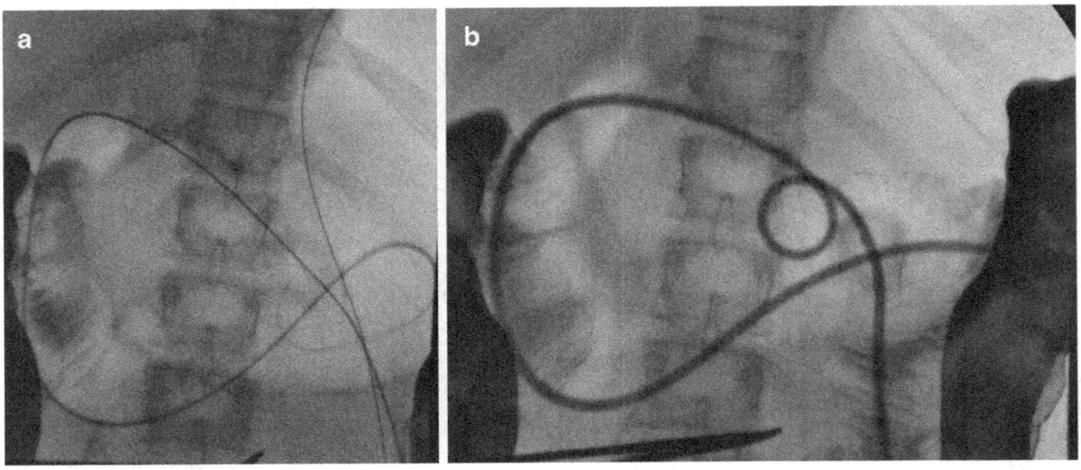

Fig. 20.17 Retrograde GJ placement. (**a**) A catheter and 0.035″ wire are used to cannulate the jejunum. (**b**) Final GJ tube position after insertion of the wire

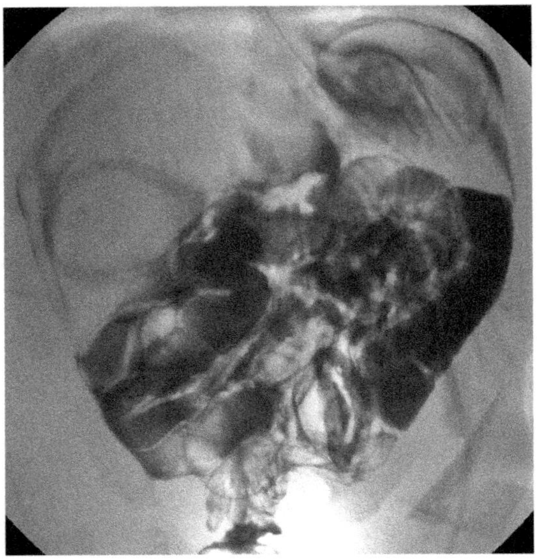

Fig. 20.18 Duodenal perforation. The initial portion of this GJ tube insertion was unremarkable. After the GJ was displaced over a normally positioned wire (see Fig. 20.17a for example), the tube was noted to project into the right upper quadrant. AP image of the abdomen demonstrates peritoneal contrast, pneumoperitoneum, and the GJ tube overlying the liver. At laparoscopy, a vertical tear of the second part of the duodenum was found

little reserve and those on beta-blockers. The use of dextrose-containing fluids can decrease the risk of hypoglycemic complications.

In cases of early tube dislodgement, access to the stomach can be attempted using the thread of the retention suture as a guide for an angiocatheter that will allow the insertion of a guidewire and reinsertion of the catheter. If this fails or there is an early migration of the catheter into the abdominal cavity, this site should be abandoned and a new G tube insertion should be scheduled when patient conditions permit.

Minor site problems are common and can be managed with conservative measures. Silver nitrate can be applied to the granulation tissue. Antibiotics are used in cases of site infection, and frequent cleaning with saline and exposure to air is used in cases of skin irritation. Other issues include gastric mucosa protruding through the tract and dilated ostomies resulted of leakage of gastric contents/feeds. The ostomy may decrease in size if the catheter is removed completely or replaced with a smaller catheter; however, surgical repair may be needed.

Intussusception can occur at any stage with the use of a GJ tube. Bilious vomiting after feeds, associated with abdominal distention and pain, is the typical clinical presentation. The diagnosis is made using ultrasound in combination with fluoroscopy. The routine approach is to remove the catheter and observe the intussusception with ultrasound. If it reduces, we reinsert a shorter catheter. If it does not resolve, a G tube can be placed for a few days for bowel rest [3, 12].

Tube Maintenance

Small-bore G and GJ tube are ideally changed every six months. Tube clogging, dislodgement, and leakage are frequent events that precipitate an early change. No analgesia or sedation is required.

The approach to management of large-bore PEG-type tubes varies by institution. Some institutions leave the catheters in place as long as needed or until there is an issue. Others electively remove the tubes and replace them with a button-type catheter after 3 months to decrease the risk of erosion of the internal fixator. Analgesia and sedation or general anesthesia may be required depending on the patient and the type of tube placed.

Cecostomy Tube Insertion

Cecostomy (C) tubes are catheters placed in the cecum to allow antegrade bowel irrigation in patients with fecal incontinence. By permitting people to evacuate their bowel in a planned manner, these catheters can significantly improve the quality of life through increased independence and social acceptance [3].

Indications/Contraindications

Spina bifida and imperforate anus are the most frequent indications for C tube insertion.

The presence of a nearby VP shunt tip is a relative contraindication—it may reposition itself if given time. The lack of safe access route and uncorrectable coagulopathy are absolute contraindications.

Preprocedure Workup

Cecostomy insertion represents a minimally invasive technique to treat fecal incontinence. As such, it carries a small but definite risk of complications (see below). In addition, creating an appropriate enema routine may take time and the tube will require ongoing interventional care. Therefore, the decision to undergo cecostomy tube insertion should not be undertaken lightly. Input from surgeons, gastroenterologists, dieticians, an encopresis team, and interventional radiologists can help guide the family during the initial evaluation and consent process.

The patient starts a clear fluid diet 2 days prior to the procedure. A bowel preparation solution is administered the day before and they are admitted the same day of the intervention. Preprocedure bloodwork (e.g., INR, PTT) is generally not required.

Equipment

- Fluoroscopy, US
- Rectal tube (Foley catheter)
- Enema inflator
- Glucagon
- Prophylactic antibiotics
- Sharp needle (such as Merit)
- 0.035″ Stiff guidewire (Amplatz)
- Retention sutures
- Dilators
- Small-bore Cope-loop catheter

Technique

The procedure is performed under general anesthesia, sedation, or local anesthesia, with the patient supine. A single dose of prophylactic antibiotics is given (cefoxitin, 30 mg/kg). The liver, gallbladder, and urinary bladder edges are marked on the skin using ultrasound. A Foley catheter is placed in the rectum that is used to insufflate air into the colon using an enema inflator. Glucagon is given intravenously to facilitate colonic distention. The cecum is localized using fluoroscopy and it is punctured using an 18-G sharp-tipped needle (Fig. 20.19). Contrast is injected to make sure that the needle is in an adequate position, and a 0.035″ Amplatz guidewire is advanced into the colon deploying two retention sutures (Cope Pediatric Gastrointestinal Suture Anchor Set, Cook). The tract is dilated with an 8-Fr dilator, and an 8-Fr

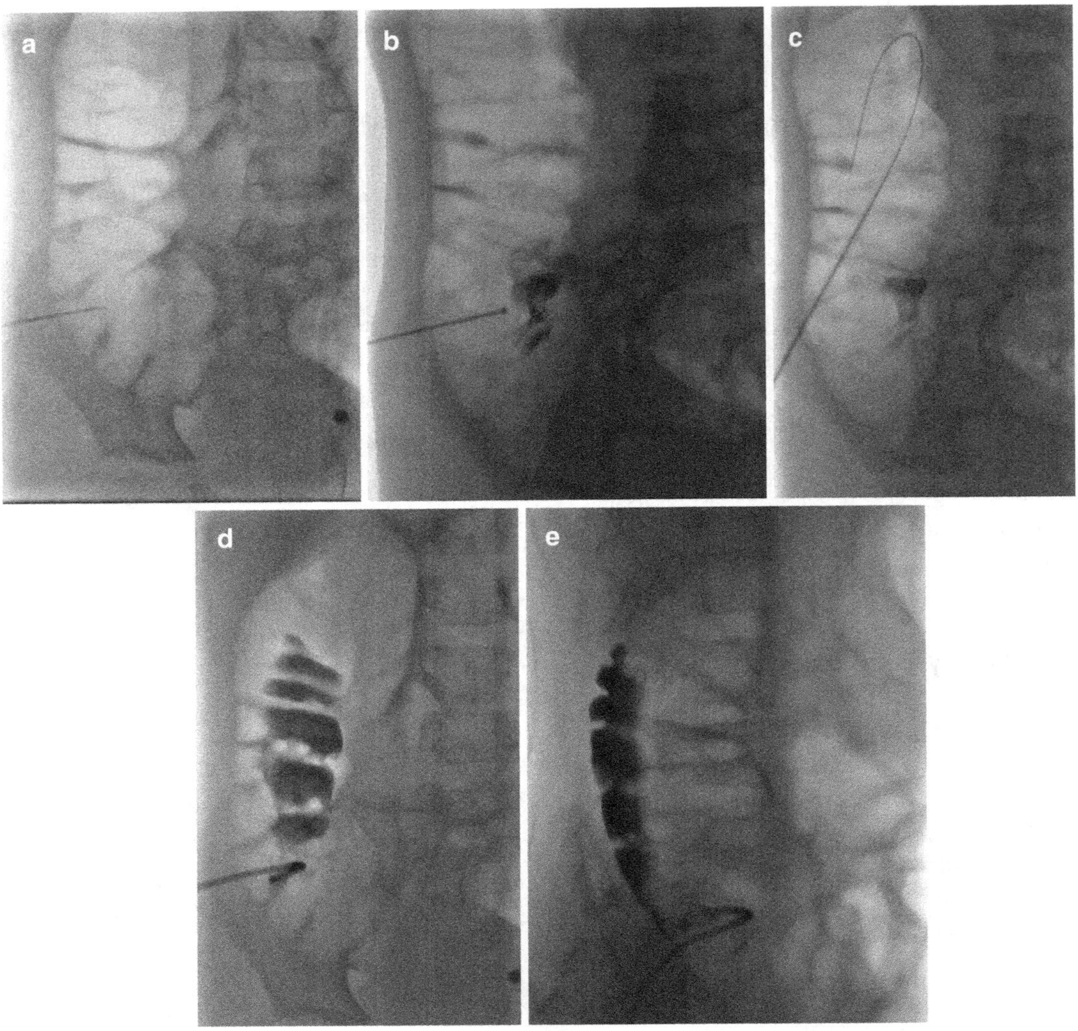

Fig. 20.19 Cecostomy tube insertion. (**a**) The cecum is localized on fluoroscopy and punctured with an 18-G needle. (**b**) Intraluminal location verified with contrast. (**c**) An 8-Fr dilator is inserted over an Amplatz wire. Intraluminal tube position is verified with (**d**) AP and (**e**) lateral projections

Cope-loop multipurpose catheter is placed in the cecum, and the guidewire is removed. A final contrast check is performed (Fig. 20.19). The tube is left open to gravity drainage.

If the colon does not distend adequately and the cecum cannot be visualized, the catheter can either be placed more distally (in the ascending or transverse colon) or the patient can be booked for a combined surgical-radiologic insertion. The cecum can be mobilized using laparoscopy to allow percutaneous cecostomy tube insertion. Cecostomy tubes inadvertently placed in the terminal ileum usually function appropriately.

Postprocedure Care

All patients are admitted to an inpatient unit after cecostomy tube insertion. Normal saline catheter flushes are started 24 h after the insertion. The patient can start slow introduction of p.o. feeds when bowel sounds are present.

Careful monitoring for fever and abdominal symptoms is mandatory as procedure-related complications include abscess formation, peritonitis, VP shunt infection, and death. If there are signs of infection, triple-antibiotic coverage is started. Special attention must be paid to symptomatic patients with VP shunts in situ—early neurosurgical consultation is warranted in these patients.

Follow-Up

The retention sutures are cut 14 days after the procedure, and the Dawson-Mueller catheter is replaced for a low-profile device (Chait Trapdoor pediatric cecostomy catheter, Cook, Bloomington, USA) 6–8 weeks after the primary insertion. To allow easy revision, our practice is to replace the C tube once a year. Tubes that are in place for longer periods become encrusted with calcified feces and can be extremely difficult to remove. For routine changes, the catheters can be removed over a hydrophilic guidewire or the trapdoor can be removed and the remaining catheter can be displaced into the cecum as the new catheter is inserted (Fig. 20.20). Fecal impaction can obstruct a catheter, blocking guidewire advancement. Blocked catheters can be displaced into the cecum, recanalized with a hydrophilic guidewire, or removed through a peelaway sheath.

There are currently three sizes of trapdoor catheters available. As patients grow and the distance from the skin to the cecum increases, insertion of longer catheters may be necessary. When a patient begins to outgrow a catheter, the loops of the pigtail can become displaced into the tract (Fig. 20.21). This causes elongation of the loops of the catheter and formation of a spiral soft tissue tract that can increase pressure at the ostomy and result in erosion of the skin. These tubes must be removed over a wire. Attempting to displace a tube with a spiral tract into the cecum can result in separation of the cecum from the abdominal wall (Fig. 20.22).

Optimally, the GI service or encopresis team works with patients and their families to develop an appropriate enema routine. This process can take several months and families need to be warned in advance.

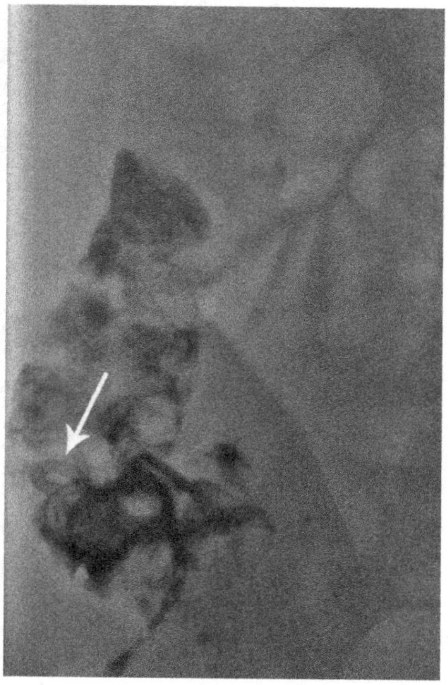

Fig. 20.20 Internal displacement of cecostomy tube. For some patients, removal of a cecostomy tube can be painful and traumatic. In the absence of a spiral soft tissue tract, a tube change can be performed by pushing the old catheter into the cecum. The new catheter is used to displace the old (after removing the trapdoor). The *arrow* demonstrates the fragment of the old tube that will be passed following the next enema

Soiling episodes following establishment of an enema routine can be secondary to a number of causes. Acute GI tract infection is a common cause. Peristaltic abnormalities of the bowel can sometimes be found. An iodinated contrast enema can be used to monitor transit through the bowel when a peristaltic abnormality is suspected.

Skin site issues are relatively common. Granulation tissue is treated with saline soaks and topical silver nitrate application. Excoriation of the site secondary to leakage of fecal contents can be treated with a barrier cream; involvement of an ostomy nurse can be helpful in severe cases. Continued leakage at the site raises the possibility of a distal colonic stenosis (Fig. 20.23).

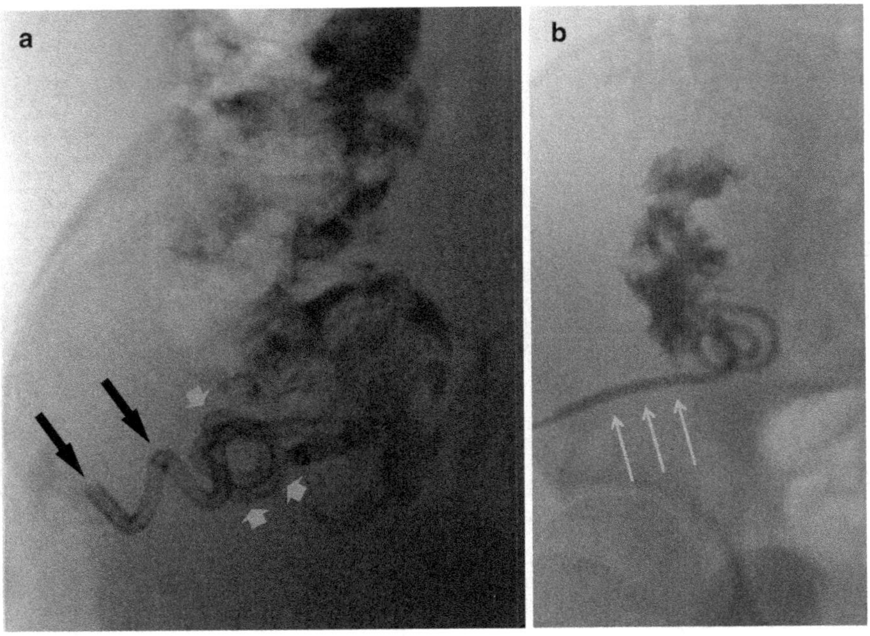

Fig. 20.21 Spiral soft tissue tract. (**a**) Short trapdoor cecostomy catheter in a patient with abdominal pain. Note the elongated coils in the soft tissues (*arrows*) and the tightly formed coils in the cecum (*arrowheads*). (The patient recently underwent a barium enema.) The tension of the catheter coils has resulted in the formation of a spiral tract in the tissues leading to the cecum. (**b**) The following day, the indwelling catheter was removed over a hydrophilic wire and a medium-length trapdoor catheter was placed under sedation. Note the straight path through the soft tissues (*arrows*)

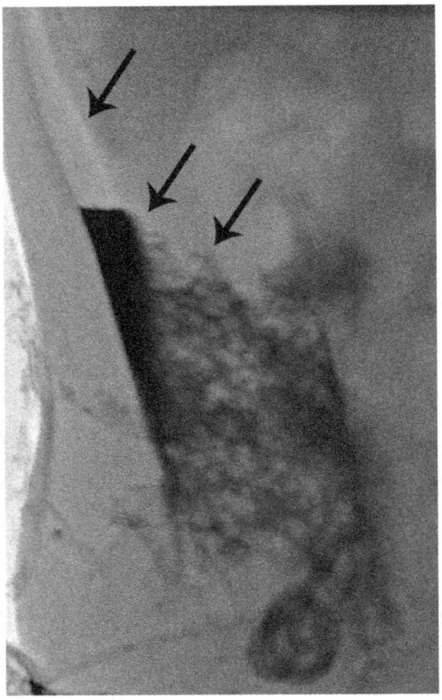

Fig. 20.22 Cecal dissection. Attempted internal displacement of a cecostomy tube in a patient with a spiral soft tissue tract resulted in loss of access to the cecum. Attempts to regain access resulted in dissection of the cecum from the abdominal wall with resultant spread of contrast and air into the soft tissues and the right paracolic gutter (*arrows*)

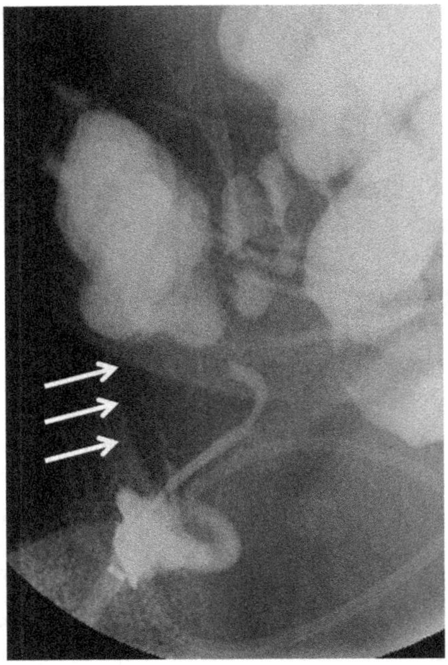

Fig. 20.23 Colonic stricture. Barium enema performed to assess massive leakage of bowel contents from cecostomy site. A tight inflammatory stricture of the ascending colon (*arrows*) was found

Chapter Summary

Esophageal Dilatation

Indications

- Tracheoesophageal fistula repair anastomosis most common
- Epidermolysis bullosa, reflux stricture, caustic ingestion, achalasia, other causes
- Swallowing issues, unable to swallow saliva

Contraindications

- Recent surgery
- Varices

Preprocedure Workup

- Upper GI or feeding study

Equipment

- 4 or 5 Fr directional catheter
- Wires—Bentson, Amplatz, glide wire, etc.
- Balloons—3–20 mm in diameter, compliant vs. noncompliant
- Inflating device if desired
- Contrast

Technique

- Delineate stenosis
- Dilate to appropriate size
- Check for complications

Pearls

- EB patients require meticulous technique
- Retrograde access (via gastrostomy site) can be used in difficult cases
- Mitomycin C has been used for resistant stenosis
- Esophageal stents are not commonly used

Postprocedure Care

- Slow introduction of feeds
- Consider admission for EB or difficult/complicated procedures

Complications

- Mucosal tear
  - Partial/submucosal—monitor
  - Full thickness—NPO, antibiotics, admit, consult surgery, and monitor closely

GAP Study

- Catheters placed into esophagus from mouth and stomach used to measure segmental gap

Gastrostomy/Gastrojejunostomy

Indications

- Inability to feed by mouth
- Inability to maintain adequate nutritional intake
- GJ for aspiration/reflux risk

Contraindications

- Uncorrectable coagulopathy
- Ascites
- Recent VP shunt insertion/revision

Workup

- Clinical assessment
- Parent teaching
- Imaging if potential access issues (multiple surgeries, severe scoliosis, etc.)
- Coagulation and CBC if clinically indicated

Equipment

- See page 313

Technique

- Prophylactic antibiotics
- Retrograde
  - Local, sedation, GA
  - Contrast enema
  - Glucagon (0.2–0.5 mg)
  - Gastric insufflation via NG tube
  - Fluoroscopy/ultrasound to puncture
  - Retention suture inserted
  - Dilate tract
  - Place and check tube
  - G and NG tubes to drainage
- Antegrade
  - Deep sedation or GA
  - Puncture as above
  - Snare and externalize wire via oral approach
  - Attach PEG tube and pull through the mouth, esophagus, and abdominal wall

- Gastrojejunostomy
  - Jejunum cannulated
  - GJ placed with retrograde technique
  - J tube placed via PEG with antegrade technique

Tips/Pearls
- Pneumoperitoneum present after insertion can be aspirated if required
- A small-gauge needle can be used to aspirate colon to facilitate gastric puncture

Postprocedure Care
- NPO until bowel sounds present
- Monitor glucose if glucagon is used
- Pain management
- Tube changes based on institutional practice

Complications
- Chemical or infections peritonitis, potentially life-threatening
- Hypoglycemia with glucagon in high-risk patients
- Tube dislodgement
- Site issues
- Intussusception with GJ tubes

Cecostomy

Indications
- Fecal incontinence
- Spina bifida, congenital rectal anomalies, and others

Workup
- Clinical assessment and family/patient teaching
- Bowel prep

Equipment
- See page 319

Technique
- Local, sedation, or GA based on patient need
- Prophylactic antibiotics (e.g., cefoxitin 30 mg/ kg)
- Mark the liver, gallbladder, and bladder location
- Note VP shunt if present
- Glucagon IV
- Insufflate colon via rectal tube
- 2 retention sutures are used
- Puncture, wire, dilate, and place catheter
- Assure appropriate intraluminal location

Postprocedure Care
- Restart feeds slowly when bowel sounds return
- Monitor for fever and pain
  - Early notification of neurosurgery in patients with VP shunt

Complications
- Infection (abscess, peritonitis, VP shunt infection, sepsis, death)
- Inappropriate tube position
- Site issues
- Bowel stenosis

Follow-Up
- Cut retention sutures after 14 days
- Can change to trapdoor catheter
- Removal vs. internal displacement for changes

References

1. Connolly BL. Gastrointestinal interventions—emphasis on children. Tech Vasc Interv Radiol. 2003;6(4):182–91 [Review].
2. Fasulakis S, Andronikou S. Balloon dilatation in children for oesophageal strictures other than those due to primary repair of oesophageal atresia, interposition or restrictive fundoplication. Pediatr Radiol. 2003; 33(10):682–7.
3. Yeming W, Somme S, Chenren S, Huiming J, Ming Z, Liu DC. Balloon catheter dilatation in children with congenital and acquired esophageal anomalies. J Pediatr Surg. 2002;37(3):398–402.
4. Mavili E, Amaral J, Healey A, Karsli C, Pope E, Connolly B. Percutaneous interventional radiology procedures in patients with epidermolysis bullosa: modifications and challenges. AJR Am J Roentgenol. 2010;195(2):468–75.
5. Roebuck DJ, McLaren CA. Gastrointestinal intervention in children. Pediatr Radiol [Review]. 2011;41(1):27–41.
6. Chung J, Connolly B, Langer J, Marcon M, Temple M, Amaral JG. Fluoroscopy-guided topical application of mitomycin-C in a case of refractory esophageal stricture. J Vasc Interv Radiol. [Case Reports] 2010;21(1):152–5.
7. Wong RF, Adler DG, Hilden K, Fang JC. Retrievable esophageal stents for benign indications. Dig Dis Sci. 2008;53(2):322–9 [Research Support, Non-U.S. Gov't].
8. Yoon CJ, Shin JH, Song HY, Lim JO, Yoon HK, Sung KB. Removal of retrievable esophageal and gastrointestinal stents: experience in 113 patients. AJR Am J Roentgenol. 2004;183(5):1437–44.
9. Kim JH, Shin JH, Song HY. Benign strictures of the esophagus and gastric outlet: interventional management. Korean J Radiol. 2010;11(5):497–506 [Review].
10. Lemberg B, Vargo JJ. Balloon dilation of colonic strictures. Am J Gastroenterol. 2007;102(10):2123–5 [Review].
11. Peer A, Klin B, Vinograd I. Balloon catheter dilatation of focal colonic strictures following necrotizing enterocolitis. Cardiovasc Intervent Radiol. 1993; 16(4):248–50 [Case Reports].
12. Luo CC, Lin JN, Wang CR. Evaluation of oesophageal atresia without fistula by three-dimensional computed tomography. Eur J Pediatr. 2002;161(11): 578–80.
13. Fitoz S, Atasoy C, Yagmurlu A, Akyar S, Erden A, Dindar H. Three-dimensional CT of congenital esophageal atresia and distal tracheoesophageal fistula in neonates: preliminary results. AJR Am J Roentgenol. 2000;175(5):1403–7.
14. Lam WW, Tam PK, Chan FL, Chan KL, Cheng W. Esophageal atresia and tracheal stenosis: use of three-dimensional CT and virtual bronchoscopy in neonates, infants, and children. AJR Am J Roentgenol. 2000;174(4):1009–12.
15. Rossi C, Domini M, Aquino A, Persico A, Lelli CP. A simple and safe method to visualize the inferior pouch in esophageal atresia without fistula. Pediatr Surg Int. 1998;13(7):535–6.
16. Preshaw RM. A percutaneous method for inserting a feeding gastrostomy tube. Surg Gynecol Obstet. 1981; 152(5):658–60.

Biliary Intervention in Children

21

Josée Dubois and Laurent Garel

Introduction

The development of magnetic resonance (MR) cholangiography has led to a decrease in the utilization of and indications for percutaneous biliary cholangiography in diagnosis of pediatric biliary diseases. However, interventional radiologists still play a central role in treatment of diseases such as biliary obstruction, choledocolithiasis, and cholecystitis.

This chapter will outline interventional techniques for performing intrahepatic and transhepatic cholangiography. Biliary diseases that are commonly diagnosed through cholangiography will then be discussed. A description of biliary interventions and associated diseases concludes the chapter.

Preprocedure Workup

An accurate history is obtained, and the previous imaging of the patient is evaluated. The imaging workup includes ultrasound, CT scan, and MR with MR cholangiography. Specific issues to be addressed include determination of allergies, renal function, coagulation status, and blood tests. The coagulation targets are platelet count over 50,000/μL, prothrombin time <18 s, partial thromboplastin time <32 s, and INR <1.2. If the blood tests are abnormal, coagulation has to be optimized to decrease the risk of procedural bleeding. Consultation with a hematologist is recommended. Depending on the case specifics, fresh plasma and/or platelet infusion may be needed. Fresh frozen plasma may be given if the prothrombin time remains >2 s above control levels.

Prophylactic antibiotic therapy should be administered 1 h before the procedure because of the high incidence of bacterial colonization of the biliary system, particularly in cases of obstruction and in patients with liver transplants. The antibiotic spectrum must cover both gram-positive and gram-negative organisms. The most common bacteria are *Escherichia coli, Enterococci, Klebsiella*, and *Streptococcus viridans*. A cephalosporin (such as ceftriaxone) is typically administered. Ciprofloxacin can be used in patients allergic to cephalosporins.

Contraindications

1. Uncorrectable coagulopathy due to the high risk of hemorrhage.
2. Ascites should be drained prior to the biliary procedure. Liver access must be performed in

J. Dubois, M.D., F.R.C.P.(C.), M.Sc. (✉)
L. Garel, M.D.
Department of Medical Imaging, Sainte-Justine Mother and Child University Hospital Center, 3175 Cote Ste-Catherine Road, Montreal, QC, Canada H3T 1C5
e-mail: josee-dubois@ssss.gouv.qc.ca; laurent_garel@ssss.gouv.qc.ca

M. Temple and F.E. Marshalleck (eds.), *Pediatric Interventional Radiology: Handbook of Vascular and Non-Vascular Interventions*, DOI 10.1007/978-1-4419-5856-3_21,

the absence of fluid between the liver margin and the abdominal wall.
3. Unsafe access route related to interposition of the bowel or lung.

Equipment

Anesthesiology and oxygen saturation monitoring devices are needed. Most biliary procedures are performed under general anesthesia. Apnea may be necessary in order to access small ducts. Dedicated modern C-arm unit equipped with pulsed fluoroscopy is required as is ultrasound.

Suggested equipment is listed under specific procedures below, and a compiled list is included in the chapter summary.

Anatomy

The liver is divided into eight segments with their own portal venous supply and biliary drainage (Fig. 21.1a). Normally, the biliary tree is adjacent and anterosuperior to the portal branch. The left hepatic biliary duct is divided into anterior (segments III and IV) and posterior (segment II) sectors separated by the left hepatic vein. The umbilical fissure and falciform ligament separate segments III and IV. The segment III biliary branch joins the segment II branch to form the left hepatic duct close to the Rex recess. Segment IV is drained by multiple biliary branches that join the left hepatic duct at the liver hilum.

The right hepatic lobe is divided into anteromedial (segments V, VIII) and posterolateral sectors (segments VI, VII) by the right hepatic vein. The right hepatic duct drains segments V, VI, VII, and VIII. The right portal vein separates the superior segments (VII and VIII) from the inferior segments (V and VI). The right posterior and anterior ducts merge close to the hilum. The right hepatic duct is shorter than the left hepatic duct. Segment I had a variable biliary drainage. Most of the time segment I drains bilaterally (80 %), in the left hepatic duct (15 %) and in the right hepatic duct (5 %).

Numerous anatomic variants are described. Most of them involve the right segments V, VI, and VIII. No anatomic variant of segment VII has been reported. On the left side, anatomic variants of segment IV have been found (Fig. 21.1b) [1].

Transhepatic Cholangiography

Percutaneous transhepatic cholangiography (PTC) is the first step for all percutaneous biliary interventions. When MR is inconclusive, cholangiography is useful to differentiate between types of neonatal cholestases treatable with surgical or noninvasive approaches.

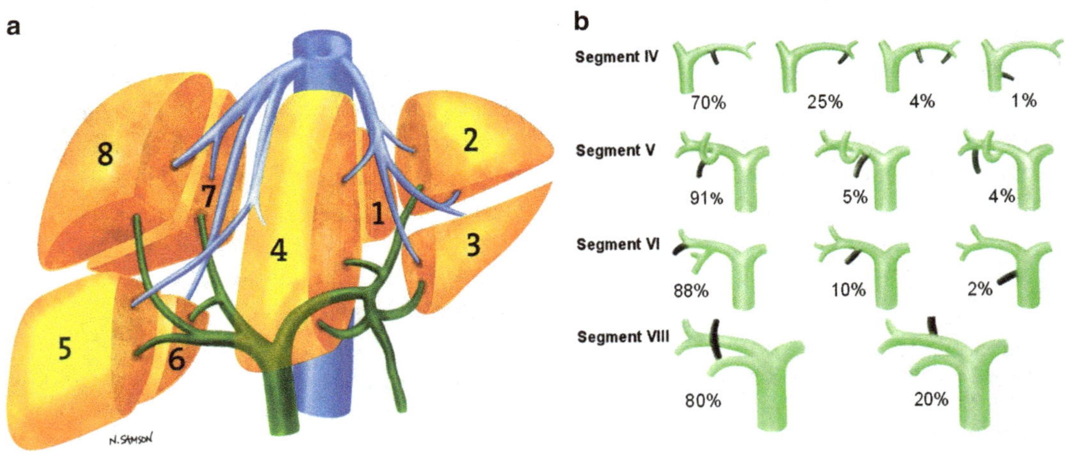

Fig. 21.1 (**a**) Segmental anatomy of the liver from Couinaud. (**b**) Common anatomic variants. Segments IV, V, VI, VIII

The initial puncture is performed with a 22-gauge Chiba needle. In case of biliary dilatation, the puncture is performed under ultrasonographic guidance. If the bile ducts are not dilated, the standard approach (described below) is recommended.

The puncture site is selected below the lateral costophrenic angle on full inspiration. The needle is inserted in the midaxillary line along the superior aspect of the lower rib to avoid the neurovascular intercostal bundle. The needle is advanced parallel to the tabletop in a 20–30° cranial direction toward a point lateral to the thoracic spine.

Classically, during the withdrawal of the needle, diluted contrast medium is gently injected until opacification of the bile ducts is seen. To minimize administration of parenchymal contrast material that will obscure the field of view, bile can be aspirated prior to injection. As an alternative technique, saline is injected while monitoring for intraluminal flow using ultrasound in order to avoid diffusion of contrast in the parenchyma and subsequent decreased visualization on fluoroscopy.

If the biliary system is not adequately opacified through the Chiba needle, a 0.018-in. mandril or hydrophilic wire can be used to insert a 3 Fr dilator through which contrast can then be injected.

The technical success of the procedure is almost 100 % if the biliary tree is dilated, but drops to 50 % when the ducts are not dilated. In pediatrics, when the biliary tree is not dilated, we frequently puncture the gallbladder for the biliary opacification. Biliary drainage is described below.

Complications

The complications of biliary access are rare (<5 %) and include sepsis, bleeding, biliary leakage, and pneumothorax [2].

Cholangiographic Diagnosis of Specific Biliary Diseases in Children

Biliary Atresia

Biliary atresia is the most common cause of neonatal cholestasis and is the main indication for liver transplantation in children. The incidence is 1/9,600 in Japan and 1/14,000 in the USA [3] with a female preponderance. The cause of the disease remains unknown [4–6]. Clinical presentation includes the presence of a hard liver and white stools. A nonsyndromic form is associated with 90 % of biliary atresia cases. In 10 %, biliary atresia can be associated with polysplenia, cardiac and pulmonary malformations, situs inversus, preduodenal portal vein, interrupted inferior vena cava, and intestinal malrotation [7]. Those abnormalities should be systematically searched for in the evaluation of biliary atresia patients.

Three types of biliary atresia are described. In type 1 (5 %), the obstruction occurs at the level of the common bile duct with the presence of a gallbladder. In type 2 (3 %), the obstruction occurs more proximally within the common hepatic duct. The small gallbladder contains no bile. In type 3 (90 %), the level of obstruction is at the porta hepatis. Examples of biliary atresia are shown in Figs. 21.2 and 21.3.

Differential diagnosis includes rare surgical causes (congenital obstructive choledochal malformations [8] and bile plug syndrome) and medical causes of neonatal cholestasis (neonatal hepatitis, α1-antitrypsin deficiency, cystic fibrosis). The diagnosis of biliary atresia is mandatory in order to delay or prevent biliary cirrhosis and the subsequent need for a liver transplantation. Accordingly, a Kasai procedure (hepatoportoenterostomy) should be performed within 40–60 days after birth [6, 8]. The majority of cases will eventually require liver transplantation.

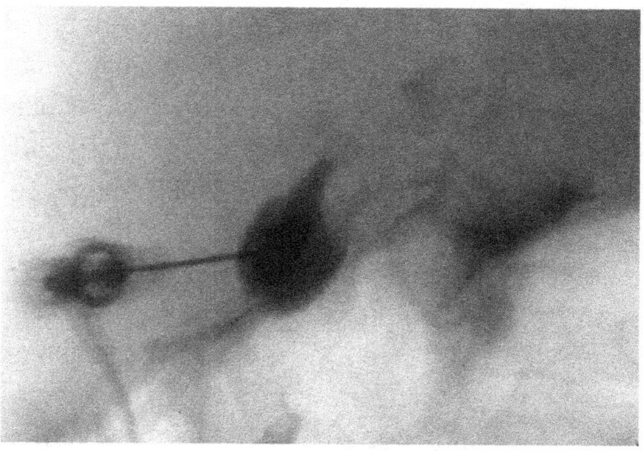

Fig. 21.2 Biliary atresia. Percutaneous transhepatic cholangiography. Puncture and opacification of the micro gallbladder demonstrate the absence of normal bile duct

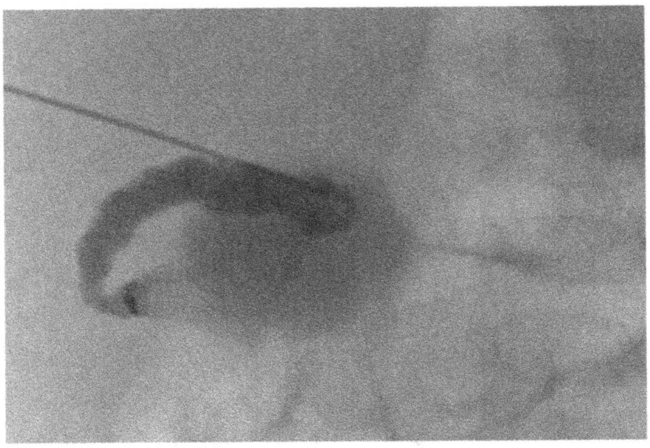

Fig. 21.3 Puncture of the gallbladder. The opacification demonstrates an abnormal gallbladder connected to a large cyst but without communication with the duodenum, indicating the biliary atresia

Choledochal Cyst

Choledochal cyst represents a rare cause of neonatal cholestatic jaundice. Development of a choledochal cyst may result from an abnormally long pancreaticobiliary duct allowing reflux of pancreatic enzymes into the biliary ducts [9–12]. Female preponderance occurs in a ratio of 4:1. Clinical manifestations such as abdominal pain, jaundice, or mass are nonspecific. Diagnosis is usually made before 10 years of age; some cases are discovered in utero and in adulthood [9, 10]. Differential diagnoses include biliary lithiasis, pancreatic pseudocyst, hepatic cyst, primary sclerosing cholangitis, enteric duplication, biliary hamartomas, microabscess, and biliary papillomatosis.

Complications include lithiasis leading to infection and even cystic rupture, biliary cirrhosis, and cholangiocarcinoma [10].

Five types of congenital biliary cysts have been described [13]. Type 1 is the most frequent (80–90 % of cases) in which the cystic malformation is confined to the extrahepatic ducts (Fig. 21.4). Three subtypes are described depending on the extension of the disease. In subtype 1a, the "diffuse type," all extrahepatic ducts are involved, and the gallbladder drains in the cyst. In subtype 1b, called "focal type," only a focal segment of the extrahepatic duct is involved, whereas subtype 1c is characterized by a fusiform enlargement of the choledochal duct, while the common hepatic duct is cylindrical. In type 2 (2 % of cases), the choledochal cyst is a diverticulum of the extrahepatic duct. In type 3 (1.4–5 % of cases), a choledochocele is located in the intraduodenal segment of the choledochal duct. In type 4, multiple cystic dilatations are encountered along both intra- and extrahepatic ducts (type 4a) (Fig. 21.5) or limited to the extrahepatic ducts (type 4b). Type 5 is known as Caroli's disease.

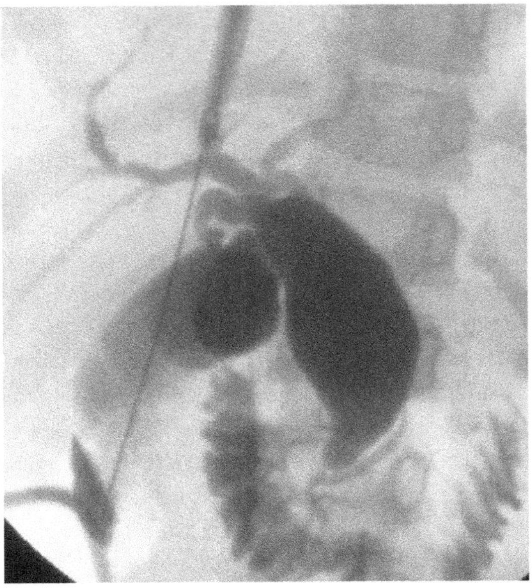

Fig. 21.4 Cholangiogram demonstrates a type 1a choledochal cyst

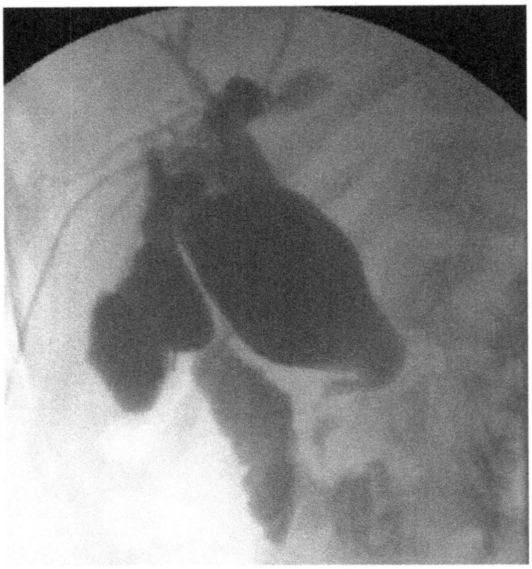

Fig. 21.5 Puncture of the gallbladder with a Chiba needle. The opacification reveals an extrahepatic and intrahepatic cystic dilatation diagnostic of type 4a choledochal cyst

This Mendelian recessive disease (same $PKHD_1$ gene as in the recessive polycystic kidney disease) is characterized by a nonobstructive cystic dilatation of the intrahepatic ducts that can be focal or diffuse.

Biliary atresia of the distal common bile duct can be associated with a choledochal cyst. When the dilated common bile duct does not communicate with the duodenum, the diagnosis is biliary atresia of the distal choledochus [8–10].

Chronic biliary stasis may lead to the same complications as listed above. Although there is no primary involvement of the extrahepatic tract, the latter can be secondarily modified in the course of recurrent infectious cholangitis.

MR cholangiography has predominantly replaced percutaneous cholangiography for diagnosis of choledochal cysts. It is useful to describe the cystic anomalies and define their type. In Caroli's disease, the "central dot sign," considered as highly suggestive, results from portal vein enhancement that is surrounded by cystic intrahepatic biliary ducts [14]. The pancreaticobiliary junction can also be analyzed by MR cholangiography.

Percutaneous or endoscopic retrograde cholangiography can be useful to confirm the diagnosis, determine the type of disease, and precisely analyze the pancreaticobiliary channel and its length.

Paucity of Intrahepatic Bile Ducts

Definitive diagnosis of this disease is histopathological requiring a liver biopsy specimen of adequate size (large) to demonstrate the paucity of bile ducts (Fig. 21.6) [15]. This is a common cause of neonatal or pediatric cholestatic jaundice. Two forms are described based on the presence or absence of other malformations. The nonsyndromic form can be idiopathic or associated with metabolic or viral diseases, chromosomal alterations, neoplasia, cystic fibrosis, and altered bile acid metabolism. The syndromic form is known as Alagille syndrome [16], an autosomal dominant inheritance disorder with variable expressivity that associates at least three of the five following major features: chronic cholestasis, characteristic facies, peripheral pulmonary artery stenosis, butterfly vertebrae (anterior rachischisis), and posterior embryotoxon. Prognosis varies, especially with the cardiovascular abnormalities. Pediatric liver transplantation is necessary in approximately 40 % of cases [17, 18].

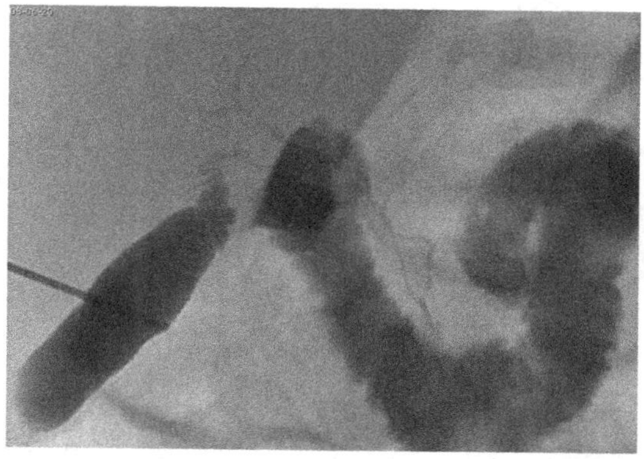

Fig. 21.6 Patient with Byler disease. Percutaneous transhepatic cholangiography demonstrates ductular hypoplasia

Infantile Sclerosing Cholangitis

Sclerosing cholangitis in children is a rare and heterogeneous condition, resulting from an inflammatory obliterative fibrosis that affects intra- and extrahepatic biliary ducts. The disease causes hepatic insufficiency and cirrhosis and carries a risk of malignant transformation into cholangiocarcinoma. Cholestatic jaundice is the main clinical finding that may occur in the early neonatal period but can be seen much later in the infant's life [19].

Etiologies vary and may remain unknown [20]. Immunodeficiency, inflammatory bowel disease, cystic fibrosis, and histiocytosis are classical etiologies of sclerosing cholangitis. Despite treatment of the underlying disease, liver transplantation is often needed.

MR cholangiography shows irregular biliary dilatation and beading which are segmental and involve multiple focal hepatic territories. The intrahepatic biliary ducts are always abnormal. The extrahepatic ducts are abnormal in 60 % of cases.

Percutaneous or endoscopic retrograde cholangiography shows intrahepatic biliary duct involvement in 100 % of cases and extrahepatic involvement in 60 % of cases [21]. There is diffuse stenosis of the bile ducts with focal dilatations between strictures providing the characteristic beaded appearance (Fig. 21.7).

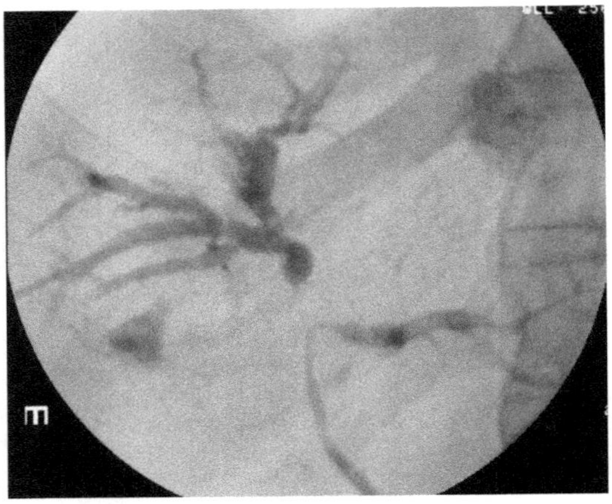

Fig. 21.7 Cholangiography in infantile sclerosing cholangitis shows irregular biliary dilatation, beading, and stenoses

Different segmental hepatic areas are involved [21, 22]. Liver biopsy is useful when cholangiography is normal [23].

Percutaneous Transhepatic Biliary Drainage

In pediatrics, percutaneous transhepatic biliary drainage is indicated in the treatment of bile plug syndrome, choledocholithiasis, tumor, and strictures associated with liver transplant. The most common obstructive tumors seen in the pediatric age group are rhabdomyosarcoma and inflammatory pseudotumor. Other causes of biliary strictures include postoperative injury after cholecystectomy, hepatic resection, laparoscopy, trauma, acute or chronic pancreatitis, primary sclerosing cholangitis, or radiation.

After opacification of the biliary tree with PTC, drain insertion is performed. When PTC is performed through a central duct, a second puncture is often needed to insert the drain into a more appropriate peripheral segmental duct. A coaxial dilator system (such as a Neff or Accustick Set) is used to traverse the hepatic parenchyma, provide stable access for biliary tract intervention, and allow upsizing of the 0.018″ mandril or hydrophilic wire to a 0.035″ system. The three components are an outer sheath, an inner tapered introducer, and an innermost metal stiffening cannula. Placement of a secondary safety wire can be considered for additional stability.

After introducing a guidewire into the biliary tract, the next step is to cross the stricture and gain access to the bowel for internal or internal–external biliary drainage. This is generally achieved with an angiographic catheter and hydrophilic guidewire. After crossing the stricture with a guidewire, balloon dilatation is performed (2–6 mm in diameter). The stricture is dilated serially until it can accommodate an appropriately sized drainage catheter (6–14 Fr). The balloon is inflated for approximately 1 min per inflation. Dilatation must usually be performed progressively to avoid laceration and massive bleeding into the biliary system. Dilatation may be repeated several times to obtain a good duct caliber. Severe fibrotic strictures can be managed with high pressure balloons. Once the inflation is initiated, a waist is seen at the stricture site that usually disappears with increasing pressure as the stenosis subsides. The hydrophilic guidewire is removed, and a stiff 0.035″ or 0.038″ Teflon-coated metallic wire is placed, and the final drainage catheter is advanced over the guidewire (Figs. 21.8 and 21.9). Standard or handmade transanastomotic internal–external biliary drainage catheters ranging from 6 to 14 Fr in size (Boston Scientific, Natick, MA) are used. Occasionally, additional side holes must be made in the catheter if the holes provided by the manufacturers do not allow adequate drainage. It is paramount to adjust the size and distribution of the holes to fit with the patient's anatomy. In other words, one must assess the exact location of the side holes to optimize the drainage without extrahepatic biliary leak. In order to do so, a guidewire is placed within a transhepatic catheter advanced in the third portion of duodenum. The ideal location of the most proximal and distal side holes is marked by bending the guidewire prior to its removal. Any necessary additional side holes are then created on the drainage catheter based on these measurements. After the placement of the catheter, contrast injection is recommended to ensure proper opacification of the biliary tree, nonopacification of the portal or hepatic venous system, and absent peritoneal extravasation.

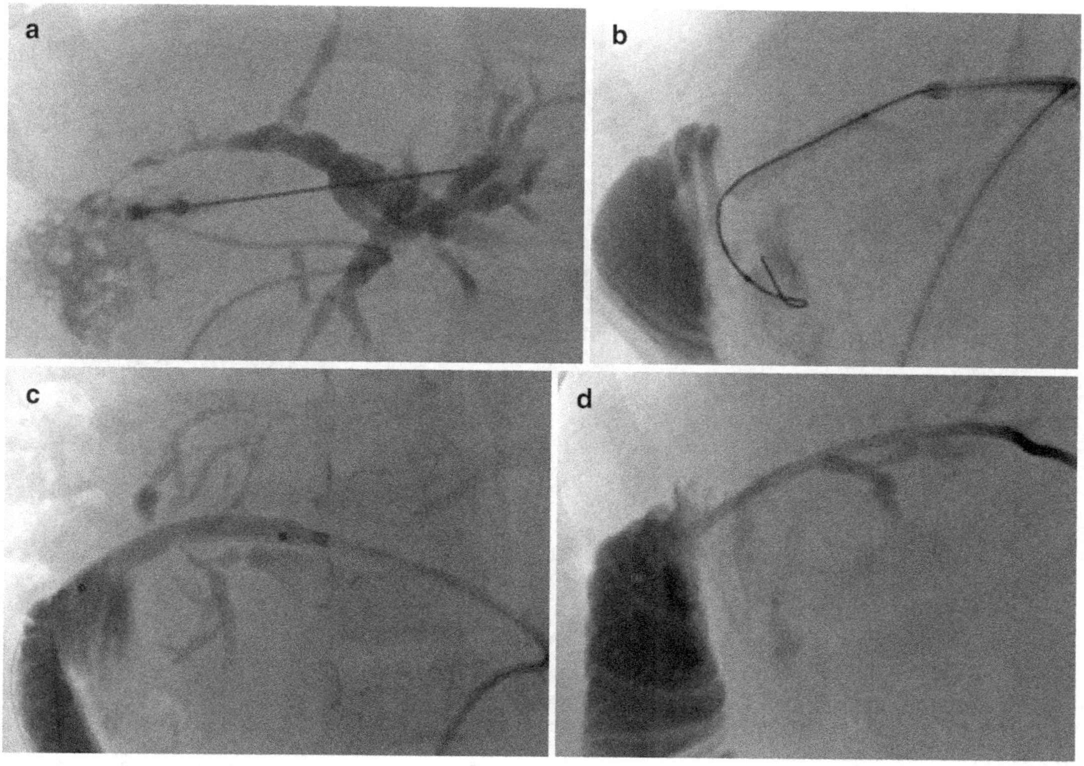

Fig. 21.8 (**a**) Puncture of the biliary branch of segment II showing a stenosis of the transplant's biliary–bowel intestinal anastomosis. (**b**) A guidewire is inserted followed by the placement of the introducer (Neff set). The end of the wire is in the blind end of the Roux-en-Y loop. The guidewire must be in the jejunal loop. (**c**) A progressive dilatation from 4 to 6 mm balloon size was performed. (**d**) An internal–external biliary catheter was placed

Sometimes a two-stage procedure is necessary. Patients with obstructed, infected biliary systems can become acutely septic as a result of bile duct manipulation. Some strictures are difficult to cross due to regional anatomy or edema of the area. In these instances, a drain is left in the biliary tree proximal to the stenosis. Secondary placement of an internal–external drain can be undertaken after a minimum of 48 h of external drainage and antibiotic treatment when the patient has defervesced.

Percutaneous cholangiogram is an effective method to identify the presence of biliary strictures. The success rate of PTC is 96 %, and the reported success rate of percutaneous biliary drainage is 89 % in pediatric liver transplant recipients [24, 25]. Sunku et al. reported a 100 % technical success rate for PTC and balloon dilatation. Stricture recurrence is a real drawback occurring in 66 % of cases in Sunku et al. series. The recurrence rate was 45 % for anastomotic strictures, 90 % for intrahepatic strictures, and 100 % for the cases with both an anastomotic and intrahepatic strictures [24].

Complications

The complications of biliary drainage are pain, bleeding, hemobilia, and infection. The incidence of bacteremia and endotoxic shock is reduced by the routine administration of prophylactic intravenous antibiotics. Pneumothorax can occur with a high right-sided puncture. It can be avoided with the fluoroscopic examination of the right costophrenic sulcus during deep inspiration. Whenever possible, the puncture site should be caudal to the sulcus. Biliary peritonitis is related

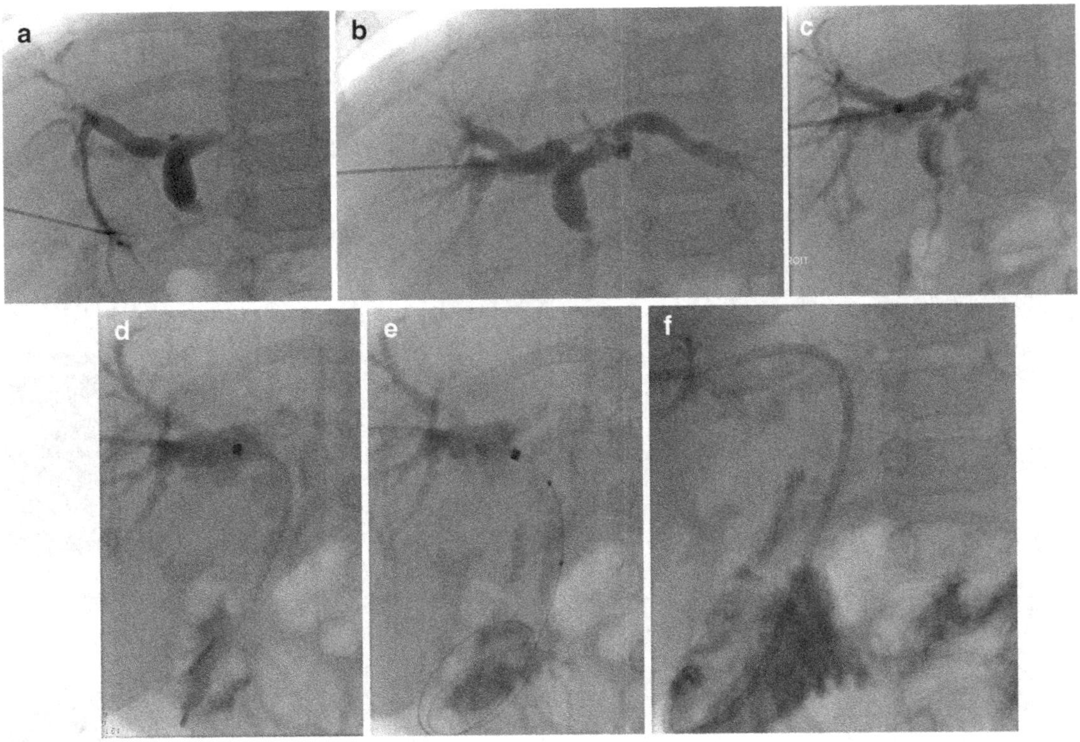

Fig. 21.9 (**a**) Image from the initial percutaneous transhepatic cholangiogram demonstrating injection into a biliary radicle with filling of the biliary tree. A severe stenosis was demonstrated without opacification of the bowel. (**b**) A distal branch of the segment VII was punctured under ultrasound. (**c**) The introducer sheath was installed. (**d**) A Terumo guidewire with a glide catheter (4 Fr) was used to cross the stenosis. (**e**) Progressive dilatation of the choledochal anastomosis was done with 4–7 mm balloons. (**f**) An internal-external biliary catheter was installed

to the catheter side holes inadvertently placed outside the liver, allowing the free flow of bile into the peritoneum. Pneumothorax, bile effusion, or subphrenic collections are rare complications that should be drained when necessary.

Postprocedure Care

In the absence of sepsis, catheters are initially flushed on a daily basis. Depending on institutional practice, catheters may or may not be flushed after discharge from hospital.

Usually, exchange of the catheter takes place every 2–3 months on an outpatient basis. If the stricture has improved and there is no bile leak, a catheter without side holes (and therefore with no draining function) is left in place above the anastomosis. This tube will preserve the biliary access. After a test period of 2–8 weeks, a normal cholangiogram, and stable LFTs, the catheter can be safely removed. Complete closure/sealing of the biliary access is advocated before surgical cholangioplasty. Sometimes the catheter is removed inadvertently resulting in biliary leak at the skin surface. Most leaks subside spontaneously during the following weeks.

Technical Remarks

1. The use of cutting balloon: Saad et al. [27] reported a success rate of 93 % ($n=22$; $p=49$).
2. Stent placement can potentially preclude or complicate definitive surgical repair. For this reason, retrievable stent graft placement is recommended.
3. Biliary leaks: Endoscopic retrograde cholangiopancreatography (ERCP) is recommended as the first option when the procedure is feasible and available.

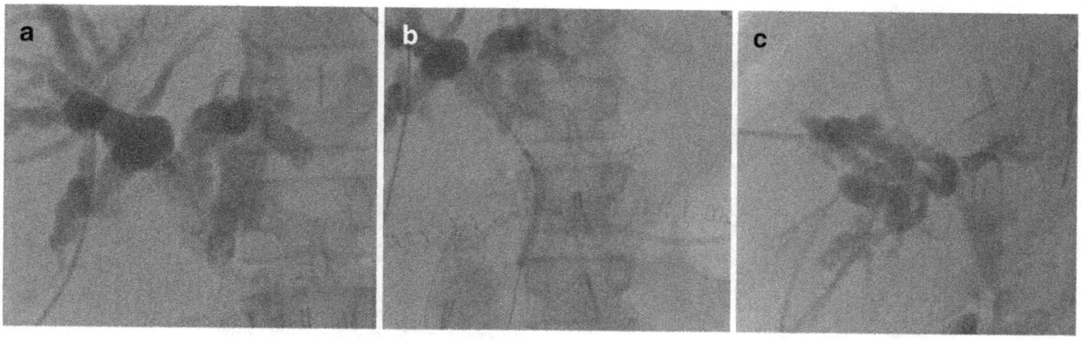

Fig. 21.10 A 17-year-old girl with whole liver transplantation complicated by artery thrombosis. (**a**) Cholangiogram demonstrates severe biliary damage with focal dilation and stenosis related to biliary necrosis. A severe obstruction was noted at the biliary anastomosis. (**b**) With a Terumo and glide catheter, the stenosis was crossed and balloon dilatation was performed. (**c**) An internal-external catheter was installed

4. Recommended timing of catheter removal is controversial ranging from a few weeks to a year. No randomized studies have compared early versus late catheter removal. No definitive advice can be given for catheter dwell time; however, removal can be considered with a normal cholangiogram, tolerance of a trial of internal drainage, and normal LFTs.

Specific Biliary Diseases Treated with Percutaneous Biliary Intervention

Benign Biliary Strictures: Liver Transplant

Biliary complications are observed in 5–34 % of pediatric liver transplant recipients [24, 26]. Complications include anastomotic leakage and stenosis with bile duct dilatation, stones, sludge or debris, and biloma. The majority of these complications occurred within the first 3 months after transplantation. However, biliary strictures and stones can occur months or even years after the procedure [25].

Strictures are commonly seen in split-liver transplantation which is frequently performed in pediatrics. Split-liver transplantation represents a technical challenge in comparison with whole liver transplantation because of the short length of the donor right (rarely left) hepatic duct available to be sutured resulting in a biliary anastomosis under tension.

Two types of biliary anastomosis are performed: choledochocholedochal (CDCD) anastomosis of the donor common bile duct to the recipient common bile duct and biliodigestive choledochojejunostomy or hepaticojejunostomy attaching the end of the common bile duct or common hepatic duct to the side of a loop of jejunum that is pulled up to the region of the porta hepatis in a Roux-en-Y configuration. The latter anastomosis is required in biliary atresia patients.

The stricture is located at the level of the anastomosis or in the intrahepatic biliary ducts. Strictures of the biliary tree are associated with hepatic artery thrombosis in liver transplant patients (Fig. 21.10). The success rate by percutaneous approach is only 78 % compared to 100 % for endoscopic approach. However, the endoscopic approach is more difficult in children, even more so in infants. Results have to be evaluated in this age group.

Biliary Rhabdomyosarcoma

This very rare pathology carries a poor prognosis. Clinical manifestations are nonspecific and include cholestatic jaundice, abdominal mass, and weight loss.

Imaging features demonstrate an infiltrative mass with proximal biliary dilatation that frequently involves the common bile duct [28, 29] (Fig. 21.11). Chemotherapy is the first choice of treatment with variable response. Liver transplantation is controversial. Prolonged drainage with an

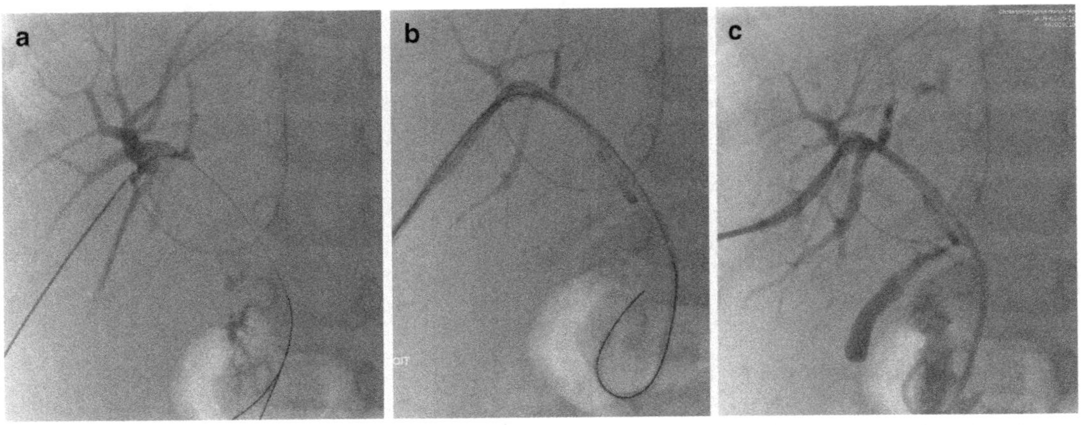

Fig. 21.11 A 20-month-old child with biliary rhabdomyosarcoma. (**a**) A puncture of biliary branch was performed with a Chiba needle. The guidewire passes easily through the tumor. (**b**) An internal-external stent was installed. (**c**) A second biliary drain was left in place proximally within the biliary tree

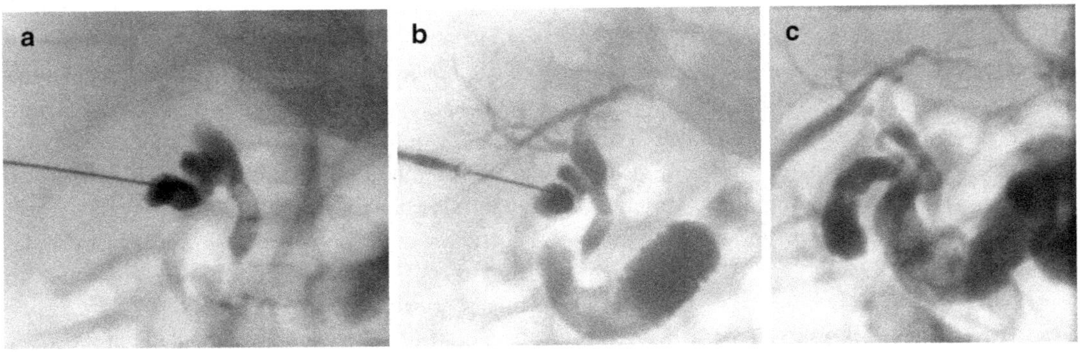

Fig. 21.12 Cholestasis in a neonate. (**a**) PTC by the gallbladder shows biliary plug. (**b**) After saline lavage, we opacified the intrabiliary tree. (**c**) Lavage was performed for 2 days. The last control showed normal biliary duct

internal–external stent is required until the tumor responds to chemotherapy or transplantation is undertaken.

Bile Plug Syndrome

Thickening of the bile often results from prematurity, hemolysis, hemorrhage, infection, cystic fibrosis, dehydration, parenteral nutrition, and intestinal atresia. Mechanical obstruction of the biliary tract leads to nonspecific symptoms such as icteric cholestasis and abdominal pain. Complications are essentially infectious with cholangitis, liver abscess, and septicemia.

Treatment is conservative in most instances. When required, treatment modalities include biliary lavage through percutaneous cholangiography approach or, rarely, surgical treatment.

Biliary Lavage

The gallbladder is usually accessed directly with a 22-gauge Chiba needle. A transhepatic approach can also be utilized. A 0.018-in. wire may be used with a coaxial dilator which allows transition to a 0.035-in. system. The biliary tree is opacified with diluted contrast. A 5 or 6 Fr drainage catheter is inserted in the gallbladder. The lavage is performed with saline. The following day, the biliary tree is reopacified and the lavage repeated if the obstruction is still present (Figs. 21.12 and 21.13). The catheter is removed when the biliary tree is free of sludge. In our institution, biliary lavage has proved safe and useful in such instances.

Cholecystostomy has also been described for the treatment of acalculous cholecystitis and obstructive jaundice in children.

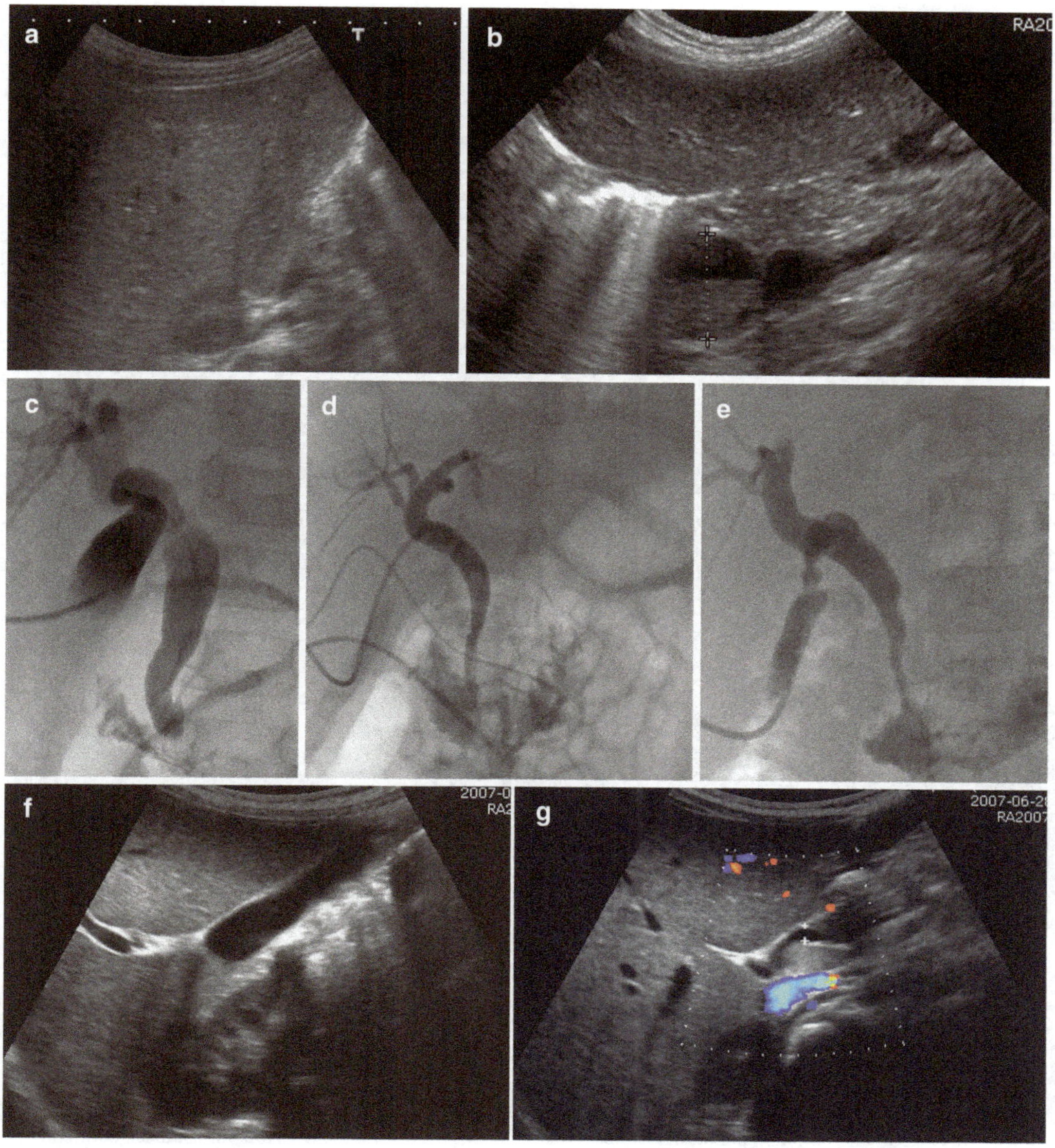

Fig. 21.13 A 3-year-old child with spherocytosis. (**a**, **b**) Abdominal pain and cholestasis were observed. An abdominal ultrasound found sludge in the gallbladder and the biliary tree. (**c**) A gallbladder puncture was performed and the biliary tree was opacified. (**d**) We crossed the cystic duct and inserted a multihole drainage catheter. (**e**) After 4 days of lavage, there is complete resolution of the sludge. (**f**) One week after the procedure, ultrasound showed a normal gallbladder and (**g**) normal biliary tree

Choledocholithiasis

Pediatric choledocholithiasis is a rare condition that is often associated with a preexisting abnormality. Prematurity, infection, dehydration, hemolysis, total parenteral nutrition, and furosemide therapy are known to be significant risk factors for lithiasis. In older children, choledochal cyst, biliary stenosis, hemolytic anemia (sickle cell), cystic fibrosis, Crohn's disease, obesity, and intestinal resection contribute to lithiasis.

Findings at ultrasonography, MR cholangiography, and percutaneous or retrograde cholangiog-

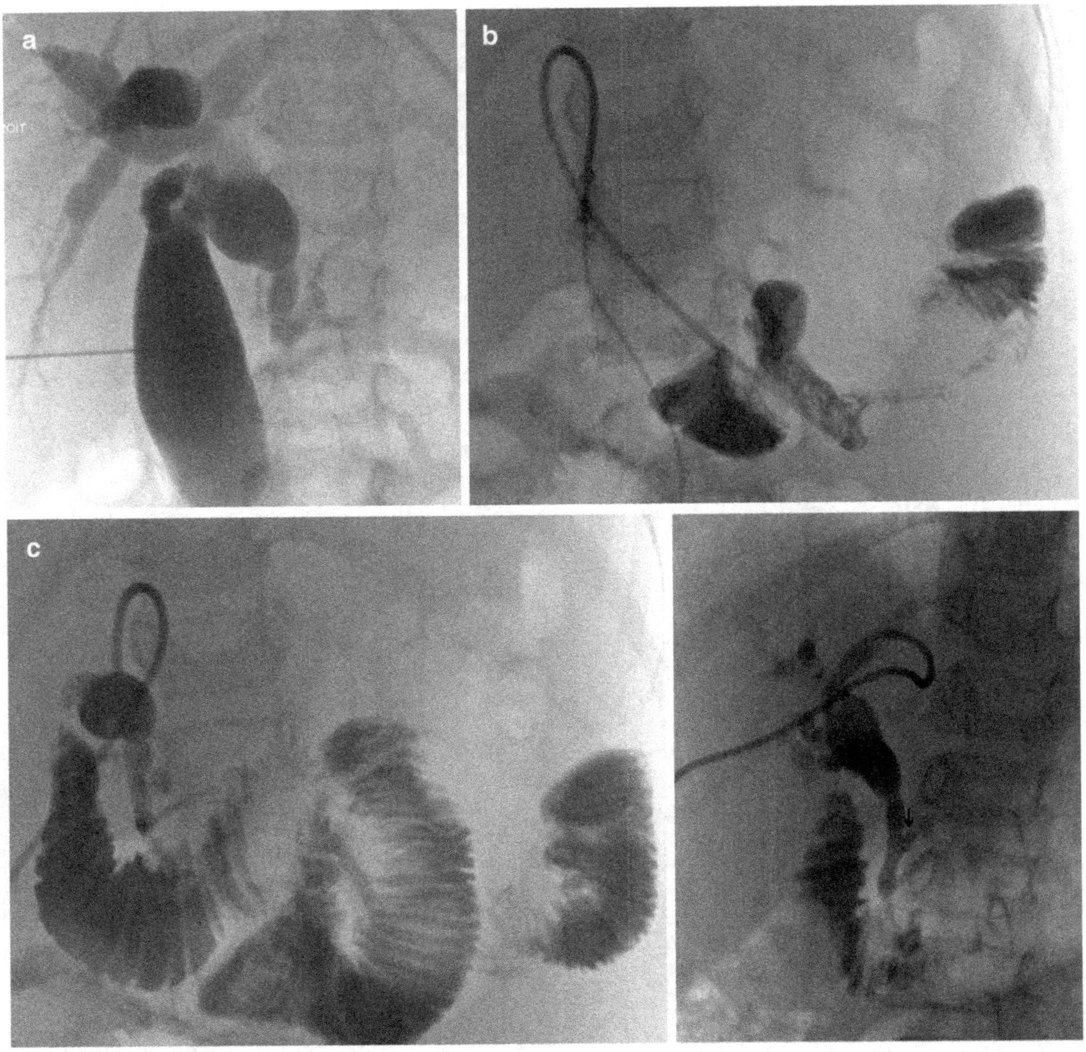

Fig. 21.14 A 4-year-old girl with cholestasis. (**a**) PTC demonstrated a choledochal stone associated with a choledochal cyst. The stone was mobilized through the biliodigestive system, and an internal-external catheter was placed. (**b**) The following day, the patient developed significant abdominal pain. Opacification of the drain demonstrated a tube-related intussusception. (**c**) The tube was removed and the intussusception subsided spontaneously. (**d**) The cholangiogram at the end of the procedure displays a diverticulum (*arrow*) of the distal common bile duct with an abnormal biliopancreatic junction as seen with choledochal cyst

raphy are quite similar, showing biliary dilatation above an impacted stone and sometimes an underlying abnormality.

Through biliary drainage and dilatation, interventional radiology plays a central role in the treatment although surgery is sometimes still required (Fig. 21.14) [30, 31]. Stones less than 1 cm can be pushed through the papilla into the bowel with balloon catheter. Stones larger than 1 cm must be fragmented to facilitate passage into the bowel.

Trauma

Trauma (Fig. 21.15) of the biliary tree can be rare or silent in the pediatric group. Three-dimensional, spiral CT cholangiography and MR cholangiography are useful in the diagnosis of bile duct injuries [32–34]. Nonsurgical management of hemodynamically stable patients with trauma has become the standard

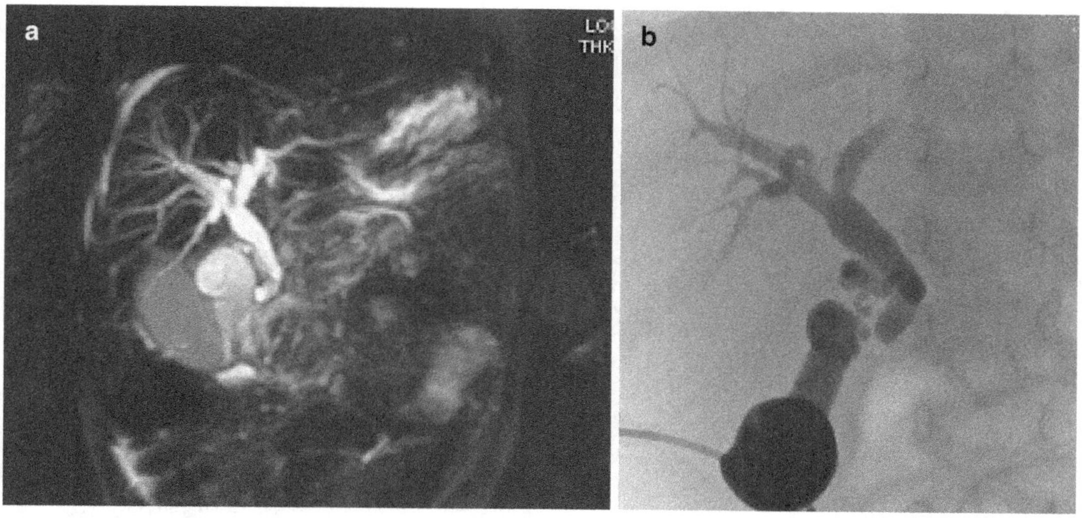

Fig. 21.15 Car accident trauma. (**a**) MR cholangiogram showed an obstruction of the distal part of the common bile duct. (**b**) The surgeon asked for cholangiography to define the anatomy. Complete occlusion of the distal part of the common bile duct was found

method of care. In pediatric hepatic trauma, 10 % of complications have been reported including rupture, hematoma, hemobilia, and biliary leaks. ERCP has been used as a diagnostic as well as therapeutic modality for extrahepatic biliary injury. Biliary stent or nasobiliary drain placement without sphincterotomy is recommended [35]. Intrahepatic biloma following blunt trauma may be more common than previously reported. They may resolve spontaneously, and many bile leaks are clinically silent [36, 37]. Most of the intrahepatic biliary leak is treated conservatively or by catheter drainage for minor leaks.

Conclusion

Diagnoses of most biliary diseases are made by MR cholangiography. However, biliary intervention is particularly useful in the treatment of biliary plug and liver transplant complications. Biliary interventions are safe and cost-effective with a low complication rate. Currently, there are no guidelines regarding the appropriate duration of biliary drainage in children, especially for liver transplant. Multidisciplinary approach is key to decide the best therapeutic option for these patients.

Chapter Summary

Background

- Performed for diagnosis and treatment of biliary disease
- Decreased role due to MRCP

Equipment

- 22 Chiba needles
- Coaxial dilator set
- Wires: 0.018″ mandril and 0.035″ hydrophilic/Teflon coated/stiff
- Balloons: 2–6 mm; use of cutting balloons has been described
- Drainage catheters: 5–14 Fr; may require creation of side holes

Indications

1. Diagnosis: neonatal cholestasis versus anatomic causes
   (a) Biliary atresia
   (b) Choledochal cyst
   (c) Paucity of intrahepatic bile ducts
   (d) Infantile sclerosing cholangitis
2. Cholestasis treatment
   (a) Faster resolution of TPN-associated cholestasis noted [37]
   (b) Treatment of biliary sludge

3. Stricture
   (a) Post liver transplant
   (b) Tumor
      (i) Biliary rhabdomyosarcoma
   (c) Idiopathic and iatrogenic
      (i) Bile plug syndrome
4. Choledolithiasis
5. Cholecystitis
6. Trauma
   (a) Consider conservative treatment and ERCP

Contraindications

1. Uncorrectable coagulopathy
2. Ascites
3. Interposed bowel or lung

Preprocedure Workup

- CBC, INR, PTT, BUN, and creatinine
- Prophylactic antibiotics (e.g., ceftriaxone, ciprofloxacin)

Technique

- Biliary access
  - Ultrasound-guided biliary access when possible
  - Standard approach (pullback contrast injection) when necessary/indicated
  - Can puncture gallbladder for diagnostic cholangiogram
- Drainage
  - Coaxial dilator provides stability for interventions
  - Minimize intervention when septic
    - Place external biliary drain and return after 48 h of antibiotics
  - Consider safety wire
  - Sequential dilatation (2–6 mm) and high pressure/cutting for resistant stenoses
  - 6–14 Fr internal–external drainage catheters
    - May require additional side holes
    - Assure adequate drainage and no peritoneal leak

Complications

1. Sepsis
2. Hemorrhage
3. Bile leak
4. Pneumothorax

Postprocedure Care

- catheters when not septic
- Catheter exchange q 2–3 months

Follow-Up

- Timing of biliary catheter removal controversial

References

1. Valette PJ, De Baere T. Anatomie biliaire et vasculaire du foie. J Radiol. 2002;83(2 Pt 2):221–32.
2. Hoevels J. Percutaneous transhepatic cholangiography and percutaneous biliary drainage. In: Dondelinger RF, Rossi P, Kurdziel JC, Wallace S, editors. Interventional radiology. New York, NY: Thieme Medical; 1990. p. 187–99.
3. Davenport M. Biliary atresia. Semin Pediatr Surg. 2005;14:42–88.
4. Fischler B, Ehrnst A, Forsgren M, Orvell C, Nemeth A. The viral association of neonatal cholestasis in Sweden: a possible link between cytomegalovirus infection and extrahepatic biliary atresia. J Pediatr Gastroenterol Nutr. 1998;27:57–64.
5. Hart MH, Kaufman SS, Vanderhoof JA, et al. Neonatal hepatitis and extrahepatic biliary atresia associated with cytomegalovirus infection in twins. Am J Dis Child. 1991;145:302–5.
6. Lachaux A, Descos B, Plauchu H, et al. Familial extrahepatic biliary atresia. J Pediatr Gastroenterol Nutr. 1988;7:280–3.
7. Kasai M, Suzuki H, Ohashi E, Ohi R, Chiba T, Okamoto A. Technique and results of operative management of biliary atresia. World J Surg. 1978; 2:571–9.
8. Pariente D, Franchi-Abella S. Cystic biliary atresia is different from choledochal cyst. Pediatr Radiol. 2009; 39:1019.
9. Wiseman K, Buczkowski AK, Chung SW, Francoeur J, Schaeffer D, Scudamore CH. Epidemiology, presentation, diagnosis, and outcomes of choledochal cysts in adults in an urban environment. Am J Surg. 2005;189:527–31.
10. Kim OH, Chung HJ, Choi BG. Imaging of the choledochal cyst. Radiographics. 1995;15:69–88.
11. Gauthier F, Brunelle F, Valayer J. Common channel for bile and pancreatic ducts. Presentation of 12 cases and discussion. Chir Pediatr. 1986;27:148–52.
12. Babbitt DP, Starshak RJ, Clemett AR. Choledochal cyst: a concept of etiology. Am J Roentgenol Radium Ther Nucl Med. 1973;119:57–62.
13. Mortelé KJ, Rocha TC, Streeter JL, Taylor AJ. Multimodality imaging of pancreatic and biliary congenital anomalies. Radiographics. 2006;26: 715–31.
14. Miller WJ, Sechtin AG, Campbell WL, Pieters PC. Imaging findings in Caroli's disease. AJR Am J Roentgenol. 1995;165:333–7.

15. Brown RM. Pathology of neonatal liver biopsy. Curr Diagn Pathol. 2006;12:202–9.
16. Hadchouel M. Le syndrome d'Alagille. www.orpha.net. May 2002.
17. Hoffenberg EJ, Narkewicz MR, Sondheimer JM, Smith DJ, Silverman A, Sokol RJ. Outcome of syndromic paucity of interlobular bile ducts (Alagille syndrome) with onset of cholestasis in infancy. J Pediatr. 1995;127:220–4.
18. Alagille D, Estrada A, Hadchouel M, Gautier M, Odièvre M, Dommergues J. Syndromic paucity of interlobular bile ducts (Alagille syndrome or arteriohepatic dysplasia): review of 80 cases. J Pediatr. 1987;110:195–200.
19. Sisto A, Feldman P, Garel L, et al. Primary sclerosing cholangitis in children: study of five cases and review of the literature. Pediatrics. 1987;80:918–23.
20. Mieli-Vergani G, Vergani D. Sclerosing cholangitis in the paediatric patient. Best Pract Res Clin Gastroenterol. 2001;15:681–90.
21. Debray D, Pariente D, Urvoas E, Hadchouel M, Bernard O. Sclerosing cholangitis in children. J Pediatr. 1994;124:49–56.
22. Wilschanski M, Chait P, Wade JA, et al. Primary sclerosing cholangitis in 32 children: clinical, laboratory, and radiographic features, with survival analysis. Hepatology. 1995;22:1415–22.
23. Pall H, Bancroft JD, Jonas M. One third of children with primary sclerosing cholangitis have normal cholangiograms at diagnosis. Gastroenterology. 2003;124 Suppl 1:A784.
24. Sunku B, Salvalaggio PR, Donaldson JS, et al. Outcomes and risk factors for failure of radiologic treatment of biliary strictures in pediatric liver transplantation recipients. Liver Transpl. 2006;12:821–6.
25. Lorenz JM, Denison G, Funaki B, Leef JA, Van Ha T, Rosenblum JD. Balloon dilatation of biliary-enteric strictures in children. AJR Am J Roentgenol. 2005;184:151–5.
26. Berrocal T, Parrón M, Alvarez-Luque A, Prieto C, Santamarıa ML. Pediatric liver transplantation: a pictorial essay of early and late complications. Radiographics. 2006;26:1187–209.
27. Saad WE, Davies MG, Saad NE, et al. Transhepatic dilatation of anastomotic biliary strictures in liver transplant recipients with use of a combined cutting and conventional balloon protocol: technical safety and efficacy. J Vasc Interv Radiol. 2006;17:837–43.
28. Donnelly LF, Bisset 3rd GS, Frush DP. Diagnosis please. Case 2: embryonal rhabdomyosarcoma of the biliary tree. Radiology. 1998;208:621–3.
29. Spunt SL, Lobe TE, Pappo AS, et al. Aggressive surgery is unwarranted for biliary tract rhabdomyosarcoma. J Pediatr Surg. 2000;35:309–16.
30. Debray D, Pariente D, Gauthier F, Myara A, Bernard O. Cholelithiasis in infancy: a study of 40 cases. J Pediatr. 1993;122:385–91.
31. Tarnasky PR, Tagge EP, Hebra A, et al. Minimally invasive therapy for choledocholithiasis in children. Gastrointest Endosc. 1998;47:189–92.
32. Wicky S, Gudinchet F, Barghouth G, Schnyder P. Three-dimensional cholangio-spiral CT demonstration of a post-traumatic bile leak in a child. Eur Radiol. 1999;9:99–102.
33. Wong YC, Wang LG, Chen RJ, Chen CJ. Magnetic resonance imaging of extrahepatic bile duct disruption. Eur Radiol. 2002;12:2488–90.
34. Youngson GG, Driver CP, Mahomed AA, Duddalwar VA. Computed tomographic cholangiography in the diagnosis of bile duct injury in children. J Pediatr Surg. 2003;38:E18–20.
35. Singh V, Narasimhan KL, Verma GR, Singh G. Endoscopic management of traumatic hepatobiliary injuries. J Gastroenterol Hepatol. 2007;22:1205–9.
36. Sharif K, Pimpalwar AP, John P, et al. Benefits of early diagnosis and preemptive treatment of biliary tract complications after major blunt liver trauma in children. J Pediatr Surg. 2002;37:1287–92.
37. Wales PW, Brindle M, Sauer CJE, et al. Percutaneous cholangiography for the treatment of parenteral nutrition-associated cholestasis in surgical neonates: preliminary experience. J Pediatr Surg. 2007;42(11):1913–8.

Section VIII

Nonvascular Interventions: Genitourinary

Genitourinary Interventions

22

Frank P. Morello

Introduction

Pediatric nonvascular genitourinary intervention may be divided into perirenal interventions, such as drainage of urinoma and urine leaks, and percutaneous nephrostomy/ureteral interventions [1–8]. Percutaneous nephrostomy is utilized for relief of urinary tract obstruction, urinary diversion for treatment of trauma, or decompression of an infected urinary tract. Percutaneous nephrostomy is also means for access for subsequent endourologic procedures.

The indications for genitourinary intervention in children differ from that in the adult in several respects. Congenital anomalies such as ureteropelvic junction (UPJ) obstruction, ureteral vesicle junction (UVJ) obstruction, and posterior urethral valves are commonly encountered conditions in children. Conditions in common with adult patients are trauma, nephrolithiasis, and drainage of complex urinary tract infections.

F.P. Morello, M.D. (✉)
Department of Radiology, University Medical Center, University of Arizona College of Medicine, 1501 N. Campbell Avenue, Tucson, AZ 85724, USA
e-mail: fmorello@kc.rr.com

Preprocedure Workup

With GU interventions in children, consideration of a pediatric sedation plan is required which includes preprocedural evaluation, drug selection, patient monitoring, and postprocedural care. See Chap. 3 for sedation information. General anesthesia is sometimes necessary, particularly for prolonged procedures or when preprocedural evaluation identifies risk or contraindications for sedation.

Coagulation parameters including PT, PTT, INR, and platelets are assessed to determine risk for bleeding. Procedures are not done with uncorrected coagulopathies. The administration of prophylactic antibiotics is controversial. However, in cases of urinary sepsis, the choice of antibiotic is based on the patient's specific risk factors for bacteriuria and bacteremia. Cefazolin, ceftriaxone, or ampicillin and gentamicin are commonly used.

Equipment

Most, if not all, interventions in the pediatric GU tract utilize ultrasound for image-guided access. A high-quality ultrasound system with a variety of linear and curved array transducers is essential.

Specific equipment for each intervention will be discussed below and is included in the chapter summary.

M. Temple and F.E. Marshalleck (eds.), *Pediatric Interventional Radiology: Handbook of Vascular and Non-Vascular Interventions*, DOI 10.1007/978-1-4419-5856-3_22,

Perinephric Fluid Collections: Urinomas and Urine Leaks

A urinoma is an encapsulated collection of extravasated urine. Urinoma in the pediatric population is most frequently due to obstructive hydronephrosis related to congenital anomalies such as UPJ obstruction, UVJ obstruction, or posterior urethral valves, where there has been calyceal perforation (Fig. 22.1). A urinoma may also occur with renal fracture following trauma. Urinomas are most often confined within the perirenal space by Gerota's fascia but may dissect along fascial planes into the peritoneal cavity or along the iliopsoas muscle extending below the inguinal ligament into the soft tissues of the thigh and buttock. A urinoma may even extend into the mediastinal and pleural spaces.

Complications associated with urinoma include hydronephrosis from mass effect, paralytic ileus, electrolyte imbalance, and abscess formation. Urinoma with active urine leak can be diagnosed with contrast-enhanced CT with delayed images, retrograde pyelography, renal scintigraphy, or IVP.

Indications/Contraindications

The indications for drainage of urinoma are large-size or persistent leak over several days and fever or sepsis, regardless of size. Also, drainage of urinoma that separates renal fragments accelerates the healing process (Fig. 22.2).

Urinoma drainage can be accomplished with ultrasound or CT guidance using standard percutaneous drainage techniques.

Percutaneous Nephrostomy

Indications

Percutaneous nephrostomy is a well-established interventional radiology procedure. The most common indications for percutaneous nephrostomy in the pediatric age group are UPJ obstruction, obstruction after pyeloplasty, UVJ obstruction, posterior urethral valves, treatment of complex urinary tract infection, and primary obstructive megaureter. Percutaneous nephrostomy may also be used as an initial step for the purpose of ureteral intervention, as discussed later in this chapter.

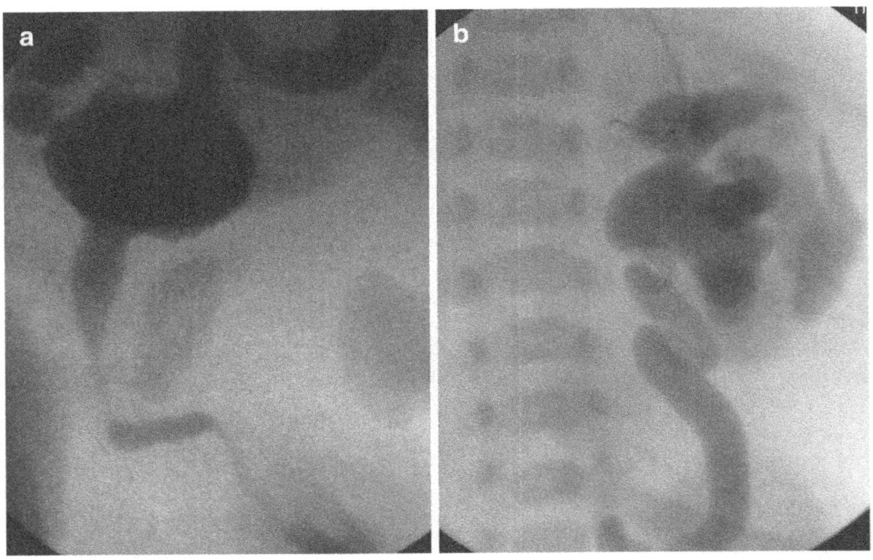

Fig. 22.1 Calyceal perforation and perirenal urinoma. (**a**) VCUG exam in newborn male with posterior urethral valves. (**b**) Vesicoureteral reflux through calyceal perforation into perirenal urinoma

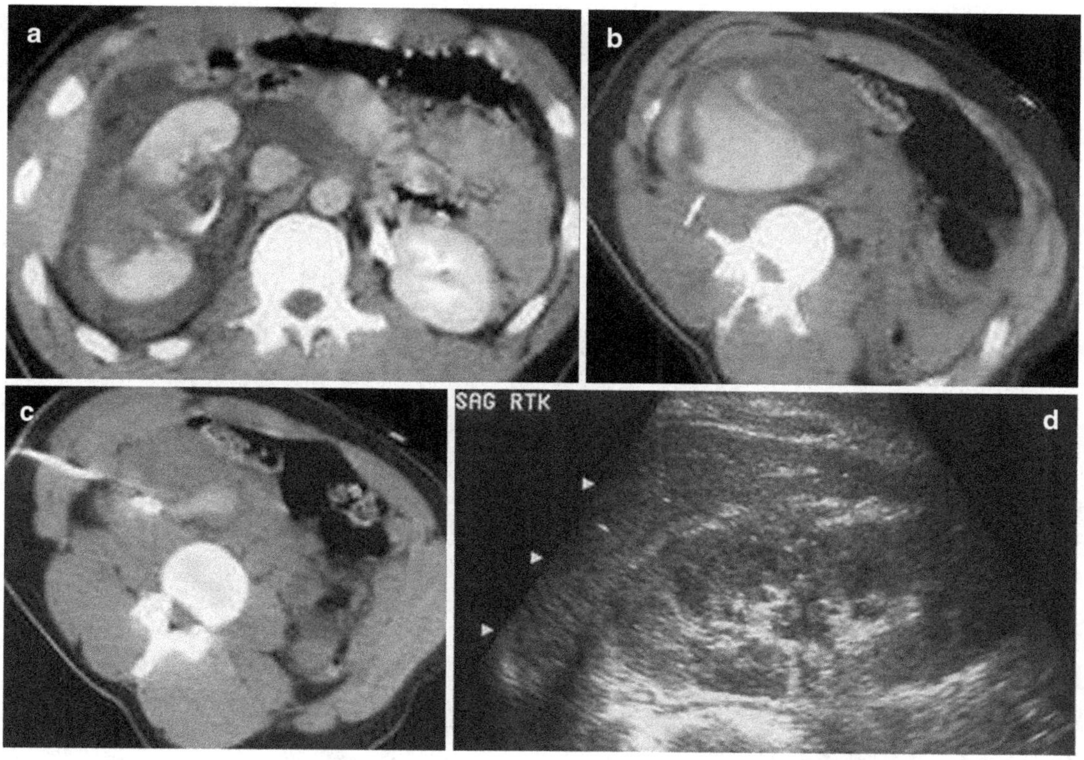

Fig. 22.2 Right renal fracture with perirenal urinoma. (**a**) Skydiver who after successful first jump was ceremoniously tossed into a pond onto a submerged rock, fracturing the right kidney. There is a sizable perinephric fluid collection around the fractured kidney. There is good enhancement of the renal fragments indicating vascular viability. (**b**) The delayed scans through the kidney show contrast collecting in the dependent portion of the perirenal space. Aspiration of the fluid yielded blood-tinged urine, indicating an active urine leak rather than active extravasation of blood. (**c**) A perirenal drainage catheter was placed and the urinoma was successfully drained. The catheter was left in place for about 10 days, over which time the catheter output gradually decreased. (**d**) A follow-up US at 1 month shows healing of the renal fracture with no re-accumulation of the urinoma

Anatomy

An understanding of renal anatomy is essential for avoiding potential complications. The main renal artery divides into the major anterior and posterior branches (Fig. 22.3) with the anterior branch supplying the anterior two-thirds and the posterior branch the posterior one-third of the kidney. Brodel's bloodless line is a zone of relative avascularity posterior to the lateral convex border at the junction of the anterior two-thirds and posterior one-third of the kidney. The posterior calyces are oriented with their long axis towards this area. This ideal nephrostomy access route minimizes vascular injury by passing parallel to the renal vessels (Fig. 22.4).

The puncture site is determined by the goal to be accomplished. A subcostal approach below the eleventh rib, into a lower pole calyx, is best for simple urinary drainage. A posterior calyx of the middle or upper collecting system is best accessed when there is expected ureteral intervention or subsequent endourologic procedures. In either instance, puncture of the renal infundibula or pelvis is avoided because there is a higher risk of vascular injury. All nephrostomy catheters should traverse the renal parenchyma before entering the collecting system. The parenchyma provides a secure seal and anchor around the catheter.

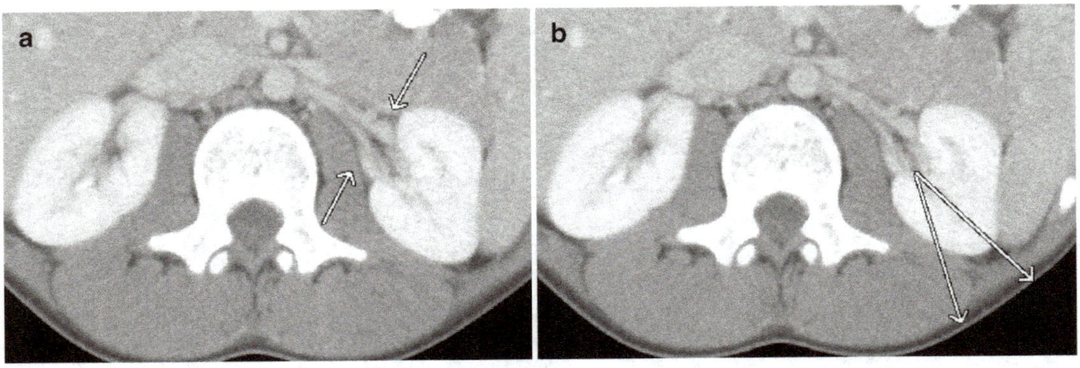

Fig. 22.3 Renal artery anatomy. (**a**) The main renal artery divides into anterior and posterior branches. (**b**) Brodel's bloodless zone, relative avascularity at the junction of the anterior two-thirds and posterior one-third of the kidney

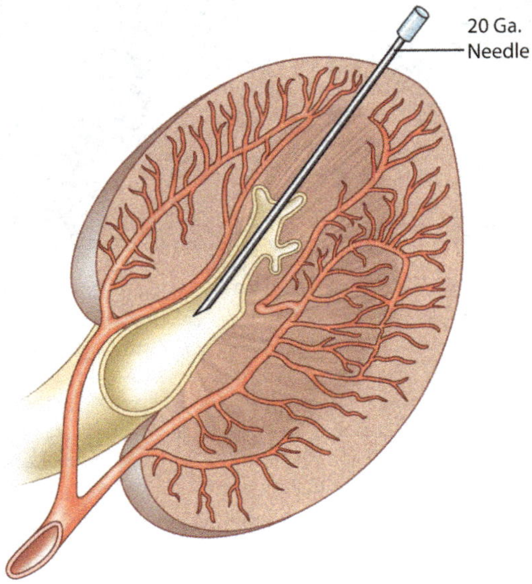

Fig. 22.4 The ideal nephrostomy access route minimizes vascular injury by passing parallel to the renal vessels

Conventional Technique

The patient is placed in a prone position on the fluoroscopy table. Aseptic technique including the use of hat, mask, and gown for the operators is performed. The patient's skin is prepped and draped. Local anesthesia with 1 % buffered lidocaine is administered at the site of the needle entry. With ultrasound guidance, a 21-gauge micropuncture needle is used to access a posterior calyx in the middle or lower pole of the kidney (Fig. 22.5). Needle placement in the collecting system is confirmed by aspirating a small amount of urine, taking care not to totally decompress the system. A small amount of contrast can be gently injected to opacify the renal collecting system. A 0.018-inch stiff guidewire is advanced under fluoroscopic observation, and the needle is removed. A small slit in the skin is made large enough to accommodate the subsequent dilators and nephrostomy catheter. A percutaneous access set is advanced over the guidewire, and the stiffener and inner dilator are removed, leaving the 0.018-inch wire in place. It is important that the guidewire, dilator, and catheter introduction is done with the C-arm angled so the beam is approximately perpendicular to the skin entry. In this way, the needle, guidewire, dilators, and catheter are seen in profile so that guidewire kinking and perforation of the collecting system is avoided.

The procedure is continued by advancing a 0.035-inch stiff hydrophilic wire through the outer dilator and coiling the wire in the renal collecting system or preferably advancing down the ureter. The 0.018-inch wire can be secured and temporarily left in place as a safety wire. The tract is serially dilated over the larger wire, and an 8-French (or larger) nephrostomy catheter is advanced over the larger wire. The larger wire is then removed and the pigtail formed in the renal pelvis. Contrast injection confirms proper catheter position without over distending the system. The catheter is connected to a drainage bag and secured to the skin with a dressing such as a Percu-Stay. The safety wire can then be removed.

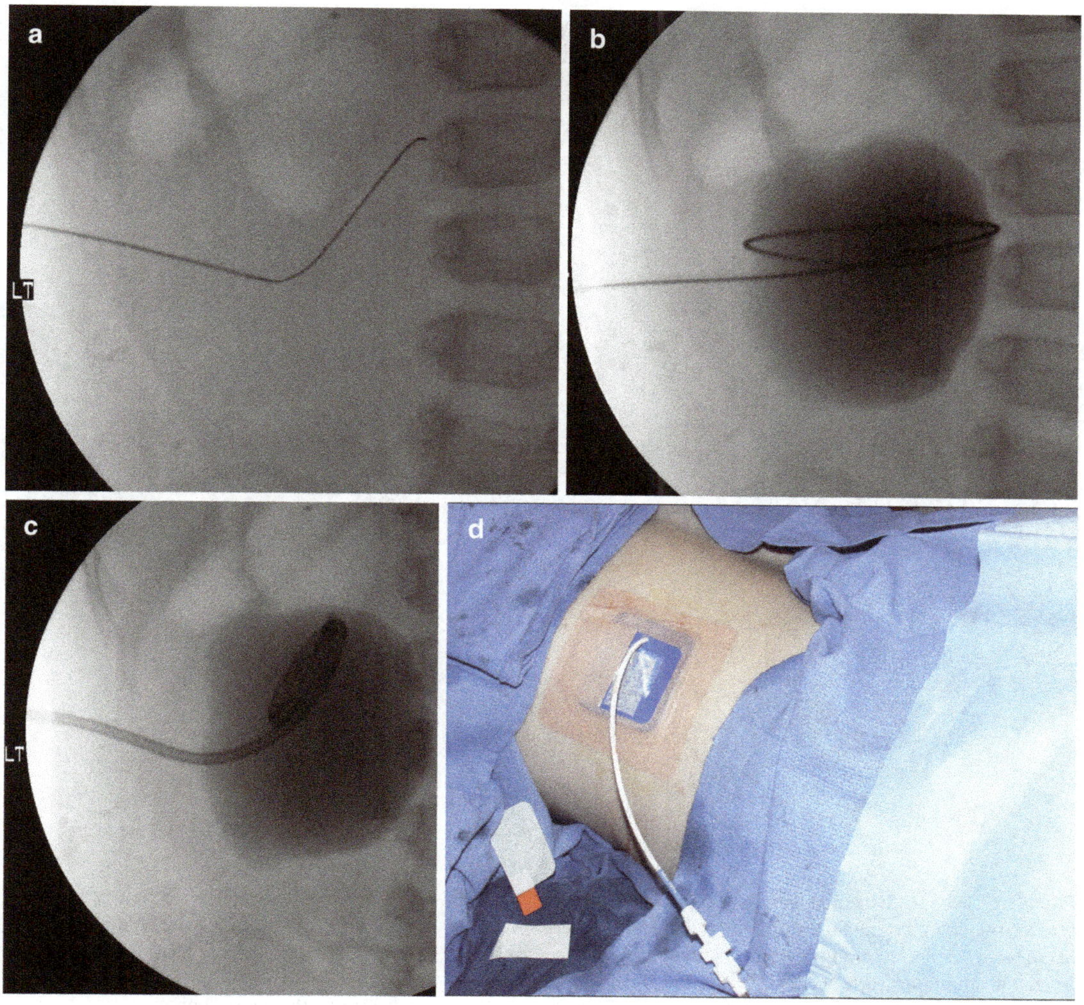

Fig. 22.5 Percutaneous nephrostomy placement using the conventional technique. (**a**) The dilated collecting system is entered with US guidance with a micropuncture needle, and a 0.018-inch Cope wire is advanced under fluoroscopic observation. (**b**) A small amount of contrast is injected to opacify the system. A 0.035-inch guidewire is coiled in the renal pelvis. (**c**) The pigtail of the nephrostomy catheter is formed in the dilated renal pelvis. (**d**) The catheter is secured with a Percu-Stay dressing and connected to gravity drainage

Modified Technique

Nephrostomy placement in neonates and young infants present unique technical challenges not encountered in older children. Renal size in a newborn or young infant is much smaller than that of an older child. Even though the collecting system may be relatively dilated, the absolute amount of urine is small, so coiling guidewires and forming a pigtail of the catheter are difficult (Fig. 22.6). The small volume also means the collecting system can decompress rapidly during the procedure. In addition, the thinner renal parenchyma and surrounding retroperitoneal fat offer less resistance and support. These factors may make it difficult to advance a micropuncture set into the collecting system; the micropuncture set indents the parenchyma but fails to traverse it. The guidewire may be in the collecting system (Fig. 22.6d); however, the dilators and nephrostomy catheter do not penetrate the cortex, resulting in extrarenal catheter placement.

The probability of catheter placement in the renal collecting system is increased with the

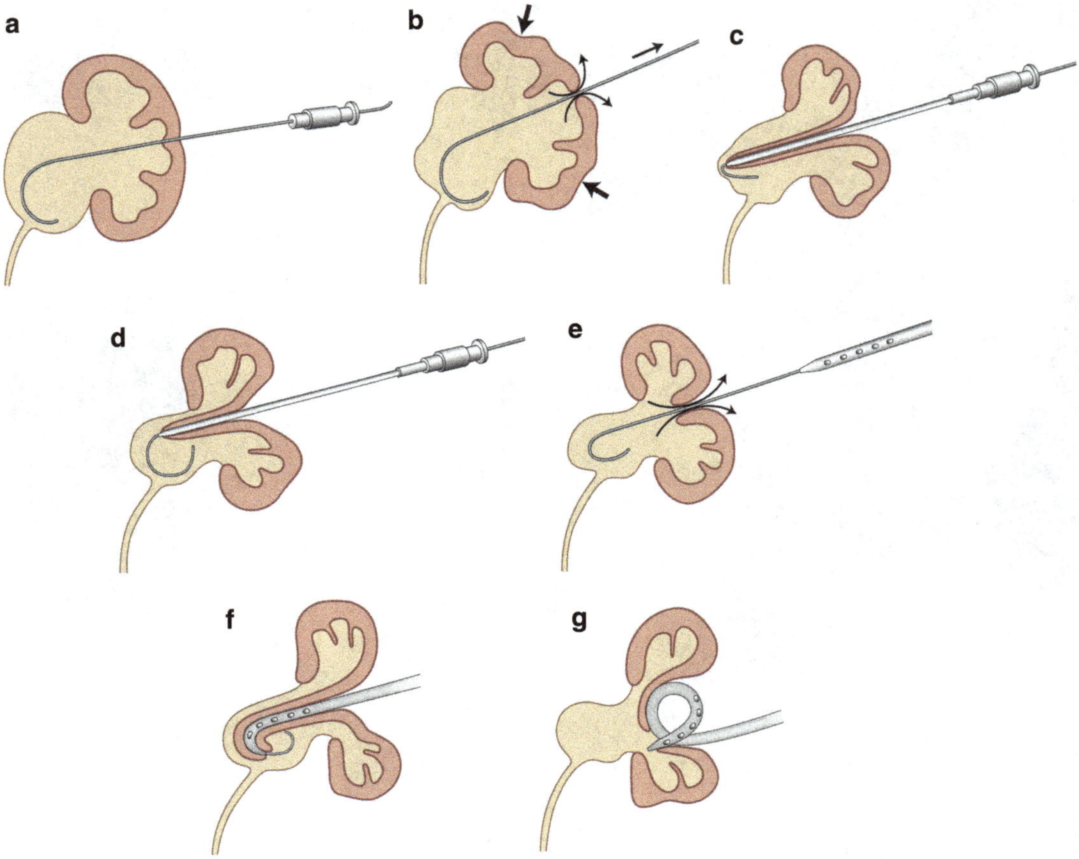

Fig. 22.6 Proposed mechanism for failed micropuncture technique in a neonatal kidney with UPJ obstruction. (**a**) The dilated collecting system is entered with a 21-gauge micropuncture needle. (**b**) As the 0.018-inch Cope wire is advanced through the needle, decompression of the collecting system begins. (**c**) An attempt is made to place a micropuncture set. The thin parenchyma offers little resistance. The small decompressing collecting system and the inability to negotiate the 0.018-inch Cope wire down the ureter, which is usually the case in severe UPJ obstruction, result in incomplete placement of the micropuncture set. (**d**) As the 0.035-inch wire is advanced through the outer sheath of the micropuncture set, the wire may or may not enter collecting system. The figure shows the floppy end of the wire in the collecting system. (**e**) The collecting system continues to decompress during each step. An attempt is made to place a nephrostomy tube over the 0.035-inch wire. (**f**) The catheter cannot be advanced into the collecting system because the wire cannot be manipulated down the ureter. The collecting system is nearly completely decompressed. On fluoroscopy, it is difficult to know whether the catheter is in the collecting system. (**g**) The wire is removed, leaving the nephrostomy catheter outside the decompressed collecting system. There is usually a urinoma around the kidney at this stage

following technique outlined by Koral et al. The initial puncture is made with an 18- to 19-gauge vascular single-wall needle, through which a 0.035-inch, 80-cm stiff guidewire is advanced. The needle is removed and a small slit is made along the guidewire down to the renal parenchyma. Under fluoroscopic observation, a 6-French hydrophilic catheter with a tapered tip and small locking pigtail is advanced over the wire. Intrarenal catheter placement is confirmed by contrast injection. This technique not only increases the success rate of nephrostomy placement in the neonate and young infant but is also quick and simple. The steps of tract manipulation and dilatation are eliminated.

Complications

Complications of percutaneous nephrostomy placement include sepsis, septic shock, vascular injury, bowel transgression, pneumothorax, and hydro/hemothorax. To avoid complications, preprocedural antibiotics, especially in the setting of pyonephrosis (Fig. 22.7), are recommended. Do not over distend an obstructed system to prevent bacteremia or perforation. A single-wall puncture of a posterior calyx from 20 to 30° oblique, below the eleventh rib and through Brodel's bloodless line, will serve to avoid vascular injury. Direct puncture of the renal pelvis is to be avoided. A preprocedural CT may be helpful in patients with distorted anatomy (Fig. 22.8).

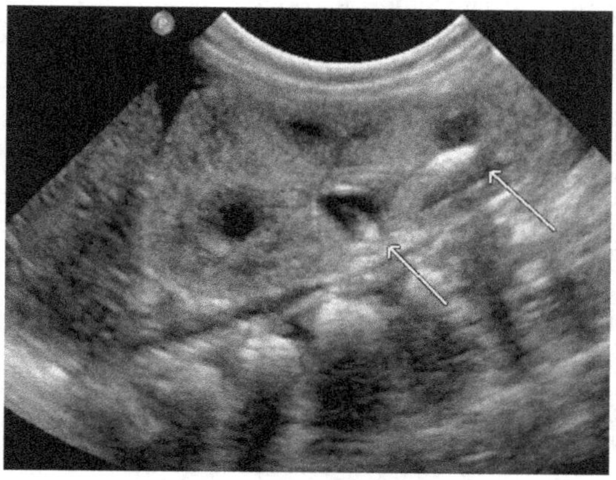

Fig. 22.7 Pyonephrosis. The pelvicalyceal system is distended with echogenic debris-ladened fluid

Ureteral Intervention

Ureteral Stents

Minimally invasive therapy in the GU tract begins with renal access by means of percutaneous nephrostomy. The most common extension of percutaneous nephrostomy is ureteral stent placement for ureteral obstruction.

Indications

Indications for ureteral stent placement include persistent UPJ obstruction following pyeloplasty, UVJ stenosis following reimplantation, ureteral calculus, and traumatic transection of the ureter.

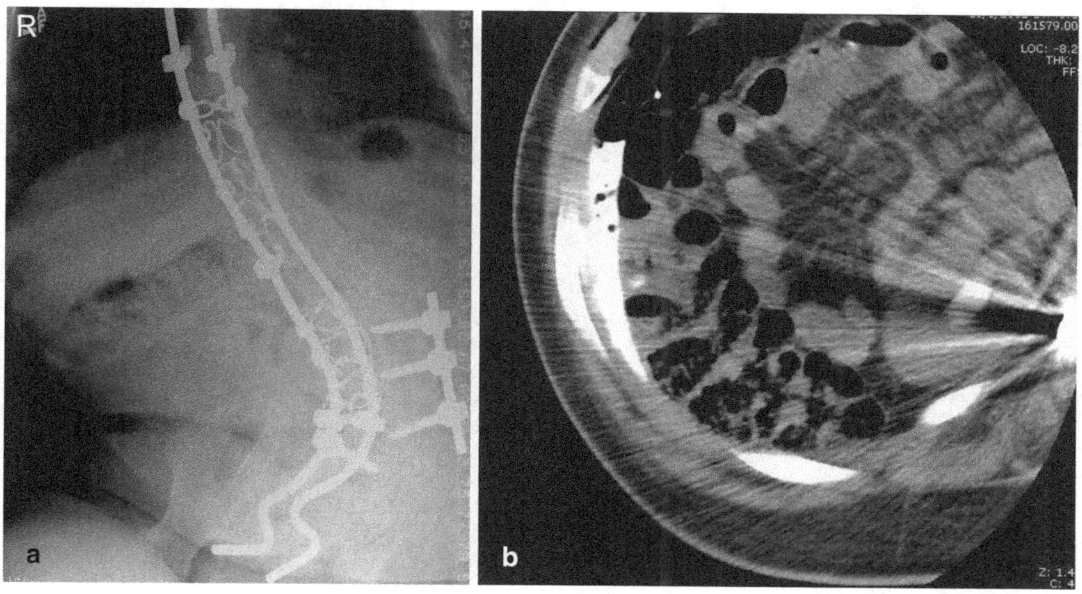

Fig. 22.8 (**a**) Neuromuscular scoliosis. (**b**) The right kidney is more medial in position with the right colon occupying the renal fossa. The kidney may be more difficult to image with US, and the colon may be inadvertently transgressed with the needle and nephrostomy catheter

Antegrade stent placement is often possible even when retrograde cystoscopic attempts are not successful.

Equipment

Ureteral stents are of two basic types: nephroureteral stents in which there is an external portion with a draining nephrostomy loop positioned in the renal pelvis and a ureteral component with distal side and end holes (Fig. 22.9) and double-J stents whose proximal and distal ends are positioned in the renal pelvis and bladder with no external component (Fig. 22.10).

The advantages of the nephroureteral stent are that it can be used for follow-up nephrostograms, a tract is maintained for possible future manipulations, it can be changed percutaneously if stent occlusion occurs, and it can be capped to function as an internal stent. The disadvantages of nephroureteral stents are that there is an external component which requires catheter care and it may get pulled on, thus dislodging the stent. The skin and subcutaneous tract may also act as a conduit for infection.

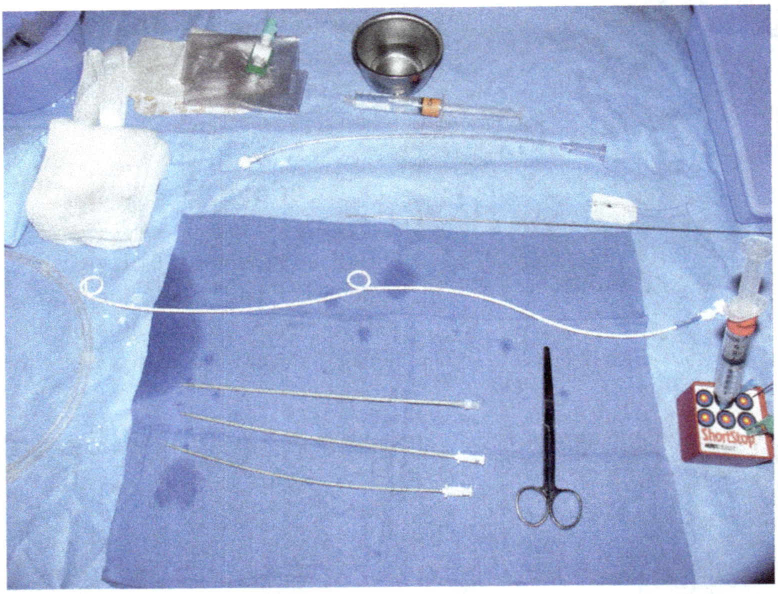

Fig. 22.9 Nephroureteral stent with the proximal self-forming renal pelvis loop and distal bladder pigtail loop. The external portion of the catheter can be left to gravity drainage or capped for internal drainage

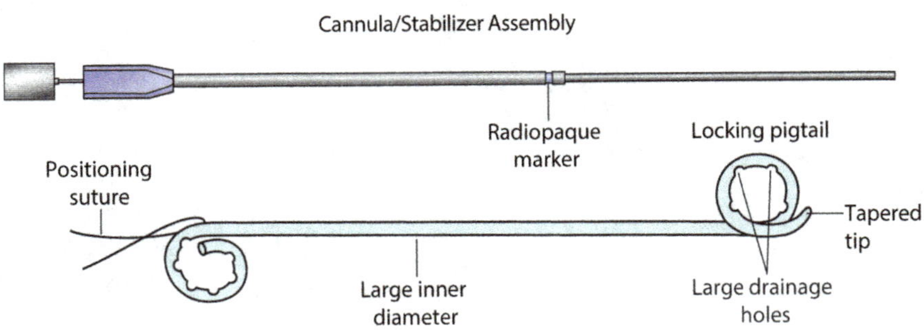

Fig. 22.10 Ureteral stent delivery system. The stent is mounted on the two-piece cannula and stabilizer for antegrade placement

If a large inventory of catheters is not available, other types of catheters can be repurposed or modified to meet your needs. For example, a biliary drainage catheter can be used in larger patients, or side holes can be created along the length of a traditional catheter to allow for drainage from the UPJ to the bladder. Double-J stents typically come in sizes of 4–6 French and are available in varying lengths.

Technique

Ureteral stent placement begins using either the conventional or modified technique for percutaneous nephrostomy as described earlier. Access through a posterior middle or upper pole calyx will facilitate access to the UPJ. The 0.018-inch safety wire and 0.035-inch stiff working wire are manipulated down the ureter and must be able to pass the segment of obstruction. When passage beyond the obstruction is not possible at the initial nephrostomy placement, it may be successful after 7–10 days of external drainage. The external drainage will often reduce proximal ureter redundancy and mucosal edema within the obstructed segment. Negotiation of the obstructed ureter is often facilitated by using an angle-tip glide catheter and hydrophilic wire. Once the obstructing segment is traversed, the wire and catheter are coiled in the bladder.

At this point, the ureteral stricture may be balloon dilated. Generally there is a good response and low morbidity associated with balloon dilatation of ureteral strictures. Dilatation with 6- to 10-mm diameter balloons for strictures at the UPJ and UVJ, and a 4- to 6-mm diameter balloons in the ureter, is recommended. After balloon dilatation, the ureteral segment is supported with a ureteral stent. Ureteral balloon dilatation supported with stent placement may be repeated two or three times before abandoning it as a primary therapy.

The procedure is continued with stent placement over the stiff guidewire. For nephroureteral stent, the stent is advanced so that 5–8 cm of distal stent is within the bladder and the nephrostomy loop is within the renal pelvis (Fig. 22.11).

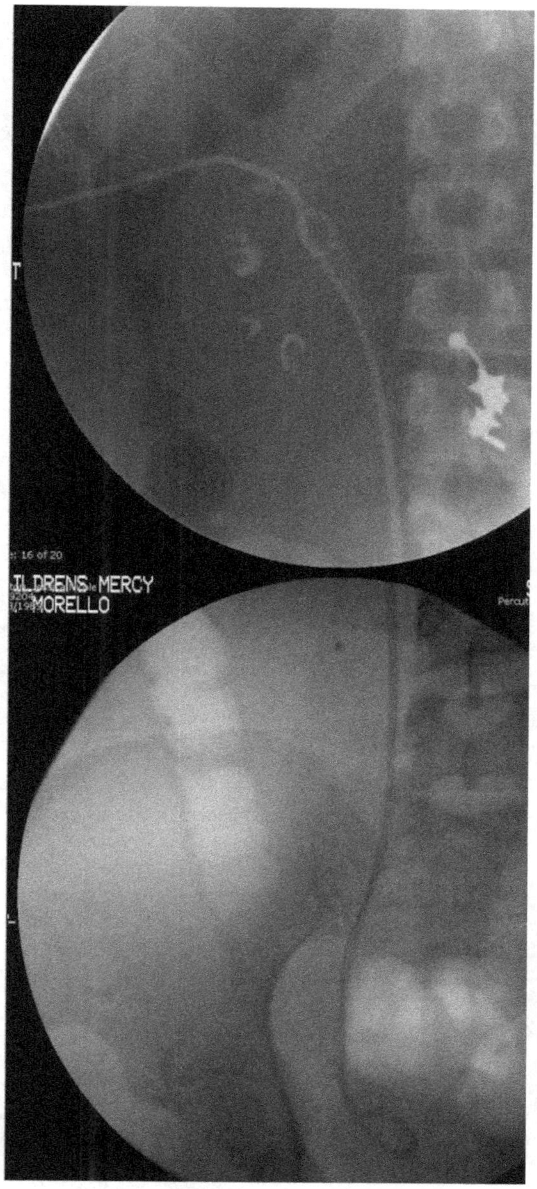

Fig. 22.11 Nephroureteral stent in place with the proximal loop in the renal pelvis and the distal loop in the urinary bladder

The nephrostomy loop is self-formed as the guidewire is removed. The tube is allowed to drain externally for 12–24 h, after which it can be capped to external drainage.

For double-J stent placement, the stent is loaded on a stiffener-pusher device and advanced over the stiff guidewire until 5–8 cm of the stent is in the bladder (Fig. 22.12). As the stiffener and guidewire

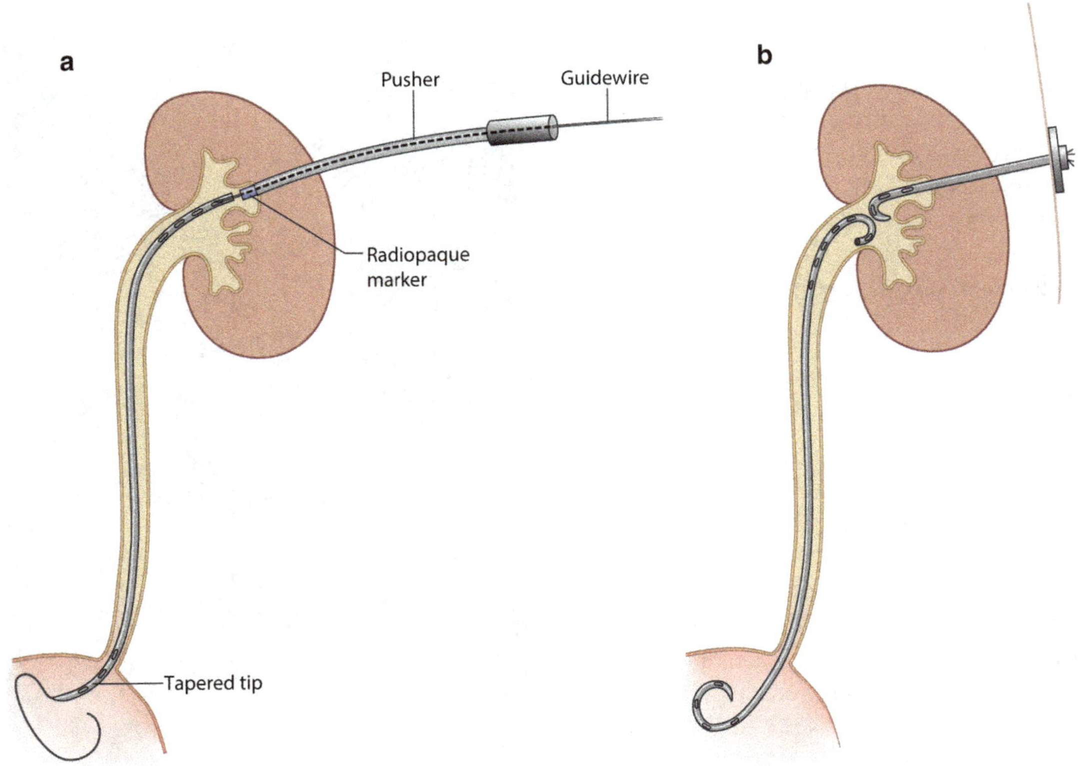

Fig. 22.12 Double-J ureteral stent placement. (**a**) The ureteral stent is loaded on the stiffener-pusher device. The system is advanced over a superstiff guidewire into the bladder. The stent is advanced several centimeters into the bladder. The stiffener and guidewire are withdrawn forming the distal pigtail in the bladder. Removing the wire from the stent allows the proximal pigtail to form. (**b**) The positioning suture is used to adjust the proximal pigtail, after which it is cut and removed. The guidewire is reintroduced into the renal pelvis via the pusher. A protective nephrostomy is left in the renal pelvis to prevent the stent from being clogged by debris and blood from the stent placement manipulations

are withdrawn, the distal pigtail is formed. The wire is entirely removed allowing the proximal pigtail to form. The positioning suture is used to adjust the position of the proximal pigtail into the renal pelvis. The suture is then cut and removed. Using the safety wire, a percutaneous nephrostomy is left within the proximal collecting system to allow temporary external urinary diversion for 12–24 h. This protective nephrostomy allows any clot or debris to drain externally. An antegrade nephrostogram is performed prior to subsequent removal of the nephrostomy tube. This will ascertain the patency and position of the double-J ureteral stent. Removal of the nephrostomy tube should be done under fluoroscopic observation over a guidewire to prevent inadvertent dislodgment of the stent.

Ureteral Calculus Removal

Indication

Percutaneous removal of symptomatic ureteral calculi is best reserved for 1 or 2 stones in a dilated distal ureter where the stone is less than 5–6 mm in size.

Technique

The approach for placement of a percutaneous nephrostomy for calculus removal is the same as the conventional or modified techniques; however, the tract will be subsequently dilated in order to except a larger flexible access sheath.

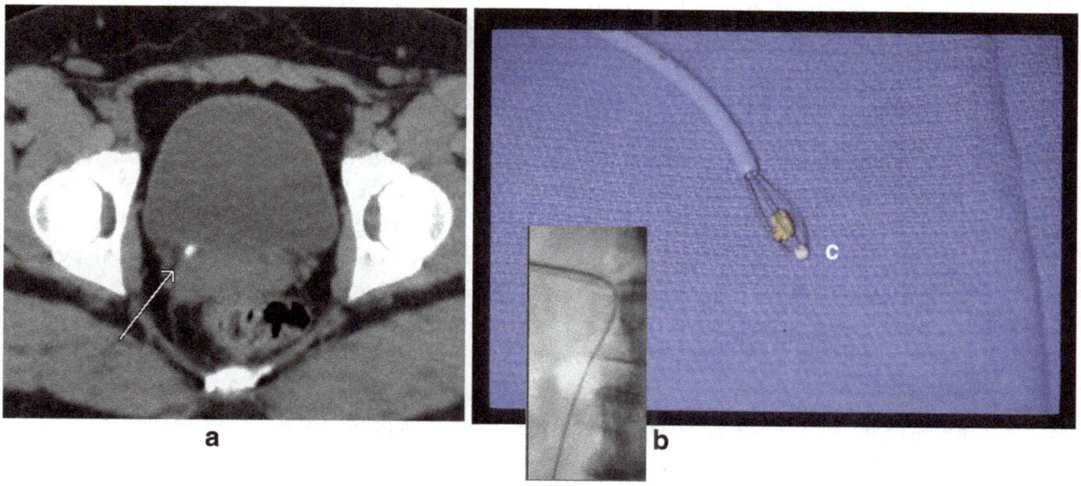

Fig. 22.13 Ureteral calculus removal. (**a**) Calculus in the distal left ureter (*arrow*). (**b**) Percutaneous sheath and guidewire extending down the ureter. (**c**) Calculus removed with a basket snare

When placed, the flexible sheath is directed down the collecting system. Through the sheath, a basket snare was used to engage and remove the stone (Fig. 22.13). A nephrostomy catheter is left to external drainage for 24 h to allow the system to decompress and the ureteral edema to resolve. An antegrade nephrostogram is performed prior to removal of the percutaneous nephrostomy catheter.

Percutaneous Nephrolithotomy

Indication

Percutaneous nephrolithotomy is a multistage procedure with the pediatric interventionalist and urologist working as a team. The procedure is indicated for large stones and staghorn calculi which can occur in young adults with spina bifida or metabolic conditions which predisposed to stone formation.

Technique

The procedure is done in an operating room environment with ultrasound, C-arm fluoroscopy, cystoscopic, and endourologic equipment. The patient is placed under general anesthesia. The collecting system is accessed through a posterior calyx using the conventional or modified technique. In this instance, an upper pole calyx access is advantageous. This may necessitate an intercostal approach, which slightly increases possible morbidity, so extra care must be taken. Once the collecting system is accessed, two 0.035-inch stiff guidewires are advanced into the bladder; one is a working wire and the other is used as a safety wire. In some instances the safety wire can be brought out through the urethra.

The fascial tract is dilated over the working wire with inflation of a 30-French dilating balloon under fluoroscopy. A 30-French sheath is then advanced into the renal collecting system. The urologist then advances a flexible endoscope and removes the clot and stone fragments. Additional stone fragmentation is accomplished with a laser. Following completion of stone fragmentation and removal, a large-caliber nephrostomy catheter is left in place for several days. A nephrostogram is then repeated to assess for contrast extravasations, residual stone fragments, and ureteral patency. If residual stone fragments are present, the nephrolithotomy procedure can be repeated using the existing access and tract. If treatment is complete and the upper tract is intact and patent, the nephrostomy catheter can be removed.

Summary

Interventional radiology plays a key role in genitourinary interventions. Treatment of urinoma and urine leaks by percutaneous drainage and/or diversion facilitates healing in the GU tract.

Knowledge of anatomy and use of good technique and technique modifications facilitate the successful completion of procedures with few complications. Finally, envision and embrace the concept that minimally invasive therapy in the genitourinary tract begins with renal access by means of percutaneous nephrostomy. Extension of the basic technique will allow ureteral intervention.

Chapter Summary

GU Interventions

Preprocedure Workup

- General anesthesia or sedation
- PT, PTT, INR, platelets
- Group and hold
- Prophylactic antibiotics

Perinephric Fluid Drainage

Indications

- Large collection
- Persistent leak
- Fever/sepsis
- Renal fragmentation

Percutaneous Nephrostomy

Indications

- Obstruction
  - UPJ
  - UVJ
  - Post pyeloplasty
  - Posterior urethral valves
  - Primary obstructive megaureter
- Complex urinary infection

Equipment—conventional Technique

- Micropuncture set
- Stiff hydrophilic wire
- Serial dilators
- Pigtail catheter—8–12 Fr.
- Drainage bag
- Dressing

Equipment—modified technique

- 18–19-gauge vascular needle
- 0.035″ stiff guidewire
- 6-Fr. hydrophilic catheter with small locking pigtail

Complications

- Sepsis
- Shock
- Vascular injury
- Bowel transgression
- Pneumothorax, hydrothorax, hemothorax

Tips/Pearls

1. Kidneys in younger patients can be quite mobile. Stabilizing the kidney by applying gentle pressure from the abdomen may make renal puncture and manipulation easier.
2. Trocar technique can be considered in massively distended systems.
3. "Body flossing" (externalizing a nephrostomy wire through the urethra and fixating both ends) can be used to stabilize the wire to allow passage of a balloon or catheter in difficult situations.

Ureteral Stenting

Indications

- UPJ obstruction
- UVJ stenosis
- Ureteral calculus
- Ureteral transection

Equipment

- Nephroureteral stents (or other modified catheters)
- Double-J stents—4–6 Fr., variable lengths
- Percutaneous nephrostomy access equipment as listed above
- 0.035″ stiff wire
- Angled glide catheter, hydrophilic wire
- Balloons—6–10 mm
- Pigtail catheter

Ureteral Calculus Removal

Indications

- 1 or 2 calculi
- 5–6 mm in size

Equipment

- Percutaneous nephrostomy access equipment as listed above
- Dilators
- Flexible sheath
- Basket snare
- Pigtail catheter

Percutaneous Nephrolithotomy

Indications

- Large stones, staghorn calculi

Equipment

- Percutaneous nephrostomy access equipment as listed above
- Fascial dilators
- 30-Fr. dilating balloon
- Surgical equipment
  - Flexible endoscope
  - Laser, etc.
- Large-caliber nephrostomy catheter

References

1. Stanley P, Bear JW, Reid BS. Percutaneous nephrostomy in infants and children. AJR. 1983;141: 473–7.
2. Hogan MJ, Coley BD, Jayanthi VR, Shiels WE, Koff SA. Percutaneous nephrostomy in children and adolescents: outpatient management. Radiology. 2001; 218:207–10.
3. Koral K, Saker MC, Morello FP, Rigsby CK, Donaldson JS. Conventional versus modified technique for percutaneous nephrostomy in newborns and infants. JVIR. 2003;14:113–6.
4. Dyer RB, Regan JD, Kavanagh PV, Khatod EG, Chen MY, Zagoria RJ. Percutaneous nephrostomy with extensions of the technique: step by step. Radiographics. 2002;22:503–25.
5. Schmidt MB, James CA. Genitourinary interventions in children. Semin Interv Radiol. 2002;19:51–7.
6. Ahmed S, Borghol M, Hugosson C. Urinoma and urine ascites secondary to calyceal perforation in neonates with posterior uretheral valves. Br J Urol. 1997; 79:991–2.
7. Mansi MK, Alkhudair WK. Conservative management with percutaneous intervention of major blunt renal injuries. Am J Emerg Med. 1997;15: 633–7.
8. Castaneda-Zuniga WR, Tadavarthy SM. In: Interventional Radiology. Baltimore: Williams and Wilkins; 1992.

Section IX

Nonvascular Interventions: Musculoskeletal

Musculoskeletal Interventions

23

Michael Temple and William E. Shiels

Introduction

Musculoskeletal interventions are composed of a large variety of procedures in bone and soft tissue. The most common procedures, biopsy and aspiration/drainage, were discussed in Chaps. 16 and 17, respectively. As such, this chapter will focus on selected procedures: osteoid osteoma and aneurysmal bone cyst (ABC) treatment and injection of corticosteroids and botulinum toxin (BTX). The section covering BTX will include both muscle and salivary gland injections.

Osteoid Osteoma

Background Information

Osteoid osteoma (OO) is a relatively common benign bone tumor measuring less than 1.5 cm in size. The lesion consists of both unmineralized osteoid and mineralized bone with loose fibrovascular tissue [1, 2]. A rim of large osteoblasts and a few scattered osteoclasts are noted histologically.

These vascular lesions produce high levels of prostacyclin and prostaglandin that is thought to sensitize the highly innervated tissue causing significant pain. The classic presentation is pain that is responsive to NSAID treatment in most patients [3]. Pain causes patients to wake during the night and can result in withdrawal from physical and social activities. Occasionally, gait changes lead to pain in secondary locations.

Males between 10 and 35 years are most commonly affected, but OO has been reported in patients as young as 7 months [4]. Any bone can be involved with the femur, digits, and spine being the most common. Lesions arise from cortical, medullary, or subperiosteal locations.

The typical radiographic appearance is a small lytic focus with a central sclerotic nidus often associated with sclerosis of the surrounding bone [5]. On CT, a sclerotic central nidus with hypodense rim is the most common appearance (Fig. 23.1). MRI is very sensitive to bone marrow changes that could result in the misdiagnosis of an aggressive lesion [6]. 3D subtraction and dynamic contrast enhancement analysis may be helpful for identification in problematic cases [7–9].

A Brodie's abscess can mimic an osteoid osteoma. Misdiagnosis can lead to inadvertent treatment and procedural complications [10].

M. Temple, M.D., F.R.C.P.(.C).
Hospital for Sick Children, University of Toronto, Toronto, ON, M5G 1X8 Canada
e-mail: michael.temple@sickkids.ca

W.E. Shiels, D.O. (✉)
Department of Radiology, Nationwide Children's Hospital, The Ohio State University College of Medicine, 700 Children's Drive, Columbus, OH 43205, USA
e-mail: william.shiels@nationwidechildrens.org

M. Temple and F.E. Marshalleck (eds.), *Pediatric Interventional Radiology: Handbook of Vascular and Non-Vascular Interventions*, DOI 10.1007/978-1-4419-5856-3_23,

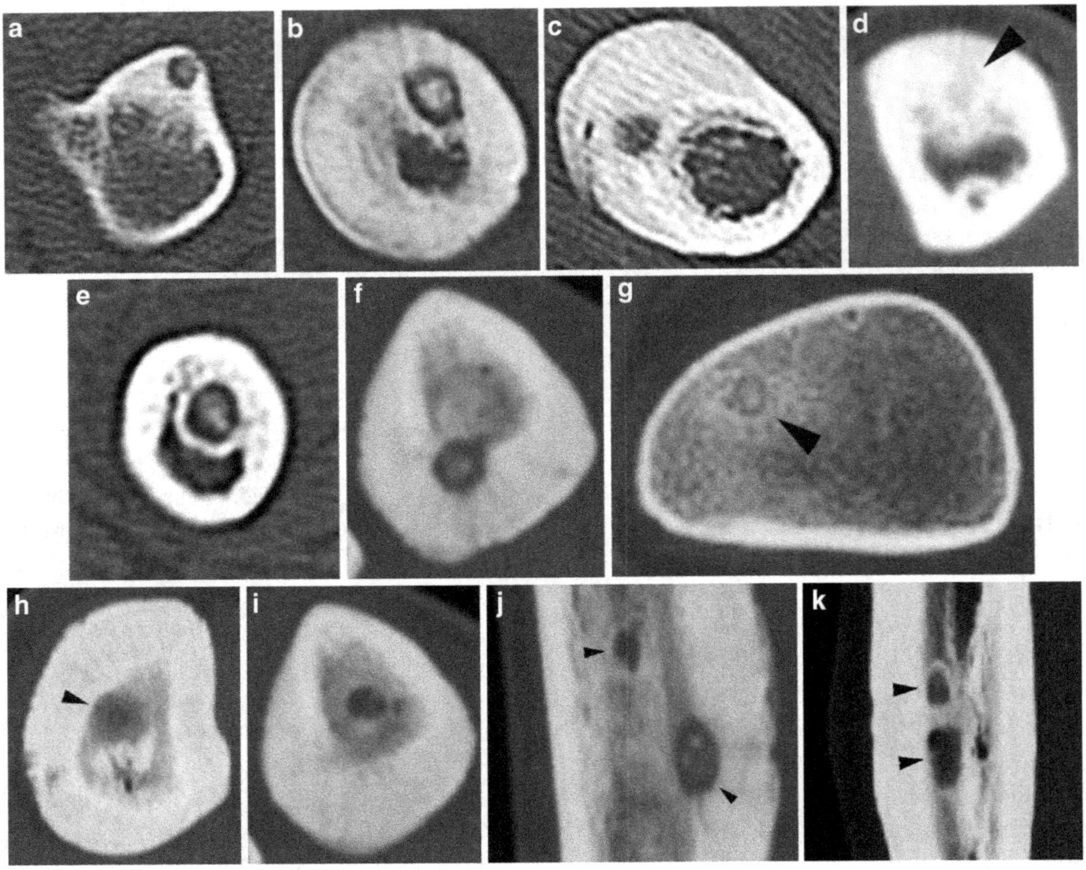

Fig. 23.1 Varying appearance of osteoid osteoma. OO tends to appear as a lytic focus with a central calcified nidus but the appearance varies. (**a**) Cortical, no sclerosis; (**b**) cortical, circumferential sclerosis; (**c**) cortical, asymmetric sclerosis; (**d**) biopsy-proven cortical OO with minimal lucency; (**e**) corticomedullary, circumferential sclerosis; (**f**) corticomedullary, asymmetric sclerosis; (**g**) medullary, no sclerosis; (**h**) medullary, circumferential sclerosis; (**i**) medullary, asymmetric sclerosis; (**j**) multifocal corticomedullary and medullary; (**k**) multifocal with two medullary foci (a third focus was present but not shown)

When a patient presents with a classic clinical history and stereotypical imaging findings, treatment can proceed in the absence of biopsy confirmation [11, 12]. When the clinical history or the imaging characteristics are in any way equivocal, a biopsy should be performed. Some operators routinely biopsy all lesions [13].

Osteoid osteomas spontaneously resolve over time but it can take several years [14–16]. Treatment options include conservative management, surgical resection or curettage, CT-guided resection (Fig. 23.2), and thermal ablation.

At the current time, thermal ablation of osteoid osteoma is the most common treatment approach. Heat applied to living cells results in cell damage or death dependent upon the temperature and the treatment time [17, 18]. Thermal therapy is most often performed using radiofrequency ablation (RFA) devices, but laser ablation has also been described [19–26]. There are single reports regarding treatment with coblation [27] and high-intensity focused ultrasound [28].

Indications/Contraindications

The most common indication for treatment is pain that is not responsive to NSAIDs. However, many families wish to undergo treatment to definitively treat a lesion and/or stop dependence on medication.

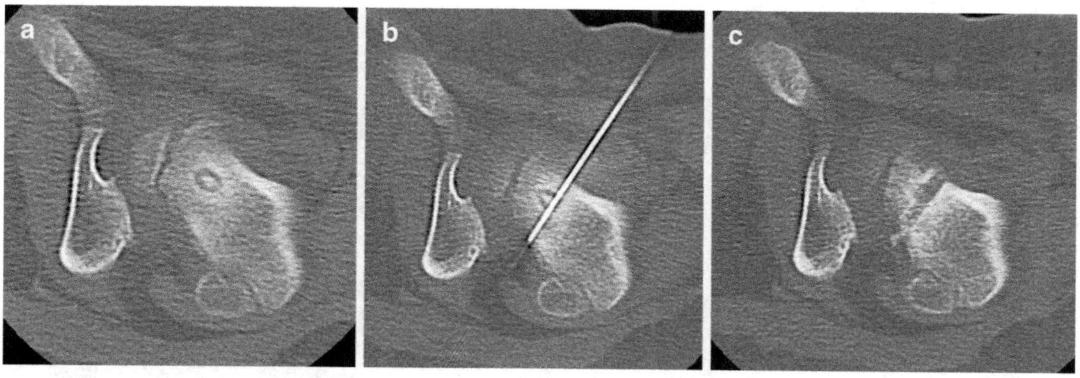

Fig. 23.2 CT-guided excision. (**a**) Axial CT showing OO of the femoral neck. (**b**) A k-wire traverses the OO. (**c**) Residual tract after removal of a bone core. A second pass was used to remove the residual nidus. A k-wire is not necessary for OO excision; a large coring needle can be used instead

Contraindications include the inability to create a tract that maintains an adequate distance from vital structures such as nerves, arteries, and skin. A distance of >1 cm is desirable [13, 29, 30].

Equipment

Imaging

While fluoroscopy can be used to localize an OO, cross-sectional imaging provides more accurate information on the extent and shape of the lesion to aid in planning and localization. CT is currently used for initial assessment and localization of the lesion although MR guidance has been described [25, 26].

RFA

Application of radiofrequency energy results in frictional tissue heating. There are numerous radiofrequency devices on the market with varying monitoring approaches that include measuring resistance or temperature. For OO treatment, single-tine electrodes are often used, but a minimally deployed umbrella-shaped device can also be utilized. It is important to know the size and shape of the active heating zone of the specific device being used in order to create a treatment plan and assure safety of surrounding structures. The pattern of heat distribution tends to be ovoid for RFA.

Traditionally, monopolar devices have been used. They require grounding pads to complete the electrical circuit and provide heating. Proper placement of the pads (over muscle and without contact between pads) can be quite difficult in small children. Bipolar RFA devices that do not require the use of grounding pads have been introduced in recent years.

Laser

A diode laser can be used to perform thermal ablation of bone. Laser tuned to ~810 nm interact with hemoglobin to create heat. The heat is generated as a point source from the fiber tip. Laser systems are used to supply low power (2 W) setting in continuous mode. The total energy deposited determines the size of the area treated.

Bone Access

A standard bone access needle or a company-specific coaxial needle is used for access. Some needles are insulated to decrease heat transmission. For RFA the access needle is approximately 11–14 gauge. Laser requires smaller 14–18 gauge needles. Bone biopsy needles are used when required.

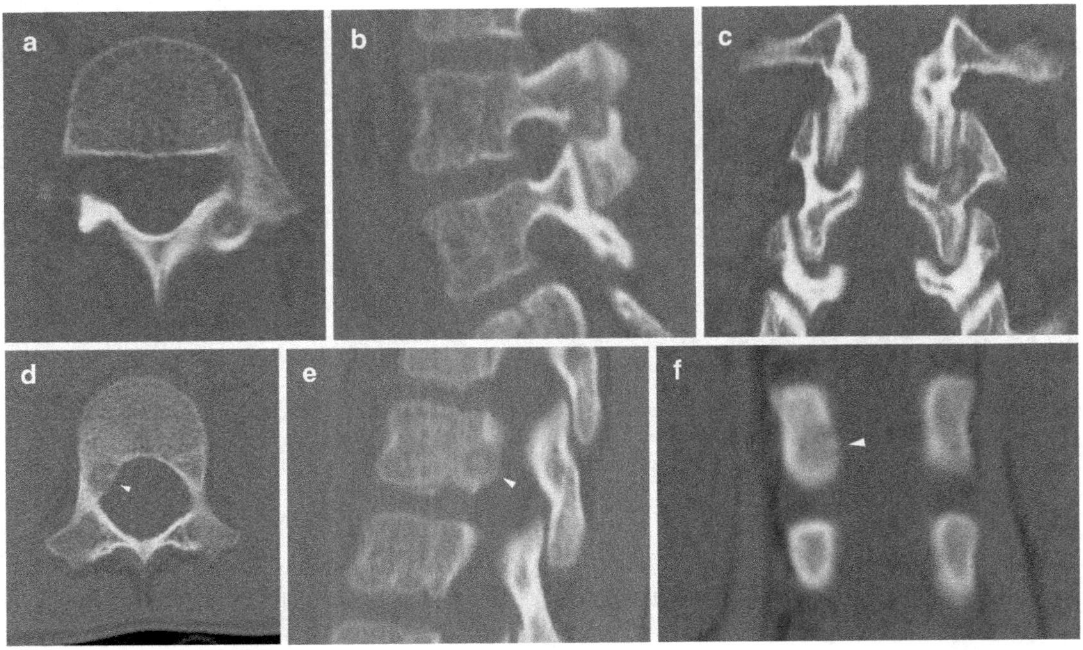

Fig. 23.3 Vertebral osteoid osteoma. (**a–c**) Axial, sagittal, and coronal images of OO of left L3 pars interarticularis and superior articular process. Intact cortex over the neural foramen protected against nerve injury. Some articular/cartilage damage was felt to be likely due to the lack of cortex in the area of the facet joint with thermal ablation, but the risk with surgical revision was felt to be greater. Laser ablation was undertaken without complication. (**d–f**) OO of right L1 pedicle (*white arrowheads*). The lesion abuts the dural sac and is within 2 mm of the exiting nerve. The lack of cortex medially raised significant concern of thermal injury to the L1 nerve. The patient's family was given the option of ablation with saline infusion and temperature monitoring but declined intervention

Preprocedure Workup

The patient's imaging should be reviewed and further studies ordered if indicated. Blood work is not necessary in otherwise healthy patients.

A clinic visit is arranged to review the patient's clinical history, discuss the treatment options (including conservative treatment), and obtain consent.

A combined approach with orthopedic surgery may be beneficial in patients with extremely thick, sclerotic overlying bone. An orthopedic bone drill can provide a large access route through the bone with minimal effort. Some access sets (Laurane, Bonopty) come with a manual drill that may also be helpful in this situation.

Procedure Technique

Treatment of OO causes significant pain so thermal ablation is performed under general anesthesia (even in adults). It is common to see an increase in heart rate and blood pressure in fully anesthetized patients when the nidus is accessed [29, 31]. Several procedural failures have been reported when ablation was attempted with sedation alone.

Antibiotic prophylaxis is used by some groups [12] but is not routinely administered.

Grounding pads are placed when necessary. The patient is positioned to allow access to the lesion keeping gantry size, instrumentation, and access during CT fluoroscopy in mind. CT is used to localize the lesion, mark the entry site, and plan the procedure.

It is essential to assure an approach that will minimize any potential risk of thermal injury to vital structures such as nerves, arteries, and skin; a distance of >1 cm should be sought [13, 29, 30]. When performing vertebral ablations, the perivenous plexus and cerebrospinal fluid can act as a heat sink. Thermal ablation in lesions with intact cortex is thought to be safe [32, 33] (Fig. 23.3) although risk of neural injury increases when using an RFA device with a 2 cm active zone [34].

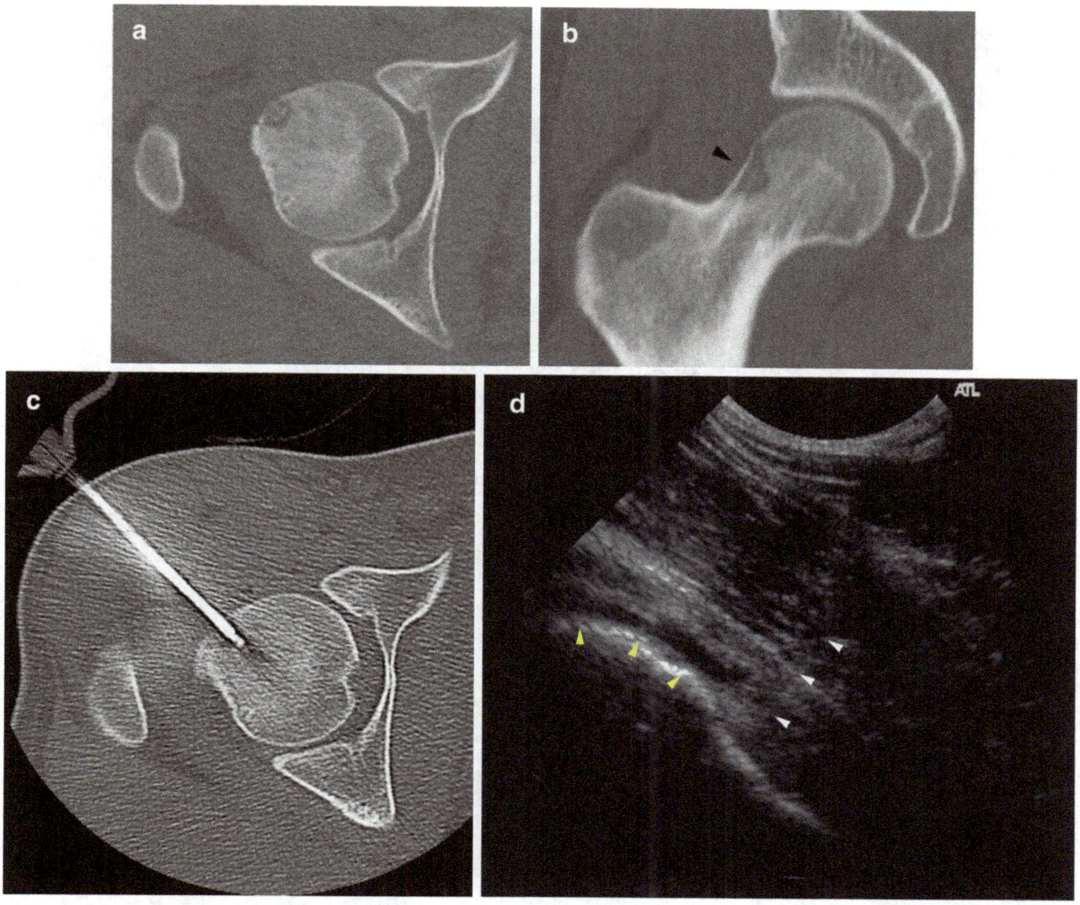

Fig. 23.4 Dextrose heat sink for RFA. (**a**, **b**) Axial and coronal CT demonstrate an OO adjacent to the femoral head. (**c**) Due to the location, a transcortical route along the femoral neck (to avoid entering the joint space) was not possible. (**d**) To minimize local heat damage to the joint capsule and cartilage, chilled dextrose was injected into the joint under ultrasound guidance. *White arrowheads* indicate the needle path. *Yellow arrowheads* outline dextrose beginning to distend the joint capsule

When performing ablations in risky areas, the thermal protocol can be modified (less time, lower temperature, lower energy deposition) to improve safety.

In areas where heat spread could result in damage to surrounding structures, direct temperature monitoring with a thermocouple or injection of fluid or gas to act as a thermal barrier or heat sink should be considered. Fluid can be injected to protect joints, overlying subcutaneous tissues, or nearby vital structures (Fig. 23.4). Saline is not recommended when using RFA due to the potential to facilitate the RF signal due to the electrolyte content. In the spine, injection of saline, dextrose, contrast, or CO_2 is used to provide protection in high-risk areas [35].

The area is prepped and draped. Fluoroscopy, CT, and/or CT fluoroscopy is used to guide insertion of the coaxial needle. A biopsy is performed when necessary. The RFA probe is then inserted and heating is commenced. If the coaxial needle is not insulated, it is pulled back over the RFA probe to decrease the chance of a tract/skin burn. The lesion is treated in accordance with the manufacturer's instructions. Reported protocols vary with most in the range of 85–95 C×4–8 min [12, 29].

There are a few differences when performing laser ablation. Prior to insertion of the coaxial bone access needle, the laser fiber is inserted and marked to show when 5 mm projects beyond the end of the coaxial needle (Fig. 23.5). Some operators use a second, smaller (18 gauge) needle to

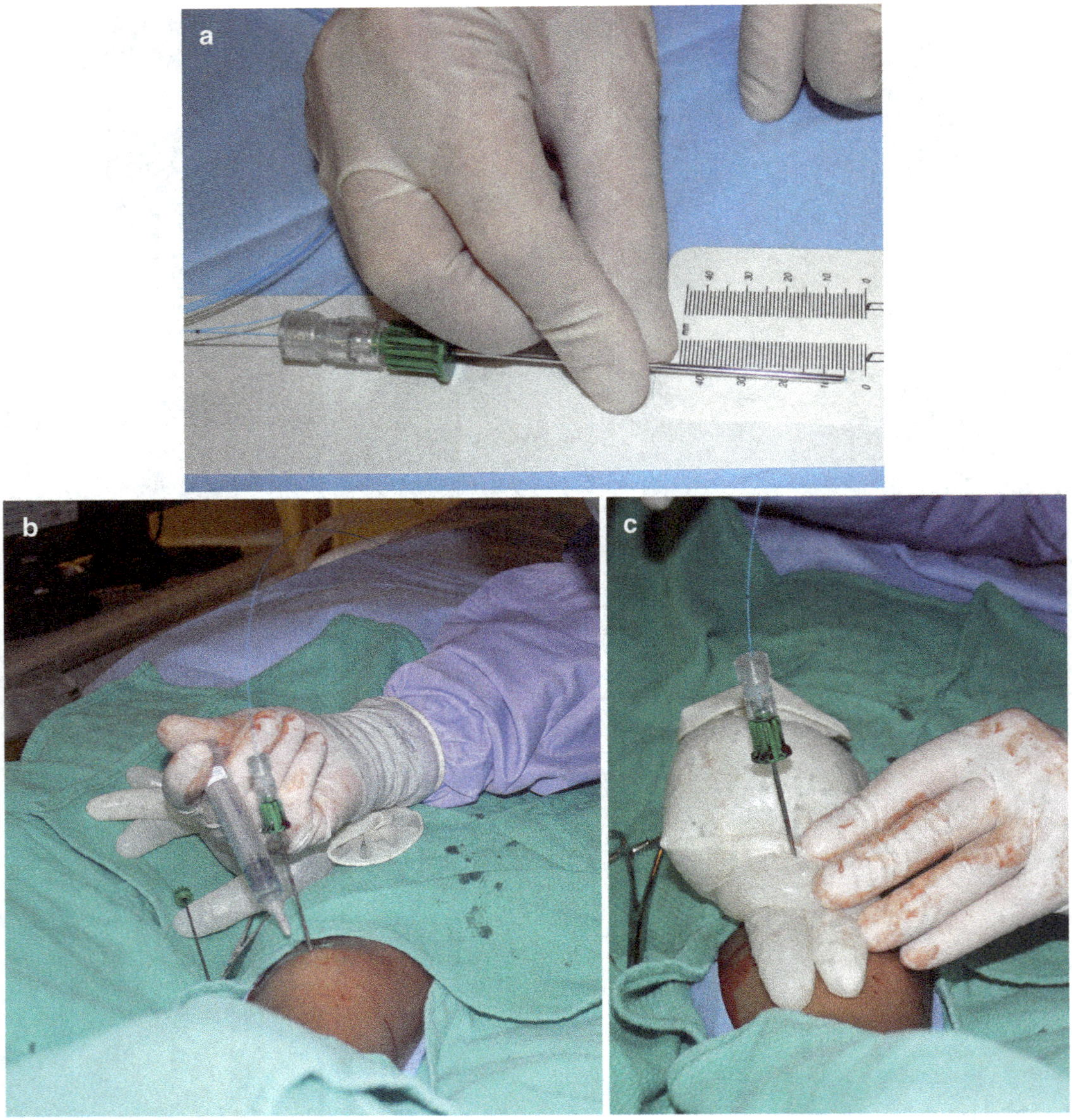

Fig. 23.5 Laser ablation. (**a**) The laser fiber (*blue*) is measured to assure that the tip projects 5 mm beyond the edge of the coaxial needle. In order to prevent a skin burn in case of heat transmission along the uninsulated coaxial needle, (**b**) saline and local anesthetic were used to "tent" the tissue overlying the tibia, and (**c**) ice was applied at the surface

protect the laser fiber during insertion [24]. The laser fiber tip is charred in a small sample of the patient's blood. In distinction to RFA, charring helps propagate laser energy. A biopsy sample is obtained to provide a path into the center of the lesion (so that the fragile glass fiber does not break during insertion). The generator is set to provide a power of 2 W in continuous mode and is activated for a specific time based on the total energy deposition desired to treat the lesion. Higher energy deposition results in a larger area (up to 1.6 cm) of ablation up to a maximum of approximately 1,000–1,200 J. When performing laser ablation in an area where there is the potential to damage surrounding structures, the desired power administered can be determined by the formula: (nidus size in mm × 100 J) + 200 J [24]. As the heat originates only from the tip, the fiber is placed centrally in the lesion. An ice pack is placed on the skin to protect against burns of the skin and tract from potential heat conduction through the uninsulated needle. For large lesions, the use of a beam splitter allows for simultaneous treatment of up to four sites.

Depending on the heat distribution characteristics of the modality used, complete treatment of larger lesions (>1 cm in *any* dimension) may require ablation in multiple locations. A report by *Vanderschueren* demonstrated that *performing more than 1 burn cycle was the best predictor of successful RFA treatment, independent of lesion size* [36].

Postprocedure Care

Immediately following the procedure, supportive care and analgesia is provided. An NSAID such as ketorolac will help decrease immediate postprocedure pain.

Following thermal ablation, some patients notice a change in the nature and/or intensity of pain immediately. In others, it can take 10–12 days.

Weight bearing is determined by the location of the intervention and the size and depth of the needle hole. For most patients with a low fracture risk, weight bearing as tolerated with no high-intensity exercise or contact sports for 4–6 weeks is an acceptable approach. In comparison, a patient who underwent an intervention in the intertrochanteric area with a long intraosseous pathway may require crutches with no weight bearing allowed for 6 weeks.

Informed discharge is performed. Signs and symptoms that would necessitate emergency treatment and a list of emergency contact numbers are discussed with the patient and their family. Ideally, a patient information sheet is given to the family.

Complications

Thermal, infectious, or lesion-related complications can occur.

Nearby structures such as arteries and nerves can be damaged during the heating process. Tracking of heat along the probe or guide needle could result in a burn to the needle tract or the skin [37]. Formation of a draining fistula has been reported following treatment of a tibial lesion [29].

Infectious complications include osteomyelitis, septic arthritis, and cellulitis.

Fracture can subsequently occur at the access site. The needle hole creates a riser concentrating stress in the area of the defect increasing the potential for fracture.

Incomplete or partial treatment can occur in approximately 10 % of patients necessitating a second treatment. Late recurrence *of OO* has been reported.

Follow-up

The patient is reassessed in the interventional radiology clinic 2 weeks following the procedure. If the patient has residual pain, a second procedure is booked.

There are no specific recommendations for imaging follow-up. While regular imaging can be performed to monitor the change in appearance of the OO, a change in the patient's clinical status will provide an indication that repeat imaging should be undertaken.

Aneurysmal Bone Cyst

ABCs are benign multiloculated, cystic, expansile bone neoplasms that are locally aggressive [38–42]. Histologically, ABCs contain a fibroproliferative mesenchymal stroma with giant cell-like osteoclasts and vascular spaces [42]. The vascular spaces do not have an epithelial lining. The lytic lesions demonstrate a "soap bubble" appearance on plain films and commonly demonstrate fluid-fluid levels on CT and MRI. A rare solid variant exists. ABCs can occur in any bone but are most commonly seen in the femur, tibia, spine, and pelvis [43].

Telangiectatic osteosarcoma has a similar appearance to ABC creating a controversy surrounding the need for biopsy prior to treatment. Some authors feel that biopsy is absolutely essential to exclude telangiectatic osteosarcoma and will postpone treatment for several months [44–46]. Others perform biopsy at the time of treatment as long as no atypical or aggressive imaging or clinical findings are present [42, 47–50]. Both surgical and percutaneous biopsies have been advocated [45, 47, 49].

The pathogenesis of ABC has been controversial. Recently it was recognized as a clonal neoplasm driven by upregulation of the USP6 oncogene [38–41]. Historical hypotheses for formation include posttraumatic reaction, intraosseous vascular anomaly, and chromosomal abnormalities [45].

Several methods of categorization exist. If the ABC is an isolated finding, it is classified as primary. Secondary ABCs are associated with other osseous abnormalities (such as a giant cell tumor, chondroblastoma, fibrous dysplasia, osteoblastoma, and osteosarcoma).

A recent paper suggests classifying ABCs as lymphatic or venous anomalies based on the appearance of aspirated fluid contents. This differentiation predicts the likelihood of venous drainage (and consequent risk of sclerotherapy). Lambot-Juhan et al. demonstrated that venous drainage correlated with the appearance of fluid aspirated from ABCs. Cysts with sanguinous fluid all demonstrated venous drainage where only 1/7 did when the fluid was clear. Fluid that was intermediate in appearance showed venous drainage in 3 of 7 cases [46].

In addition to venous and lymphatic components, ABCs demonstrate variable arterial perfusion. Treatment-related deaths have been reported secondary to intraoperative bleeding in one patient [51] and retrograde arterial embolization of Ethibloc following treatment of a cervical ABC in another [52].

The lack of consensus in the literature makes specific treatment recommendations difficult. Surgical methods such as curettage or resection are associated with a recurrence rate as high as 71 % [42, 53]. Cryotherapy and radionuclide treatment have also been described [54, 55]. Interventional radiologists are involved when embolization or percutaneous sclerotherapy is undertaken.

Indications/Contraindications

ABC are routinely treated to stop potential expansion and instability of the involved osseous segment. The need for treatment is more urgent when there is a risk of fracture or the lesion threatens a growth plate or joint space. Nonaggressive lesions that do not threaten surrounding structures can be (closely) followed as spontaneous regression can occur [56–58].

There are no absolute contraindications to ABC treatment. Arterial embolization may not be possible in hypovascular lesions. Sclerosing agents can escape through draining veins resulting in systemic complications. When dealing with vertebral ABCs, some favor embolization as a primary treatment method [59, 60], and others specify that Ethibloc is contraindicated [45, 50].

Embolization

Embolization has been used both as a primary treatment method and as an adjunct to decrease blood loss prior to surgical intervention [59, 61, 62]. Arterial supply is variable with hypervascular, hypovascular, and combined perfusion patterns described.

Glue, polyvinyl alcohol (PVA) particles, and Gelfoam have been used as embolic agents. When the risks of nontarget embolization are low and deep penetration into small arteries is desired, 150–250 μm particles have been used. In the spinal area, where the risks of nontarget embolization are high, 250–350 μm particles have been used. Coils are not recommended in case repeat embolization is required.

When successful, symptoms resolved in days to weeks and ossification occurred within 2–4 months [59].

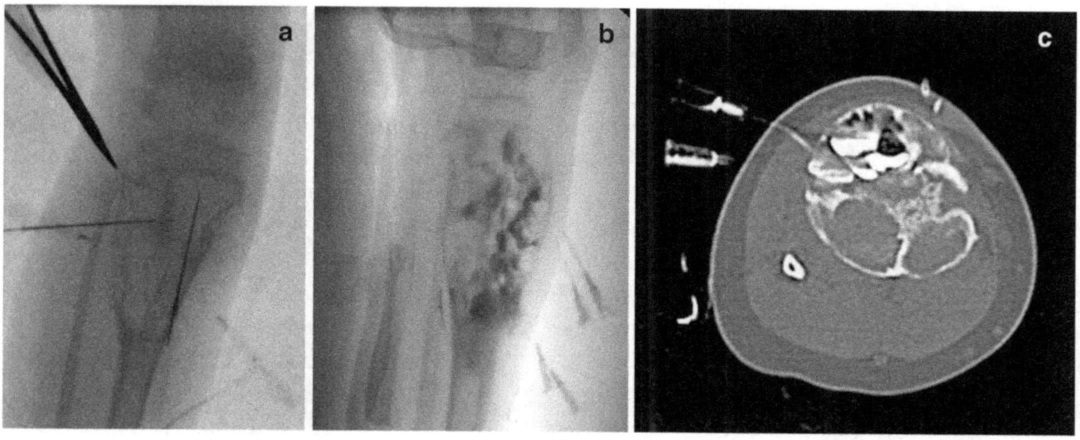

Fig. 23.6 Sclerosis of aneurysmal bone cyst. (**a**) Right tibial ABC prior to injection of sclerosing agent. (**b**) Lateral image demonstrates locules filled with doxycycline foam (that includes contrast). The tourniquet (seen at the top of the image) has been released. (**c**) CT imaging identified several posterior locules that have not yet been filled with sclerosant

Sclerotherapy

Many interventional radiologists feel that sclerotherapy is the method of treatment of choice for most ABCs.

Numerous sclerosing agents have been used in the treatment of ABCs. The most common agents are described below.

Regardless of the agent used, sclerotherapy follows the basic approach described below. See Fig. 23.6.

1. *General anesthesia*. Due to the pain associated with bone access and sclerosis, ABC treatment is performed under general anesthesia.
2. *Access lesion*. Depending on the cortical thickness, a 12–16 gauge needle is introduced into the lesion using ultrasound, CT, or fluoroscopy. Biopsy specimens can be obtained at this time.
3. *Aspirate lesional fluid*. The fluid is aspirated to assess appearance and volume.
4. *Inject contrast* to determine volume, distribution pattern within locules, and the presence of venous drainage. Aspirate contrast when finished.
5. *Place secondary needles* (if necessary). Multiple needles can be placed to maximize likelihood of treating entire lesion and/or to allow drainage of sclerosant.
   (a) Success treatment is dependent on sclerosant reaching every locule. This may be achieved by placement of multiple needles or repositioning of one needle in order to access all areas of the lesion.
   (b) A second needle is placed to allow drainage, decompression and a decrease in intralesional pressure (decreasing the risk of venous escape or extravasation of sclerosant).
6. *Apply tourniquet*. Hand-tied tourniquets or orthopedic tourniquet machines can be used. The tourniquet pressure should not exceed systolic in order to maintain arterial inflow. A repeat contrast study is performed to assess for any change in vascular drainage. The tourniquets are left in place for approximately 10 min after sclerosis is finished to decrease risk of escape by allowing time for thrombosis and drainage from secondary needles to occur.
7. *Inject sclerosant*. The sclerosant is injected slowly taking care that it fills the cavity gradually and does not leak out. The effluent from the other needle(s) is monitored for appearance. Depending on the location and sclerosant, the injection may be monitored during administration with ultrasound (especially doxycycline foam injection into

solid tumor nodules), fluoroscopy, or CT. Cross-sectional imaging may be helpful in assuring that all locules are treated.

8. *Remove needles.* Consider methods to decrease the risk of leakage of sclerosant as described below.
9. *Remove tourniquet.* The tourniquet can be removed 5–10 min following completion of sclerosant administration. If the chance of venous escape of sclerosant is high, systemic effects can be seen with ethanol as a sclerosant. Gradually decreasing the pressure in an orthopedic tourniquet (e.g., 10 mmHg every 1–2 min) allows time for thrombosis and controlled release of any nontarget embolic.
10. *Follow-up imaging.* The ABC is followed with serial radiographs (often at 1, 3, 6, and 12 months) and cross-sectional imaging (either MRI or CT).
11. *Repeat treatment as necessary.* Repeat procedures may be necessary to completely treat locules not previously accessed or large or poorly responding lesions.

Doxycycline Foam +/– Tricalcium Phosphate Bone Graft

Doxycycline is tetracycline antibiotic that is effective as a direct tumor ablation agent. Tetracyclines have been associated with photosensitization and teeth yellowing in pediatric patients. Mild tooth discoloration from doxycycline has been seen rarely following large IV doses in children under 8 years of age. Discoloration can be treated with cleaning or bleaching. Photosensitivity has not been reported following doxycycline sclerosis in ABCs or lymphatic malformations.

The maximum dose for sclerosis has not been determined. A maximum dose of 300–500 mg in neonates and 1,000–1,200 mg in older patients has been suggested.

Doxycycline foam has been successfully used in the treatment of ABC [42]. Doxycycline injection treatment of ABCs can be routinely performed on an outpatient basis. The use of a bone graft substitute can increase effectiveness in larger locules.

Protein foam delays release of doxycycline for a longer antineoplastic effect, creates greater viscosity than a simple liquid embolic agent, and provides more contact between the doxycycline and cyst walls (tumoral elements).

To create 10 mg/mL doxycycline foam:

1. Reconstitute doxycycline in normal saline or 0.5 % lidocaine with epinephrine (1:200,000) to create a 40 mg/mL solution.
2. Combine:
   (a) 5 mL of prepared doxycycline solution (200 mg)
   (b) 5 mL of 25 % human serum albumin (if operators desire positive contrast in the foam, substitute 2.5 mL of water soluble contrast medium and 2.5 mL human serum albumin)
   (c) 10 mL of air
3. The mixture is then agitated with 2 syringes and a 3-way stopcock (at least 30 times) to produce the foam. Repeat agitation may be required due to settling throughout the procedure.

The foam is injected to fill the cyst or until the solution comes out through the other needle. Ultrasound can be used to inject the foam into solid ABC components.

When larger locules are present, a tricalcium phosphate bone graft substitute with doxycycline is subsequently used.

To create a Vitoss Flow (tricalcium phosphate) slurry:

1. Break 5 mL block of *Vitoss Foam Flow (Stryker Orthobiologics, Malvern, USA)* into 1–2 mm fragments.
2. Mix fragments with:
   (a) 1 mL of contrast
   (b) 4 mL of doxycycline/albumin solution (20 mg/mL)
3. After sitting for at least a minute, pass the mixture back and forth between 2 syringes through a 3-way stopcock.

Cavities are filled to between 50 and 70 % of their volume leaving the second needle in place to clear the indwelling original doxycycline mixture. To minimize bleeding, Gelfoam pledgets can be inserted through needles as they are withdrawn.

Follow-up imaging with plain film is performed at 10-week intervals prior to subsequent treatment. Treatment is repeated every 12 weeks until full new bone healing and elimination of the cystic spaces or until residual lucent spaces show no evidence of further growth. Due to the slow growth of the ABC neoplastic cells, surveillance is maintained annually for 5 years in order to detect residual foci of ABC expansion that require focused percutaneous treatment.

Ethanol

The use of alcohol as a sclerosant for ABC was recently described [46]. Alcohol is a powerful sclerosant with a low viscosity that can cause significant morbidity or even mortality [63]. As a general rule, alcohol should only be administered by experienced operators utilizing meticulous technique.

When administering alcohol, use of the double (multiple) needle access technique is essential. Administering ethanol through one needle while simultaneously draining through another allows a greater volume of sclerosant to be delivered and decreases the intralesional pressure, making escape into venous structures less likely.

After accessing the lesion, anhydrous ethanol (96–98 % after exposure to air) is instilled to a maximum dose of 1 mL/kg. The tourniquet is deflated after 10 min. The patient is monitored in the hospital for 24 h.

Ethibloc

Ethibloc is a sclerosing agent available in Europe and Australia that includes alcohol, radiopaque contrast, and zein, a maize-derived protein [48–50, 64, 65]. When exposed to fluid, the viscous emulsion solidifies and the alcohol is slowly released.

When used for treatment of ABCs, it is injected through large-bore needles (14–18 gauge). A second needle is often used to allow evacuation of cyst contents or provide access to isolated locules. Depending on lesion size, up to 7.5 mL is injected. Some groups mix the 7.5 mL syringe of Ethibloc with an additional 1–5 mL of pure alcohol [48, 49]. Injections can be repeated every 1–2 months for large lesions that cannot be entirely treated with one procedure. The injection can be actively monitored with fluoroscopy or CT. Histacryl can be used to embolize the tract [66] or pressure is held for 10 min at the site [49].

Plain films and CT are obtained after the procedure. Patients are followed with plain films at 1, 3, 6, and 12 months and either CT or MRI at 6 and 12 months.

Local complications of Ethibloc injection include inflammation, sterile abscess formation, and soft tissue extrusion.

Pulmonary embolism and a high complication rate resulted in one group abandoning the use of Ethibloc [66]. However, the pulmonary embolism occurred following injection of 12 mL of Ethibloc into a pelvic ABC, 60 % more than the maximum volume of 7.5 mL recommended by the manufacturer [49].

As mentioned previously, death has been reported secondary to retrograde arterial embolization during treatment of a C2 ABC [52].

Injections

Steroid Injections

Background

Corticosteroids are a family of powerful anti-inflammatory medications. Corticosteroid injections are used in the treatment of juvenile arthritides and other inflammatory conditions. Injections can be performed to treat joints, tendon sheaths, bursae, neuromas, and ganglia or as a part of an invasive pain procedure, such as a celiac plexus block. This section will focus on joint and tendon injections.

In arthritis, steroid injections are often undertaken when oral anti-inflammatory medication does not provide adequate symptom relief.

Accurate delivery of corticosteroid into the affected area results in better symptom relief [67]. The accuracy of joint localization using clinical landmarks is as low as 50 %. Image guidance increases the accuracy of injection [67, 68]. This may be particularly helpful for complex or difficult-to-access joints such as the subtalar, sacroiliac, shoulder, and temporomandibular. While ultrasound is the most commonly used guidance modality, fluoroscopy, arthrography, CT, and MRI localization have all been described.

Contraindications

Contraindications to steroid administration include infectious arthritis, sepsis, joint instability, severe periarticular osteoporosis, and coagulopathy [69].

Equipment

Corticosteroids: Numerous corticosteroid preparations are commercially available. The dose, concentration, and duration vary by product. Steroids can be either soluble or insoluble. Insoluble corticosteroids form microcrystalline structures that vary in size and aggregation characteristics [70]. Soluble steroids, such as dexamethasone sodium phosphate, provide a rapid onset but a shorter duration in comparison with insoluble corticosteroids [69].

Preprocedure Workup

Patients are referred after assessment by a rheumatologist. Patients may require reassessment on the day of the procedure if there has been a recent change in their symptoms.

Review of the pertinent imaging is helpful. MRI can be used to identify the exact location of inflammation in areas of complex anatomy where localization through clinical examination is difficult (such as the feet).

Injections can be performed with local anesthesia only, sedation, or general anesthesia. The choice depends on the location and number of joints being injected and patient need.

No specific blood work or patient preparation is required.

Procedure

The patient is positioned to allow access to the targeted area(s). The appropriate imaging modality is used to introduce a small needle into the area to be injected. Depending on the anatomy of the joint, ultrasound, fluoroscopy, or CT are commonly used for access. Arthrography can be performed to assure an intra-articular location if desired (Fig. 23.7). When a joint effusion is present, fluid is collected to perform a cell count.

No scientifically determined dose parameters exist. As such, the dose is usually determined based on the product being used and institutional and personal preference by the rheumatologist and radiologist. Young et al. [71] recently proposed a dose protocol for triamcinolone acetonide and triamcinolone hexacetonide that is based on the patient age and the joint to be injected (Table 23.1). The doses in this study were calculated based on typical adult doses and scaled according to the body surface area based on weight/age. It should be noted that the radiologist may choose to decrease the prescribed dose/volume at the time of injection due to technical or anatomic concerns.

Active monitoring during injection assures the needle tip is in an appropriate location and the steroid is injected into the targeted space/fluid without intra-pannus injection or extravasation (Fig. 23.8).

The corticosteroid can be mixed with local anesthetic or administered on its own and then followed by local anesthetic injection based on operator or institutional preference. It is thought that there may be less chance of leakage of corticosteroid into the surrounding tissues when it is "pushed in" with local anesthetic. However, when injecting a combined mixture, there is no need to change syringes leading to better needle stability.

Ultrasound examination at the time of procedure is also used to identify enlarged tendon sheaths that require injection. The steroid is injected into the tendon sheath taking care not to inject the tendon itself. Synechiae are sometimes identified at the time of injection (Fig. 23.9). There are anecdotal reports of attempted disruption of synechiae with a needle.

When injections are being performed in areas where any possibility of arterial embolization carries high risk (e.g., spinal injections, especially transforaminal or intercostal nerve blocks), contrast injection with high-quality fluoroscopy or DSA should be used to monitor the injection [72].

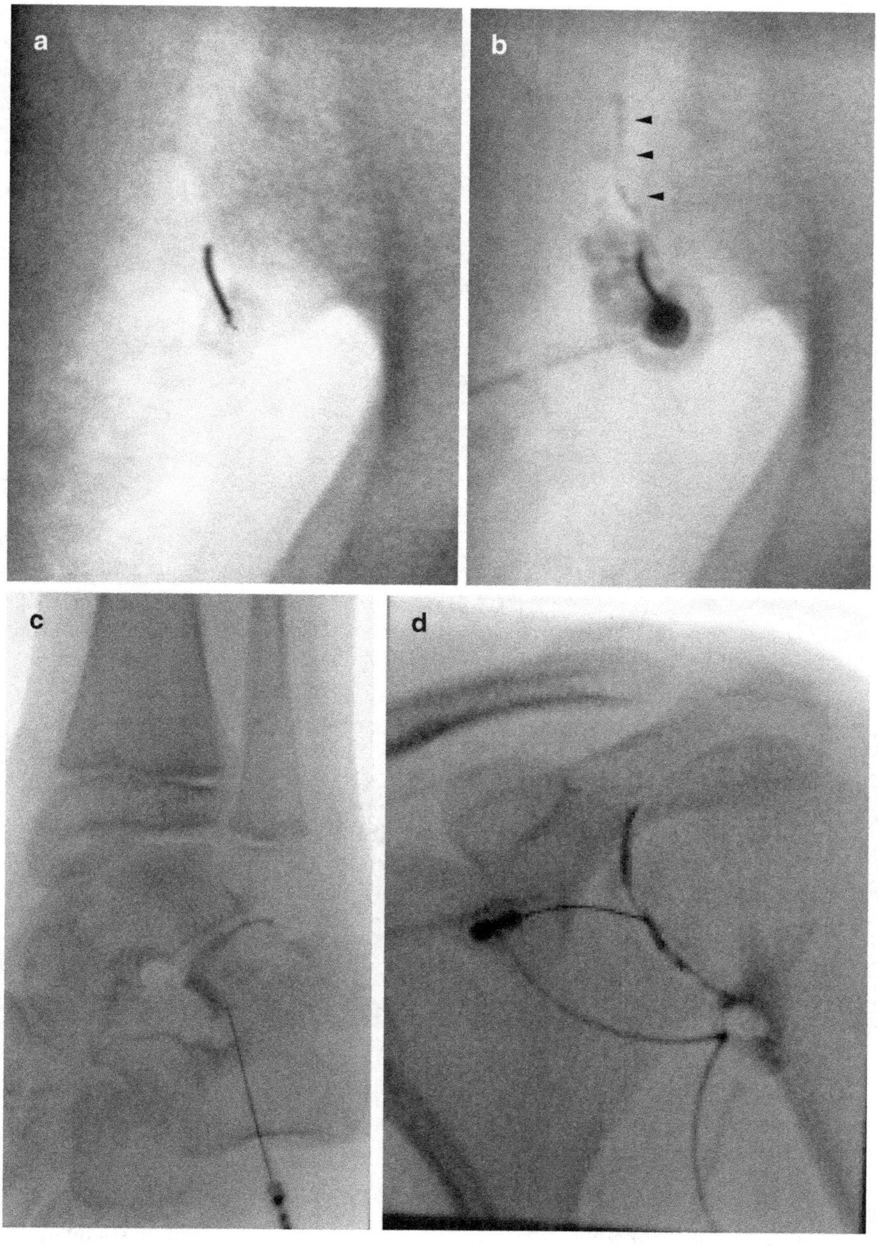

Fig. 23.7 Arthrography. Arthrography can be used to assure the needle is in an intra-articular location prior to injection. (**a**) Fluoroscopy was used to insert needle into the lower portion of the sacroiliac joint. (**b**) Linear contrast outlines the SI joint (*arrowheads*) indicating an appropriate intra-articular position. The needle was repositioned after the initial contrast injection did not flow into the joint. CT guidance and arthrography are commonly used to access the SI joint. (**c**) Arthrogram of the posterior subtalar joint. (**d**) Shoulder arthogram

Postprocedure Care

Patients may experience pain from the injection tract, from joint distension, or from the steroid itself. The latter is called postinjection or steroid flare and is thought to be secondary to the use of microcrystalline steroid preparations [69]. These causes of pain are self-limited and can be controlled with analgesics such as acetaminophen.

Patients and parents should be informed of the signs and symptoms of septic arthritis and

Table 23.1 Dose range for triamcinolone joint injections based on age in children

Location	Adult	12 years old	8 years old	4 years old
Knee Hip Shoulder	20–40	15–30	10.6–21.2	7.8–15.6
Tibiotalar	16–30	12–22.5	8.5–16	6.2–11.7
Elbow	8–20	6–15	4.2–10.6	3.1–7.8
Radiocarpal	8–20	6–15	4.2–10.6	3.1–7.8
Subtalar	8–16	6–12	4.2–8.5	3.1–6.2
Cuboid-cuneiform	8–14	6–10.5	4.2–7.4	3.1–5.5
Talonavicular	8–12	6–9	4.2–6.4	3.1–4.7
Navicular-cuneiform	8–12	6–9	4.2–6.4	3.1–4.7
Mid-cuneiform	8	6	4.2	3.1
Intercarpal	8	6	4.2	3.1
MCP/MTP	6–8	4.5–6	3.2–4.2	2.3–3.1
PIP	4–6	3–4.5	2.1–3.2	1.6–2.3
DIP	2	1.5	1.1	0.8

The doses for use in children were tabulated for triamcinolone hexacetonide and triamcinolone acetonide are based on adult doses were suggested in a recent paper [71]. Doses are reported in milligrams. The injection volume will vary depending on steroid concentration. *MCP* metacarpal-phalangeal, *MTP* metatarsal-phalangeal, *PIP* proximal interphalangeal, *DIP* distal interphalangeal. Reprinted with permission © Springer 2012

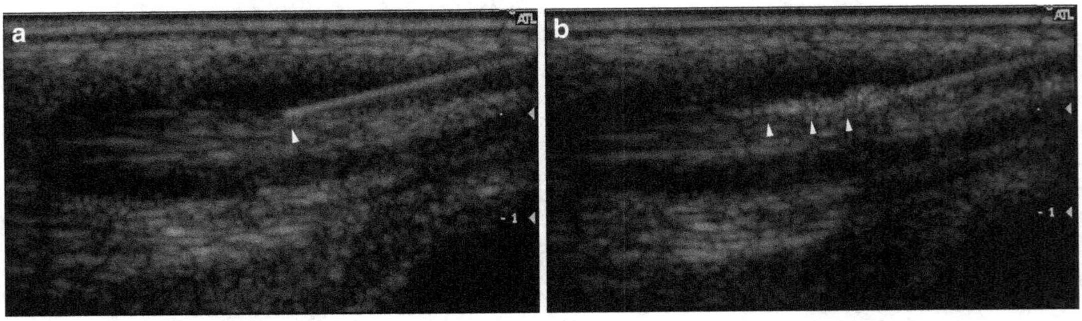

Fig. 23.8 Proper needle positioning. (**a**) Longitudinal ultrasound image shows the tip of a needle (*white arrowhead*) within a fluid-filled tendon sheath. (**b**) Ultrasound monitoring of the injection demonstrates corticosteroid flowing appropriately through the tendon sheath (*yellow arrowheads*). Active monitoring allows the injection to be halted and the needle repositioned if there is a problem

given clear instructions to immediately contact their rheumatologist or the interventional radiology call service or go to the emergency room.

Complications

Septic arthritis is a rare but important complication of joint injections. Due to the potential for joint destruction, septic arthritis is a surgical emergency and requires lavage in addition to intravenous antibiotics.

Pain related to steroid flare is usually self-limited, lasting 24–48 h. It tends to be milder in severity than the pain associated with septic arthritis.

Intra-articular steroid administration has been associated with avascular necrosis (AVN) [73, 74]. However, attributing AVN directly to steroid injection is often not possible as it can also be caused by arthritis or oral steroid use.

Diabetic patients should be informed that elevation of blood glucose levels can occur several days after corticosteroid administration [69].

Leakage of steroid into the soft tissues can result in calcification, atrophy, discoloration, and

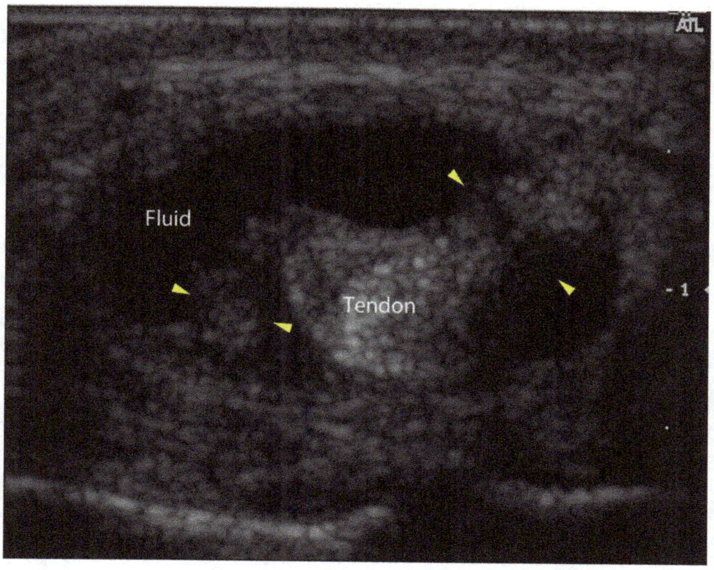

Fig. 23.9 Transverse ultrasound image demonstrates the central tendon surrounded by an enlarged, fluid-filled tendon sheath (labeled). Strands extending from the tendon to the edge of the tendon sheath (*yellow arrowheads*) are consistent with synechiae

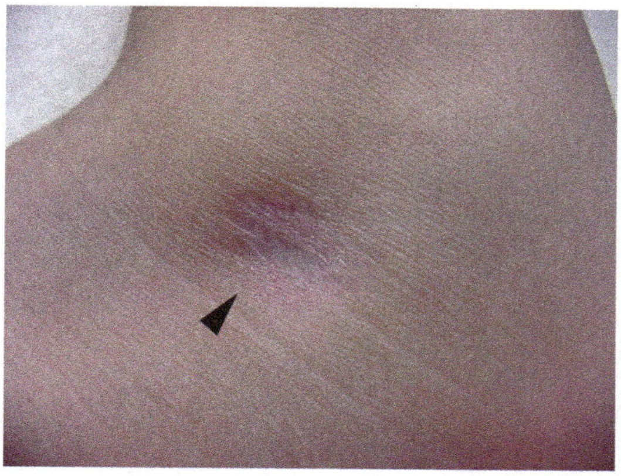

Fig. 23.10 Lateral ankle with an area of tissue atrophy and discoloration (*arrowhead*) that developed as a result of leakage of corticosteroid after tendon injection

scar formation (Fig. 23.10). In addition, tendon sheath injections carry a risk of tendon rupture. Injection of the Achilles tendon [75] is considered contraindicated by some authors.

Arterial embolization is a rare complication of steroid injection (Fig. 23.11) [76]. Blindness, stroke, and infarction of the brainstem and spine have been reported following corticosteroid injection in the spinal area [77–82]. If embolization occurs and treatment is necessary, intra-arterial iloprost infusion +/– thrombolysis can be considered [83, 84]. Iloprost, a prostacyclin analogue, is a potent vasodilator used in the treatment of pulmonary hypertension and Raynaud's phenomenon.

Botulinum Toxin Injections

Since the introduction of BOTOX® (Botox) in the 1980s, numerous approved and off-label uses have been developed. In pediatrics, Botox is used primarily to treat muscle spasticity and drooling. While not technically part of the MSK system, salivary Botox injection will be covered in this section.

Background Information

The anaerobic bacteria, *Clostridium botulinum*, produce endotoxins responsible for the food-borne disease, botulism. The symptoms of botulism include vomiting, diarrhea, and muscle paralysis. Potential therapeutic use of BTX was suggested by Justinus Kerner in 1817 [85].

The bacteria secrete seven active neurotoxins denoted by the letters A–G. Each has a different mechanism of action and pharmacokinetic profile. Types A, B, C, and F are thought to have potential for use in humans [86]. The serotypes approved

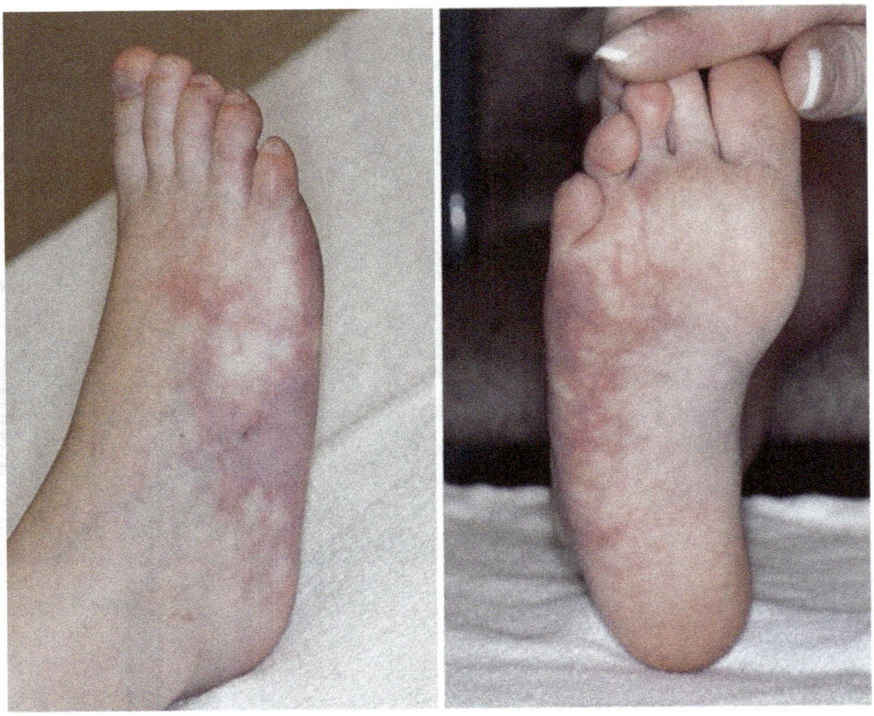

Fig. 23.11 Arterial corticosteroid embolization. This clinical image demonstrates findings consistent with arterial embolization following after the uneventful ultrasound-guided injection of a cystic extension of the calcaneocuboid joint. Transient mottling of the foot appeared in the recovery room but resolved elevation and warming. Pain and discoloration recurred the following day leading to immediate reassessment and referral to plastic surgery. The signs and symptoms resolved over the next 7–10 days without intervention

for clinical use in humans are BTX-A (BOTOX®, Allergan Pharmaceuticals, USA; Dysport®, Ipsen Limited, UK; and Xeomin®, Merz Pharmaceuticals, USA) and BTX-B (Myobloc®, Soltice Neurosciences Inc., USA). BTX temporarily inhibits release of acetylcholine at neuromuscular and neuroglandular junctions. BTX precludes presynaptic fusion of vesicles with the axonal endplate membrane preventing acetylcholine release. BTX-A affects SNAP-25 (synaptosomal-associated protein), and BTX-B affects VAMP (vesicle-associated membrane protein/synaptobrevin). Other neurotransmitters, such as nitric oxide, may be affected by BTX [87].

It is important to note that the available commercial products each have a different potency and, as such, doses are not equivalent and cannot be directly converted between brands [1]. As Botox is by far the most commonly used neurotoxin, other formulations of BTX will not be discussed further in this chapter.

Some authors have attempted to assess dose response [88], but clinical trials to determine optimal dose of Botox have not been performed. As such, doses quoted relate to consensus opinion and those published in previous studies [1].

Table 23.2 outlines a selection of the currently approved uses for Botox in countries that have published specific prescribing information.

Muscle Injections

Botox is used to improve the quality of life of children with spasticity and dystonia, most commonly in cerebral palsy [89]. Specific indications for use include the desire to improve gait and function, relieve pain, reduce the burden of care, and delay hip subluxation [1].

At the current time, ultrasound-guided muscle injections are most often performed by neurologists and rehabilitation medicine specialists. However, access to high-end imaging equipment and anesthesiologists has resulted in interventional

Table 23.2 Approved uses (selected) and lower age limits for Botox

Country	Cervical dystonia	Spasticity	Equinus foot deformity	Focal spasticity	Sialorrhea drooling	Hyperhydrosis
USA	16	18	–	–	X	18
Canada	16	18	2*	–	X	18
Australia	NS	–	2**	2**	X	NS
UK	12	–	2	NS	X	NS

The countries listed have made specific recommendations for the use of Botox. Compiled October 2012 using country-specific package inserts and/or federal health agency recommendations. Please refer to the country's newest prescribing information to assure accuracy as recommendations are updated on an ongoing basis

The numbers reflect the lower approved age limit in years

NS = approved but age not specified or specified as "adults"

– = not included or covered by other recommendations

* = in cerebral palsy patients

** = upper or lower limb spasticity in cerebral palsy patients

X = not approved

radiologist becoming increasingly involved at some centers.

The decision to inject specific muscles or muscle groups is based on the physical findings and needs of the patient. The dose used is based on patient motor function and risk factors [1]. An injection plan is created that outlines the number and location of injections and a standardized Botox dilution used for each muscle. The plan is based on the muscle shape, presynaptic receptor density, and amount of diffusion expected. This complex decision-making process is beyond the scope of this book.

Depending on patient need, the procedure is performed with local anesthesia, sedation, or general anesthesia. No preprocedure blood work is required.

Ultrasound guidance is used to perform the injections as outlined in the injection plan. Exact targeting is essential as injection into the wrong muscle can result in greater muscular imbalance and worsening of symptoms (Fig. 23.12). When the needle tip is difficult to visualize, a nerve-stimulating needle can be used to cause the muscle to contract, ensuring appropriate localization of the target muscle (Fig. 23.13).

In muscle, Botox begins taking effect in 2–4 days with the peak effect taking 1–2 weeks and a duration of 3–4 months. Patients are followed by their neurologist or rehabilitation medicine specialist.

Salivary Gland Injection

Drooling in the neurologically impaired child can result in social and emotional difficulties. In cerebral palsy, drooling is usually caused by swallowing issues rather than excessive saliva production (sialorrhea) [90]. Traditional treatment options include diet modification, behavioral therapy, surgery (gland excision, tympanic neurectomy, diversion, and mechanical ligation/occlusion), radiation (historical), and administration of systemic parasympatholytics [91, 92]. In recent years, Botox has been used for the treatment of drooling in pediatric patients. Botox is not currently approved for the treatment of drooling/sialorrhea in any jurisdiction.

BTX-A inhibits production/release of the fluid component of saliva by interrupting parasympathetic innervation. Cholinergic receptors are responsible for the fluid and electrolyte component of saliva. Adrenergic receptors control the excretion of proteinaceous and mucinous components [87, 93]. It has been theorized that continued excretion of thick, proteinaceous, intraoral saliva better protects the patient's dentition in distinction to surgical intervention where salivary ducts are ligated or rerouted.

Numerous studies have been performed in both adults [94–98] and children [99–106] using Botox. There is a huge variation in the reported dose and volume administered in both adults and children indicating that there is no scientifically

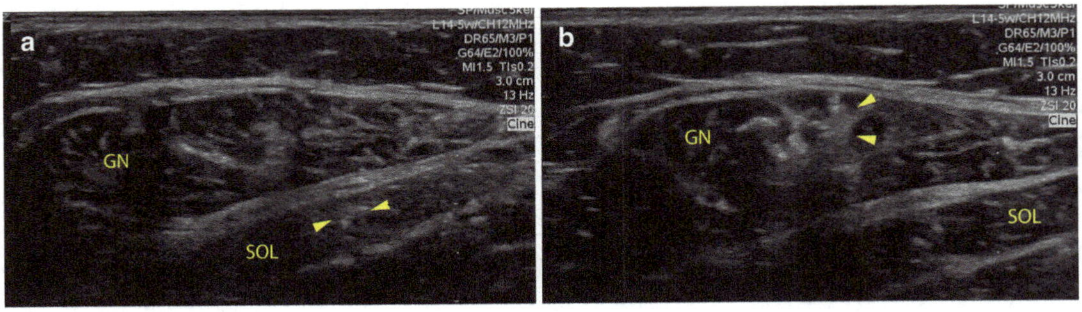

Fig. 23.12 Botox injection for muscle spasticity. When performing muscle injection, accuracy is essential for a successful outcome. Injection of the wrong muscle can exacerbate symptoms. (**a**) A 25 gauge needle was introduced into the soleus (*arrowheads*) in transverse orientation. (**b**) Similarly, the gastrocnemius muscle was targeted (*arrowheads*) and injection was monitored with ultrasound. *GN* gastrocnemius, *SOL* soleus

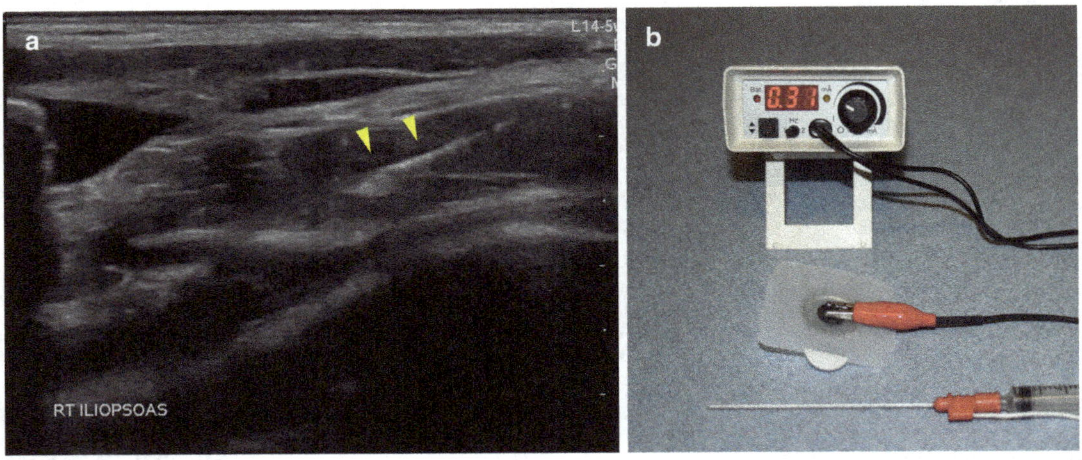

Fig. 23.13 (**a**) Ultrasound can be used to guide superficial muscle injections. The needle (*arrowheads*) is easily seen in the iliopsoas injection. (**b**) When attempting to access the deep, intra-abdominal portion of the psoas, the tip is not easily identified with ultrasound. In such cases, a nerve stimulator needle is introduced. The ground lead (middle of picture) is placed over a distal muscle to complete the electrical circuit. The current is slowly increased until muscle movement is identified

based consensus at this time. In adult patients, doses ranged from 2.5 to 450 U per gland. In children, doses ranged from 5 to 65 U/gland and injection volumes ranged from 0.05 to 2 mL. Recent papers use a weight-based approach of 0.5–1 units/kg/gland and a maximum dose of 50–100 units in total [106–109].

Reported responses were variable in onset and duration [110]. Most patients notice an effect after 1–2 weeks lasting from several weeks to 7 months. In addition, primary nonresponders are found.

Preliminary studies have shown that BTX-B can be used for control of salivation [111, 112]. BTX-B may offer an alternative for primary nonresponders and those who develop antibodies to other botulinum serotypes.

Botox injections can be used as a primary treatment method for drooling or following failed duct ligation or relocation. Some families opt for a trial of Botox treatment prior to making a decision to proceed with surgical intervention.

In most patients, bilateral parotid and submandibular gland injection is performed leaving the sublingual and numerous small glands to produce saliva. The parotid and submandibular glands are estimated to be responsible for approximately 75 % of saliva production. For a more targeted

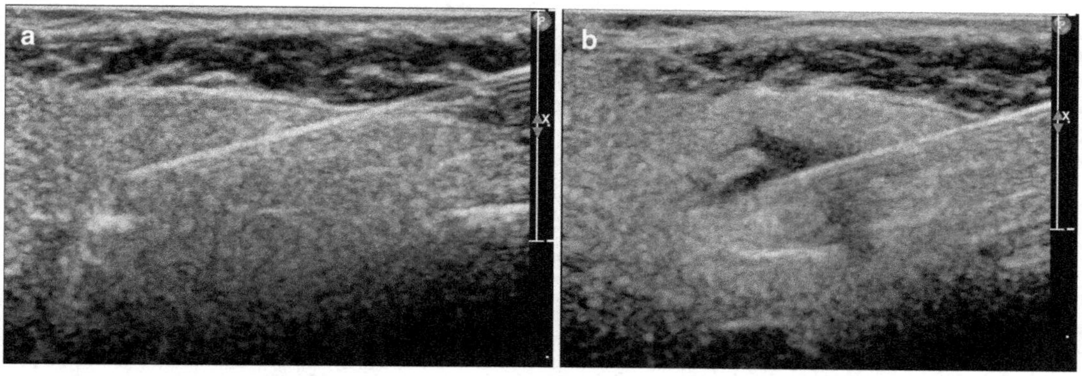

Fig. 23.14 Salivary gland injection. (**a**) A needle was introduced into the parotid gland parenchyma avoiding the nearby facial artery (not shown). (**b**) A small volume of Botox-containing solution is injected. Constant monitoring assures the medication is delivered into the central portion of the gland without extravasation or unexpected spread

approach, salivary gland scintigraphy can be used to identify the source of ongoing salivary production in patients following failed surgery.

Preprocedure Workup

Treatment options and risks of injection are discussed at an IR clinic visit. No specific blood work is necessary. An anesthesia consult may be necessary for complex patients.

Procedure Technique

Injections can be performed using local anesthesia, sedation, or general anesthesia. When injected, Botox locally diffuses through tissues. As such, accurate injection technique is essential to decrease the risk of regional, non-target effects.

Botox is reconstituted with normal saline or sterile water based on the dose and volume of solution desired. For example, to perform injection of 25 units of Botox in 0.25 mL of solution into 4 glands, 1 mL of solution is added to a 100 unit bottle (100 units/mL). If only 12.5 units in 0.25 mL were to be injected into each gland, 2 mL of solution would be added to a 100 unit bottle (50 units/mL). The manufacturer recommends gently swirling the liquid to dissolve the cryoprecipitate as agitation can denature the BTX-A molecule.

Ultrasound is used to identify the target gland. A small volume of solution is injected into the central portion of gland (Fig. 23.14). If a large dose (>25–50 units) or a large volume (>0.5 mL) is used, multiple locations can be injected (Table 23.3).

Table 23.3 Commonly reported Botox doses in children

Muscle [1]
– 6–24 units/kg
• GFMCS I–IV, no risk factors: 16–20 units/kg; max. < 300 units
• GFMCS V, with risk factors: 12–16 units/kg; max. <400–600 units
Salivary glands: (parotid, submandibular)
– 4–5 units/kg
– 1–1.25 units/kg/gland
– Maximum total dose 50–100 units
– Maximum dose per site 25–50 units
– Maximum dose per gland 25–50 units

GFMCS gross motor function classification system for cerebral palsy. Ranges from “walks without limitations” (I) to “transported in manual wheelchair” (V)

Postprocedure

Patients may require acetaminophen for minor discomfort. Patients who undergo salivary gland injections will occasionally have blood-tinged saliva immediately after the procedure.

Informed discharge is performed when the patient has recovered from sedation/GA. The signs and symptoms that should prompt immediate emergency contact should be reviewed with the patient and/or caregivers.

Complications

Complications include those related to local diffusion or distal effects, xerostomia, allergy, antibody formation, and death.

Diffusion of Botox into the surrounding soft tissues can cause unwanted local effects [113]. For example, chewing and swallowing difficulties have been attributed to local diffusion following salivary gland injection. However, it can be difficult to attribute minor changes in perceived muscle function as a change in saliva viscosity can change the perception of swallowing.

Distal effects, potentially attributable to Botox injection, have been noted. Bloodstream absorption is thought to be responsible for identification of the botulinum-receptor complex in mouse diaphragm after calf injection. Experimental models have shown that Botox affects axonal function and can be transported in a retrograde transport through neurons [114, 115] although this has not been demonstrated clinically. Reported cases of pneumonia following Botox administration illustrate the difficulty in determining an exact cause. The pneumonia could be attributed to the patient's underlying neurologic condition, aspiration from drooling/sialorrhea, anesthetic administration, or distal Botox effect (related to absorption or CNS effects).

Children form antibodies to Botox more readily than adults [116] that can affect efficacy. To minimize risk of antibody formation, it seems prudent to use the lowest effective dose possible and repeat the injections only after symptoms return.

Death has been reported secondary to a probable anaphylactic reaction in one patient [117].

In 2008, the FDA and Health Canada released warnings related to symptoms of botulism (requiring insertion of feeding tubes and ventilator support) and death in patients after receiving Botox or Myobloc®. Affected pediatric patients were less than 16 years old and received high doses (up to 32 units/kg Botox) for muscle injections. FDA recommendations include that physicians understand potency determinations of the products they administer, be alert for side effects (as early as one day up to several weeks), provide patients and caregivers with information regarding signs and symptoms of side effects, and discuss the need for immediate medical attention when there is any muscle weakness, difficulty swallowing, or respiratory issues [118]. In addition, off-label use should be disclosed during the consent process.

Chapter Summary

Osteoid Osteoma

Background

- Benign tumor
- Males, 10–35 years old
- Any bone
- <1.5 cm
- Central calcified nidus in lucent area often with surrounding sclerosis
  - Brodie's abscess main differential diagnosis
- Classic history: pain, relieved by NSAIDs, waking at night
- Conservative treatment, surgical excision/curettage, CT-guided excision, and thermal ablation possible

Indications

- Inadequate pain control
- Desire to definitively treat

Contraindications

- Inability to create safe access route
  - >1 cm from vital structures ideally

Equipment

- CT guidance commonly used
- Radiofrequency ablation
  - Various devices and probes available
  - Grounding pads required with monopolar machines
- Laser
  - 810 nm laser
- Bone access/biopsy needles
  - 11–18 gauge depending on system used

Preprocedure Workup

- Review imaging.
- IR clinic visit.
- Blood work not necessary unless high-risk area or patient.

Procedure Technique

- General anesthesia.
- Not all steps below are used for all procedures. Exact procedural approach depends on method of thermal ablation, system used, and location-specific need.

- Place grounding pads.
- Position to allow appropriate access in CT gantry.
- Place access needle.
- Place monitoring device and/or administer thermal protection (fluid, CO_2).
- Perform biopsy.
- Insert RFA probe or laser fiber.
- Pull back uninsulated coaxial needle.
- Heat.
  - RFA: 85–95 C×4–8 min.
  - Laser: 1,000–1,200 J or (lesion diameter (mm)×100)+200 J.
  - Can decrease dosimetry in high-risk areas.
  - Multiple locations may be necessary for lesions >1 cm.

• Place ice on skin.

Postprocedure Care

• Analgesia
  - NSAID (ketorolac) is helpful.

• Weight bearing dependent on specific region and size of access defect(s)
  - "Activity as tolerated" for most patients.
  - High-risk areas may require crutches without weight bearing.

• Informed discharge

Complications

• Thermal
  - Burn of surrounding structures, needle tract
  - Draining fistula reported

• Infectious
  - Osteomyelitis
  - Septic arthritis
  - Cellulitis

• Incomplete/partial treatment response

Follow-Up

• IR clinic visit in 2 weeks
  - Rebook if there is residual lesion-related pain.

Aneurysmal Bone Cyst

Background

• Locally aggressive, benign neoplasm.
  - Related to upregulation of USP6 oncogene

• "Soap bubble" on CT/X-ray; fluid-fluid levels.
• Rare solid variant exists.
• Telangiectatic osteosarcoma main differential diagnosis.
  - Need for biopsy is controversial.

• Secondary ABC associated with giant cell tumor, chondroblastoma, osteoblastoma, and osteosarcoma.
• Lymphatic, venous, and arterial components are present.
• Treatment includes embolization and sclerotherapy.

Indications

• Stop expansion and instability.
• Nonaggressive lesions in low-risk areas could be followed.

Contraindications

• Ethibloc listed as contraindicated in spinal ABC by some

Equipment

• Fluoroscopy, CT, ultrasound
• Access/biopsy needles
  - 12–16 gauge

• Embolic agent (glue, PVA, Gelfoam)
• Sclerotherapy agent
  - Doxycycline
    - Albumin, Gelfoam powder
  - Tricalcium phosphate
  - Ethanol
  - Ethibloc
  - Contrast

Embolization

• Treatment method or adjunct to surgery
• Glue, PVA, and Gelfoam described
• PVA
  - 150–250 μm in low-risk area
  - 250–350 μm in spine or high-risk area

• Suggested as treatment of choice in spine ABC by some
• Complications
  - Nontarget embolization

Sclerotherapy

• Numerous agents described
• General procedure technique
  - General anesthesia
  - Access lesion +/– biopsy
  - Aspirate fluid
  - Inject contrast
    - Assess volume, distribution, and venous drainage.
    - Aspirate.
  - Place secondary needles for treatment and drainage.
  - Apply tourniquet.

- Inject sclerosant.
  - Avoid extravasation.
  - Monitor with imaging.
- Remove needles.
  - Consider site pressure, Gelfoam, and glue injection.
- Remove tourniquet.
  - Consider gradual release if there is high risk of venous escape of embolic agent.
- Follow up imaging.
  - X-rays; CT/MRI
- Repeat treatment as necessary.

- *Doxycycline foam*
  - Foam provides better contact, longer effect, and easier administration.
  - To create doxycycline foam (10 mg/mL):
    - Reconstitute doxycycline to 40 mg/mL with NS or 0.5 % lidocaine.
    - Agitate mixture containing:
      - 5 mL of 40 mg/mL doxycycline solution (200 mg)
      - 5 mL of albumin *or* 2.5 mL albumin with 2.5 mL contrast
      - 10 mL air
      - Can be scaled proportionally
    - Inject foam until fill cyst or until exits through secondary needle.
    - Can be injected directly into solid components.
    - Maximum dose: 300–500 mg for neonates.
- *Tricalcium phosphate bone graft*
  - Used in combination with doxycycline foam to treat larger locules.
  - Inject to fill cavity between 50 and 70 % of cyst volume; indwelling doxycycline foam drains through secondary needle.
  - Vitoss Flow slurry:
    - Break 5 mL Vitoss Flow block in 1–2 mm fragments.
    - Add 1 mL contrast and 4 mL doxycycline/albumin solution (20 mg/mL) and leave for >1 min.
    - Pass through a 3-way stopcock.
- *Ethanol*
  - Powerful sclerosant with narrow safety margin
  - Absolute alcohol administered using multiple needle technique
    - Minimizing potential for venous escape essential
  - Maximum dose 1 mL/kg
  - Monitored in the hospital for 24 h
- *Ethibloc*
  - Viscous sclerosant mixture containing alcohol
  - Maximum dose 7.5 mL
- Complications
  - Extravasation or arterial/venous escape
    - Skin necrosis
    - Systemic effects (acute pulmonary hypertension, right heart failure, death)
    - Death related to basilar thrombosis report

Corticosteroid Injections

- Background
- Powerful anti-inflammatory medication.
- Joint and tendon injections for arthritis.
- Accurate injection improves outcomes.

Indications

- Inadequate response oral medications

Contraindications

- Infectious arthritis
- Sepsis
- Joint instability
- Severe periarticular osteoporosis
- Coagulopathy

Equipment

- Ultrasound most often used.
  - CT, fluoroscopy, MRI, arthrography possible
- Steroids.
  - Soluble/insoluble
  - Better response with insoluble steroids
- Local anesthetic may be used.
  - Lidocaine, bupivacaine, etc.

Preprocedure Workup

- Rheumatology assessment.
- Review imaging.
  - MR helpful for identifying targets in areas of complex anatomy
- Local, sedation, or GA based on patient need, number of injections, and difficulty of access.

Procedure Technique

- Position to allow access.
- Target joint with imaging.
  - Consider arthrography for difficult areas.

- Injection corticosteroid/local anesthetic.
  - Combined with local anesthetic vs. steroid first and LA second.
  - Dose varies with product and institutional/personal preference.
    - Table 23.1—recently recommended dose protocol
- Monitor during injection when possible.
  - Use high-quality fluoroscopy or DSA in high-risk areas.
- Postprocedure Care
- Analgesia
- Informed discharge

Complications
- Septic arthritis
- Steroid flare
- Avascular necrosis
- Hyperglycemia (in diabetics)
  - Soft tissue calcification, atrophy, discoloration, scar
- Tendon rupture
- Arterial embolization
  - Thrombolysis, Iloprost if necessary

Botulinum Toxin Injections

Background
- Botulinum toxins A and B are most commonly used.
  - Botox is discussed in this chapter.
- BTX-A blocks presynaptic acetylcholine release.
- Diffuses through tissues.
- Cannot covert doses between commercial brands.
- Approved uses are listed in Table 23.2.

Muscle Injections
- Most often used for spastic cerebral palsy (CP).
- Injection protocol based on muscle shape, receptor density, and degree of diffusion expected.
- Inaccurate injection can worsen symptoms.
- Onset, 2–4 days; peak effect, 1–2 weeks; duration, 3–4 months.

Salivary Gland Injections
- Usually used to control drooling in CP patients.
- Off-label use of Botox.
- Botox decreases fluid component of saliva while maintaining protein/mucus.
- Effect variable.
  - Onset, 1–2 weeks; duration, up to 7 months
- Usually parotid and submandibular glands injected.

Preprocedure Workup
- Clinic visit to discuss treatment options and risks.
- Consider anesthesia consult for complex patients.

Procedure Technique
- Saline or sterile water added to achieve desired dilution.
  - Do not agitate when mixing.
- Ultrasound for guidance.
  - Consider nerve-stimulating needle for difficult to visualize areas (muscle injection).
- Reported doses are listed in Table 23.3.

Postprocedure Care
- Analgesia
- Informed discharge

Complications
- Local
  - Salivary: swallowing, chewing difficulties
  - Muscle: imbalance, increased pain
- Distal
  - Theoretical central effects possible
  - Pneumonia reported
- Xerostomia
- Anaphylaxis
- Antibody formation
- Death
  - FDA and Health Canada warning

References

1. Love SC, Novak I, Kentish M, Desloovere K, Heinen F, Molenaers G, et al. Botulinum toxin assessment, intervention and after-care for lower limb spasticity in children with cerebral palsy: international consensus statement. Eur J Neurol. 2010;17 Suppl 2:9–37.
2. Kransdorf MJ, Stull MA, Gilkey FW, Moser RP. Osteoid osteoma. Radiographics. 1991;11(4):671–96.
3. Healey JH, Ghelman B. Osteoid osteoma and osteoblastoma. Current concepts and recent advances. Clin Orthop Relat Res. 1986;204:76–85.
4. Virayavanich W, Singh R, O'Donnell RJ, Horvai AE, Goldsby RE, Link TM. Osteoid osteoma of

the femur in a 7-month-old infant treated with radiofrequency ablation. Skeletal Radiol. 2010; 39(11):1145–9.
5. Chai JW, Hong SH, Choi JY, Koh YH, Lee JW, Choi JA, et al. Radiologic diagnosis of osteoid osteoma: from simple to challenging findings. Radiographics. 2010;30(3):737–49.
6. Hosalkar HS, Garg S, Moroz L, Pollack A, Dormans JP. The diagnostic accuracy of MRI versus CT imaging for osteoid osteoma in children. Clin Orthop Relat Res. 2005;433:171–7.
7. von Kalle T, Langendorfer M, Fernandez FF, Winkler P. Combined dynamic contrast-enhancement and serial 3D-subtraction analysis in magnetic resonance imaging of osteoid osteomas. Eur Radiol. 2009;19(10):2508–17.
8. Liu PT, Chivers FS, Roberts CC, Schultz CJ, Beauchamp CP. Imaging of osteoid osteoma with dynamic gadolinium-enhanced MR imaging. Radiology. 2003;227(3):691–700.
9. Zampa V, Bargellini I, Ortori S, Faggioni L, Cioni R, Bartolozzi C. Osteoid osteoma in atypical locations: the added value of dynamic gadolinium-enhanced MR imaging. Eur J Radiol. 2009;71(3):527–35.
10. Chan R, Abdullah B, Aik S, Tok C. Radiofrequency ablation of a misdiagnosed Brodie's abscess. Biomed Imaging Interv J. 2011;7(2):e17.
11. Lindner NJ, Ozaki T, Roedl R, Gosheger G, Winkelmann W, Wortler K. Percutaneous radiofrequency ablation in osteoid osteoma. J Bone Joint Surg Br. 2001;83(3):391–6.
12. Hoffmann RT, Jakobs TF, Kubisch CH, Trumm CG, Weber C, Duerr HR, et al. Radiofrequency ablation in the treatment of osteoid osteoma-5-year experience. Eur J Radiol. 2010;73(2):374–9.
13. Motamedi D, Learch TJ, Ishimitsu DN, Motamedi K, Katz MD, Brien EW, et al. Thermal ablation of osteoid osteoma: overview and step-by-step guide. Radiographics. 2009;29(7):2127–41.
14. Jackson RP, Reckling FW, Mants FA. Osteoid osteoma and osteoblastoma. Similar histologic lesions with different natural histories. Clin Orthop Relat Res. 1977;128:303–13.
15. Yanagawa T, Watanabe H, Shinozaki T, Ahmed AR, Shirakura K, Takagishi K. The natural history of disappearing bone tumours and tumour-like conditions. Clin Radiol. 2001;56(11):877–86.
16. Feletar M, Hall S. Osteoid osteoma: a case for conservative management. Rheumatology (Oxford). 2002;41(5):585–6.
17. Ahmed M, Brace CL, Lee Jr FT, Goldberg SN. Principles of and advances in percutaneous ablation. Radiology. 2011;258(2):351–69.
18. Heisterkamp J, van Hillegersberg R, Ijzermans JNM. Critical temperature and heating time for coagulation damage: implications for interstitial laser coagulation (ILC) of tumors. Lasers Surg Med. 1999;25(3):257–62.
19. Aschero A, Gorincour G, Glard Y, Desvignes C, Paris M, Bourliere-Najean B, et al. Percutaneous treatment of osteoid osteoma by laser thermocoagulation under computed tomography guidance in pediatric patients. Eur Radiol. 2009;19(3):679–86.
20. Gangi A, Gasser B, De Unamuno S, Fogarrassy E, Fuchs C, Siffert P, et al. New trends in interstitial laser photocoagulation of bones. Semin Musculoskel Radiol. 1997;1(2):331–8.
21. Gangi A, Basile A, Buy X, Alizadeh H, Sauer B, Bierry G. Radiofrequency and laser ablation of spinal lesions. Semin Ultrasound CT MR. 2005; 26(2):89–97.
22. Gangi A, Alizadeh H, Wong L, Buy X, Dietemann JL, Roy C. Osteoid osteoma: percutaneous laser ablation and follow-up in 114 patients. Radiology. 2006;2007;242:293–301.
23. Gangi A, Buy X. Percutaneous bone tumor management. Semin Intervent Radiol. 2010;27(2):124–36.
24. Moser T, Giacomelli MC, Clavert JM, Buy X, Dietemann JL, Gangi A. Image-guided laser ablation of osteoid osteoma in pediatric patients. J Pediatr Orthop. 2008;28:265–70.
25. Sequeiros R, Hyvönen P, Sequeiros A, Jyrkinen L, Ojala R, Klemola R, et al. MR imaging-guided laser ablation of osteoid osteomas with use of optical instrument guidance at 0.23 T. Eur Radiol. 2003;13(10):2309–14. Epub 2003 May 7.
26. Streitparth F, Teichgraber U, Walter T, Schaser KD, Gebauer B. Recurrent osteoid osteoma: interstitial laser ablation under magnetic resonance imaging guidance. Skeletal Radiol. 2010;39(11):1131–7.
27. Dasenbrock HH, Gandhi D, Kathuria S. Percutaneous plasma mediated radiofrequency ablation of spinal osteoid osteomas. J Neurointerv Surg. 2012;4: 226–8.
28. Napoli A, Mastantuono M, Marincola BC, Anzidei M, Zaccagna F, Moreschini O, et al. Osteoid osteoma: MR-guided focused ultrasound for entirely noninvasive treatment. Radiology. 2013;267(2): 514–21. doi: 10.1148/radiol.13120873. Epub 2013 Feb 7.
29. Pinto CH, Taminiau AH, Vanderschueren GM, Hogendoorn PC, Bloem JL, Obermann WR. Technical considerations in CT-guided radiofrequency thermal ablation of osteoid osteoma: tricks of the trade. AJR Am J Roentgenol. 2002;179(6): 1633–42.
30. Rosenthal DI, Hornicek FJ, Torriani M, Gebhardt MC, Mankin HJ. Osteoid osteoma: percutaneous treatment with radiofrequency energy. Radiology. 2003;229(1):171–5.
31. Rosenthal DI, Marota JJ, Hornicek FJ. Osteoid osteoma: elevation of cardiac and respiratory rates at biopsy needle entry into tumor in 10 patients. Radiology. 2003;226(1):125–8.
32. Dupuy DE, Hong R, Oliver B, Goldberg SN. Radiofrequency ablation of spinal tumors: temperature distribution in the spinal canal. AJR Am J Roentgenol. 2000;175(5):1263–6.
33. Hadjipavlou AG, Tzermiadianos MN, Kakavelakis KN, Lander P. Percutaneous core excision and radio-

frequency thermo-coagulation for the ablation of osteoid osteoma of the spine. Eur Spine J. 2009;18(3): 345–51.
34. Adachi A, Kaminou T, Ogawa T, Kawai T, Takaki Y, Sugiura K, et al. Heat distribution in the spinal canal during radiofrequency ablation for vertebral lesions: study in swine. Radiology. 2008;247(2):374–80.
35. Rybak LD, Gangi A, Buy X, La Rocca Vieira R, Wittig J. Thermal ablation of spinal osteoid osteomas close to neural elements: technical considerations. AJR Am J Roentgenol. 2010;195(4):W293–8.
36. Vanderschueren GM, Taminiau AH, Obermann WR, van den Berg-Huysmans AA, Bloem JL. Osteoid osteoma: factors for increased risk of unsuccessful thermal coagulation. Radiology. 2004;233(3):757–62.
37. Lyon C, Buckwalter J. Case report: full-thickness skin necrosis after percutaneous radio-frequency ablation of a tibial osteoid osteoma. Iowa Orthop J. 2008;28:85–7.
38. Oliveira AM, Chou MM, Perez-Atayde AR, Rosenberg AE. Aneurysmal bone cyst: a neoplasm driven by upregulation of the USP6 oncogene. J Clin Oncol. 2006;24(1):e1; author reply e2.
39. Oliveira AM, Perez-Atayde AR, Inwards CY, Medeiros F, Derr V, Hsi BL, et al. USP6 and CDH11 oncogenes identify the neoplastic cell in primary aneurysmal bone cysts and are absent in so-called secondary aneurysmal bone cysts. Am J Pathol. 2004;165(5):1773–80.
40. Dal Cin P, Kozakewich HP, Goumnerova L, Mankin HJ, Rosenberg AE, Fletcher JA. Variant translocations involving 16q22 and 17p13 in solid variant and extraosseous forms of aneurysmal bone cyst. Genes Chromosomes Cancer. 2000;28(2):233–4.
41. Panoutsakopoulos G, Pandis N, Kyriazoglou I, Gustafson P, Mertens F, Mandahl N. Recurrent t(16;17)(q22;p13) in aneurysmal bone cysts. Genes Chromosomes Cancer. 1999;26(3):265–6.
42. Shiels WE, Mayerson JL. Percutaneous doxycycline treatment of aneurysmal bone cysts with low recurrence rate. Clin Orthop Relat Res. 2013;471(8):2675–83. doi: 10.1007/s11999-013-3043-2. Epub 2013 May 14.
43. Cottalorda J, Kohler R, Sales de Gauzy J, Chotel F, Mazda K, Lefort G, et al. Epidemiology of aneurysmal bone cyst in children: a multicenter study and literature review. J Pediatr Orthop B. 2004;13(6): 389–94.
44. Adamsbaum C, Mascard E, Guinebretiere JM, Kalifa G, Dubousset J. Intralesional Ethibloc injections in primary aneurysmal bone cysts: an efficient and safe treatment. Skeletal Radiol. 2003;32(10): 559–66.
45. Cottalorda J, Bourelle S. Modern concepts of primary aneurysmal bone cyst. Arch Orthop Trauma Surg. 2007;127(2):105–14.
46. Lambot-Juhan K, Pannier S, Grevent D, Pejin Z, Breton S, Berteloot L, et al. Primary aneurysmal bone cysts in children: percutaneous sclerotherapy with absolute alcohol and proposal of a vascular classification. Pediatr Radiol. 2012;42(5):599–605.
47. Crocoli A, Fassari FM, Natali GL, La Rosa G, Devito R, Falappa P. Sclerotherapy of primary aneurysmal bone cysts: comment to Lambot-Juhan et al. Pediatr Radiol. 2013;43(3):385–6.
48. Dubois J, Chigot V, Grimard G, Isler M, Garel L. Sclerotherapy in aneurysmal bone cysts in children: a review of 17 cases. Pediatr Radiol. 2003;33(6): 365–72.
49. Falappa P, Fassari FM, Fanelli A, Genovese E, Ascani E, Crostelli M, et al. Aneurysmal bone cysts: treatment with direct percutaneous Ethibloc injection: long-term results. Cardiovasc Intervent Radiol. 2002;25(4):282–90.
50. Garg NK, Carty H, Walsh HP, Dorgan JC, Bruce CE. Percutaneous Ethibloc injection in aneurysmal bone cysts. Skeletal Radiol. 2000;29(4):211–6.
51. Papagelopoulos PJ, Currier BL, Shaughnessy WJ, Sim FH, Ebsersold MJ, Bond JR, et al. Aneurysmal bone cyst of the spine. Management and outcome. Spine (Phila Pa 1976). 1998;23(5):621–8.
52. Peraud A, Drake JM, Armstrong D, Hedden D, Babyn P, Wilson G. Fatal ethibloc embolization of vertebrobasilar system following percutaneous injection into aneurysmal bone cyst of the second cervical vertebra. AJNR Am J Neuroradiol. 2004;25(6):1116–20.
53. Marcove RC, Sheth DS, Takemoto S, Healey JH. The treatment of aneurysmal bone cyst. Clin Orthop Relat Res. 1995;311:157–63.
54. Peeters SP, Van der Geest IC, de Rooy JW, Veth RP, Schreuder HW. Aneurysmal bone cyst: the role of cryosurgery as local adjuvant treatment. J Surg Oncol. 2009;100(8):719–24.
55. Bush CH, Adler Z, Drane WE, Tamurian R, Scarborough MT, Gibbs CP. Percutaneous radionuclide ablation of axial aneurysmal bone cysts. AJR Am J Roentgenol. 2010;194(1):W84–90.
56. Malghem J, Maldague B, Esselinckx W, Noel H, De Nayer P, Vincent A. Spontaneous healing of aneurysmal bone cysts. A report of three cases. J Bone Joint Surg Br. 1989;71(4):645–50.
57. McQueen MM, Chalmers J, Smith GD. Spontaneous healing of aneurysmal bone cysts. A report of two cases. J Bone Joint Surg Br. 1985;67(2):310–2.
58. Cottalorda J, Chotel F, Kohler R, de Gauzy JS, Louahem D, Lefort G, et al. Aneurysmal bone cysts of the pelvis in children: a multicenter study and literature review. J Pediatr Orthop. 2005;25(4):471–5.
59. De Cristofaro R, Biagini R, Boriani S, Ricci S, Ruggieri P, Rossi G, et al. Selective arterial embolization in the treatment of aneurysmal bone cyst and angioma of bone. Skeletal Radiol. 1992;21(8):523–7.
60. Koci TM, Mehringer CM, Yamagata N, Chiang F. Aneurysmal bone cyst of the thoracic spine: evolution after particulate embolization. AJNR Am J Neuroradiol. 1995;16(4 Suppl):857–60.
61. Wathiong J, Brys P, Samson I, Maleux G. Selective arterial embolization in the treatment of an aneurysmal bone cyst of the pelvis. Jbr-Btr. 2003;86(6):325–8.
62. Yildirim E, Ersozlu S, Kirbas I, Ozgur AF, Akkaya T, Karadeli E. Treatment of pelvic aneurysmal bone

cysts in two children: selective arterial embolization as an adjunct to curettage and bone grafting. Diagn Interv Radiol. 2007;13(1):49–52.
63. Yakes WF, Luethke JM, Parker SH, Stavros AT, Rak KM, Hopper KD, et al. Ethanol embolization of vascular malformations. Radiographics. 1990;10(5): 787–96.
64. Guibaud L, Herbreteau D, Dubois J, Stempfle N, Berard J, Pracros JP, et al. Aneurysmal bone cysts: percutaneous embolization with an alcoholic solution of zein–series of 18 cases. Radiology. 1998;208(2):369–73.
65. de Gauzy JS, Abid A, Accadbled F, Knorr G, Darodes P, Cahuzac JP. Percutaneous Ethibloc injection in the treatment of primary aneurysmal bone cysts. J Pediatr Orthop B. 2005;14(5):367–70.
66. Topouchian V, Mazda K, Hamze B, Laredo JD, Pennecot GF. Aneurysmal bone cysts in children: complications of fibrosing agent injection. Radiology. 2004;232(2):522–6.
67. Naredo E, Cabero F, Beneyto P, Cruz A, Mondejar B, Uson J, et al. A randomized comparative study of short term response to blind injection versus sonographic-guided injection of local corticosteroids in patients with painful shoulder. J Rheumatol. 2004;31(2):308–14.
68. Daley EL, Bajaj S, Bisson LJ, Cole BJ. Improving injection accuracy of the elbow, knee, and shoulder: does injection site and imaging make a difference? A systematic review. Am J Sports Med. 2011;39(3): 656–62.
69. MacMahon PJ, Eustace SJ, Kavanagh EC. Injectable corticosteroid and local anesthetic preparations: a review for radiologists. Radiology. 2009;252(3): 647–61.
70. Kahn CB, Hollander JL, Schumacher HR. Corticosteroid crystals in synovial fluid. JAMA. 1970;211(5):807–9.
71. Young CM, Shiels II WE, Coley BD, Hogan MJ, Murakami JW, Jones K, et al. Ultrasound-guided corticosteroid injection therapy for juvenile idiopathic arthritis: 12-year care experience. Pediatr Radiol. 2012;42(12):1481–9.
72. Baker R, Dreyfuss P, Mercer S, Bogduk N. Cervical transforaminal injection of corticosteroids into a radicular artery: a possible mechanism for spinal cord injury. Pain. 2003;103(1–2):211–5.
73. Sparling M, Malleson P, Wood B, Petty R. Radiographic followup of joints injected with triamcinolone hexacetonide for the management of childhood arthritis. Arthritis Rheum. 1990;33(6):821–6.
74. Gunal I, Karatosun V. Avascular necrosis of the femoral heads after single corticosteroid injection. CMAJ. 2006;175(1):31.
75. Astrom M. Partial rupture in chronic achilles tendinopathy. A retrospective analysis of 342 cases. Acta Orthop Scand. 1998;69(4):404–7.
76. Swindells MG, Tehrani H, Goodwin-Walters A, Sassoon EM. Acute radial artery ischemia following therapeutic steroid injection. Ann Plast Surg. 2007;58(4):461–2.
77. Suresh S, Berman J, Connell DA. Cerebellar and brainstem infarction as a complication of CT-guided transforaminal cervical nerve root block. Skeletal Radiol. 2007;36(5):449–52.
78. Kennedy DJ, Dreyfuss P, Aprill CN, Bogduk N. Paraplegia following image-guided transforaminal lumbar spine epidural steroid injection: two case reports. Pain Med. 2009;10(8):1389–94.
79. Edlow BL, Wainger BJ, Frosch MP, Copen WA, Rathmell JP, Rost NS. Posterior circulation stroke after C1-C2 intraarticular facet steroid injection: evidence for diffuse microvascular injury. Anesthesiology. 2010;112(6):1532–5.
80. Ruttum MS, Abrams GW, Harris GJ, Ellis MK. Bilateral retinal embolization associated with intralesional corticosteroid injection for capillary hemangioma of infancy. J Pediatr Ophthalmol Strabismus. 1993;30(1):4–7.
81. Kushner BJ, Lemke BN. Bilateral retinal embolization associated with intralesional corticosteroid injection for capillary hemangioma of infancy. J Pediatr Ophthalmol Strabismus. 1993;30(6):397–9.
82. Mabry RL. Visual loss after intranasal corticosteroid injection. Incidence, causes, and prevention. Arch Otolaryngol. 1981;107(8):484–6.
83. Tait IS, Holdsworth RJ, Belch JJ, McCollum PT. Management of intra-arterial injection injury with iloprost. Lancet. 1994;343(8894):419.
84. Andreev A, Kavrakov T, Petkov D, Penkov P. Severe acute hand ischemia following an accidental intraarterial drug injection, successfully treated with thrombolysis and intraarterial Iloprost infusion. Case report. Angiology. 1995;46(10):963–7.
85. Erbguth FJ, Naumann M. Historical aspects of botulinum toxin: Justinus Kerner (1786–1862) and the "sausage poison". Neurology. 1999;53(8):1850–3.
86. Eleopra R, Tugnoli V, Quatrale R, Rossetto O, Montecucco C. Different types of botulinum toxin in humans. Mov Disord. 2004;19 Suppl 8:S53–9.
87. Ellies M, Laskawi R, Schutz S, Quondamatteo F. Immunohistochemical evidence of nNOS and changes after intraglandular application of botulinum toxin A in cephalic salivary glands of adult rats. ORL J Otorhinolaryngol Relat Spec. 2003;65(3):140–3.
88. Kawamura A, Campbell K, Lam-Damji S, Fehlings D. A randomized controlled trial comparing botulinum toxin A dosage in the upper extremity of children with spasticity. Dev Med Child Neurol. 2007;49(5):331–7.
89. Jankovic J, Esquenazi A, Fehlings D, Freitag F, Lang AM, Naumann M. Evidence-based review of patient-reported outcomes with botulinum toxin type A. Clin Neuropharmacol. 2004;27(5):234–44.
90. Senner JE, Logemann J, Zecker S, Gaebler-Spira D. Drooling, saliva production, and swallowing in cerebral palsy. Dev Med Child Neurol. 2004;46(12): 801–6.

91. Ellies M, Laskawi R, Gotz W, Arglebe C, Tormahlen G. Immunohistochemical and morphometric investigations of the influence of botulinum toxin on the submandibular gland of the rat. Eur Arch Otorhinolaryngol. 1999;256(3):148–52.
92. Blasco PA. Management of drooling: 10 years after the Consortium on Drooling, 1990. Dev Med Child Neurol. 2002;44(11):778–81.
93. Ellies M, Laskawi R, Rohrbach-Volland S, Arglebe C. Up-to-date report of botulinum toxin therapy in patients with drooling caused by different etiologies. J Oral Maxillofac Surg. 2003;61(4):454–7.
94. Bushara KO. Sialorrhea in amyotrophic lateral sclerosis: a hypothesis of a new treatment—botulinum toxin A injections of the parotid glands. Med Hypotheses. 1997;48(4):337–9.
95. Ellies M, Laskawi R, Rohrbach-Volland S, Arglebe C, Beuche W. Botulinum toxin to reduce saliva flow: selected indications for ultrasound-guided toxin application into salivary glands. Laryngoscope. 2002;112(1):82–6.
96. Friedman A, Potulska A. Quantitative assessment of parkinsonian sialorrhea and results of treatment with botulinum toxin. Parkinsonism Relat Disord. 2001;7(4):329–332.
97. Mancini F, Zangaglia R, Cristina S, Sommaruga MG, Martignoni E, Nappi G, et al. Double-blind, placebo-controlled study to evaluate the efficacy and safety of botulinum toxin type A in the treatment of drooling in parkinsonism. Mov Disord. 2003; 18(6):685–8.
98. Winterholler MG, Erbguth FJ, Wolf S, Kat S. Botulinum toxin for the treatment of sialorrhoea in ALS: serious side effects of a transductal approach. J Neurol Neurosurg Psychiatry. 2001;70(3):417–8.
99. Ellies M, Rohrbach-Volland S, Arglebe C, Wilken B, Laskawi R, Hanefeld F. Successful management of drooling with botulinum toxin A in neurologically disabled children. Neuropediatrics. 2002;33(6): 327–30.
100. Bothwell JE, Clarke K, Dooley JM, Gordon KE, Anderson R, Wood EP, et al. Botulinum toxin A as a treatment for excessive drooling in children. Pediatr Neurol. 2002;27(1):18–22.
101. Jongerius PH, Rotteveel JJ, van den Hoogen F, Joosten F, van Hulst K, Gabreels FJ. Botulinum toxin A: a new option for treatment of drooling in children with cerebral palsy. Presentation of a case series. Eur J Pediatr. 2001;160(8):509–12.
102. Suskind DL, Tilton A. Clinical study of botulinum-A toxin in the treatment of sialorrhea in children with cerebral palsy. Laryngoscope. 2002;112(1): 73–81.
103. Savarese R, Diamond M, Elovic E, Millis SR. Intraparotid injection of botulinum toxin A as a treatment to control sialorrhea in children with cerebral palsy. Am J Phys Med Rehabil. 2004;83(4):304–11; quiz 12–4, 36.
104. Hassin-Baer S, Scheuer E, Buchman AS, Jacobson I, Ben-Zeev B. Botulinum toxin injections for children with excessive drooling. J Child Neurol. 2005;20(2): 120–3.
105. Jongerius PH, Rotteveel JJ, van Limbeek J, Gabreels FJ, van Hulst K, van den Hoogen FJ. Botulinum toxin effect on salivary flow rate in children with cerebral palsy. Neurology. 2004;63(8):1371–5.
106. Jongerius PH, van den Hoogen FJ, van Limbeek J, Gabreels FJ, van Hulst K, Rotteveel JJ. Effect of botulinum toxin in the treatment of drooling: a controlled clinical trial. Pediatrics. 2004;114(3):620–7.
107. Jeong HS, Lee JW, Kim SH, Myung JS, Kim JH, Kang HS. Effectiveness of transforaminal epidural steroid injection by using a preganglionic approach: a prospective randomized controlled study. Radiology. 2007;245(2):584–90.
108. Kim H, Lee Y, Weiner D, Kaye R, Cahill AM, Yudkoff M. Botulinum toxin type a injections to salivary glands: combination with single event multilevel chemoneurolysis in 2 children with severe spastic quadriplegic cerebral palsy. Arch Phys Med Rehabil. 2006;87(1):141–4.
109. Pena AH, Cahill AM, Gonzalez L, Baskin KM, Kim H, Towbin RB. Botulinum toxin A injection of salivary glands in children with drooling and chronic aspiration. J Vasc Interv Radiol. 2009;20(3): 368–73.
110. Reid SM, Johnstone BR, Westbury C, Rawicki B, Reddihough DS. Randomized trial of botulinum toxin injections into the salivary glands to reduce drooling in children with neurological disorders. Dev Med Child Neurol. 2008;50(2):123–8.
111. Ondo WG, Hunter C, Moore W. A double-blind placebo-controlled trial of botulinum toxin B for sialorrhea in Parkinson's disease. Neurology. 2004;62(1):37–40.
112. Racette BA, Good L, Sagitto S, Perlmutter JS. Botulinum toxin B reduces sialorrhea in parkinsonism. Mov Disord. 2003;18(9):1059–61.
113. Reid SM, Walstab JE, Chong D, Westbury C, Reddihough DS. Secondary effects of botulinum toxin injections into salivary glands for the management of pediatric drooling. J Craniofac Surg. 2013; 24(1):28–33.
114. Restani L, Giribaldi F, Manich M, Bercsenyi K, Menendez G, Rossetto O, et al. Botulinum neurotoxins A and E undergo retrograde axonal transport in primary motor neurons. PLoS Pathog. 2012;8(12): e1003087.
115. Curra A, Trompetto C, Abbruzzese G, Berardelli A. Central effects of botulinum toxin type A: evidence and supposition. Mov Disord. 2004;19 Suppl 8:S60–4.
116. Herrmann J, Geth K, Mall V, Bigalke H, Schulte Monting J, Linder M, et al. Clinical impact of antibody formation to botulinum toxin A in children. Ann Neurol. 2004;55(5):732–5.

117. Li M, Goldberger BA, Hopkins C. Fatal case of BOTOX-related anaphylaxis? J Forensic Sci. 2005; 50(1):169–72.
118. FDA. Early Communication about an Ongoing Safety Review of Botox and Botox Cosmetic (Botulinum toxin Type A) and Myobloc (Botulinum toxin Type B) 2008 [cited 2013 2013/02/21]. http://www.fda.gov/Drugs/DrugSafety/PostmarketDrugSafetyInformationforPatientsandProviders/DrugSafetyInformationforHeathcareProfessionals/ucm070366.htm.

Section X

Nonvascular Interventions: Oncology

24 Thermal Therapies

Fredric A. Hoffer

Introduction

The general work-up for thermal ablation of malignant tumors includes a review of the imaging, pathology, and clinical history by the pediatric or interventional radiologist and presentation to a local tumor board. If chemotherapy, radiotherapy, or surgery is not preferred, then thermal ablation is indicated. It is helpful but difficult to have a prospective institutional review board-approved protocol available at your institution for thermal ablation of malignant lesions. Most pediatric cancer patients will have been treated on chemotherapy protocols. You will increase your accrual and get more information out of a prospective protocol.

Radiofrequency Ablation

Indications

Radiofrequency ablation (RFA) has mainly been used for benign lesions of bone in children. It is the treatment of choice for osteoid osteoma as covered in the musculoskeletal chapter (see Chap. 22) and has also been used to cure Langerhans cell histiocytosis of bone and to palliate desmoid tumor of the soft tissues [1].

RFA has been used to palliate and rarely cure malignant tumors in children. The largest experience reported prospectively was from St. Jude Children's Research Hospital [1]. A recurrence rate of 50 % within the pulmonary/pleural incision has been reported after surgical resection of pediatric pulmonary osteosarcoma metastases [2]. The St. Jude RFA series mainly involved lung metastases recurring after initial pulmonary resections of osteosarcoma.

The other large group of pediatric patients that may benefit from RFA are those with multifocal primary or metastatic hepatic lesions, for example, fibrolamellar hepatoma, desmoplastic round cell tumor, pancreatoblastoma, colon carcinoma (Fig. 24.1), and rhabdomyosarcoma. Indications for RFA include hepatic lesions that would require a larger hepatic resection than a curative RF ablation zone. These lesions would typically be central but not in contact with the common hepatic or first-order branch bile ducts.

The third group of malignant lesions in children that may be amenable to RFA are soft tissue or bone lesions. Examples include rhabdomyosarcoma in the breast and maxilla, leiomyosarcoma of the chest wall, and metastatic osteosarcoma to the humerus [1].

F.A. Hoffer, M.D., F.A.A.P., F.S.I.R. (✉)
Department of Radiology, University of Washington, 3904 Northeast Belvoir Place, Seattle, WA 98105, USA
e-mail: fhoffer@gmail.com; fred.hoffer@seattlechildrens.org

M. Temple and F.E. Marshalleck (eds.), *Pediatric Interventional Radiology: Handbook of Vascular and Non-Vascular Interventions*, DOI 10.1007/978-1-4419-5856-3_24,

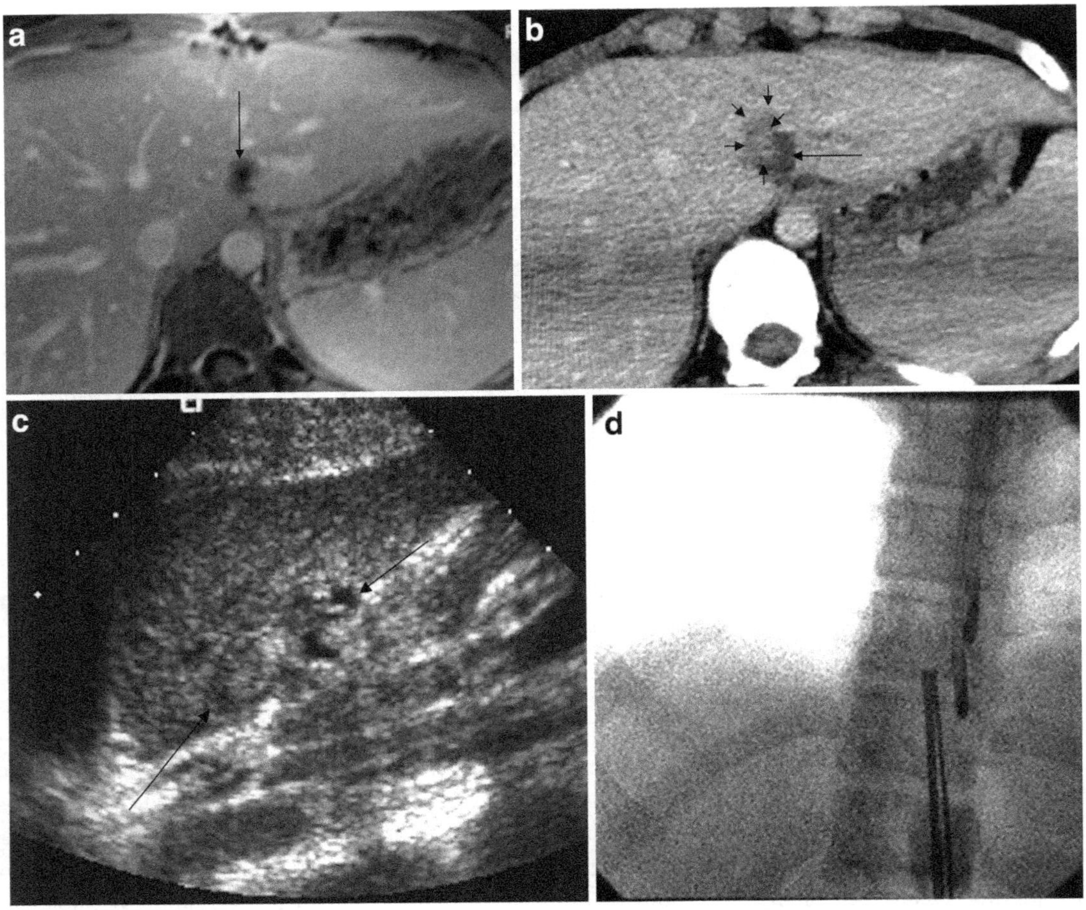

Fig. 24.1 This 16-year-old had colon cancer discovered when he had a laparotomy after a motor vehicle accident. (**a**) Because of the scarring from the prior surgery, the surgeon did not want to resect the segment II hepatic metastasis (*arrow*) as noted on this contrast-enhanced fat-suppressed T1-weighted MR. (**b**) After RFA the left hepatic lesion was partially ablated. Note the hyperdense burn zone (*short arrows*) is not completely covering the hypodense lesion (*long arrow*) on this contrast-enhanced CT. (**c**) A sagittal US image shows the RF target (*arrows*) for re-ablation in the left lobe of the liver. (**d**) Because this lesion was so close to the esophagus, this procedure was done under fluoroscopy and US guidance. A triple (cluster) Cool-tip RF probe was placed. Two catheters were placed in the esophagus, which was only 8 mm away from the RF probe. One catheter was perfused with cold water and the other was placed to wall suction. This was done to protect the esophagus during RFA

Contraindications

Contraindications are listed in Table 24.1.

Preprocedure Work-Up

Cross-sectional imaging with PET/CT is preferred prior to pulmonary RFA. MR of the head and neck, pelvic, or extremity lesion is preferred. MR (Fig. 24.1a) or CT (Fig. 24.1b) of hepatic or retroperitoneal lesions is sufficient. If US guidance is going to be used such as in hepatic (Fig. 24.1c), retroperitoneal, or soft tissue lesions, then US should be performed prior to the ablation by the interventionalist that will perform the ablation. A radiograph of a bone lesion is also necessary to rule out a pathological fracture.

A complete blood count, electrolytes, BUN, creatinine, liver function, and coagulation testing should be performed. Thrombocytopenia, anemia, coagulation disorders, and electrolyte derangements should be corrected. Pulmonary

Table 24.1 Contraindications to radiofrequency ablation

1. Proximity of intended target tumor to adjacent vital structures
a. Tumor < 1 cm from the main bile duct
b. Tumor < 1 cm from the portal vessel (without adjunct technique to minimize heat sink effect)
c. Tumor < 1 cm from the colon, small bowel, or stomach (without adjunct technique to displace)
2. Intrahepatic bile duct dilatation (poor prognostic indicator) or presence of biliary-enteric anastomosis
3. Exophytic tumor (risk of tumor seeding)
4. Untreatable/unmanageable coagulopathy
5. Lack of safe access route to tumor
6. Active infection
7. Pulmonary insufficiency (for lung RFA)

RFA radiofrequency ablation

function testing should be performed prior to RFA of the lung.

A history and physical examination is performed in the clinic to include a pain intensity assessment. Consent during an unhurried clinic visit is warranted so the patient and family are fully aware of the risks and potential complications of this procedure.

Equipment and Procedure Technique

General anesthesia is necessary for all RF ablations in children. There are multiple types of RFA systems available that include mono- and bipolar devices. The control methods for energy deposition vary depending on the manufacturers. Common approaches include monitoring of impedance or temperature. It is important to be familiar with the specific control of your institutional RFA system.

The author is most familiar with using Radionics, ValleyLab, and Covidien (Boulder, CO) as progressive vendors for the same RF ablation system. A Cool-tip RF system has a 200 W 480 kHz generator with continuous internal cycling of chilled saline to minimize charring of tissues and to increase tissue impedance. It works using either manual control or impedance control. Grounding pads are placed transversely typically over the thighs. If a single RFA probe is used, two grounding pads are sufficient. If more probes are used, four grounding pads are necessary (anterior and posterior on each thigh). The linear 17 gauge RFA probes are cooled at the active tips. This prevents charring and gas formation and increases the burn volume by more effectively conducting the current to the periphery of the tumor. An impedance-controlled system also aids in conduction of the energy to a larger volume by shutting off the energy if the baseline impedance rises more than 20 Ω. The active tip length varies from 1 to 4 cm. For most malignant lesions, a cluster probe with three linear probes separated by 5 mm and with 2.5 cm active tips can be used (Fig. 24.1d). The probe is placed percutaneously under CT/CT fluoroscopy guidance for lung lesions and by US for most other lesions. The probe is placed in the deepest portion of the tumor. Typically the lesion is burned for 12 min, and then the energy and cold perfusion is turned off. A temperature of ≥60 °C at the tip of the probe indicates adequate tumor ablation in that zone. If, however, the temperature does not reach 60 °C, measures such as stopping cooling and impedance control can be used to reach a temperature of 90 °C for 1 min. Then the probe is pulled back to a location that registers 55 °C. If this is inside of the tumor, the cool perfused impedance-controlled ablation is repeated. If the 55 °C is outside the tumor, then the percutaneous tract is ablated by a series of manual burns avoiding burning the skin. To cover a larger burn volume, a switch controller allows three probes with 3 or 4 cm active tips to be placed farther apart and at different angles during a single ablation. The switch controller allows for each probe to be turned on sequentially and thus avoids the interference and incomplete ablation zones between probes. The ablation time with the switch controller is often 18 min. Having the manufacturer's representative with you for your ablations is recommended until you are quite familiar with the technique.

Complications and Their Preventions

It is important to keep up to date on the complications of all thermal therapies. The US Food and Drug Administration (FDA) mandates reporting of all serious and fatal complications in the Manufacturer and User Facility Device Experience

(MAUDE) database: http://www.accessdata.fda.gov/scripts/cdrh/cfdocs/cfMAUDE/search.cfm?searchoptions=1. To search for fatal complications of thermal ablations, enter: Event Type—Death and Product Code—GEI.

Significant complications such as fatal hemoptysis have been reported after pulmonary RFA. This MAUDE database revealed 19 deaths related to RFA, five related to pulmonary RFA, one included massive fatal hemoptysis. Two other cases of massive hemoptysis, 7 and 17 days post RFA, respectively, have been recently reported to be associated with pulmonary pseudoaneurysms treated successfully with coil embolization [3, 4]. In one large series, there was a 3 % incidence of procedural-related deaths after pulmonary RFA [5], with an increased risk of hemoptysis in patients receiving prior radiotherapy. Nonfatal hemoptysis can occur in 9 % of patients after RFA of lung lesions [6]. Treatment of nodules near large pulmonary arteries was thought to be safe but not effective [7]. One is taught that vessels over 4 mm in diameter are spared by RFA due to their internal cooling of normal blood flow. However, if the ventilation is compromised in the lung during RFA, pulmonary artery perfusion may decrease by as much as 84 % allowing larger pulmonary arteries to be thermally injured [8]. Delayed pseudoaneurysms and hemoptysis have been reported at 2 weeks post ablation of central pulmonary lesions. The lesions that involve the main or intermediate branch pulmonary arteries therefore should be avoided.

Left diaphragmatic herniation after pulmonary RFA in children has also been reported [1] after RFA of left lower lobe pulmonary metastases in contact with the diaphragm. RFA of lesions abutting the right diaphragm did not result in herniation possibly due to the large liver surface.

Pulmonary insufficiency including shortness of breath at rest can occur after RFA of the lung. Patients considered for pulmonary RFA may have already received pulmonary irradiation, chemotherapy, bone marrow transplantation, or prior thoracotomy or thoracostomy. Patients already dependent on supplemental oxygenation are at high risk of pulmonary insufficiency post RFA. Pulmonary function testing is performed on cooperative patients (age 5 and older), and the author suggests a forced vital capacity ≥33 % of normal to consider pulmonary RFA. Poor pulmonary compliance also may predispose the patient to air embolization through a bronchopulmonary vein fistula during forced ventilation during [9] or after RFA.

When dealing with small children and large or central lesions, a rise in core body temperature must be controlled by cooling blankets, or the procedure should be stopped when the core body temperature reaches 40 °C [10].

Also if there are unexpendable nerves or spinal cord within 1 cm of the ablation zone, a separate temperature probe near the vital nerve can be placed. If the temperature reaches above 45 °C, nerve damage may occur and the ablation should be halted [11].

It is wise to deliver twice maintenance fluid replacement during and after the ablation to prevent renal damage from tumor lysis [12]. Dipstick urine to detect blood will reveal the presence of hemoglobinuria or myoglobinuria. The twice maintenance fluid replacement should be maintained until the urine is clear.

Pain is a significant problem following ablation of large malignant lesions especially near the pleura, chest wall, subcutaneous tissues, and diaphragm. General anesthesia during the procedure and patient-controlled or parent-controlled analgesia in the recovery room may alleviate much of this temporary pain. Most patients with malignant lesions require only overnight admission for pain control.

Bile duct injury will occur when treating contiguous hepatic lesions. Peripheral lesions can also be RF ablated, but if they are in contact with the GI tract, the GI tract wall needs to be separated from the ablation zone by fluid or a balloon catheter. The esophageal gastric junction can be protected by infusing cold liquid into the lumen during RFA (Fig. 24.1d). Patients with biliary-enteric anastomoses are prone to bile sepsis after RFA. Either RFA should be avoided in these patients or prophylactic antibiotics and careful post-RFA care should be given.

Treating lesions under 3 cm is most successful. If treating over four lesions, one may consider chemoembolization as an alternative to thermal ablation. Large hepatic lesions may also be more effectively RF ablated by pre-ablation chemoembolization. This will decrease the cooling effect from the hypervascularity within the tumors and allow complete heating and tumor destruction.

Skin burns are a frequent problem especially on small or emaciated children. It is important to place the grounding pads with the broad portion of the rectangle transversely over the muscle or fat and separated from bony protuberances to avoid burns under the grounding pad. Small or patients with amputated limbs have a higher risk of burns with RFA in the groin. Also one must completely cover the upper extremities to avoid a hand or arm touching the flank or thigh as that may cause a reentry burn [1]. Skin burns over the superficially treated lesions can be avoided by placing ice in the fingers and palm of a sterile glove and covering the skin access site. If one uses a metallic coaxial needle outside the RF probe and if the active tip of the probe comes in contact with the coaxial needle, a serious skin burn can occur which may require surgery. This can be avoided by having a coaxial needle shorter than the insulated portion of the RF probe and pulling back the coaxial needle fully. The operator can touch the coaxial needle at the skin surface during ablation to assure that heating is not occurring at that location.

RFA of head and neck and extremity malignancies is challenging. The lesions are often far removed from the grounding pads, and the available energy to ablate these peripheral tumors is often insufficient due to high impedance. Bipolar RFA, cryotherapy, microwave, or irreversible electroporation may be more efficient at treating peripheral malignant lesions.

Postprocedure Care and Follow-Up

After RFA, the patient is admitted until the urine is clear of hemoglobin or myoglobin, and the patient's pain is controlled to a level of <4 out of 10 of severity on oral medications. Electrolytes post RFA should be stable and not show evidence of tumor lysis. Pain control may exacerbate pulmonary insufficiency. Patients may be discharged on supplemental oxygen with the goal to get them back to room air by 1 month.

Patients are followed in interventional radiology clinic at 1 month, 3 months, 6 months, and 1 year. After pulmonary RFA, pulmonary function tests, pulse oximetry, and PET/CT are performed. Liver function tests and contrast-enhanced MR or CT are obtained after hepatic RFA. Following musculoskeletal lesion ablation, contrast-enhanced MR is performed. All patients have a pain score reevaluated at each visit.

Cryotherapy

Cryotherapy has been used on adults for prostate and renal tumor ablation. There is a 17 gauge system available that delivers up to 28×28×55 mm −20 °C ablation zone per probe (www.galilmedical.com) (Galil Medical Inc., Plymouth Meeting, PA). No grounding pads are necessary. Multiple probes may be used to decrease the time but increase the cost. A freeze-thaw-refreeze cycle is necessary for tumor ablation. CT accurately determines the freezing edges of the zone. Membranes may be spared offering some advantage when close to cystic structures such as the renal collecting system or urethra. The intraprocedural and postprocedural pain is often less with cryotherapy than with RFA [13]. The skin over subcutaneous or musculoskeletal lesions may have to be protected by directly warming the skin to prevent frostbite.

Microwave

Microwave ablation [14] can be delivered without a grounding pad using 1–3 percutaneously placed probes (Evident NWA system, www.covidien.com, Covidien AG, Boulder, CO). Internal cooling of the shaft proximal to the ablation zone protects the skin or other adjacent tissues from being damaged by the microwave. The active tips are either 2 or 3.7 cm producing a 28×28×40 mm ablation zone per probe at 45 W for 10 min. The probes are really antennas, and the distribution of the energy is not affected or blocked by the cooling effect of passing vessels or airway. Therefore, there is a theoretical advantage in ablating tumors near large vessels that may be incompletely treated by RFA.

Irreversible Electroporation

Irreversible electroporation is able to cause complete tumor cell apoptosis (progression to irreversible cell death) in tumor tissue even in areas where contiguous supporting structures such as blood vessels and bile ducts are completely spared [15]. It is marketed as NanoKnife (www.Angiodynamics.com, AngioDynamics, Queensbury, NY). It uses 1–6 percutaneous devices. Single 1 mm diameter (19 gauge) electrode probe requiring at least one other probe is available with an active length of 0–40 mm. When two probes are placed 1.5 cm apart and the active length is set at 2 cm, then the dimensions of ablation will be 25 × 17 × 30 mm. Maximum current is 50 A. The single bipolar 1.5 mm diameter (16 gauge) probes are not yet available. No grounding pads are necessary.

Chapter Summary

Radiofrequency Ablation

- Indications
  - Pulmonary osteosarcoma mets
  - Hepatic neoplasms
  - Soft tissue/bone lesions

Contraindications

- See page Table 24.1, page 393

Preprocedure Workup

- PET CT, MRI, ultrasound, plain film based on location
- CBC, electrolytes, BUN, creatinine, liver function and coagulation
- Pulmonary function tests for lung RFA
  - Suggest forced vital capacity > 33 %
- Pain intensity assessment
- IR clinic visit

Equipment

- RFA unit with appropriate single, multi-tined or multiple probes
- Chilled saline for infusion for some RFA units
- Coaxial needle
- Temperature probe
- Grounding pads
- CT, CT fluoroscopy, US

Technique

- All cases under GA
- Cell death related to combination of time and temperature
- Burn protocol as per manufacturer
- Consider protective methods (carbon dioxide, fluid administration, displacement, ice, etc.) when near vital structures
- Consider double maintenance fluid infusion
- Consider pre RFA chemoembolization for large hepatic lesions

Complications

- Lung
  - Hemoptysis
  - Pseuodaneurysm
  - Diaphragmatic herniation
  - Pulmonary insufficiency
  - Air embolization
- Increased core body temperature
- Nerve damage
- Renal damage—hemoglobinuria/myogobinuria
- Pain
- Bile duct injury
- Burns
  - Grounding pad
  - Coaxial needle
  - Reentry
  - Superficial lesion

Postprocedure Care

- Urine monitoring
- Pain control
- Electrolytes

Followup

- IR clinic—1, 3, 6 and 12 months.

- Lung: pulmonary function tests, pulse oximetry and PET CT
- Liver: LFT's, MR or CT
- MSK lesions: MR

Cryotherapy

- 17 gauge system commercially available
- Freeze–thaw–refreeze cycle used for ablation
- Membrane sparing

Microwave

- No grounding pads
- Burn zone not affected by air or flowing blood

Electroporation

- Electrical current results in cell apoptosis sparing blood vessels and bile ducts
- No grounding pads
- Recent introduction of commercial unit

References

1. Hoffer FA, Daw NC, Xiong X, Anghelescu D, Krasin M, Yan X, Davidoff AM, Furman WL, Carlos Rodriguez-Galindo C, Spunt SL. A phase I/pilot study of radiofrequency ablation for the treatment of recurrent pediatric solid tumors. Cancer. 2009;115: 1328–37.
2. McCarville MB, Kaste SC, Cain AM, Goloubeva O, Rao BN, Pratt CB. Prognostic factors and imaging patterns of recurrent pulmonary nodules after thoracotomy in children with osteosarcoma. Cancer. 2001; 91:1170–6.
3. Sakurai J, et al. Pulmonary artery pseudoaneurysm related to RFA of lung tumor. Cardiovasc Intervent Radiol. 2010;33(2):413–6.
4. Yamakado K, et al. Massive hemoptysis from pulmonary artery pseudoaneurysm caused by lung RFA: successful treatment by coil embolization. Cardiovasc Intervent Radiol. 2010;33(2):410–2.
5. Simon CJ, Dupuy DE, DiPetrillo TA, et al. Pulmonary radiofrequency ablation: long term safety and efficacy in 153 patients. Radiology. 2007;243:268–75.
6. Okuma T, et al. Frequency & risk of various complications after CT guided radiofrequency ablation of lung tumors. Cardiovasc Intervent Radiol. 2008;31:122–30.
7. Nomori H, Imazu Y, Watanabe K, Ohtsuka T, Naruke T, Kobayashi T, Suemasu K. Radiofrequency ablation of pulmonary tumors and normal lung tissue in swine and rabbits. Chest. 2005;127(3):973–7.
8. Oshima F, Yamakado K, Akeboshi M, et al. Lung radiofrequency ablation with and without bronchial occlusion: experimental study in porcine lungs. J Vasc Interv Radiol. 2004;15:1451–6.
9. Burgoyne LL, Pereiras LA, Laningham F, Shearer JR, Bikhazi GB, Hoffer FA. Near-fatal acute bronchovenous fistula in a child undergoing radiofrequency ablation of a metastatic lung tumor. Paediatr Anaesth. 2008;18:131–3.
10. Hoffer FA, Campos A, Xiong X, Wu S, Oigbokie N, Proctor K. Core body temperature regulation of pediatric patients during radiofrequency ablation. Pediatr Radiol. 2007;37:297–300.
11. Dupuy DE, Hong RJ, Oliver B, Goldberg SN. Radiofrequency ablation of spinal tumors: temperature distribution within the spinal canal. Am J Roentgenol. 2000;175:1263–6.
12. Keltner JR, Donegan E, Hynson JM, Shapiro WA. Acute renal failure after radiofrequency liver ablation of metastatic carcinoid tumor. Anesth Analg. 2001;93: 587–9.
13. Allaf ME, Varkarakis IM, Bhayani SB, Inagaki T, Kavoussi LR, Solomon SB. Pain control requirements for percutaneous ablation of renal tumors: cryoablation versus radiofrequency ablation—initial observations. Radiology. 2005;237:366–70.
14. Wolf FJ, Grand DJ, Machan JT, DiPetrillo TA, Mayo-Smith WW, Dupuy DE. Microwave ablation of lung malignancies: effectiveness, CT findings, and safety in 50 patients. Radiology. 2008;247:871–9.
15. Lee EW, Chen C, Prieto VE, Dry SM, Loh CT, Kee ST. Advanced hepatic ablation technique for creating complete cell death: irreversible electroporation. Radiology. 2010;255:426–33.

Transarterial Chemoembolization (TACE) for Malignant Hepatic Tumors in Children

25

Nghia-Jack Vo, Fredric A. Hoffer, and Sandeep S. Vaidya

Introduction

Primary malignant liver cancers in children have an overall incidence of two cases per million. Hepatoblastoma (HB) is the most common, and the majority will present in infants and toddlers within the first 2 years of life. On the other hand, hepatocellular carcinoma (HCC) which is the second most frequent malignant liver tumor will present later, typically in school-aged children or adolescents [1, 2].

The fundamental principle for treatment is complete surgical resection of the tumor. Unfortunately 50 % of children with HB and 70 % of those with HCC present initially as inoperable due to the extent of tumor involvement, vascular invasion, or distant metastasis. The prognosis for children that cannot ultimately achieve a complete tumor resection or transplant is dismal [3]. HB is generally chemosensitive, particularly to platinum-based agents such as cisplatin. Following systemic chemotherapy up to 85 % are appropriate candidates for surgical resection [4]. However, HCC remains relatively chemoresistant, and the fibrolamellar type of HCC most often attributable to children (13–22 % of HCC in children) does not respond any differently than the typical HCC with current therapeutic regimens, having an overall survival rate below 25 % at 3 years [5].

Treatment can be challenging, and the options for children with these malignant liver tumors have increased to include local regional treatment options such as transarterial chemoembolization (TACE) and radiofrequency ablation (RFA) procedures. Both TACE and RFA can be incorporated individually or in conjunction as complimentary treatments. RFA is further discussed earlier in this chapter.

The normal liver parenchyma with its dual blood supply is appropriately situated for TACE. TACE takes advantage and is premised upon the basis that malignant tumors are hypervascular and draw upon supply from the arterial component, while normal liver parenchyma draws the vast majority of its blood supply (70–80 %) from the portal vein. With this dual supply the tumor can be selectively targeted with minimal risk of inducing hepatic insufficiency [6]. Combining the embolic component along with

N.-J. Vo, M.D. (✉)
Department of Radiology, Pediatric Imaging and Interventional Radiology, Children's Hospital of Wisconsin, Medical College of Wisconsin
9000 W. Wisconsin Ave M/S 721, Milwaukee, WI 53226, USA
e-mail: nvo@chw.org

F.A. Hoffer, M.D., F.A.A.P., F.S.I.R.
Department of Radiology, University of Washington, 3904 NE Belvoir Place, Seattle, WA 98105, USA
e-mail: fred.hoffer@seattlechildrens.or

S.S. Vaidya, M.D.
Department of Radiology, Vascular and Interventional Radiology, Seattle Children's Hospital and the University of Washington, 4800 Sand Point Way NE, Seattle, WA 98105, USA
e-mail: svaidya@uw.edu

M. Temple and F.E. Marshalleck (eds.), *Pediatric Interventional Radiology: Handbook of Vascular and Non-Vascular Interventions*, DOI 10.1007/978-1-4419-5856-3_25,

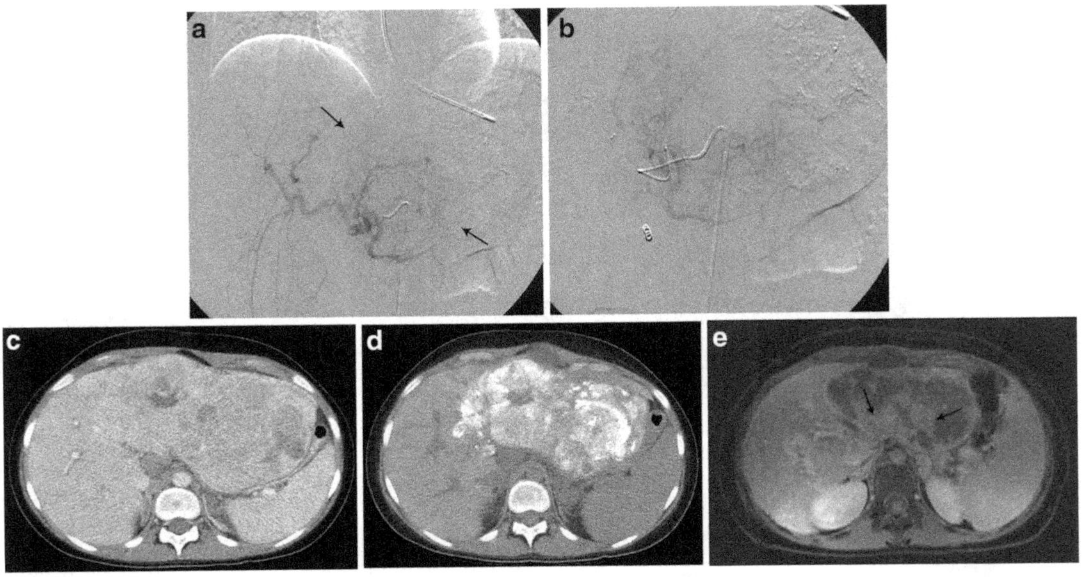

Fig. 25.1 (**a**) A 15-year-old girl with fibrolamellar HCC. Angiogram performed from the celiac trunk demonstrates the hypervascular character of the tumor involving the left hepatic lobe (*arrows*). (**b**) Microcatheter was used to select a dominant feeding artery to the tumor. The chemoembolic emulsion was infused from this selective position. Evident are the oily contrast beads collecting into the tumor. Note a coil was placed into the gastroduodenal artery (GDA) to protect against reflux into the gastric and proximal small bowel supply. (**c**) Baseline CT demonstrating tumor involving the left lobe. (**d**) Post-TACE CT without IV contrast demonstrates the distribution of the chemoembolic emulsion throughout the tumor. (**e**) MRI 3 months following the initial TACE demonstrates tumor necrosis and retraction of the tumor following four rounds of triple drug TACE. There remains residual enhancing tumor (*arrows*)

the chemotherapy offers the opportunity to highly concentrate the agent directly into the tumor, reduce the systemic effects, and increase the dwell time and effects of the chemotherapy. Biologically active chemoembolic material has been shown to remain in the tumor tissue for up to 3 weeks from surgical resection specimens [7–10]. Furthermore, embolization induces ischemic necrosis of the tumor with the benefit of not only tumor size reduction but also devascularization, which has been shown to reduce blood loss during subsequent surgical resections (Fig. 25.1) [6, 8, 11].

Indications and Role of TACE in Children

In that HB is generally chemosensitive, systemic neoadjuvant chemotherapy is typically the preferred initial treatment course prior to or following surgical resection [2]. However, in up to 30 % of children, the tumor will not respond adequately to systemic chemotherapy, and TACE can be considered as an additional treatment option. TACE has been shown to be effective as a salvage preoperative technique to convert unresectable tumor into a resectable tumor [12]. Children that have bilobar or multicentric disease and despite an apparent effective response of the tumor to the systemic or localized regional chemotherapy, surgery may not be able to achieve an adequate resection and still maintain sufficient tissue volume to preserve function. In these circumstances liver transplantation is increasingly considered a viable option, and TACE can serve as a bridging technique until an appropriate organ is available (Fig. 25.2) [13, 14].

Less than 30 % of children with HCC present with a primarily resectable tumor. Liver transplantation has been shown to be much more

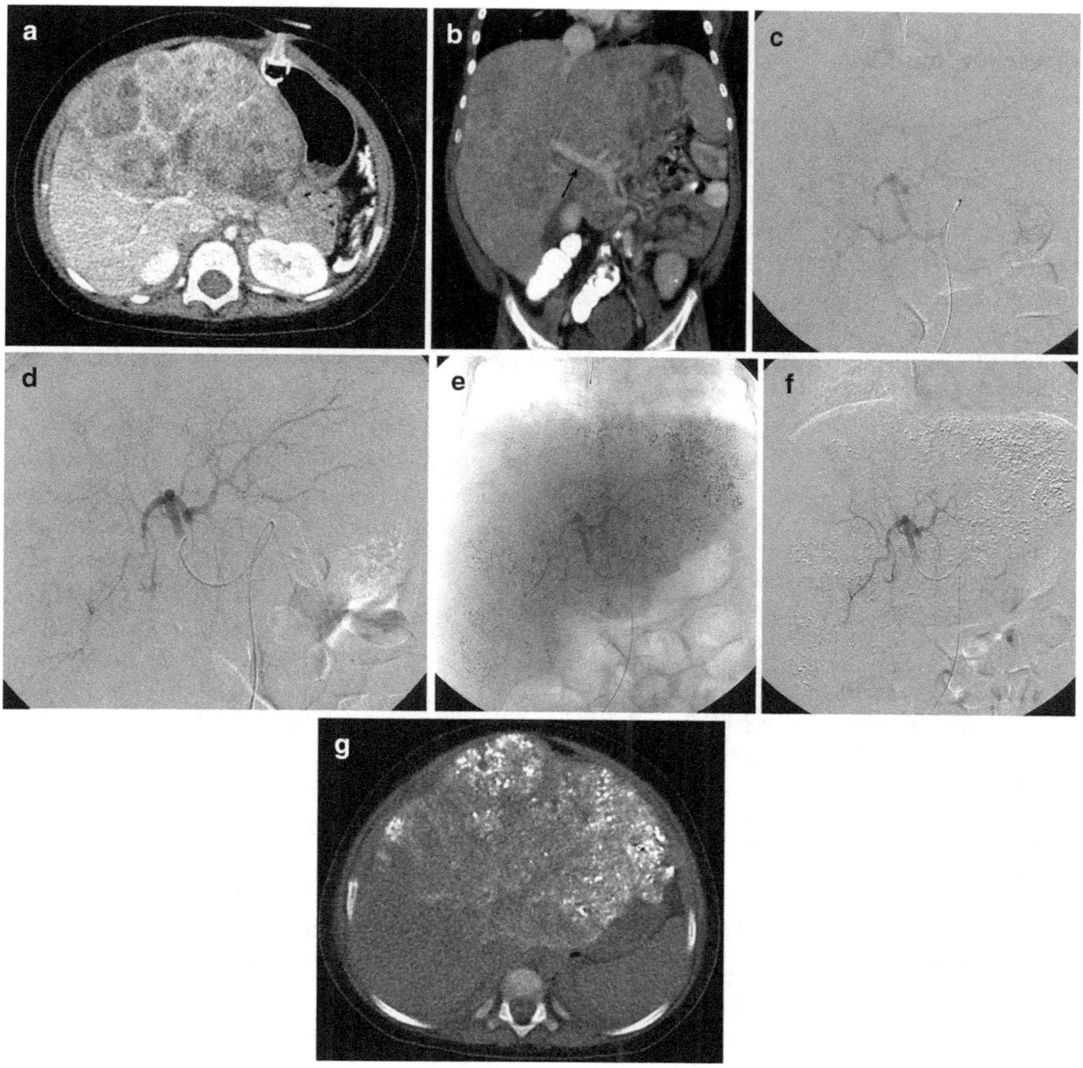

Fig. 25.2 A 23-month-old boy with hepatoblastoma, nonresponsive to systemic chemotherapy, had a TACE performed as a bridge for transplant. The child was transplanted after a single session of TACE when an organ became available. (**a**) CT demonstrates tumor involving the left hepatic lobe with minimal necrosis (response) to systemic chemotherapy. (**b**) Coronal image demonstrates patency of the main portal vein (*arrow*) and extent of left hepatic lobe involvement. (**c**) Angiogram performed from the celiac trunk. (**d**) Selective angiogram of the left hepatic lobe demonstrates innumerable enhancing nodules throughout the left lobe. (**e**) Unsubtracted image demonstrates the distribution of the chemoembolic mixture throughout the nodular masses occupying the left hepatic lobe. (**f**) Subtracted image demonstrating pruned appearance of the arterial vasculature following particle embolization. (**g**) Non-contrast CT demonstrating distribution of the chemoembolic mixture within nodules throughout the left lobe and sparing the right

successful than conventional systemic chemotherapy in children with HCC, even if they were outside the Milan transplant criteria (adult basis for liver transplantation) [15]. In these circumstances TACE clearly has a role as a bridging technique until an organ is available.

Finally TACE has a role as a palliative treatment option for those with symptoms related to the mass effect caused by the tumor burden. TACE has been shown with randomized controlled trials to prolong survival compared to conservative medical management in the adult population [16, 17].

Contraindications

Contraindications are listed in Table 25.1.

There are three major categories that relate to contraindications for TACE. First are those issues related to the angiographic procedure (see Chap. 4). Second are contraindications related to the chemotherapeutic agents such as severe thrombocytopenia, neutropenia, and cardiac or renal dysfunction. Finally, there are issues related to hepatic function and vascular involvement. The child must have adequate reserves and sufficient hepatic function following the embolization of the hepatic artery. This requires adequate portal venous support at baseline. An occluded portal vein is not necessarily a contraindication to TACE as long as there is sufficient collateral flow from cavernous transformation to support the liver should the arterial supply become compromised as is the case with an effective TACE (Fig. 25.3). In these circumstances the tumor should be embolized as selectively as possible to minimize risk of inducing hepatic failure. Children with biliary obstruction should have this relieved prior to a TACE due to the increased risk of developing a post-TACE hepatic abscess, sepsis, or hepatic failure [18]. Tumors that have excessive arterial venous shunting may not be appropriate for TACE treatment due to the risk of developing clinically significant pulmonary emboli as a result of the embolic material.

Table 25.1 Contraindications

1. Decompensated liver disease with inadequate synthetic function as indicated by:
(a) Jaundice
(b) Encephalopathy
(c) Refractory ascites
2. Persistent biliary obstruction or untreated varices at risk for hemorrhage
3. Extensive bilobar tumor infiltration and replacement with tumor (>50 % of liver; inadequate volume to preserve hepatic function)
4. Inadequate portal vein flow (portal vein occlusion is not a contraindication if there is sufficient cavernous portal flow)
5. Technical contraindications
(a) Contraindication to angiography (see Chap. 4)
(b) Arteriovenous shunting that would result in embolization to the lung
6. Renal insufficiency (creatinine >2 mg/dL or creatinine clearance <30 mL/min)

Preprocedure Workup

The workup before the actual procedure is an extremely important step in the entire process. This includes not only imaging and laboratory

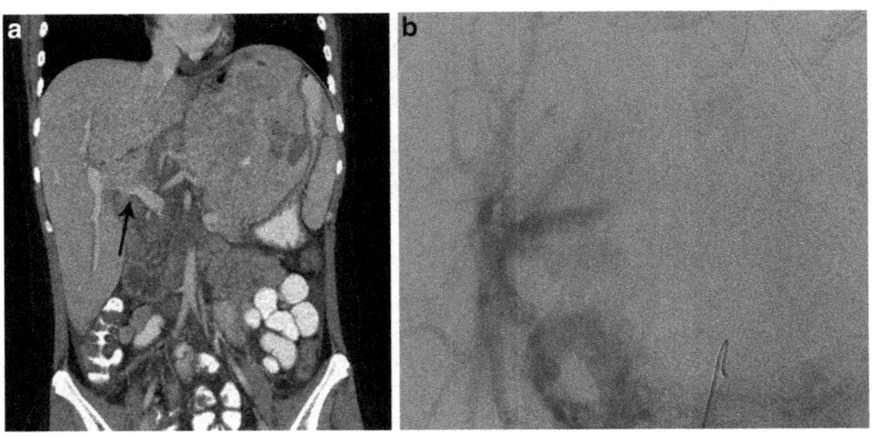

Fig. 25.3 Child with HCC involving the left lobe of the liver and portal vein thrombosis. (**a**) Coronal CT image demonstrates portal vein occlusion from tumor invasion (*arrow*). (**b**) Mesenteric angiogram imaged during the portal venous phase confirms portal vein occlusion, but demonstrates adequate portal supply to the right lobe secondary to cavernous transformation

values but also a frank discussion at tumor board and a clinic visit for the child and family.

Typically, when a patient is to be worked up for a chemoembolization procedure, by the time referral is made to the interventional radiology service, a definitive diagnosis along with the necessary imaging and lab workup has been completed. However it must be kept in mind that the imaging and labs should be relatively recent prior to the procedure. The imaging modality preferred is usually a multiphase contrast-enhanced MRI. This is especially helpful compared to a CT in the event that there has been prior percutaneous therapy. However if an MRI is not available or obtainable for various reasons, then a multiphase CT with contrast is sufficient.

Along with the imaging, the bloodwork is undertaken to assess for ability to tolerate TACE. The standard bloodwork performed should include a CBC, liver and renal function, coagulation profile, serum electrolytes, and tumor markers. A differential white count and an absolute neutrophil count may be required for those children previously treated with systemic chemotherapy. Once these facts are in hand, the case is discussed in the multidisciplinary tumor board. This is the forum to clarify the ultimate goal of the TACE, i.e., whether this is being done as a primary preoperative procedure, salvage, bridge to transplant, or palliative procedure.

Having made the decision to offer a TACE, the candidacy of the patient needs to be determined. This is done based on the performance status of the patient, the imaging findings, and the lab values. Usually patients with an Eastern Cooperative Oncology Group (ECOG) Performance Status score of more than 2 are poor candidates (see Table 25.2). However, ECOG scoring is always challenging in the pediatric population. On imaging one needs to ascertain the degree of the liver parenchyma replaced. If more than 70 % of the liver is replaced by tumor, then the patient is a poor candidate in terms of tolerating the procedure due to the risk of inducing hepatic failure. Tumor distribution, i.e., unilobar or bilobar, also plays a role in the planning of the procedure. Bilobar disease will need good documentation of the areas treated at each session to make sure that all lesions are treated. Unilobar disease consisting of a solitary lesion is the best scenario as it allows a more targeted delivery of the chemoembolic agent with the best results.

Next, one needs to assess the lab values. The coagulation parameters and the total bilirubin are critical values to consider. A total bilirubin of more than 2 mg/dL can suggest increased risk for complications, and proceeding with treatment should be taken into careful consideration with the care team. Also remember that when using Adriamycin, since it has cardiac side effects, it requires that cardiac function be evaluated in advance. Some of the lab value cutoffs are mentioned in the Table 25.3.

Table 25.2 Eastern Cooperative Oncology Group (ECOG) Performance Status[a]

Grade	ECOG
0	Fully active, able to carry on all pre-disease performance without restriction
1	Restricted in physically strenuous activity but ambulatory and able to carry out work of a light or sedentary nature, e.g., light house work, office work
2	Ambulatory and capable of all self-care but unable to carry out any work activities. Up and about more than 50 % of waking hours
3	Capable of only limited self-care, confined to bed or chair more than 50 % of waking hours
4	Completely disabled. Cannot carry on any self-care. Totally confined to bed or chair
5	Dead

[a]As published in Oken, M.M., Creech, R.H., Tormey, D.C., Horton, J., Davis, T.E., McFadden, E.T., Carbone, P.P.: Toxicity And Response Criteria Of The Eastern Cooperative Oncology Group. Am J Clin Oncol 1982;5:649–655

Table 25.3 Lab values for TACE

1. T. Bilirubin less than 2 mg/dL
2. LDH less than 425 units/L
3. Creatinine less than 2 mg/dL
4. Platelets more than 50,000/dL
5. Neutrophils greater than 1,500/μL

If there is a cardiac history, then document an ejection fraction of >50 %

The final step in the workup is the clinic visit. This is the time when the patient and the family get to know the interventionalist. Explanation of the procedure, the goals of the plan (palliation or bridge to transplant, etc.), the potential side effects, and the complications need to be explained to them. It is essential to make them aware of the "tumor lysis syndrome" which inevitably follows. Essentially this is where the patient–doctor relationship is consolidated and prepares the family for the TACE.

Procedure Technique

In that TACE is essentially an angiographic endovascular procedure, standard pediatric access techniques, sheaths, catheters, and precautions should be utilized based upon the child's physical characteristics [19]. We perform all TACE procedures in children with the benefit of a general anesthetic. *Preprocedure medications* include antibiotic prophylaxis consisting of a first-generation cephalosporin and metronidazole. In an attempt to minimize the postprocedure inflammatory reaction, the child is given a single preprocedure IV dose of 250 mg/m^2 of methylprednisolone (maximum of 260 mg) [20].

The initial TACE procedure should include a well-performed *visceral angiogram* of both the celiac and superior mesenteric artery (SMA) to fully map the vascular anatomy supplying the liver and specifically the tumor (Fig. 25.1). This is followed by selective catheterization and angiogram of both the right and left hepatic artery; a microcatheter can be used to decrease the risk of inducing arterial spasm. Spasm is a pitfall that can produce the false appearance of early adequate embolization or worse inhibit the ability to instill the entire aliquot of the chemoembolic emulsion. The SMA arteriogram should be imaged through the portal venous phase to ensure patency of the portal vein (if not recently cleared by ultrasound, CT, or MRI). A replaced hepatic artery originating from the SMA or left gastric artery is a common anatomical variant that should be looked for. The vascular catheter should be positioned as selectively as reasonable to treat the greatest volume of tumor. It is through this position that the chemoembolic emulsion is instilled under live fluoroscopy to look for emulsion distribution and persistent antegrade flow or reflux.

Table 25.4 Chemotherapeutic agents

Cisplatin	60 mg/m^2
Adriamycin	30 mg/m^2
Mitomycin C	20 mg/m^2

The *chemotherapeutic agent(s)* should be prepared by the oncologic pharmacy into a 10 mL solution that can be drawn up in the IR suite into a glass or polycarbonate syringe. At our children's hospital, in conjunction with the pediatric oncologists, we have preferred a triple drug cocktail (Table 25.4). The chemotherapy is then vigorously mixed with 5–10 mL of the *ethiodized oily contrast* (Guebert LLC, Bloomington IN) using a metallic 3-way stopcock just prior or immediately upon the final positioning of the angiographic catheter. Initially, mix the chemotherapy with only 5 mL of ethiodized oily contrast; after half of the emulsion is instilled, additional contrast (up to 5 mL) will be mixed if there is persistent adequate antegrade flow. A 3 mL polycarbonate syringe is used to facilitate introduction of the chemoembolic emulsion if a microcatheter is used. *Caution*: standard syringes and plastic stopcocks are susceptible to erosion due to the chemotherapy.

Particle embolization is performed following the complete introduction of the chemotherapeutic emulsion mixture. Various particles have been described for use to include Gelfoam, trisacryl gelatin particles, and polyvinyl alcohol (PVA) embolization particles. Particle embolization should proceed until cessation of antegrade arterial flow into the vasculature that supplies the tumor (Fig. 25.2). Metallic coils are not used to embolize the hepatic artery due to the potential future need for repeat TACE procedures. Studies have shown that particle embolization at the conclusion (along with our own University Hospital experience) is more effective than only relying upon the ethiodized oily contrast portion of the emulsion mixture as the sole embolic component [21].

Note that protective eyewear and double gloving when working with chemotherapeutic agents is highly recommended. All materials are disposed in specially labeled waste containers.

Postprocedure Patient Care and Follow-up

The child should be aggressively treated with supportive care for an expected *post-embolization syndrome* (*tumor lysis syndrome*). This consists of pain, nausea and vomiting, and fevers. Fevers <102 F (38.9 °C) are not unusual in the first week and should not automatically trigger a sepsis workup [22]. However, as prophylaxis against gram-negative bacteremia, we initiate a 5-day course of antibiotics consisting of amoxicillin-clavulanate or ciprofloxacin. IV narcotics along with antiemetics should be liberally utilized in the first 24–48 h following the TACE procedure. Various chemotherapeutic agents, particularly cisplatin, can induce dehydration along with the fevers, and therefore aggressive hydration should be considered to maintain adequate fluid status until the child is able to maintain sufficient oral intake volumes.

The day following the TACE, a non-contrast abdominal CT is performed to identify distribution of the chemoembolic mixture (Fig. 25.1). Labs to include CBC, electrolytes, and liver function tests (LFTs) are obtained. It is expected that the LFTs will be dramatically elevated in this post-TACE period. This set of labs serves as a baseline for subsequent follow-up comparisons. Labs are redrawn in 3 weeks following the TACE, and the LFTs should be expected to have significantly improved compared with the baseline post TACE. Multiple TACE procedures can be performed (every 4–5 weeks) based upon the tumor response, the patient's laboratory and clinical tolerance, and the surgical or transplant status.

Tumor response can be followed by imaging and the serum AFP. Follow-up imaging for tumor response is best performed with contrast-enhanced MRI. The Ethiodol staining in the tumor limits the ideal ability to visualize tumor enhancement with CT (Fig. 25.1).

Complications Related to TACE

The development of post-embolization syndrome is common following TACE in children. This can be addressed with aggressive postprocedure supportive care. One of the keys to its management is actually in preparing the family and child for its occurrence in advance during the initial consultative and consenting process.

Major potential complications that can arise as a result of a TACE procedure include the induction of hepatic failure or insufficiency. It is important to assess the liver function prior to a TACE to help ensure adequate post-embolization hepatic perfusion. Infections and the development of a hepatic abscess can be minimized with the use of antibiotic prophylaxis. A hepatic abscess can be addressed with a percutaneous drain. Careful technique will minimize nontarget embolization as well as careful review of the angiogram for anatomical variants that could lead to unintended embolic material occluding gastric or bowel vasculature. Pulmonary embolus as a result of shunting from the tumor has also been described [23]. The use of IV steroids can also significantly alter the glucose control of a child, and this should be monitored and aggressively treated to minimize both the acute and long-term effects of hyperglycemia [24].

Conclusion

The fundamental principle of treatment for children with primary malignant liver tumors is complete surgical resection. TACE is technically achievable and has been shown to be effective as an additional treatment technique for children that do not respond adequately to systemic chemotherapy. Its role can be as a salvage procedure, a bridge to eventual transplant, or palliative.

Chapter Summary

Introduction

- Pediatric liver cancer uncommon
  - Hepatoblastoma (HB) (<2 years old)
  - Fibrolamellar HCC (adolescents)
- Outcomes without complete surgical resection/transplant dismal
  - 50 % HB and 70 % HCC inoperable
  - HB more chemosensitive than HCC

Indications

- Inadequate response to systemic chemotherapy (HB)
- Bridge to transplant (HB, TACE)
- Palliation—decrease tumor burden/pain

Contraindications

- Inability to undergo angiogram
- Chemotherapy associated issues:
  - Severe thrombocytopenia
  - Neutropenia
  - Renal/cardiac dysfunction
- Suspected inadequate hepatic function post embolization
- Portal vein occlusion (without sufficient collateral flow)
- Biliary obstruction
- Arteriovenous shunting

Preprocedure Workup

- Review imaging and bloodwork.
  - MRI and CT
  - CBC with differential, liver function, renal function, coagulation, electrolytes, and tumor markers
- Review at tumor board.
- Clinic visit with family.
- Determine eligibility.
  - ECOG status
  - % liver affected (>70 % poor candidate)
  - Lab values (Table 25.1)

Equipment

- Angiography supplies
  - Microcatheters
- Chemotherapy (see Table 25.2)
- Protective eyewear
- Double gloves
- Ethiodized oil contrast
- Metallic 3-way stopcock
- Polycarbonate syringe
- Embolic agent
  - Gelfoam, PVA, tris-acryl gelatin
- Appropriate disposal container

Technique

- GA
- Antibiotic prophylaxis (cephalosporin and metronidazole)
- Methylprednisolone (250 mg/m^2; 260 mg max)
- Determine hepatic and tumor vascular anatomy
  - Celiac/SMA
  - Both hepatic arteries
- Place catheter into appropriate branch
- Monitor chemotherapy administration under fluoroscopy
- Embolize

Postprocedure Care

- Supportive care
  - Pain, nausea, vomiting, fever, and fluid intake
- Antibiotic coverage (amoxicillin/clavulanate or ciprofloxacin)
- CT used to identify distribution
- CBC, electrolytes, glucose, LFTs, POD#1, and #21

Complications

- Post-embolization syndrome
- Hepatic failure/insufficiency
- Nontarget embolization
  - Stomach and duodenum
  - Pulmonary embolization

References

1. Pham TH, Iqbal CW, Grams JM, et al. Outcomes of primary liver cancer in children: an appraisal of experience. J Pediatr Surg. 2007;42:834–9.
2. Meyers RL. Tumors of the liver in children. Surg Oncol. 2007;16:195–203.
3. Malogolowkin MH, Stanley P, Steele DA, et al. Feasibility and toxicity of chemoembolizations for children with liver tumors. J Clin Oncol. 2000; 18(6):1279–84.
4. Tannuri ACA, Tannuri U, Givelli NEM, et al. Surgical treatment of hepatic tumors in children: lessons learned from liver transplantation. J Pediatr Surg. 2009; 44:2083–7.
5. Cruz O, Laguna A, Vancells M, et al. Fibrolamellar hepatocellular carcinoma in an infant and literature review. J Pediatr Hematol Oncol. 2008;30(12):968–71.
6. Xuewu J, Jianhong L, Xianliang H, et al. Combined treatment of hepatoblastoma with transcatheter arterial chemoembolizations and surgery. J Pediatr Hematol Oncol. 2006;23:1–9.
7. Chou FI, Fang KC, Chung C, et al. Lipiodol uptake and retention by human hepatoma cells. Nucl Med Biol. 1995;22(3):379–86.
8. Vogl TJ, Scheller A, Jakob U, et al. Transarterial chemoembolizations in the treatment of hepatoblastoma in children. Eur Radiol. 2006;16:1393–6.
9. Ohtsuka Y, Matsunaga T, Yoshida H, et al. Optimal strategy of preoperative transcatheter arterial chemoembolizations for hepatoblastoma. Surg Today. 2004;34:127–33.
10. Nakamura H, Hashimoto T, Oi H, et al. Transcatheter oily chemoembolizations of hepatocellular carcinoma. Radiology. 1989;170:783–6.
11. Tashjian DB, Moriarty KP, Courtney RA, et al. Preoperative chemoembolization for unresectable hepatoblastoma. Pediatr Surg Int. 2002;18:187–9.
12. Li J, Chu J, Yang J, et al. Preoperative transcatheter selective arterial chemoembolizations in treatment of unresectable hepatoblastoma in infants and children. Cardiovasc Intervent Radiol. 2008;31:1117–23.
13. Czuaderna P, Abrzezniak G, Narozanski W, et al. Preliminary experience with arterial chemoembolizations for hepatoblastoma and hepatocellular carcinoma in children. Pediatr Blood Cancer. 2006; 46:825–8.
14. Avila LF, Luis AL, Hernandez F, et al. Liver transplantation for malignant tumours in children. Eur J Pediatr Surg. 2006;16:411–4.
15. Ismail H, Broniszczak D, Kalicinski P, et al. Liver transplantation in children with hepatocellular carcinoma Do Milan Criteria apply to pediatric patients? Pediatr Transplant. 2008;13(6):682–92.
16. Llovet JM, Real MI, Montana X, et al. Arterial embolization or chemoembolizations versus symptomatic treatment in patients with unresectable hepatocellular carcinoma: a randomized controlled trail. Lancet. 2002;359:1734–9.
17. Lo CM, Nhan H, Tso WK, et al. Randomized controlled trial of transarterial lipiodol chemoembolizations for unresectable hepatocellular carcinoma. Hepatology. 2002;35(5):1164–71.
18. Chung JW, Park JH, Han JK, et al. Hepatic tumors: predisposing factors for complications of transcatheter oily embolization. Radiology. 1996;198:33–40.
19. Heran MKS, Marshalleck F, Temple M, et al. Joint quality improvement guidelines for pediatric arterial access and arteriography: from the Society of Interventional Radiology and Pediatric Radiology. Pediatr Radiol. 2010;40:237–50.
20. Bissler JJ, Racadio J, Donnelly LF, et al. Reduction of postembolization syndrome after ablation of renal angiomyolipomas. Am J Kidney Dis. 2002; 39:966–71.
21. Arcement CM, Towbin RB, Meza MP, et al. Intrahepatic chemoembolizations in unresectable pediatric liver malignancies. Pediatr Radiol. 2000; 30:779–85.
22. Li CP, Chao Y, Chen LT, et al. Fever after transcatheter arterial chemoembolizations for hepatocellular carcinoma: incidence and risk factor analysis. Scand J Gastroenterol. 2008;43:992–9.
23. Yamaura K, Higashi M, Akiyoshi K, et al. Pulmonary lipiodol embolism during transcatheter arterial chemoembolizations for hepatoblastoma under general anesthesia. Eur J Anaesthesiol. 2000;17(11):704–8.
24. Moghissi ES, Korytkowski MT, DiNardo M, et al. American association of clinical endocrinologists and American Diabetes Association consensus statement on inpatient glycemic control. Diabetes Care. 2009;32(6):1119–31.

Index

M. Temple and F.E. Marshalleck (eds.), *Pediatric Interventional Radiology: Handbook of Vascular and Non-Vascular Interventions*, DOI 10.1007/978-1-4419-5856-3,

D

CPSIA information can be obtained
at www.ICGtesting.com
Printed in the USA
LVHW062020160622
721323LV00002B/17

9 781441 958556